AF715258

Network Pharmacology

Network Pharmacology

Editor: Lida Murdock

AMERICAN
MEDICAL PUBLISHERS
www.americanmedicalpublishers.com

AMERICAN
MEDICAL PUBLISHERS
www.americanmedicalpublishers.com

Cataloging-in-Publication Data

Network pharmacology / edited by Lida Murdock.
p. cm.
Includes bibliographical references and index.
ISBN 979-8-88740-299-4
1. Pharmacology--Data processing. 2. Pharmacology--Computer network resources.
3. Pharmacology--Computer simulation. 4. Bioinformatics. 5. Information storage and retrieval systems--Pharmacology. 6. Pharmaceutical technology. I. Murdock, Lida.
RM301 .N48 2023
615.1--dc23

© American Medical Publishers, 2023

American Medical Publishers,
41 Flatbush Avenue,
1st Floor, New York,
NY 11217, USA

ISBN 979-8-88740-299-4 (Hardback)

This book contains information obtained from authentic and highly regarded sources. Copyright for all individual chapters remain with the respective authors as indicated. All chapters are published with permission under the Creative Commons Attribution License or equivalent. A wide variety of references are listed. Permission and sources are indicated; for detailed attributions, please refer to the permissions page and list of contributors. Reasonable efforts have been made to publish reliable data and information, but the authors, editors and publisher cannot assume any responsibility for the validity of all materials or the consequences of their use.

Trademark Notice: Registered trademark of products or corporate names are used only for explanation and identification without intent to infringe.

Contents

Preface

Network pharmacology is an emerging discipline focused on understanding drug interactions and actions within multiple targets. It systematically lists the molecular interactions of a drug that take place in a living cell, by making use of computational techniques. It studies the effect of a drug on the body and the biological system. It comprises chemical properties, sources, biological effects and use of drugs for therapeutics. Bioinformatics, high-throughput histology and system biology are utilized by network pharmacology, which combines information network and pharmacology. Pharmacokinetics and pharmacodynamics are the two main branches of pharmacology. Pharmacokinetics is concerned with the supply, absorption, metabolism and excretion of drugs, while pharmacodynamics is related with the physiological, molecular and biochemical effects of drugs. It integrates polypharmacology and network biology, which helps in the identification of drugs and disease targets, simultaneously understanding pathways and mechanisms between them. This book is a compilation of chapters that discuss the most vital concepts in the field of network pharmacology. The topics covered herein offer the readers new insights into this field.

All of the data presented henceforth, was collaborated in the wake of recent advancements in the field. The aim of this book is to present the diversified developments from across the globe in a comprehensible manner. The opinions expressed in each chapter belong solely to the contributing authors. Their interpretations of the topics are the integral part of this book, which I have carefully compiled for a better understanding of the readers.

At the end, I would like to thank all those who dedicated their time and efforts for the successful completion of this book. I also wish to convey my gratitude towards my friends and family who supported me at every step.

Editor

1

Confirmation of Inhibiting TLR4/MyD88/NF-κB Signalling Pathway by Duhuo Jisheng Decoction on Osteoarthritis: A Network Pharmacology Approach-Integrated Experimental Study

Linglong Liu[1†], Limei Xu[1,2†], Shengjie Wang[3†], Lili Wang[2,4], Xiaoning Wang[1,2], Huifeng Xu[2,4], Xihai Li[1,4] and Hongzhi Ye[2,4]*

[1]College of Integrative Medicine, Fujian University of Traditional Chinese Medicine, Fuzhou, China, [2]Academy of Integrative Medicine, Fujian University of Traditional Chinese Medicine, Fuzhou, China, [3]College of Pharmacy Science, Fujian University of Traditional Chinese Medicine, Fuzhou, China, [4]Fujian Key Laboratory of Integrative Medicine on Geriatrics, Fuzhou, China

***Correspondence:**
Xihai Li
lixihaifz@163.com

[†]These authors have contributed equally to this work

This study was conducted to identify whether the TLR4/MyD88/NF-κB signalling pathway plays a vital role in osteoarthritis (OA) treatment with Duhuo Jisheng Decoction (DHJSD) on the basis of a network pharmacology approach (NPA)-integrated experiment. Two experiments were conducted as follow: NPA for DHJSD using six OA-related gene series and the key pathway was screened out using NPA. NPA identified a vital role for the TLR4/MyD88/NF-κB signalling pathway in OA treatment with DHJSD, the conventional western blot analysis and qPCR confirmed it. Furthermore, changes of miR-146a-5p and miR-34a-5p in the cellular models were recovered by DHJSD administration, which synergistically contributed to OA therapy. The toll-like receptor signalling pathway and the NF-κB signalling pathway were meaningfully enriched by the miRNA-regulated gene pathways. This study identified and confirmed the TLR4/MyD88/NF-κB signalling pathway is an essential inflammatory signalling pathway in the DHJSD underlying OA treatment. The results provide a basis for further evaluation of the regulatory mechanism of the drug's efficacy in treating OA.

Keywords: network pharmacology approach, complex herbal formulations, molecular targets, osteoarthritis, Duhuo Jisheng decoction, inflammatory

INTRODUCTION

Osteoarthritis (OA) is a progressive, degenerative disease characterised by inflammation-driven cartilage degradation in the elderly (Kwon et al., 2018; Funck-Brentano et al., 2019; Peat and Thomas, 2021). OA resulting in joint chronic pain and disability can lead to remarkable reduction of the quality of life, which poses an increasing socioeconomic and healthcare burden. However, prolonged use of non-steroidal anti-inflammatory drugs for OA treatment may lead to cardiovascular and gastrointestinal side effects (UK NCGC, 2014; Latourte et al., 2020). Pharmacological treatments for OA are aimed at alleviating the clinical symptoms rather than treating the underlying causes. Hence it is in desperate need of more effective and safer therapeutic approaches to reduce chronic pain and functional recovery of joint in patients with OA.

In the field of traditional Chinese medicine (TCM), Chinese herbal medicine has a deep history and special features for OA treatment, and it has been explored to be effective in improving clinical symptoms with few side effects. Duhuo Jisheng Decoction (DHJSD) has been widely used to treat OA in China, and has been confirmed to relieve OA-related symptoms in several clinical trials (Zhang et al., 2016). Studies have shown that DHJSD could alleviate OA by suppressing inflammation and chondrocyte apoptosis (Liu et al., 2018; Liu et al., 2020). Our previous studies shown that DHJSD inhibits chondrocyte apoptosis by affect the mitochondrial-dependent apoptotic pathway (Liu et al., 2014) and suppresses the endoplasmic reticulum stress-mediated apoptosis (Lin et al., 2015). Some clues about the pharmacological mechanism of DHJSD have been provided, indicating that its pharmacological efficacy may through the synergistic actions of the multi-ingredients modulating multi-pathways. Nevertheless, the specific pharmacological mechanisms of DHJSD and their interaction with OA-related targets and pathways is not yet elucidated and require further investigation.

Network pharmacology approach (NPA), a novel and powerful strategy, integrates chemo-informatics, bio-informatics, network biology, network analysis and traditional pharmacology, which conforms to an organic whole or the holistic view of TCM theory and elucidates the active compounds and potential mechanisms of TCM formulas. Classical network pharmacology explores molecular targets from the ingredients of the complex herbal formulation and the target disease, simultaneously and refines the intersections between the formulations and disease to identify the therapeutic molecular targets (Lai et al., 2020). NPA has been beneficial in elucidating the interrelationship of the compounds and construct the compound, compound target, and target disease networks to exploring the possible mechanisms of multi-component and multi-target drugs (Liu et al., 2016). Jian et al. used NPA to investigate the effects of Eucommia ulmoides-Radix Achyranthis Bidentatae (EU-RAB) in OA, showed that TNF, MAPK, PI3K/AKT and IL-17 signalling pathways may be pathway that EU-RAB affects in OA (Jian et al., 2020). Zhu et al. reported that cell cycle, cell apoptosis, immune modulation, inflammation and drug metabolism maybe the pathway that Shaoyao Gancao (SGD) affects in OA by NPA analysis (Zhu et al., 2019). Recently, Zhang et al. found that virus-related, apoptotic, IL-17 and PI3K/Akt signalling pathway are involved in the mechanisms of Radix Achyranthis Bidentatae in treating acute OA using NPA (Zhang et al., 2020), Huang et al. used NPA and found that Simiao may exert its effect on multi-pathway such as IL-17 signalling pathway, HIF-1 signalling pathway, Toll-like receptor signalling pathway and TNF signalling pathway (Huang et al., 2020). In our previous study, we also used NPA and OA in a cellular model and found that the NF-κB signalling pathway was the important inflammatory signalling pathway involved in the mechanism of Bushen Zhuangjin Decoction (BZD) in treating OA (Xu et al., 2021). These studies had focused on investigating the potential molecular targets and mechanisms of a certain herbal formulation using NPA. Therefore, using NPA-integrated experimental to acquire the bioactive components, targets and the underlying mechanisms of DHJSD in treating OA. The following two experiments were designed: 1) network pharmacology for DHJSD and 2) variation of the pathway detected from network pharmacology and confirming the key signalling pathway of DHJSD on a lipopolysaccharide (LPS) induced OA cellular model. This study provides a newish approach to understand the theoretical basis of DHJSD in treating OA.

METHODS AND MATERIALS

Preliminary Exploration of the Bioactive Components of DHJSD

Preparation of DHJSD

DHJSD is formed from 15 Chinese medical plants, including Duhuo (DH) [Angelica biserrata (Shan et Yuan) Yuan et Shan], Sang Ji Sheng (SJS) [Taxillus chinensis (DC.) Danser], Qin Jian (QJ) [Gentiana Macrophylla Pall.], Fang Feng (FF) [Saposhnikovia divaricata (Turcz.) Schischk.], Xi Xin (XX) [Manchurian Wildginger], Chuan Xiong (CX) [Szechuan Lovage Rhizome], Dang Gui (DG) [Angelica sinensis (Oliv.) Diels.], Shu Di Huang (SDH) [Rehmanniaglutinosa (Gaertn.) DC.], Bai Shao (BS) [Paeonia lactiflora Pall], Rou Gui (RG) [Cortex Cinnamomi Cassiae], Fu Ling (FL) [Smilax glabra Roxb], Du Zhong (DZ) [Eucommia ulmoides Oliv], Niu Xi (NX) [Radix Achyranthis Bidentatae], Dang Shen (DS) [Root of Pilose Asiabell], Gan Cao (GC) [Glycyrrhiza uralensis Fisch.], were obtained from the Third People's Hospital affiliated to the Fujian University of TCM (Fuzhou, China). Regarding the ratio of DHJSD (**Supplementary Table S1**), 90 g of herbal powder was soaked in 720 ml distilled water and boiled three times for 2 h, and the extracts were filtered. The filtrate was completely evaporated on a rotary evaporator (RE-2000; Shanghai Yarong Biochemistry Instrument Factory, Shanghai, China), dried in vacuum drying oven until it was constant weight, and then stored at −20 °C (DZF-300; Shanghai Yiheng Scientific Instrument Co., Shanghai, China). The DHJSD solid dry matter was dissolved in Dulbecco's modified Eagle's medium (HyClone, Logan, UT, United States) and then filtered through a 0.22 μm filter. When used, was prepared as necessary. The extracts of DHJSD were detected by high performance liquid chromatography (HPLC) fingerprint on an Agilent 1200 HPLC system (Agilent, Santa Clara, CA,United States) using an Agilent 5 TC-C_{18} (250 × 4.6 mm). The conditions for the analysis were acetonitrile (A) 0.2% phosphoric acid water (B) as a mobile phase, a detection wavelength at 230 nm for paeoniflorin (peak 1) (purity 98%), ligustrazine hydrochloride (peak 2) (purity 98%) and osthole (peak 3) (purity 98%) (China Institute of

TABLE 1 | The final selected compounds of DuHuo JiSheng Decoction for analysis.

ID	Name	OB	DL	Herb
MOL003608	O-Acetylcolumbianetin	60.04	0.26	DH
MOL004777	Angelol D	34.85	0.34	DH
MOL004778	[(1R,2R)-2,3-dihydroxy-1-(7-methoxy-2-oxochromen-6-yl)-3-methylbutyl] (Z)-2-methylbut-2-enoate	46.03	0.34	DH
MOL004780	Angelicone	30.99	0.19	DH
MOL004782	[(1R,2R)-2,3-dihydroxy-1-(7-methoxy-2-oxochromen-6-yl)-3-methylbutyl] 3-methylbutanoate	45.19	0.34	DH
MOL004792	Nodakenin	57.12	0.69	DH
MOL000011	(2R,3R)-3-(4-hydroxy-3-methoxy-phenyl)-5-methoxy-2-methylol-2,3-dihydropyrano[5,6-h][1,4]benzodioxin-9-one	68.83	0.66	FF
MOL011730	11-hydroxy-sec-o-beta-d-glucosylhamaudol_qt	50.24	0.27	FF
MOL011732	Anomalin	59.65	0.66	FF
MOL011737	Divaricatacid	87	0.32	FF
MOL011740	Divaricatol	31.65	0.38	FF
MOL011747	Ledebouriellol	32.05	0.51	FF
MOL011749	Phelloptorin	43.39	0.28	FF
MOL011753	5-O-Methylvisamminol	37.99	0.25	FF
MOL002644	Phellopterin	40.19	0.28	FF
MOL003588	Prangenidin	36.31	0.22	FF
MOL013077	Decursin	39.27	0.38	FF
MOL012140	4,9-dimethoxy-1-vinyl-$b-carboline	65.3	0.19	XX
MOL012141	Caribine	37.06	0.83	XX
MOL001460	Cryptopin	78.74	0.72	XX
MOL001558	Sesamin	56.55	0.83	XX
MOL002501	[(1S)-3-[(E)-but-2-enyl]-2-methyl-4-oxo-1-cyclopent-2-enyl] (1R,3R)-3-[(E)-3-methoxy-2-methyl-3-oxoprop-1-enyl]-2,2-dimethylcyclopropane-1-carboxylate	62.52	0.31	XX
MOL002962	(3S)-7-hydroxy-3-(2,3,4-trimethoxyphenyl)chroman-4-one	48.23	0.33	XX
MOL009849	ZINC05223929	31.57	0.83	XX
MOL002135	Myricanone	40.6	0.51	CX
MOL002151	Senkyunone	47.66	0.24	CX
MOL002157	Wallichilide	42.31	0.71	CX
MOL000433	FA	68.96	0.71	CX
MOL001918	Paeoniflorgenone	87.59	0.37	BS
MOL001925	Paeoniflorin_qt	68.18	0.4	BS
MOL001928	Albiflorin_qt	66.64	0.33	BS
MOL001910	11alpha,12alpha-epoxy-3beta-23-dihydroxy-30-norolean-20-en-28,12beta-olide	64.77	0.38	BS
MOL000492	(+)-catechin	54.83	0.24	BS
MOL001924	Paeoniflorin	53.87	0.79	BS
MOL001921	Lactiflorin	49.12	0.8	BS
MOL001919	(3S,5R,8R,9R,10S,14S)-3,17-dihydroxy-4,4,8,10,14-pentamethyl-2,3,5,6,7,9-hexahydro-1H-cyclopenta [a] phenanthrene-15,16-dione	43.56	0.53	BS
MOL001930	Benzoyl paeoniflorin	31.27	0.75	BS
MOL000273	(2R)-2-[(3S,5R,10S,13R,14R,16R,17R)-3,16-dihydroxy-4,4,10,13,14-pentamethyl-2,3,5,6,12,15,16,17-octahydro-1H-cyclopenta [a]phenanthren-17-yl]-6-methylhept-5-enoic acid	30.93	0.81	FL
MOL000275	Trametenolic acid	38.71	0.8	FL
MOL000276	7,9 (11)-dehydropachymic acid	35.11	0.81	FL
MOL000279	Cerevisterol	37.96	0.77	FL
MOL000280	(2R)-2-[(3S,5R,10S,13R,14R,16R,17R)-3,16-dihydroxy-4,4,10,13,14-pentamethyl-2,3,5,6,12,15,16,17-octahydro-1H-cyclopenta [a]phenanthren-17-yl]-5-isopropyl-hex-5-enoic acid	31.07	0.82	FL
MOL000282	Ergosta-7,22E-dien-3beta-ol	43.51	0.72	FL
MOL000283	Ergosterol peroxide	40.36	0.81	FL
MOL000285	(2R)-2-[(5R,10S,13R,14R,16R,17R)-16-hydroxy-3-keto-4,4,10,13,14-pentamethyl-1,2,5,6,12,15,16,17-octahydrocyclopenta [a]phenanthren-17-yl]-5-isopropyl-hex-5-enoic acid	38.26	0.82	FL
MOL000287	3beta-Hydroxy-24-methylene-8-lanostene-21-oic acid	38.7	0.81	FL
MOL000289	Pachymic acid	33.63	0.81	FL
MOL000290	Poricoic acid A	30.61	0.76	FL
MOL000291	Poricoic acid B	30.52	0.75	FL
MOL000292	Poricoic acid C	38.15	0.75	FL
MOL000296	Hederagenin	36.91	0.75	FL
MOL000300	Dehydroeburicoic acid	44.17	0.83	FL
MOL002058	40957-99-1	57.2	0.62	DZ
MOL004367	Olivil	62.23	0.41	DZ
MOL000443	Erythraline	49.18	0.55	DZ
MOL005922	Acanthoside B	43.35	0.77	DZ
MOL006709	AIDS214634	92.43	0.55	DZ
MOL000073	Ent-Epicatechin	48.96	0.24	DZ

(Continued on following page)

TABLE 1 | (*Continued*) The final selected compounds of DuHuo JiSheng Decoction for analysis.

ID	Name	OB	DL	Herb
MOL007563	Yangambin	57.53	0.81	DZ
MOL009007	Eucommin A	30.51	0.85	DZ
MOL009009	(+)-medioresinol	87.19	0.62	DZ
MOL009015	(-)-Tabernemontanine	58.67	0.61	DZ
MOL009027	Cyclopamine	55.42	0.82	DZ
MOL009029	Dehydrodiconiferyl alcohol 4,gamma'-di-O-beta-D-glucopyanoside_qt	51.44	0.4	DZ
MOL009030	Dehydrodieugenol	30.1	0.24	DZ
MOL009031	Cinchonan-9-al, 6′-methoxy- (9R)-	68.22	0.4	DZ
MOL009038	GBGB	45.58	0.83	DZ
MOL009042	Helenalin	77.01	0.19	DZ
MOL009047	(+)-Eudesmin	33.29	0.62	DZ
MOL009053	4-[(2S,3R)-5-[(E)-3-hydroxyprop-1-enyl]-7-methoxy-3-methylol-2,3-dihydrobenzofuran-2-yl]-2-methoxy-phenol	50.76	0.39	DZ
MOL009055	Hirsutin_qt	49.81	0.37	DZ
MOL009057	Liriodendrin_qt	53.14	0.8	DZ
MOL002773	Beta-carotene	37.18	0.58	DZ
MOL008240	(E)-3-[4-[(1R,2R)-2-hydroxy-2-(4-hydroxy-3-methoxy-phenyl)-1-methylol-ethoxy]-3-methoxy-phenyl]acrolein	56.32	0.36	DZ
MOL011604	Syringetin	36.82	0.37	DZ
MOL012461	28-norolean-17-en-3-ol	35.93	0.78	NX
MOL012505	Bidentatoside, ii_qt	31.76	0.59	NX
MOL012542	β-ecdysterone	44.23	0.82	NX
MOL001454	Berberine	36.86	0.78	NX
MOL001458	Coptisine	30.67	0.86	NX
MOL002643	Delta 7-stigmastenol	37.42	0.75	NX
MOL002714	Baicalein	33.52	0.21	NX
MOL002776	Baicalin	40.12	0.75	NX
MOL002897	Epiberberine	43.09	0.78	NX
MOL003847	Inophyllum E	38.81	0.85	NX
MOL000785	Palmatine	64.6	0.65	NX
MOL000085	Beta-daucosterol_qt	36.91	0.75	NX
MOL012537	Spinoside A	41.75	0.4	NX
MOL008406	Spinoside A	39.97	0.4	DS
MOL002879	Diop	43.59	0.39	DS
MOL003036	ZINC03978781	43.83	0.76	DS
MOL004492	Chrysanthemaxanthin	38.72	0.58	DS
MOL005321	Frutinone A	65.9	0.34	DS
MOL000006	Luteolin	36.16	0.25	DS
MOL006554	Taraxerol	38.4	0.77	DS
MOL006774	Stigmast-7-enol	37.42	0.75	DS
MOL008391	5alpha-Stigmastan-3,6-dione	33.12	0.79	DS
MOL008393	7-(beta-Xylosyl)cephalomannine_qt	38.33	0.29	DS
MOL008397	Daturilin	50.37	0.77	DS
MOL008400	Glycitein	50.48	0.24	DS
MOL008407	(8S,9S,10R,13R,14S,17R)-17-[(E,2R,5S)-5-ethyl-6-methylhept-3-en-2-yl]-10,13-dimethyl-1,2,4,7,8,9,11,12,14,15,16,17-dodecahydrocyclopenta [a]phenanthren-3-one	45.4	0.76	DS
MOL008411	11-Hydroxyrankinidine	40	0.66	DS
MOL001484	Inermine	75.18	0.54	GC
MOL001792	DFV	32.76	0.18	GC
MOL002311	Glycyrol	90.78	0.67	GC
MOL000239	Jaranol	50.83	0.29	GC
MOL002565	Medicarpin	49.22	0.34	GC
MOL000354	Isorhamnetin	49.6	0.31	GC
MOL003656	Lupiwighteone	51.64	0.37	GC
MOL000392	Formononetin	69.67	0.21	GC
MOL000417	Calycosin	47.75	0.24	GC
MOL004328	Naringenin	59.29	0.21	GC
MOL004805	(2S)-2-[4-hydroxy-3-(3-methylbut-2-enyl)phenyl]-8,8-dimethyl-2,3-dihydropyrano [2,3-f]chromen-4-one	31.79	0.72	GC
MOL004806	Euchrenone	30.29	0.57	GC
MOL004808	Glyasperin B	65.22	0.44	GC
MOL004810	Glyasperin F	75.84	0.54	GC
MOL004811	Glyasperin C	45.56	0.4	GC
MOL004814	Isotrifoliol	31.94	0.42	GC
MOL004815	(E)-1-(2,4-dihydroxyphenyl)-3-(2,2-dimethylchromen-6-yl)prop-2-en-1-one	39.62	0.35	GC
MOL004820	Kanzonols W	50.48	0.52	GC

(Continued on following page)

TABLE 1 | (*Continued*) The final selected compounds of DuHuo JiSheng Decoction for analysis.

ID	Name	OB	DL	Herb
MOL004824	(2S)-6-(2,4-dihydroxyphenyl)-2-(2-hydroxypropan-2-yl)-4-methoxy-2,3-dihydrofuro [3,2-g]chromen-7-one	60.25	0.63	GC
MOL004827	Semilicoisoflavone B	48.78	0.55	GC
MOL004828	Glepidotin A	44.72	0.35	GC
MOL004829	Glepidotin B	64.46	0.34	GC
MOL004833	Phaseolinisoflavan	32.01	0.45	GC
MOL004835	Glypallichalcone	61.6	0.19	GC
MOL004838	8-(6-hydroxy-2-benzofuranyl)-2,2-dimethyl-5-chromenol	58.44	0.38	GC
MOL004841	Licochalcone B	76.76	0.19	GC
MOL004848	Licochalcone G	49.25	0.32	GC
MOL004849	3-(2,4-dihydroxyphenyl)-8-(1,1-dimethylprop-2-enyl)-7-hydroxy-5-methoxy-coumarin	59.62	0.43	GC
MOL004855	Licoricone	63.58	0.47	GC
MOL004856	Gancaonin A	51.08	0.4	GC
MOL004857	Gancaonin B	48.79	0.45	GC
MOL004860	Licorice glycoside E	32.89	0.27	GC
MOL004863	3-(3,4-dihydroxyphenyl)-5,7-dihydroxy-8-(3-methylbut-2-enyl)chromone	66.37	0.41	GC
MOL004864	5,7-dihydroxy-3-(4-methoxyphenyl)-8-(3-methylbut-2-enyl)chromone	30.49	0.41	GC
MOL004866	2-(3,4-dihydroxyphenyl)-5,7-dihydroxy-6-(3-methylbut-2-enyl)chromone	44.15	0.41	GC
MOL004879	Glycyrin	52.61	0.47	GC
MOL004882	Licocoumarone	33.21	0.36	GC
MOL004883	Licoisoflavone	41.61	0.42	GC
MOL004884	Licoisoflavone B	38.93	0.55	GC
MOL004885	Licoisoflavanone	52.47	0.54	GC
MOL004891	Shinpterocarpin	80.3	0.73	GC
MOL004898	(E)-3-[3,4-dihydroxy-5-(3-methylbut-2-enyl)phenyl]-1-(2,4-dihydroxyphenyl)prop-2-en-1-one	46.27	0.31	GC
MOL004903	Liquiritin	65.69	0.74	GC
MOL004904	Licopyranocoumarin	80.36	0.65	GC
MOL004905	3,22-Dihydroxy-11-oxo-delta (12)-oleanene-27-alpha-methoxycarbonyl-29-oic acid	34.32	0.55	GC
MOL004907	Glyzaglabrin	61.07	0.35	GC
MOL004908	Glabridin	53.25	0.47	GC
MOL004910	Glabranin	52.9	0.31	GC
MOL004911	Glabrene	46.27	0.44	GC
MOL004912	Glabrone	52.51	0.5	GC
MOL004913	1,3-dihydroxy-9-methoxy-6-benzofurano [3,2-c]chromenone	48.14	0.43	GC
MOL004914	1,3-dihydroxy-8,9-dimethoxy-6-benzofurano [3,2-c]chromenone	62.9	0.53	GC
MOL004915	Eurycarpin A	43.28	0.37	GC
MOL004917	Glycyroside	37.25	0.79	GC
MOL004924	(-)-Medicocarpin	40.99	0.95	GC
MOL004935	Sigmoidin-B	34.88	0.41	GC
MOL004941	(2R)-7-hydroxy-2-(4-hydroxyphenyl)chroman-4-one	71.12	0.18	GC
MOL004945	(2S)-7-hydroxy-2-(4-hydroxyphenyl)-8-(3-methylbut-2-enyl)chroman-4-one	36.57	0.32	GC
MOL004948	Isoglycyrol	44.7	0.84	GC
MOL004949	Isolicoflavonol	45.17	0.42	GC
MOL004957	HMO	38.37	0.21	GC
MOL004959	1-Methoxyphaseollidin	69.98	0.64	GC
MOL004961	Quercetin der	46.45	0.33	GC
MOL004966	3′-Hydroxy-4′-O-Methylglabridin	43.71	0.57	GC
MOL000497	Licochalcone a	40.79	0.29	GC
MOL004974	3′-Methoxyglabridin	46.16	0.57	GC
MOL004978	2-[(3R)-8,8-dimethyl-3,4-dihydro-2H-pyrano [6,5-f]chromen-3-yl]-5-methoxyphenol	36.21	0.52	GC
MOL004980	Inflacoumarin A	39.71	0.33	GC
MOL004985	Icos-5-enoic acid	30.7	0.2	GC
MOL004988	Kanzonol F	32.47	0.89	GC
MOL004989	6-prenylated eriodictyol	39.22	0.41	GC
MOL004990	7,2′,4′-trihydroxy-5-methoxy-3-arylcoumarin	83.71	0.27	GC
MOL004991	7-Acetoxy-2-methylisoflavone	38.92	0.26	GC
MOL004993	8-prenylated eriodictyol	53.79	0.4	GC
MOL004996	Gadelaidic acid	30.7	0.2	GC
MOL000500	Vestitol	74.66	0.21	GC
MOL005000	Gancaonin G	60.44	0.39	GC
MOL005001	Gancaonin H	50.1	0.78	GC
MOL005003	Licoagrocarpin	58.81	0.58	GC
MOL005007	Glyasperins M	72.67	0.59	GC
MOL005008	Glycyrrhiza flavonol A	41.28	0.6	GC
MOL005012	Licoagroisoflavone	57.28	0.49	GC

(Continued on following page)

TABLE 1 | *(Continued)* The final selected compounds of DuHuo JiSheng Decoction for analysis.

ID	Name	OB	DL	Herb
MOL005013	18α-hydroxyglycyrrhetic acid	41.16	0.71	GC
MOL005016	Odoratin	49.95	0.3	GC
MOL005017	Phaseol	78.77	0.58	GC
MOL005018	Xambioona	54.85	0.87	GC
MOL005020	Dehydroglyasperins C	53.82	0.37	GC
MOL000098	Quercetin	46.43	0.28	DZ/SJS
MOL000098	Quercetin	46.43	0.28	GC/NX
MOL000173	Wogonin	30.68	0.23	FF/NX
MOL000211	Mairin	55.38	0.78	BS/DZ/GC
MOL000358	Beta-sitosterol	36.91	0.75	DH/QJ/FF/DG/BS/DZ/NX
MOL000359	Sitosterol	36.91	0.75	SJS/QJ/FF/CX/SDH/BS/GC
MOL000422	Kaempferol	41.88	0.24	XX/BS/DZ/NX/GC
MOL000449	Stigmasterol	43.83	0.76	DG/SDH/NX/DS
MOL001006	poriferasta-7,22E-dien-3beta-ol	42.98	0.76	NX/DS
MOL001494	Mandenol	42	0.19	FF/CX
MOL001941	Ammidin	34.55	0.22	DH/FF
MOL001942	Isoimperatorin	45.46	0.23	DH/FF
MOL002140	Perlolyrine	65.95	0.27	CX/DS
MOL003896	7-Methoxy-2-methyl isoflavone	42.56	0.2	DS/GC
MOL004355	Spinasterol	42.98	0.76	NX/DS
MOL007059	3-beta-Hydroxymethyllenetanshiquinone	32.16	0.41	DZ/DS
MOL007514	Methyl icosa-11,14-dienoate	39.67	0.23	FF/DS

OB, oral bioavailability; DL, drug-likeness; DH, Du Huo; SJS, Sang Ji Sheng; QJ, Qin Jiao; FF, Fang Feng; XX, Xi Xin; CX, Chuan Xiong; DG, Dang Gui; SDH, Shu Di Huanga; BS, Bai Shao; RG, Rou Gui; FL, Fu Ling; DZ, Du Zhong; NX, Niu Xi; DS, Dang Shen; GC, Gan Cao.

Food and Drug Test, Beijing, China) (**Supplementary Figure S1**), with flow rate of 0.8 ml/min under column temperature.

Screening of the Bioactive Components of DHJSD

All DHJSD components were explored using the TCM systems pharmacology database and analysis platform (TCMSP, https://tcmspw.com/tcmsp.php). The chemical composition of TCM was screened based on oral bioavailability (OB ≥ 30%) and drug-likeness (DL ≥ 0.18). The OB value describe the relative amount drug which was absorbed into the systemic blood circulation, through the extravascular route. DL means the degree of similarity between bioactive component and a known drug, and the class of compounds with the potential for drug development. Moreover, 206 eligible DHJSD compounds were obtained from the TCM systems pharmacology database, and considered as candidate compounds (**Table 1**), including 9 for DH, 2 for QJ, 2 for SJS, 8 for XX, 0 for RG, 18 for FF, 15 for FL, 2 for SDH, 20 for NX, 21 for DS, 28 for DZ, 7 for CX, 2 for DG, 13 for BS and 92 for GC.

Animals

Sprague Dawley rats aged 4 weeks (BW: 90–120g, n = 24) were purchased from Shanghai Slack Laboratory Animal Co. (Shanghai, China). Rats were raised in the SPF-class housing of laboratory at 60% humidity, 23°C room temperature and 12 h rhythm (8:00 a.m.-8:00 p.m.) with food and water freely available. The animals were carefully treated according to the National Institutes of Health Guidelines for the Care and Use of Laboratory Animals, and the Animal Care and Use Committee of the Fujian University of TCM play a major role in approved and supervised the experimental (approval number: 2020015).

Preparation of Chondrocytes and LPS-Exposed Model

Chondrocytes were harvested and produced to an LPS-exposed cellular model as done in our previous studies (Liang et al., 2019; Li et al., 2020a; Li et al., 2020b). Briefly, chondrocytes were harvested from the knee joints of four Sprague Dawley rats at a time, six times in total. Cells were identified with collagen II antibody by immunohistochemistry. The cellular model was built by exposed Chondrocytes under10 ng/mL of LPS (Sigma-Aldrich, United States) for 8 h.

Identification of the Key Pathway Concerning DHJSD in Treating OA by NPA

Predicting the Molecular Targets of OA

Genetic date on patients with OA acquisition from the Gene Expression Omnibus database (GEO, https://www.ncbi.nlm.nih.Gov/geo/). The series GSE46750 was an analysis of synovial cells from OA patients' local tissue of inflammatory (I) or normal/reactive (N/R). Differential expression patterns were identified in two regions of the synovium in 12 patients undergoing total knee arthroplasty. The series GSE82107 was an analysis of synovial biopsies that were obtained from the synovium of patients with OA to identify genes upregulated during OA. A total of 10 microarrays of end-stage OA synovial biopsies were compared with 7 microarrays of synovial biopsies obtained from individuals without a joint disease. The series GSE51588 was isolated from total RNA from the regions of interest from OA (n = 20) and non-OA (n = 5) patients, samples were got from knee lateral (LT) and medial tibial (MT) plateaus. This profile was obtained by performing whole-genome microarray profiling of the human osteoarthritic subchondral bone. The series GSE117999 was an analysis of cartilage tissues obtained from 12 OA patients 12 normal patients. The series GSE32317 characterised analyse the synovial membranes from early-stage or end-stage OA patients. A total of 10 samples of early-stage knee OA synovial membranes from the patients undergoing arthroscopic procedures for degenerative meniscal tears and 9 samples of end-stage knee OA synovial membranes. The series GSE29746 was used to identify difference expression gene between human synovial fibroblasts (SF) from OA synovial tissues and normal SF from healthy individuals (HSF). Synovial fibroblasts were obtained from 11 sex-matched and age-matched adult healthy donors (HSF) and 11 sex-matched and age-matched patients with OA (OASF). The raw file was processed by a robust multi-array average algorithm with normalisation of matrix data, and then filtered using the Limma package to analyse twice. The genes with $p < 0.05$ and $|\log 2 \text{ (fold change)}| > 0.263$ were screened as significantly differentially expressed genes. The analysis data obtained from the two series GSE46750 and GSE82107 were integrated as series 1, the analysis data obtained from the two series GSE51588 and GSE117999 were integrated as series 2 and the analysis data obtained from the two series GSE32317 and GSE29746 were integrated as series 3.

Construction of the Active Component-Target Network of DHJSD

The compound target network of DHJSD was constructed and visualised by the Cytoscape 3.7.2 software. Protein–protein interaction (PPI) data that contain many database including the Database of Interacting Proteins (DIP™), Biological General Repository for Interaction Datasets, Human Protein Reference Database, IntAct Molecular Interaction Database (IntAct), Molecular Interaction database (MINT) and the Biomolecular Interaction Network Database. The Cytoscape3.7.2 software provides a visual for the PPI networks for DHJSD putative targets and OA-related targets.

Construction of PPI Networks and Screening of Key Targets

In this study, the Biogenet plugin was used to construct the PPI networks for DHJSD and OA targets, and Cytoscape was further to intersection of the two networks, screened the direct or indirect target regulatory network for DHJSD in OA treatment. Key genes were identified based on the network topology analysis plugin CytoNCA and filter out by degree centrality (DC), betweenness centrality (BC) and closeness centrality (CC) and explored for the core genes for DHJSD activity against OA.

Gene Ontology and KEGG Analysis

The Gene Ontology (GO) database (http://geneontology.org/) includes biological process (BP), molecular function (MF) and cellular component (CC) data, and it was used to identify the biological mechanisms of a number of large genomes. The top 20 functional categories of each category were selected (FDR< 0.05). The KEGG database (https://www.kegg.jp/) was used to explore possible function and biological correlation with candidate target genes. The Cluster Profiler R package was used to visualise the result of GO and KEGG pathway enrichment. Pathways with an FDR of <0.05 were selected for the next step analysis. The gene pathway network analysis was used to determine significantly regulated pathways. To screen key target genes involved in DHJSD activity, we constructed the gene pathway network.

Component-Target Molecular Docking

The 3D structure of the key target genes was downloaded from the RSCB PDB database (https://www.rcsb.org/), the Auto Dock Tools 1.5.6 software was used to remove water and ligands and add hydrogen and stored as PDBQT file. The 2D structures of the top nine compounds of DHJSD were downloaded from the PubChem database (https://pubchem.ncbi.nlm.nih.gov/), processed, transformed into PDB format by Chem3D and stored as PDBQT file. The key target genes were provided as receptors, and the active compounds were provided as ligands. Finally, Autodock vina 1.1.2 was used to dock compounds with key target genes and protein.

Venn Analysis

The key target genes of intersections among series 1, series 2 and series 3 were screened by Venn analysis. The results of the key target genes of DHJSD, interactive PPI network topological analysis were submitted for Venn analysis. KEGG was performed to further analysis the genes dropped in the intersections of the target genes of DHJSD along with PPI network topological analysis. Finally, the key pathways concerning DHJSD in OA treatment were identified.

Verification of the Involvement of Targeted Pathways

Verification of the Efficacy of DHJSD on OA Related miRNA and Regulatory Pathway Prediction

Total RNA was extracted from chondrocytes using the TRIZOL reagent (Life, United States) and reverse transcribed into cDNA using RevertAid First Strand cDNA Synthesis kit (PrimeScript™ RT reagent kit). The mRNA expressions of miR-146a-5p and miR-34a-5p were detected using the ABI 7500 Fast Real-time PCR system. The primers used for amplification were as follows: miR-146a-5p (sequence UGA GAA CUG AAU UCC AUG GGU U, forward TGA GAA CTG AAT TCC ATG GGT T) and miR-34a-5p (sequence UGG CAG UGU CUU AGC UGG UUG U, forward TGG CAG TGT CTUT AGC TGG TTG T). The DIANA Tools (http://www.microrna.gr) was used to predict miRNA target mRNAs (Vlachos and Hatzigeorgiou, 2017), and we also analysed the miRNA target mRNA regulatory pathways.

Verification of the Efficacy of DHJSD by Western Blotting

It is found that the protein expression of MMP-9 in chondrocytes (LPS 10 ng/ml) was significantly reduced after culture under

300 μg/ml of DHJSD for 8 h in our previous research (Xu et al., 2019). Therefore, we selected 300 μg/ml of DHJSD and a duration of 8 h as the experimental conditions. According to NPA results, we also performed standard western blot analysis was used to confirm the involvement of the targeted pathway. We confirmed the involvement of the NF-κB signalling pathway and the toll-like receptor signalling pathway (Please refer to the Results and Discussion section). Chondrocytes were subjected to four treatment group, namely, control, model (LPS 10 ng/ml), DHJSD (DHJSD 300 μg/ml + LPS 10 ng/ml) and PDTC (an inhibitor of the NF-κB signalling pathway) (PDTC 10 μM + LPS 10 ng/ml) or TAK 242 (an inhibitor of the toll-like receptor four signalling pathway) (TAK 242 1 μM + LPS 10 ng/ml) for 8 h. Cell were lysed immediately in lysis buffer (Beyotime Institute of Biotechnology, Haimen, China) for 30 min on ice, and total proteins were collected and quantified by the bicinchoninic acid assay. Protein sample (20 μg) was run on a 10% SDS-PAGE gel and then transferred protein onto polyvinylidene fluoride membranes (Sigma-Aldrich, United States). Then, 5% non-fat milk was used to block the membranes before incubation with primary antibodies against NF-κB p65 (ab16502, abcam, United States), IKK-β (ab124957, abcam, United States), TLR4 (ab22048, abcam, United States), MyD88 (ab 2064, abcam, United States), TRAF6 (ab40675, abcam, United States), IKK-α (ab32041, abcam, United States), IKB-α (ab32518, abcam, United States), *p*-IKB-α (ab2859, abcam, United States), ADAMTS-4 (ab185722, abcam, United States), ADAMTS-5 (ab41037, abcam, United States), MMP-3 (ab52915, abcam, United States), MMP-13 (ab39012, abcam, United States), MMP-14 (ab51074, abcam, United States), collagen II (ab34712, abcam, United States) and *β*-actin (ab8226, Cambridge, UK) at 4°C overnight. Goat anti-rabbit horseradish peroxidase-conjugated secondary antibody IgG (bs-0295G-HRP, Bioss, China) or goat anti-mouse horseradish peroxidase-conjugated secondary antibody IgG (bs-0296G-HRP, Bioss, China) was added to the membranes at 30°C column temperature. The enhanced chemiluminescence method was used to visualize the immunocomplexes. Protein bands were quantified by densitometry scanning (X-ray Spectroscopy System, cat. no. 170-8070; Bio-Rad). The Blots was analyzed using the Image Lab software, *β*-actin used as the control.

Quantitative Real-Time PCR (qPCR) Assay

The mRNA expression levels of TLR4, TRAF-6, MyD88, NF-κB p65, IKK-α, IKK-β, MMP-3, MMP-13, MMP-14, IL-1β and TNF-α were detected by using the ABI 7500 Fast Real-time PCR system. The primers used for amplification were as follows: TLR4 (forward 5′-CCG CTC TGG CAT CAT CTT CA-3′, reverse 5′-CTC CCA CTC GAG GTA GGT GT-3′); TRAF-6 (forward 5′-TGG TCA TTC ATA GCC CTG GAT-3′, reverse 5′-AGG ATC GTG AGG CGT ATT GTA-3′); MyD88 (forward 5′-CGG AGG AGA TGG GTT TCG AG-3′, reverse 5′-CCA GGC ATC CAA CAA ACT GC-3′); NF-κB p65 (forward 5′-AGA GAA GCA CAG ATA CCA CTA AGA-3′, reverse 5′-GTT CAG CCT CAT AGA AGC CAT C-3′); IKK-α (forward 5′-TGG AGT GAG AGG CTG TGA TAG-3′, reverse 5′-TTG AGT TGC TGT GAT GCT GAG-3′); IKK-β (forward 5′-CAT CAA GCA ATG CCG ACA GG-3′, reverse 5′-CAT TGG GTG CCA AGT TCT GC-3′); MMP-3 (forward 5′-ATG ATG ATG AAC GAT GGA CAG ATG-3′, reverse 5′-TGC TAC ACA TTG GTA AGG TCT CAG-3′); MMP-13 (forward 5′-GGA GTA ATC GCA TTG TGA GAG TC-3′, reverse 5′-GGT TCC AGC CAC GCA TAG TC-3′); MMP-14 (forward 5′-GCA CTT CGT GTT GCC TGA TGA C-3′, reverse 5′-GCC AGA ACC ATC GCT CCT TGA-3′); IL-1β (forward 5′-GCA CAG TTC CCC AAC TGG TA-3′, reverse 5′-AAG ACA CGG GTT CCA TGG TG-3′); TNF-α (forward 5′-ACT GAA CTT CGG GGT GAT CG-3′, reverse 5′-GCT TGG TGG TTT GCT ACG AC-3′). GAPDH was used as an internal control.

Statistical Analysis

All statistical data were analysed by SPSS 20.0 software (SPSS Inc., Chicago, IL, United States) and expressed as mean ± standard deviation (SD). Data obtained from three independent experiments were analysed by two-way analysis of variance, through Bonferroni's post-hoc correction for multiple comparisons. $P < 0.05$ was considered to indicate a significant difference.

RESULTS

Screening of the Key Pathway of DHJSD Using NPA

Compound Target Network Analysis

Differential analysis of the GEO database gene series GSE46750, GSE82107, GSE51588, GSE117999, GSE32317 and GSE29746 identified 538, 2,161, 4,531, 93, 433, and 2341 OA-related targets respectively. The heatmaps and volcano plot of OA-related targets are depicted in **Figure 1A–1F** and **Supplementary Figure S1A–1F**. A total of 2,638, 4,598 and 2715 OA-related targets were identified from series 1, 2 and 3, respectively. Altogether there were 85 OA-related targets at the intersection of series 1, 2 and 3 (**Figure 1G**).

Using the screened compounds and their targets, the compound-target network for DHJSD was constructed (**Figure 2**). For series 1, the network consisted of 175 nodes (131 compounds for DHJSD and 44 compound targets) and 358 edges (**Figure 2A**). For series 2, the network consisted of 201 nodes (121 compounds for DHJSD and 80 compound targets) and 486 edges (**Figure 2B**). For series 3, the network consisted of 188 nodes (129 compounds for DHJSD and 59 compound targets) and 563 edges (**Figure 2C**).

Screening of Candidate Targets for DHJSD Against OA

To investigate the possible mechanisms that correlated with the effect of DHJSD on OA, the PPI networks of the OA-related targets and putative DHJSD targets were merged to identify a set of candidate targets. The first network of series 1 consisted of 2,785 nodes and 64,777 edges (**Figure 3A**), with a median of 27° among all nodes, and identified nodes with more than 61° as significant targets. A secondary network consisting of significant (DC > 61) targets from the first network, which contained 635 nodes and 24,605 edges (**Figure 3B**). The median values for BC and CC

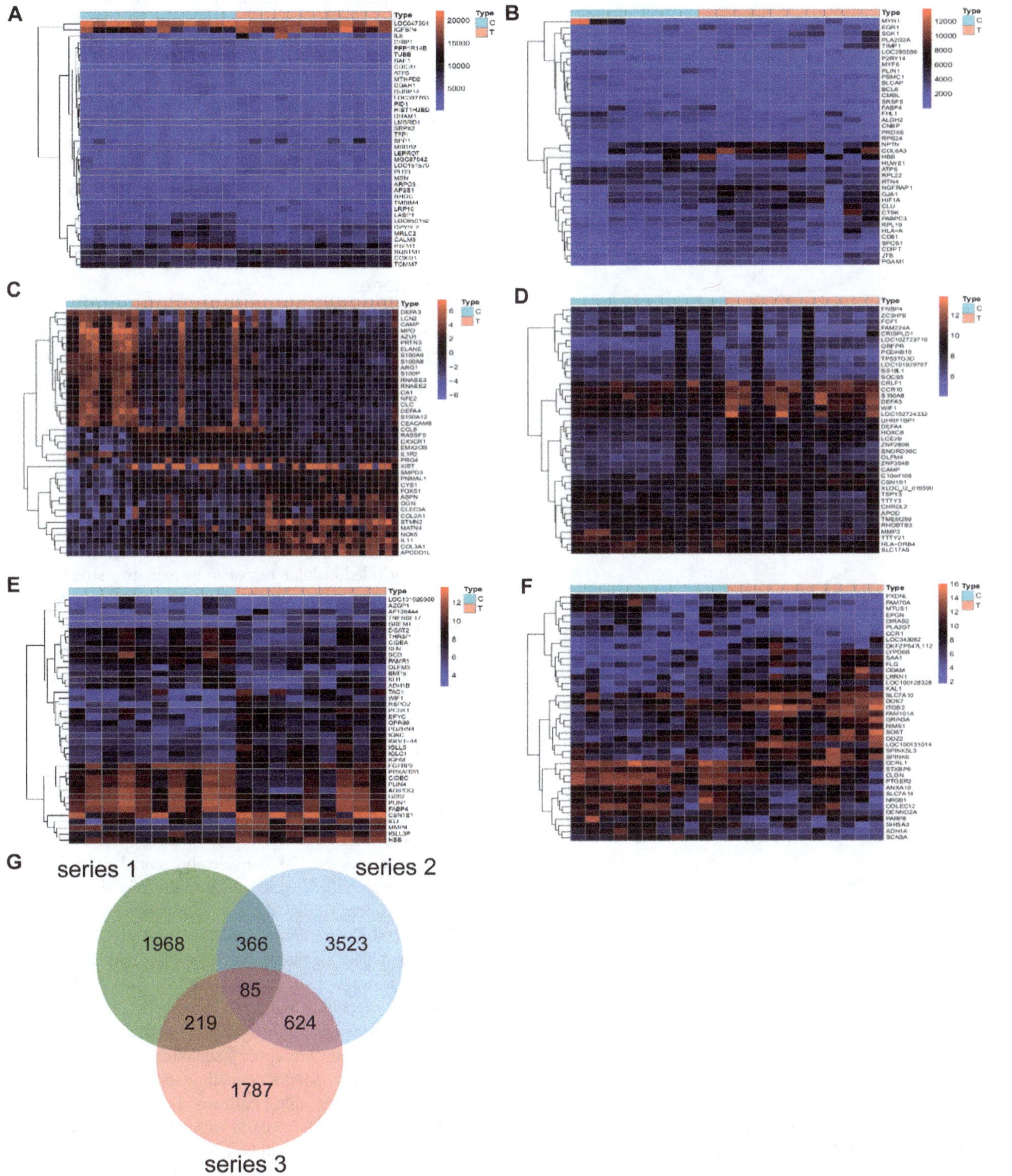

FIGURE 1 | Differentially expressed genes in series 1, series 2 and series 3. The heatmap of series 1 (GSE46750 and GSE82107) **(A,B)**, series 2 (GSE51588 and GSE117999) **(C,D)**, series 3 (GSE32317 and GSE29746) **(E,F)**. **(G)** There are a total of 85 gene intersection in the three series, including PITPNC1, GYPC, AK5, DOK7, KLK3, DRG1, SIGLEC10, PHLDB1, ZCCHC5, TFPI, NUF2, LTC4S, CENPM, RBX1, DKC1, PRPS1, TMEM217, EXO1, ARHGAP11A, ELL2, FANCI, NAMPT, LPPR4, CDK2AP2, RARG, CERCAM, SPTAN1RAB20, MFNG, FKBP10, MARC1, TMEM35, MXD1, ISM1, BGN, SPATA18, FMNL3, LTBP3, CD300C, SPATA19, ABLIM3, RSPO2, STXBP2, CPLX1, ZBTB7B, BCL2L1, PNPLA2, SLC22A4, ANO3, SHROOM2, CRIP2, HPRT1, HBB, PRUNE2, SCRG1, WISP2, CCDC86, PDZRN4, HTR2A, RNF150, PCSK1, ZFP14, CCNB1, ANGPTL2, ZFAND5OGN, SLC11A1, KCNJ15, P2RY14, FABP4, SLC2A1, ALOX12, SF3A3, TCF7, TUSC3, C15orf26, SPATA17, LCAT, SLC16A6, SMOC2, LIMK2, CCDC136, PLA2G5, CKS2 and CCR5.

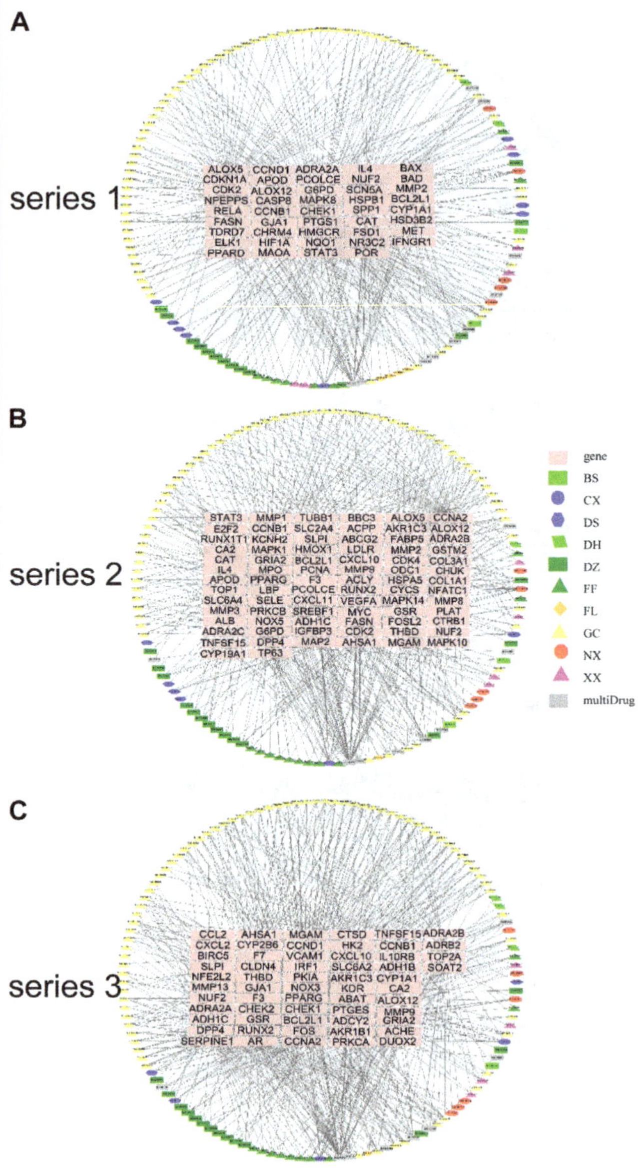

FIGURE 2 | Compound-target network for DHJSD. The pink rectangle represents targets; the green rectangle, blue ellipse, blue hexagon, green parallelogram, cyan rectangle, cyan triangle, orange diamond, yellow triangle, red octagon, purple triangle and gray rectangle represent the compounds from BS, CX, DS, DH, DZ, FF, FL, GC, NX, XX and 22 multi-Drug.

were 255.456929 and 0.567514, respectively. In order to construct the final network, additional screened to identify candidate targets, 163 targets with BC > 255.456929 and CC > 0.567514 were selected (**Figure 3C**). A total of 163 target genes were eventually identified for DHJSD activity against OA in series 1. The same process was used for series 2, and the network consisted of 3,652 nodes and 90,109 edges (**Figure 3D**), with a median of 29° among all nodes. The secondary network consisted of 898 nodes and 38,683 edges (**Figure 3E**). The median values for BC and CC were 360.002407 and 0.544242, respectively. In order to construct the final network, additional screened to identify candidate targets, 228 targets with BC > 360.002407 and CC > 0.544242 were selected (**Figure 3F**). Thus, 228 target genes were eventually identified for DHJSD activity against OA in series 2. For series 3, the network consisted of 2,462 nodes and 57,944 edges (**Figure 3G**) with a median 27° among all nodes. The secondary network contained 580 nodes and 23,359 edges (**Figure 3H**). The median values for BC and CC were 236.991554 and 0.556917, respectively. In order to construct the final network, additional screened to identify candidate targets, 150 targets with BC > 236.991554 and CC > 0.556917 were selected (**Figure 3I**). Finally, 150 target genes were eventually identified for DHJSD activity against OA in series 3.

KEGG and GO Enrichment Analysis of Compound Target Genes

GO and KEGG pathway analysis was conducted to examine the 44 compound targets from series 1, 80 compound targets from series 2 and 59 compound targets from series 3. For series 1, 790 GO terms were significantly enriched (FDR <0.05) (734 BP categories, 14 CC categories and 42 MF categories). The highly enriched GO terms for BP, CC and MF included response to alcohol, response to antibiotic, cyclin-dependent protein kinase holoenzyme complex, mitochondrial outer membrane, NADP binding and histone kinase activity. For series 2, 695 GO terms were significantly enriched (FDR <0.05) (616 BP categories, 32 CC categories and 47 MF categories). The highly enriched GO terms for the BP, CC, and MF included cellular response to oxidative stress, response to oxidative stress, secretory granule lumen, cytoplasmic vesicle lumen, serine-type endopeptidase activity and serine-type peptidase activity. For series 3, 607 GO terms were significantly enriched (FDR <0.05) (551 BP categories, 19 CC categories and 37 MF categories). The highly enriched GO terms for the BP, CC, and MF included regulation of wound healing, regulation of response to wounding, apical part of cell, collagen-containing extracellular matrix, adrenergic receptor activity and histone kinase activity. The top 20 terms are depicted in **Supplementary Figures S2–S4**.

Figure 4 shows the pathways significantly correlation with DHJSD and OA, which were identified by the KEGG pathway analysis. For series 1, 93 considerably enriched pathways (FDR <0.05) were identified, which include the p53 signalling pathway, Pancreatic cancer, PI3K-Akt signalling pathway, IL-17 signalling pathway, Toll-like receptor signalling pathway, MAPK signalling pathway and TNF signalling pathway. For series 2, 88 significantly enriched pathways (FDR <0.05) were identified, which include the AGE-RAGE signalling pathway in diabetic complications, IL-17 signalling pathway, p53 signalling pathway, TNF signalling pathway, Toll-like receptor signalling pathway, PI3K-Akt signalling pathway, MAPK signalling pathway, NF-κB signalling pathway and Ras signalling pathway. For series 3, 21 significantly enriched pathways (FDR <0.05) were identified, which include the AGE-RAGE signalling pathway in diabetic complications, p53 signalling pathway, TNF signalling pathway and IL-17 signalling pathway. Series 1 and 2 contained 72 identical pathways, series 2 and 3 contained 14 identical pathways and series 1 and 3 consisted of 13 identical pathways.

Gene Pathway Network Analysis

The gene pathway network based on the significantly enriched pathways and genes were constructed (**Figure 5**). For series 1,

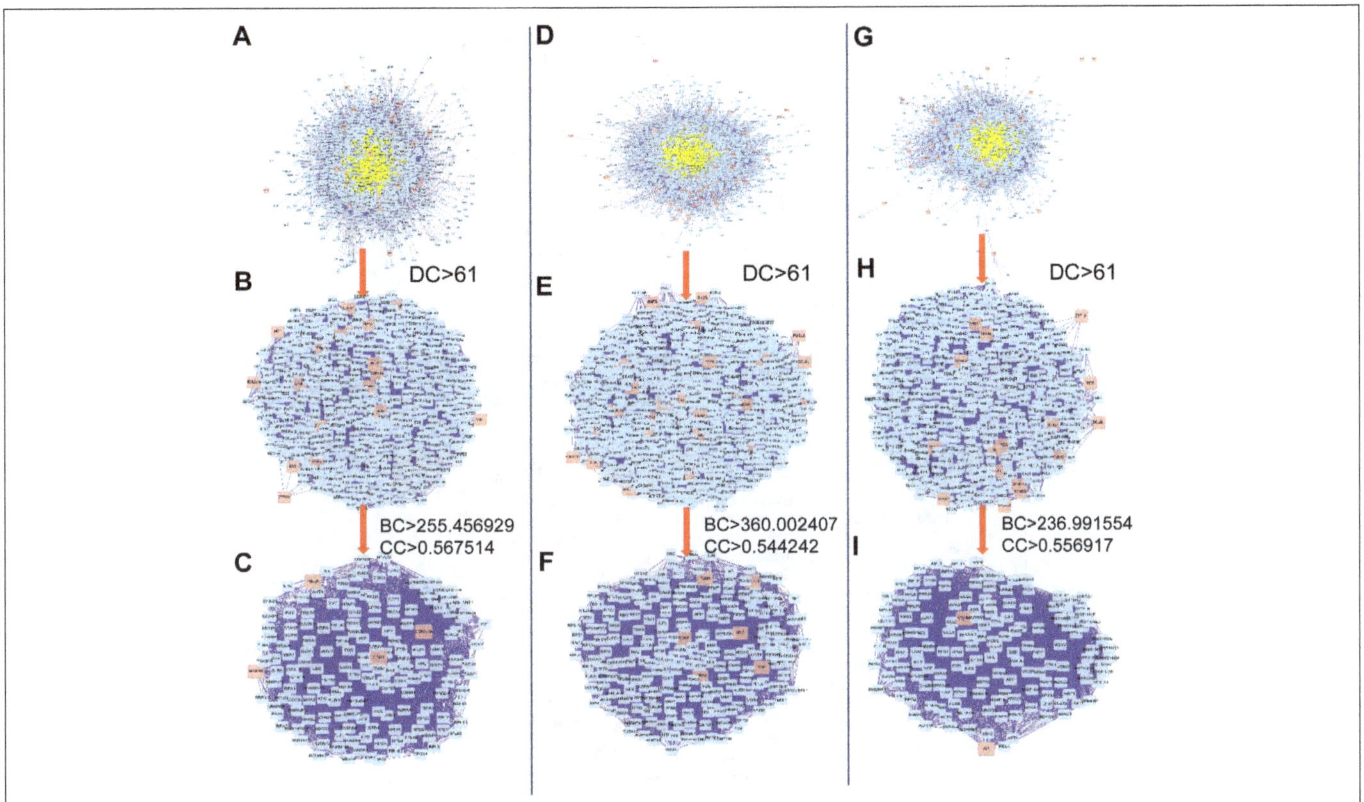

FIGURE 3 | The candidate targets for DHJSD activity against OA. The interactive PPI network topology analysis of DHJSD putative targets and OA-related targets were constructed for series 1 **(A, B, C)**, series 2 **(D, E, F)** and series 3 **(G, H, I)**. DC, degree centrality; BC, betweenness centrality; CC, closeness centrality.

based on the topological analysis and degree 20 pathways was performed. The network diagram showed that MAPK8, CCND1, RELA and CDKN1A had the highest degree, and selected as the core target gene. Moreover, BAD, STAT3, BCL2L1, CASP8 and CDK2 also exhibited a large degree (**Figure 5A**). For series 2, based on the topological analysis and degree 20 pathways was performed. The network diagram showed that MAPK1, MAPK14, MAPK10, CHUK had the highest degree, and selected as the core target gene. Moreover, STAT3, MMP9, MYC, CDK2, CYCS, CDK4 and E2F2 also exhibited a large degree (**Figure 5B**). For series 3, based on the topological analysis and degree 20 pathways was performed. The network diagram indicated that FOS had the highest degree, and selected as the core target gene. Moreover, ADCY2, MMP13, PRCKA, CCL2, MMP9, CCND1 and SERPINE1 also exhibited a high degree (**Figure 5C**).

The intersection of DHJSD and the three chip targets and the core targets obtained after the topological analysis of the three chips were selected for KEGG analysis. DHJSD was analysed for the union of the three chip targets and 77 KEGG pathways were detected. After the topological analysis of the three chips, 126 core targets were selected for KEGG analysis to obtain 41 KEGG pathways. The intersection of 77 and 41 pathways and 22 KEGG pathways are shown in **Figure 6**. Based on these results, the NF-κB signalling pathway and the toll-like receptor signalling pathway were chosen as the key pathways for further research.

Molecular Docking Analysis

The results of molecular docking analysis to confirm the top nine compounds (quercetin, baicalein, beta-carotene, isorhamnetin, kaempferol, licochalcone a, luteolin, naringenin and wogonin) related to TLR4 showed that all compounds had strong binding affinity to TLR4, as shown in **Table 2**. The top three compounds strongly associated with TLR4 were beta-carotene, quercetin and luteolin (**Figure 7**). In addition, the top nine compounds also showed tightly bound to RELA (also known as NF-κB3), CHUK (also known as IKKα) (**Supplementary Table S2, Figure S5, S6**), RELA and CHUK were the core target genes obtained from the topological analysis. Verification of the involvement of targeted pathways in the therapeutic effects of DHJSD against OA.

DHJSD Inhibited the Expression of miR-146a-5p and miR-34a-5p in LPS-Exposed Chondrocytes

LPS exposure increased the expressions of miR-146a-5p (**Figure 8A**) and miR-34a-5p (**Figure 8B**), whereas DHJSD downregulated these expressions in LPS-exposed chondrocytes. The miRNA-regulated gene-pathway analysis (**Figure 8C**) showed that the toll-like receptor signalling pathway (p = 0.012) and the NF-κB signalling pathway (p = 0.042) were significantly enriched, which was consistent with the NPA analysis.

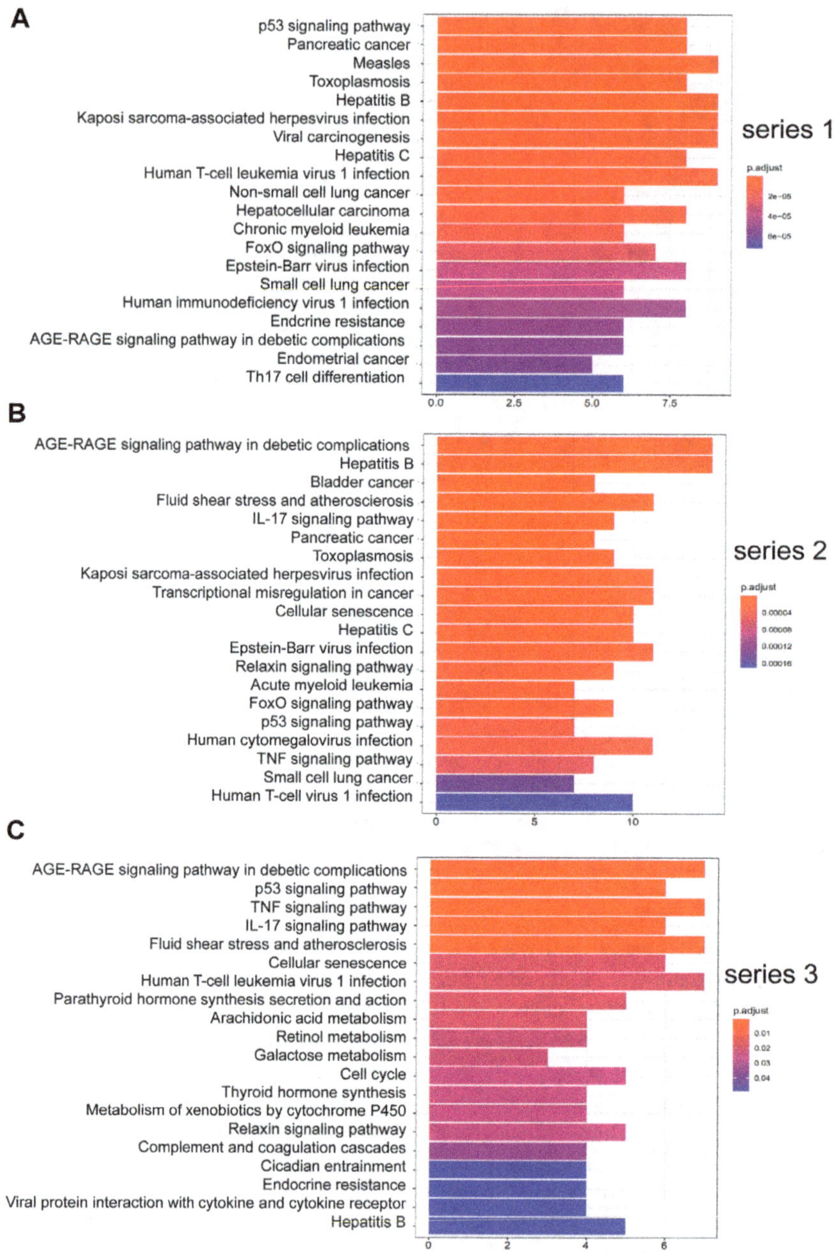

FIGURE 4 | Top 20 KEGG pathway enrichment candidate targets for DHJSD activity against OA for each expression profile. Pathways with significant changes (FDR <0.05) were identified. KEGG pathway labels the vertical axis, and number of differentially expressed genes marks the horizontal. The colour of the bar graph indicates the significance of the enriched KEGG pathway, and the colour gradient represents the size of the *p*-value. Inflammatory signalling pathways are underlined with a red bar. **(A)** series 1, **(B)** series 2 and **(C)** series 3.

DHJSD Suppressed the Expression of Inflammatory Proteins and Genes

The expression of collagen II protein was upregulated by DHJSD or TAK-242. Chondrocytes were treated with or without LPS and DHJSD and TAK-242 in the presence of LPS for 8 h (**Figure 9A**). The protein expressions of ADAMTS-4, ADAMTS-5, MMP-3, MMP-13 and MMP-14 were downregulated by DHJSD or TAK-242 treatment (**Figures 9B–F**). The mRNA expressions of MMP-3, MMP-13, IL-1β and TNF-α upregulated after LPS treatment and downregulated after DHJSD or TAK-242 treatment (**Figures 9I–K**).

DHJSD Effects Were Associated With the TLR4/MyD88/NF-κB Pathway

All the biomarkers of the LPS-exposed cells exhibited significant differences compared with intact cells. The protein expressions of NF-κB p65 and IKK-β were significantly upregulated after LPS exposure but

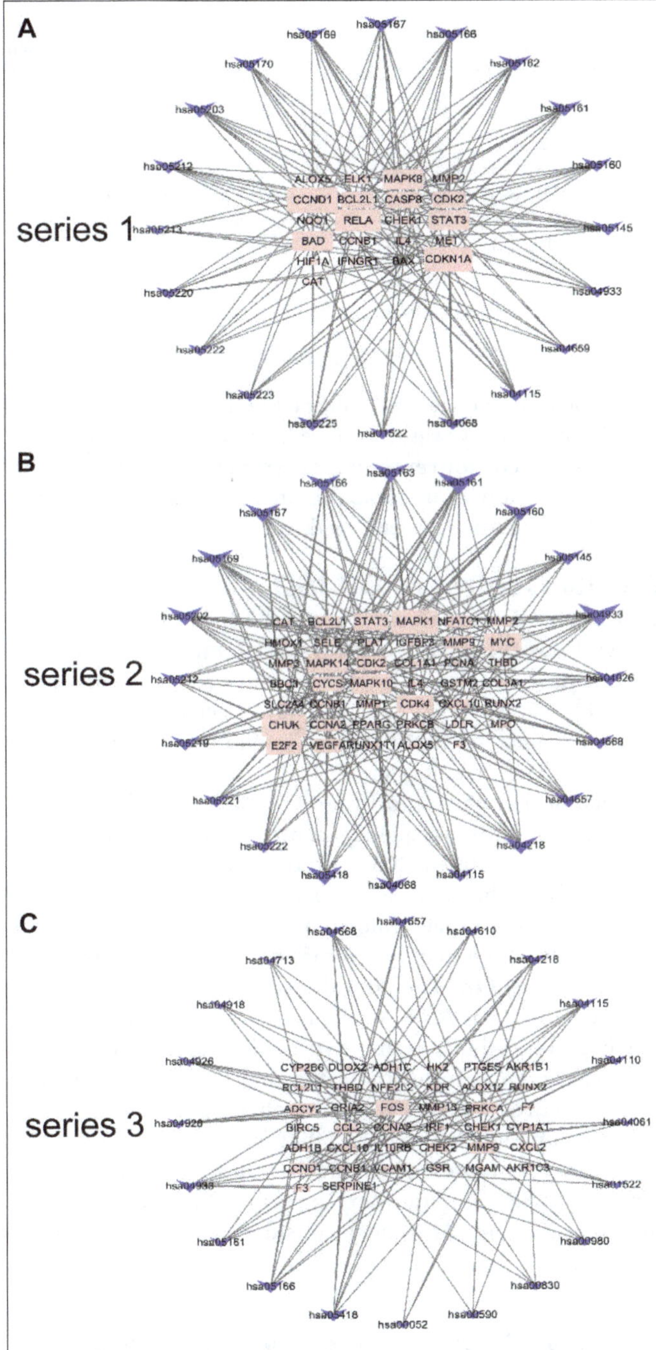

FIGURE 5 | Gene pathway network for DHJSD activity against OA. Top 20 pathways was performed with degree according to the topological analysis for series 1**(A)**, series 2**(B)** and series 3**(C)**.

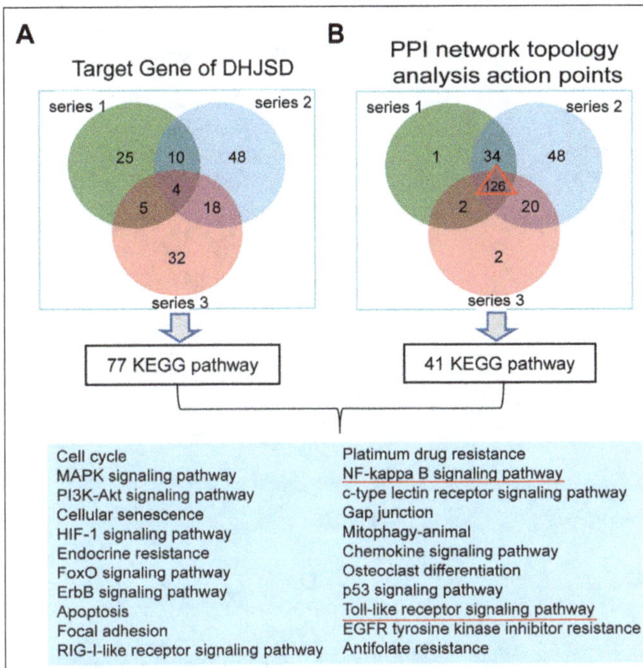

FIGURE 6 | Results of the KEGG enrichment analysis. **(A)** KEGG analysis of the union of the three series target genes of DHJSD, 77 KEGG pathways were significantly enriched. **(B)** KEGG analysis of the Venn of three series' PPI network topology analysis action points. The result showed that there are a total of 126 genes and 41 KEGG pathways. Venn analysis showed that 22 KEGG pathways were identified after the intersection of A and B.

significantly downregulated under DHJSD and PDTC treatment (**Figures 10A–C**). In the DHJSD and TAK-242 treatment groups, the protein expressions of TLR4, MyD88, TRAF-6, NF-κB p65, IKK-α, IKK-β and *p*-IκB-α were downregulated, and the mRNA expressions of TLR4, MyD88, TRAF-6, NF-κB p65, IKK-α and IKK-βwere downregulated (**Figure11**). In the DHJSD or PDTC treatment groups, the protein expressions of NF-κB p65 and IKK-β were downregulated, and the mRNA expressions of NF-κB p65 and IKK-β were downregulated (**Figure 10**). These changes have close correlation with changes in the TLR4/MyD88/NF-κB pathway mediated chondrocyte apoptosis, indicating that chondrocyte inflammation is a vital mechanisms of the effects of DHJSD.

DISCUSSION

In this research, we confirmed the utility of NPA for investigating the molecular targets of a complex herbal formulation using two sequential experiments. DHJSD is a typical widely-used complex herbal formulation with complicated ingredients (15 herbs), and research involving DHJSD is limited. We identified the quality control of DHJSD using conventional HPLC and identified 206 candidate compounds related to OA by TCM. In experiment 1, we constructed a standard NPA for DHJSD. The KEGG and GO enrichment analyses identified several inflammatory signalling pathways highly associated with DHJSD, and the results of Venn analysis between the target gene and PPI network topology analysis action point supported that the NF-κB signalling pathway and the toll-like signalling

TABLE 2 | The binding free energy between the top nine compounds and TLR4.

Compound	Molecular formula	CAS	docking score (kcal/mol)
Quercetin	$C_{15}H_{10}O_7$	117-39-5	−8.1
Baicalein	$C_{15}H_{10}O_5$	491-67-8	−7.5
Beta-carotene	$C_{40}H_{56}$	7,235-40-7	−8.3
Isorhamnetin	$C_{16}H_{12}O_7$	480-19-3	−7.7
Kaempferol	$C_{15}H_{10}O_6$	520-18-3	−7.6
Licochalcone a	$C_{21}H_{22}O_4$	58749-22-7	−7.0
Luteolin	$C_{15}H_{10}O_6$	491-70-3	−8.0
Naringenin	$C_{15}H_{12}O_5$	480-41-1	−7.6
Wogonin	$C_{16}H_{12}O_5$	632-85-9	−7.4

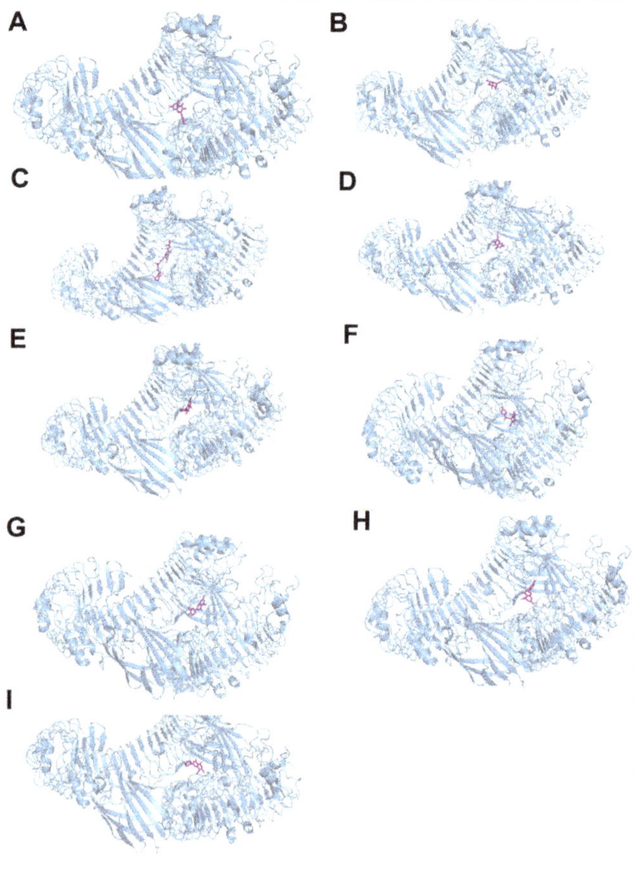

FIGURE 7 | The docking between the top nine compounds [quercetin **(A)**, baicalein **(B)**, beta-carotene **(C)**, isorhamnetin **(D)**, kaempferol **(E)**, licochalcone a **(F)**, luteolin **(G)**, naringenin **(H)** and wogonin **(I)**]of Duhuo Jisheng Decoction (DHJSD) and Osteoarthritis target TLR4. The crystal structures of TLR4 was shown in blue and the compound was shown in purple.

pathway play a key role in the effects of DHJSD, which were then subjected to experiment 2. We confirmed the involvement of miR-146a-5p and miR-34a-5p, the TLR4/MyD88/NF-κB signalling pathway and inflammatory-related genes by western blotting and qPCR. We found that DHJSD in fact contributed suppression of the expression of miR-146a-5p and miR-34a-5p, the TLR4/MyD88/NF-κB signalling pathway-related genes and inflammatory-related genes, which were upregulated upon LPS exposure. Hence, the role of the TLR4/MyD88/NF-κB signalling pathway was confirmed. In the present study we first performed conventional experiments combined with NPA and obtained an intact chain of evidence of DHJSD; thus, the value of NPA emerged.

Quality Control of DHJSD

Ligustrazine hydrochloride, paeoniflorin and osthole were chosen to be the quality control markers for DHJSD extract since it have been confirmed as quality control markers of CX, BS and DH, respectively, according to the pharmacopoeia of the People's Republic of China (2015 version). The results of HPLC identified ligustrazine hydrochloride, paeoniflorin and osthole, confirming the three compounds as quality control markers for DHJSD extract. We identified 206 candidate compounds from the NPA analysis that may be associated with DHJSD activity against OA. Only paeoniflorin was one of these candidate compounds which may play a major role in the treatment of DHJSD against OA. The OB values of paeoniflorin was 53.87 and DL values was 0.79. Whereas the candidate compounds which excludes ligustrazine hydrochlorideand and osthole. The experimental result indicated that the pharmacological quality control markers from the pharmacopoeia may be a stable components of DHJSD but have some limitations, which were not present in the list of effective compound from NPA. Hence, in our next experiment the core bioactive compounds from NPA may considered as new candidate markers.

Bioactive Components and Molecular of DHJSD Construction by NPA Analysis

In this study, we first used three OA-related gene series for NPA. The compound-target networks of DHJSD were constructed using 131, 121 and 129 compounds and 44, 80 and 59 compound targets in the three series, respectively. Quercetin, luteolin, wogonin and baicalein acted on 23, 11, 9 and 8 targets in series 1; quercetin, luteolin, baicalein, and kaempferol acted on 41, 18, 13 and 12 targets in series 2; and quercetin, luteolin, kaempferol and wogonin acted on 36, 14, 12 and 10 targets in series 3, respectively. Therefore, quercetin, luteolin and kaempferol were probably the vital pleiotropically active compounds for DHJSD.

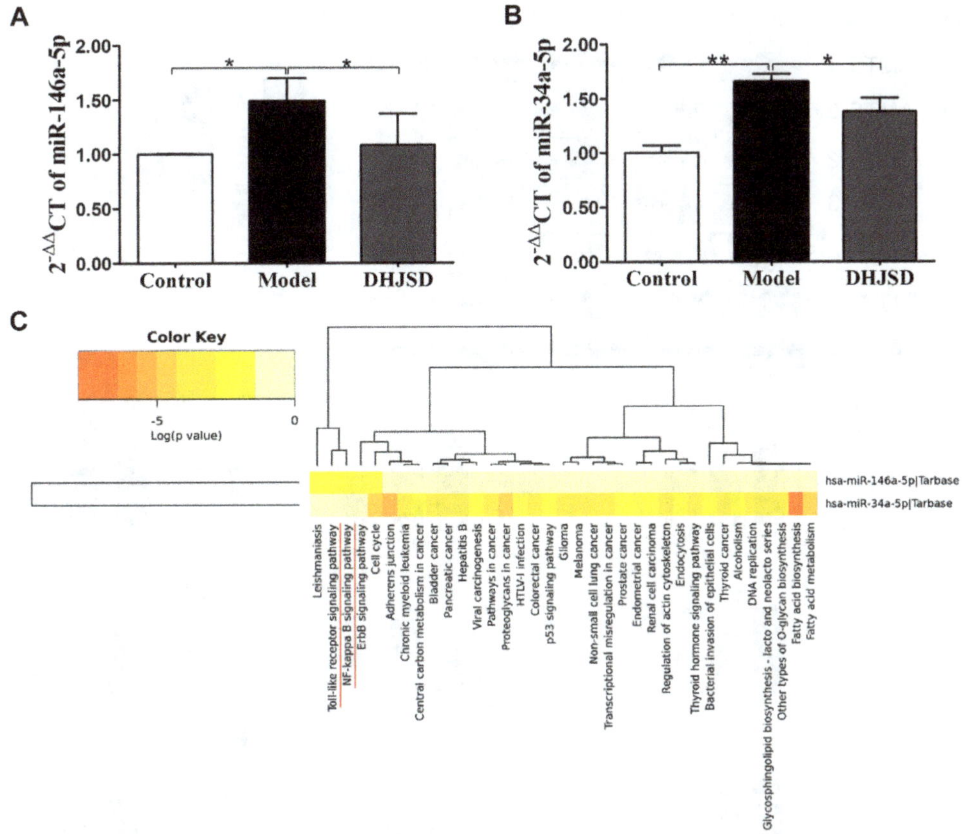

FIGURE 8 | DHJSD suppresses the mRNA expression of miR-146a-5p **(A)** and miR-34a-5p **(B)**. Chondrocytes were treated with or without LPS and DHJSD for 8 h. The expressions of miR-146a-5p and miR-34a-5p were upregulated after LPS exposure and downregulated after DHJSD treatment. β-actin was selected as internal standards. miRNA-regulated gene-pathway analysis **(C)** found that the toll-like receptor signalling pathway and the NF-κB signalling pathway were significantly enriched. Values are mean ± standard deviation (SD), and SD is shown as vertical bars. ** indicates $p < 0.01$ and * indicates $p < 0.05$ compared with control or LPS-exposed chondrocytes.

The candidate targets for DHJSD activity against OA were obtained by merging the three series PPI networks of DHJSD putative targets and OA-related targets. Furthermore, to achieve more accurate targets and structure a new network, we set 3, 6, 5 parameters, including DC and BC to further screen the nodes. Finally, 163, 228 and 150 targets were identified in series 1, 2 and 3, respectively, with 85 common action point targets.

To investigate the biological information of the targets of DHJSD activity against OA, we performed GO analysis. Results showed that DHJSD was involved in the regulation of some biological processes, indicating that the reduction of cartilage degeneration by DHJSD might related to the inflammatory response. The three series target genes related to the gene pathway network was constructed, and Venn analysis was performed to identify the intersections of the three OA-related pathway to identify key pathways for DHJSD activity against OA. The results of the gene pathway network analysis suggested that MAPK8, MAPK1 and FOS had the maximum degree, and it might be the core target in series 1, 2 and 3. The other top three genes were CCND1, RELA and CDKN1A in series 1; MAPK14, MAPK10 and CHUK in series 2; and ADCY2, MMP13 and PRCKA in series 3. In our previous study, the level of MMP-9 in LPS exposed chondrocytes was upregulated, and DHJSD reduced the MMP-9 level. MMP-9 was the key target genes in series 2 and series 3; furthermore the MMP family of genes, including MMP-1, MMP-2, MMP-3 and MMP-13, were also the key target genes of DHJSD in all the series. The MMP family participates in degradation of the extracellular matrix and basement membrane such as collagen II and collagen IV, which leads to joint integrity and function (Lewis et al., 1997; Van Doren, 2015). Further verification is needed in future investigation.

Verification of the Key Role of the NF-κB Signalling Pathway of DHJSD in OA

Inflammation has an important and close relationship with the pathogenesis of OA (Shen et al., 2017). MMP-9 is one of the

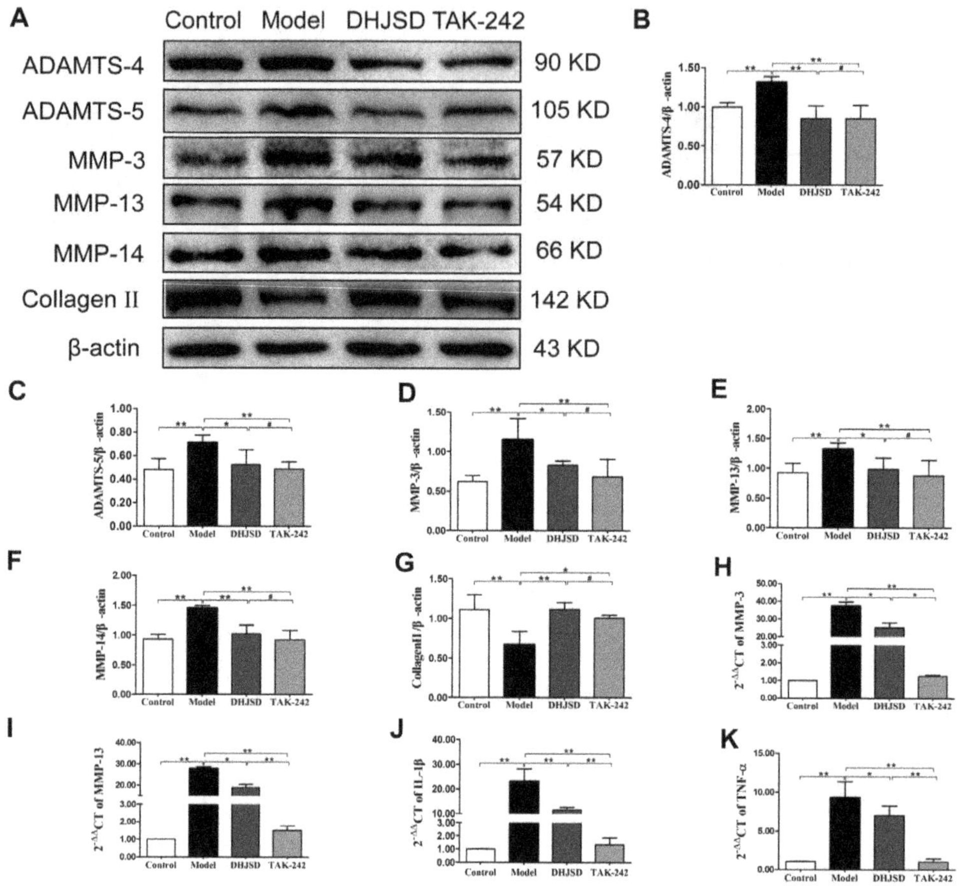

FIGURE 9 | DHJSD suppresses the expression of inflammatory proteins and genes. Chondrocytes were cultivation with or without LPS and DHJSD or TAK-242 treatment in the presence of LPS for 8 h, and the associated protein level was conformed by western blot analysis **(A)**. Protein levels of ADAMTS-4 **(B)**, ADAMTS-5 **(C)**, MMP-3 **(D)**, MMP-13 **(E)**, MMP-14 **(F)** and collagen-II **(G)**. β-actin was used as the internal control for normalisation. MMP-3 **(H)**, MMP-13 **(I)**, IL-1β **(J)** and TNF-α **(K)** mRNA expressions were detected by RT-PCR. GAPDH was selected as internal standards. Values are mean ± standard deviation (SD), and SD is shown as vertical bars. $N = 3$. **Indicates $p < 0.01$ and *indicates $p < 0.05$ compared with control or LPS-exposed chondrocytes. #Implies $p > 0.05$ compared with TAK-242.

cartilage degradation biomarkers that is directly affected. Previous research has shown that the expression of MMP-9 is under the control of NF-κB signalling pathway (Alves et al., 2014; Nambi, 2021). In our experiments, the MMP-9 levels were significantly increased after LPS exposure, consistent with our previous study (Xu et al., 2021), but remarkably decreased after DHJSD treatment (Xu et al., 2019). NF-κB p65 and IKK-β expressions were significantly upregulated after LPS exposure and downregulated after DHJSD or PDTC treatment. IKK-β is a vital upstream activator that participates in the active and release cytosolic sequestration of NF-κB p65 subunits and nuclear repositioning (Durand and Baldwin, 2017; Jimi et al., 2019). The expression of these genes is altered after DHJSD or PDTC treatment, we hypothesised that the NF-κB signalling pathway plays a distinctive role in the effects of DHJSD on OA.

Verification of the Key Role of the TLR4/MyD88/NF-κB Signalling Pathway of DHJSD in OA

Regarding the involvement of miR-146a-5p and miR-34a-5p in OA development, Shao et al. found that miR-146a-5p would activated NF-κB signalling pathway through TRAF6 which contribute to the chondrocyte apoptosis (Shao et al., 2020). MiR-34a-5p induced joint destruction and miR-34a-5p ASO injection protection cartilage damage (Endisha et al., 2021). Another recent study also showed that miRNA-regulated neuronal inflammation and apoptosis through NF-κB 1-induced LINC00665, and the inhibition of miR-34a-5p would restrain NF-κB-1 expression (Deng et al., 2021). In addition, the prediction target of miR-146a-5p showed that the NF-κB signalling pathway and the toll-like receptor signalling pathway were closely related pathways. Our experiment

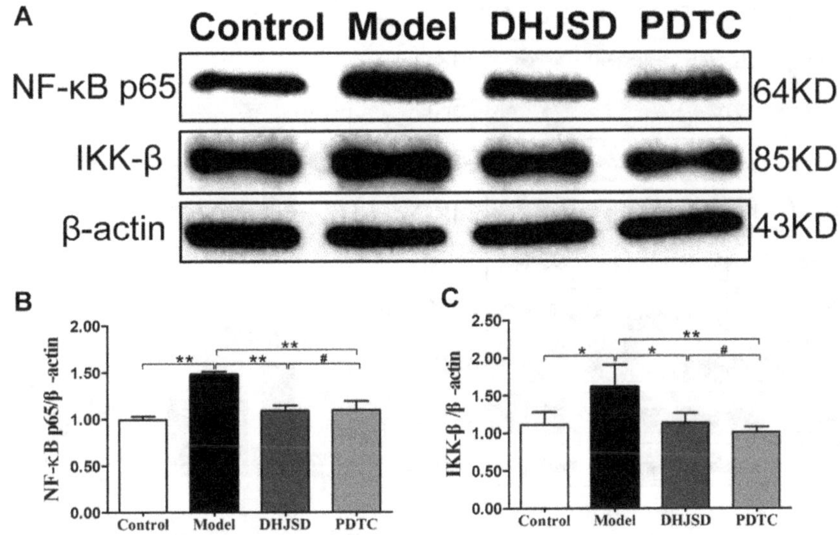

FIGURE 10 | DHJSD administration effects the NF-κB signalling pathway genes in LPS-exposed chondrocytes. The protein expression of NF-κB p65 and IKK-β after treatment with different concentrations of DHJSD for 8 h. Western blot analysis of protein expression levels **(A)**; the protein expressions of NF-κB p65 **(B)** and IKK-β **(C)** were significantly upregulated after LPS exposure and downregulated after DHJSD or PDTC treatment. Data are expressed as mean ± standard deviation (SD), and SD is shown as vertical bars. N = 3. *Indicates $p < 0.05$, **Indicates $p < 0.01$, #implies $p > 0.05$ compared with PDTC.

showed that after the LPS exposure of chondrocytes, the expressions of miR-146a-5p and miR-34a-5p increased in the OA cell model group. Moreover, the miRNA-regulated gene-pathway analysis revealed that the toll-like receptor signalling pathway and the NF-κB signalling pathway were significantly enriched, which was consistent with the NPA analysis.

The venn analysis between the KEGG pathway enrichment analysis of target gene and PPI network topology analysis action point found 22 identical pathways, and the NF-κB signalling pathway and the toll-like receptor signalling pathway were in the lists of both analysis. The toll-like receptor (TLR) family has primary sensors that are essential for eliciting innate immune responses (Akira et al., 2006). The TLR signalling pathway controls the expression of inflammatory cytokine genes by the activation of NF-κB (Hayden et al., 2006). TLR4 recruits the MyD88 adaptor triggering the MyD88-dependent pathway, and the TLR4 MyD88 complex interacts with TRAF6. Next, IκB kinase is regulated by two kinases IKK-α and IKK-β, followed by phosphorylation and degradation, resulting in NF-κB p65 release from cytosolic sequestration and nuclear repositioning (Wang et al., 2015). Based on the above described results, we finally determined the TLR4/MyD88/NF-κB signalling pathway for further verification in experiment 2, in which we observed the effects of LPS, DHJSD, PDTC and TAK-242 on the expression of proteins related to the TLR4/MyD88/NF-κB signalling pathway. The expressions of NF-κB p65 and IKK-β were downregulated after DHJSD or PDTC treatment. The expressions of TLR4, MyD88, TRAF-6, NF-κB p65, IKK-α, IKK-β, P-IKB-α and IKB-α were affected by DHJSD and TAK-242 treatment, confirming the key role of the TLR4/MyD88/NF-κB signalling pathway in the effects of DHJSD treating OA.

Collagen II was significantly downregulated after LPS exposure and increased with DHJSD or TAK-242 treatment, whereas the expressions of ADAMTS-4, ADAMTS-5, MMP-3, MMP-13 and MMP-14 showed opposite results. Collagen II plays a pivotal role in regulating cartilage matrix degeneration in OA progression (Hao et al., 2019), and the synthesis of collagen II would inhibited by MMPs including MMP-3 and MMP-13, while upregulated by IL-1β or other pro-inflammatory cytokines (Kapoor et al., 2011; Fei et al., 2019). MMP-3, MMP-13 and MMP-14 are crucial enzymes that directly degrade the extracellular matrix (Honsawek et al., 2013). ADAMTS-4 and ADAMTS-5 were identified as the major cartilage aggrecanases in arthritis (Cooper et al., 2000). These proteins play vital role in cartilage matrix degeneration, confirming that DHJSD, PDTC or TAK-242 therapy would influence OA development. Furthermore, molecular docking showed that beta-carotene, quercetin and isorhamnetin had strong affinity for TLR4, implying that TLR4 plays an important role in the DHJSD treatment of OA. In addition the top nine compounds also showed strong affinity with TLR4/MyD88/NF-κB-related genes. As proved by the above-result, the TLR4/MyD88/NF-κB-related genes, inflammatory gene transcription and various inflammatory factors function together to regulate the inflammatory reaction in the DHJSD treatment of OA.

Altogether, the results of NPA and conventional experiments suggested that the mechanisms of the action of DHJSD include comprehensive effects of several compounds and pathways, and

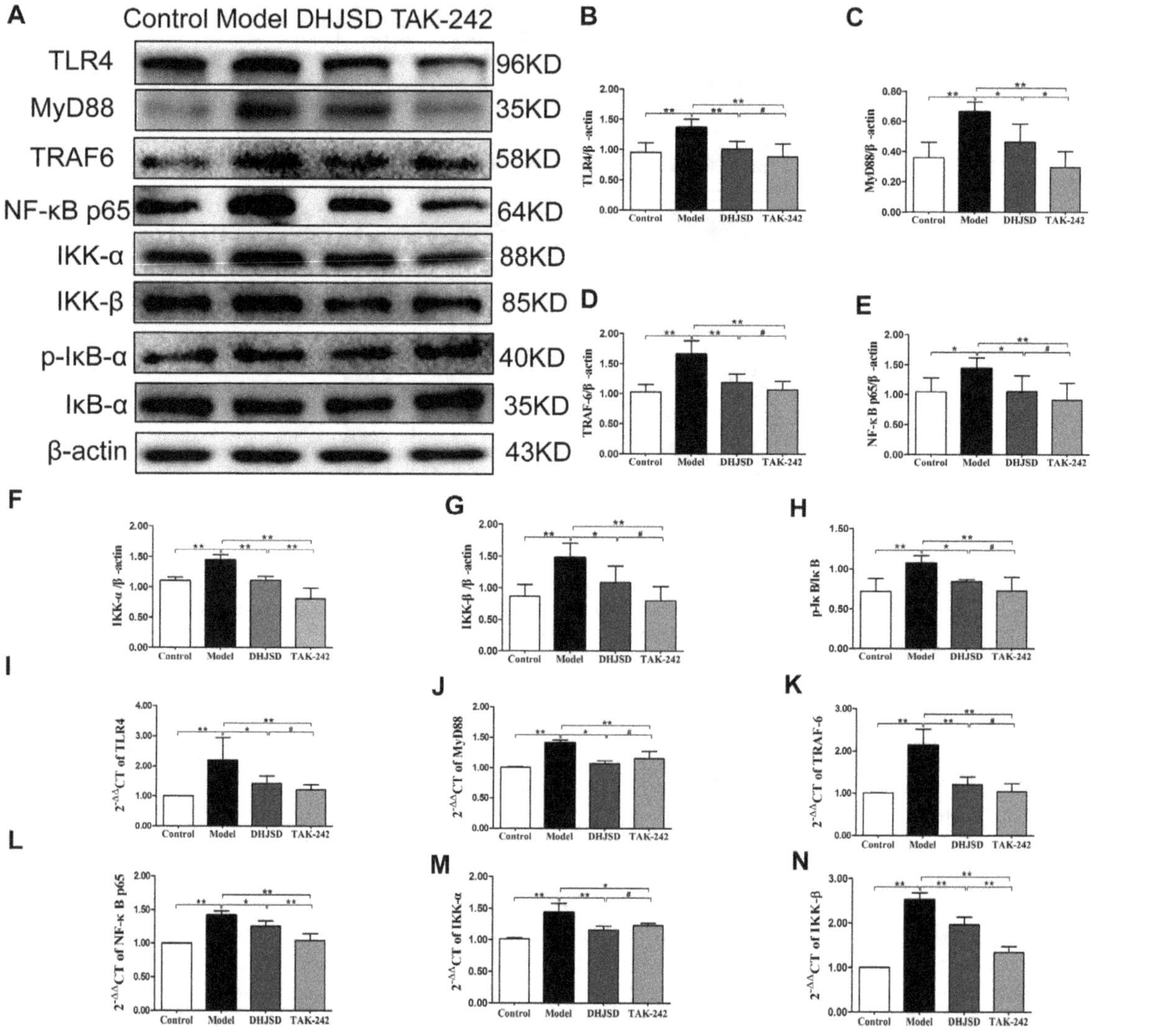

FIGURE 11 | DHJSD inhibits the TLR4 signalling pathway-induced apoptosis of LPS-exposed chondrocytes. Chondrocytes were cultivation with or without LPS and DHJSD or TAK -242 treatment in the presence of LPS for 8 h, and the associated protein level was tested by western blot **(A)**. Protein levels of TLR4 **(B)**, MyD88 **(C)**, TRAF-6 **(D)**, NF-κB p65 **(E)**, IKK-α **(F)**, KK-β **(G)** and *p*-IκB-α **(H)**. *β*-actin was selected as internal standards. TLR4 **(I)**, MyD88 **(J)**, TRAF-6 **(K)**, NF-κB p65 **(L)**, IKK-α **(M)** and IKK-β **(N)** mRNA expressions were detected by qPCR. GAPDH was selected as internal standards. Values are means ± standard deviation (SD), and SD is shown as vertical bars. **indicates $p < 0.01$ and *indicates $p < 0.05$ compared with control or LPS-exposed chondrocytes. # implies $p > 0.05$ compared with TAK-242.

the TLR4/MyD88/NF-κB signalling pathway plays a key role. Suppression of the inflammatory response involved in the chondrocyte apoptosis, which may relevant to cartilage degeneration, is the key mechanism.

CONCLUSION

To explore the molecular targets of DHJSD in treating OA, we used NPA and designed two experiments, including the angles of compounds, genes and pathways. The results of this study suggest that NPA requires a powerful tool to investigate the molecular targets of the complex herbal formulations such as DHJSD and revealed the TLR4/MyD88/NF-κB signalling pathway as a key therapeutic target, although requiring and further investigation.

AUTHOR CONTRIBUTIONS

All authors listed have made a substantial, direct, and intellectual contribution to the work and approved it for publication.

FUNDING

This study was supported by the National Natural Science Foundation of China (Grant No. 82074461), the Science and Technology Programs Pilot Project of Fujian Province (Grant No. 2021Y0032).

REFERENCES

Akira, S., Uematsu, S., and Takeuchi, O. (2006). Pathogen Recognition and Innate Immunity. *Cell* 24124 (4), 783–801. doi:10.1016/j.cell.2006.02.015

Alves, A. C., Albertini, R., dos Santos, S. A., Santana, E., Serra, A. J., Silva, J. A., et al. (2014). Effect of Low-Level Laser Therapy on Metalloproteinase MMP-2 and MMP-9 Production and Percentage of Collagen Types I and III in a Papain Cartilage Injury Model. *Lasers Med. Sci.* 29 (3), 911–919. May. doi:10.1007/s10103-013-1427-x

Cooper, C., Snow, S., McAlindon, T. E., Kellingray, S., Stuart, B., Coggon, D., et al. (2000). Risk Factors for the Incidence and Progression of Radiographic Knee Osteoarthritis. *Arthritis Rheum.* 43 (5), 995–1000. doi:10.1002/1529-0131(200005)43:5<995:AID-ANR6>3.0.CO;2-1

Deng, Q., Ma, L., Chen, T., Yang, Y., Ma, Y., and Ma, L. (2021). NF-κB 1-induced LINC00665 Regulates Inflammation and Apoptosis of Neurons Caused by Spinal Cord Injury by Targeting miR-34a-5p. *Neurol. Res.* 43 (5), 418–427. doi:10.1080/01616412.2020.1866373

Durand, J. K., and Baldwin, A. S. (2017). Targeting IKK and NF-Kb for Therapy. *Adv. Protein Chem. Struct. Biol.* 107, 77–115. doi:10.1016/bs.apcsb.2016.11.006

Endisha, H., Datta, P., Sharma, A., Nakamura, S., Rossomacha, E., Younan, C., et al. (2021). MicroRNA-34a-5p Promotes Joint Destruction during Osteoarthritis. *Arthritis Rheumatol.* 73 (3), 426–439. doi:10.1002/art.41552

Fei, J., Liang, B., Jiang, C., Ni, H., and Wang, L. (2019). Luteolin Inhibits IL-1β-induced Inflammation in Rat Chondrocytes and Attenuates Osteoarthritis Progression in a Rat Model. *Biomed. Pharmacother.* 109, 1586–1592. doi:10.1016/j.biopha.2018.09.161

Funck-Brentano, T., Nethander, M., Movérare-Skrtic, S., Richette, P., and Ohlsson, C. (2019). Causal Factors for Knee, Hip, and Hand Osteoarthritis: A Mendelian Randomization Study in the UK Biobank. *Arthritis RheumatolOct* 71 (10), 1634–1641. doi:10.1002/art.40928

Hao, H. Q., Zhang, J. F., He, Q. Q., and Wang, Z. (2019). Cartilage Oligomeric Matrix Protein, C-Terminal Cross-Linking Telopeptide of Type II Collagen, and Matrix Metalloproteinase-3 as Biomarkers for Knee and Hip Osteoarthritis (OA) Diagnosis: a Systematic Review and Meta-Analysis. *Osteoarthritis Cartilage* 27 (5), 726–736. May. doi:10.1016/j.joca.2018.10.009

Hayden, M. S., West, A. P., and Ghosh, S. (2006). NF-kappaB and the Immune Response. *Oncogene* 25 (51), 6758–6780. doi:10.1038/sj.onc.1209943

Honsawek, S., Malila, S., Yuktanandana, P., Tanavalee, A., Deepaisarnsakul, B., and Parvizi, J. (2013). Association of MMP-3 (-1612 5A/6A) Polymorphism with Knee Osteoarthritis in Thai Population. *Rheumatol. Int.* 33 (2), 435–439. doi:10.1007/s00296-012-2371-y

Huang, Z., Shi, X., Li, X., Zhang, L., Wu, P., Mao, J., et al. (2020). Network Pharmacology Approach to Uncover the Mechanism Governing the Effect of Simiao Powder on Knee Osteoarthritis. *Biomed. Res. Int.* 2020, 6971503. doi:10.1155/2020/6971503

Jian, G. H., Su, B. Z., Zhou, W. J., and Xiong, H. (2020). Application of Network Pharmacology and Molecular Docking to Elucidate the Potential Mechanism of Eucommia Ulmoides-Radix Achyranthis Bidentatae against Osteoarthritis. *BioData Min* 13, 12. doi:10.1186/s13040-020-00221-y

Jimi, E., Takakura, N., Hiura, F., Nakamura, I., and Hirata-Tsuchiya, S. (2019). The Role of NF-Kb in Physiological Bone Development and Inflammatory Bone Diseases: Is NF-Kb Inhibition "Killing Two Birds with One Stone". *Cells* 8 (12), 8. Dec 14. doi:10.3390/cells8121636

Kapoor, M., Martel-Pelletier, J., Lajeunesse, D., Pelletier, J. P., and Fahmi, H. (2011). Role of Proinflammatory Cytokines in the Pathophysiology of Osteoarthritis. *Nat. Rev. Rheumatol.* 7 (1), 33–42. doi:10.1038/nrrheum.2010.196

Kwon, J. Y., Lee, S. H., Na, H. S., Jung, K., Choi, J., Cho, K. H., et al. (2018). Kartogenin Inhibits Pain Behavior, Chondrocyte Inflammation, and Attenuates Osteoarthritis Progression in Mice through Induction of IL-10. *Sci. Rep.* 8 (1), 13832. Sep 14. doi:10.1038/s41598-018-32206-7

Lai, X., Wang, X., Hu, Y., Su, S., Li, W., and Li, S. (2020). Editorial: Network Pharmacology and Traditional Medicine. *Front. Pharmacol.* 11, 1194. doi:10.3389/fphar.2020.01194

Latourte, A., Kloppenburg, M., and Richette, P. (2020). Emerging Pharmaceutical Therapies for Osteoarthritis. *Nat. Rev. Rheumatol.* 16 (12), 673–688. doi:10.1038/s41584-020-00518-6

Lewis, E. J., Bishop, J., Bottomley, K. M., Bradshaw, D., Brewster, M., Broadhurst, M. J., et al. (1997). Ro 32-3555, an Orally Active Collagenase Inhibitor, Prevents Cartilage Breakdown *In Vitro* and *In Vivo*. *Br. J. Pharmacol.* 121 (3), 540–546. Jun. doi:10.1038/sj.bjp.0701150

Li, L., Liu, H., Shi, W., Liu, H., Yang, J., Xu, D., et al. (20172017). Insights into the Action Mechanisms of Traditional Chinese Medicine in Osteoarthritis. *Evidence-Based Complement. Altern. Med.* 2017, 1–13. doi:10.1155/2017/5190986

Li, X., Zhang, Z., Liang, W., Zeng, J., Shao, X., Xu, L., et al. (2020a). Data on Tougu Xiaotong Capsules May Inhibit P38 MAPK Pathway-Mediated Inflammation *In Vitro*. *Data BriefFeb* 28, 105023. doi:10.1016/j.dib.2019.105023

Li, X., Zhang, Z., Liang, W., Zeng, J., Shao, X., Xu, L., et al. (2020b). Tougu Xiaotong Capsules May Inhibit P38 MAPK Pathway-Mediated Inflammation: *In Vivo* and *In Vitro* Verification. *J. Ethnopharmacol* 249, 112390. doi:10.1016/j.jep.2019.112390

Liang, W., Li, X., Hu, L., Ding, S., Kang, J., Shen, J., et al. (2019). An *In Vitro* Validation of the Therapeutic Effects of Tougu Xiaotong Capsule on Tunicamycin-Treated Chondrocytes. *J. Ethnopharmacol* 229, 215–221. doi:10.1016/j.jep.2018.10.022

Lin, P., Weng, X., Liu, F., Ma, Y., Chen, H., Shao, X., et al. (2015). Bushen Zhuangjin Decoction Inhibits TM-Induced Chondrocyte Apoptosis Mediated by Endoplasmic Reticulum Stress. *Int. J. Mol. Med.* 36 (6), 1519–1528. doi:10.3892/ijmm.2015.2387

Liu, F., Liu, G., Liang, W., Ye, H., Weng, X., Lin, P., et al. (2014). Duhuo Jisheng Decoction Treatment Inhibits the Sodium Nitroprussiate-induced A-poptosis of C-hondrocytes through the M-itochondrial-dependent S-ignaling P-athway. *Int. J. Mol. Med.* 34 (6), 1573–1580. doi:10.3892/ijmm.2014.1962

Liu, H., Zeng, L., Yang, K., and Zhang, G. (2016). A Network Pharmacology Approach to Explore the Pharmacological Mechanism of Xiaoyao Powder on Anovulatory Infertility. *Evid. Based Complement. Alternat Med.* 2016, 2960372. doi:10.1155/2016/2960372

Liu, W., Jin, S., Huang, M., Li, Y., Wang, Z., Wang, P., et al. (2020). Duhuo Jisheng Decoction Suppresses Matrix Degradation and Apoptosis in Human Nucleus Pulposus Cells and Ameliorates Disc Degeneration in a Rat Model. *J. Ethnopharmacol* 250, 250112494. doi:10.1016/j.jep.2019.112494

Liu, Z. C., Wang, Z. L., Huang, C. Y., Fu, Z. J., Liu, Y., Wei, Z. C., et al. (2018). Duhuo Jisheng Decoction Inhibits SDF-1-Induced Inflammation and Matrix Degradation in Human Degenerative Nucleus Pulposus Cells *In Vitro* through the CXCR4/NF-Kb Pathway. *Acta Pharmacol. Sin* 39 (6), 912–922. doi:10.1038/aps.2018.36

Nambi, G. (2021). Does Low Level Laser Therapy Has Effects on Inflammatory Biomarkers IL-1β, IL-6, TNF-α, and MMP-13 in Osteoarthritis of Rat Models- A Systemic Review and Meta-Analysis. *Lasers Med. Sci.* 36 (3), 475–484. Apr. doi:10.1007/s10103-020-03124-w

Peat, G., and Thomas, M. J. (2021). Osteoarthritis Year in Review 2020: Epidemiology & Therapy. *Osteoarthritis and Cartilage* 29 (2), 180–189. doi:10.1016/j.joca.2020.10.007

Shao, J., Ding, Z., Peng, J., Zhou, R., Li, L., Qian, Q., et al. (2020). MiR-146a-5p Promotes IL-1β-induced Chondrocyte Apoptosis through the TRAF6-Mediated NF-kB Pathway. *Inflamm. Res.* 69 (6), 619–630. Jun. doi:10.1007/s00011-020-01346-w

Shen, J., Abu-Amer, Y., O'Keefe, R. J., and McAlinden, A. (2017). Inflammation and Epigenetic Regulation in Osteoarthritis. *Connect. Tissue Res.* 58 (1), 49–63. Jan;. doi:10.1080/03008207.2016.1208655

UK NCGC (2014). *Osteoarthritis: Care and Management in Adults.* London: National Institute for Health and Care Excellence (UK)Feb.

Van Doren, S. R. (2015). Matrix Metalloproteinase Interactions with Collagen and Elastin. *Matrix Biol.* 44-46, 224–231. May-Jul. doi:10.1016/j.matbio.2015.01.005

Vlachos, I. S., and Hatzigeorgiou, A. G. (2017). Functional Analysis of miRNAs Using the DIANA Tools Online Suite. *Methods Mol. Biol.* 1517, 25–50. doi:10.1007/978-1-4939-6563-2_2

Wang, P. F., Xiong, X. Y., Chen, J., Wang, Y. C., Duan, W., and Yang, Q. W. (2015). Function and Mechanism of Toll-like Receptors in Cerebral Ischemic Tolerance: from Preconditioning to Treatment. *J. Neuroinflammation* 12, 1280. Apr 28. doi:10.1186/s12974-015-0301-0

Xu, L., Li, H., Xu, Y., Wang, S., Zeng, J., Wang, L., et al. (2019). An Experimental Study of Mechanism of Action of Duhuo Jisheng Tang in Inhibiting Inflammatory Reaction Induced by Lipopolysaccharide in Chondroytes Based on NF-Kb Signalling Pathway. *J. Traditional Chin. Orthopedics Traumatol.* 31 (07), 9–14+20.

Xu, Y., Li, H., He, X., Huang, Y., Wang, S., Wang, L., et al. (2021). Identification of the Key Role of NF-Kb Signaling Pathway in the Treatment of Osteoarthritis with Bushen Zhuangjin Decoction, a Verification Based on Network Pharmacology Approach. *Front. Pharmacol.* 12, 637273. doi:10.3389/fphar.2021.637273

Yang, M., Jiang, L., Wang, Q., Chen, H., and Xu, G. (2017). Traditional Chinese Medicine for Knee Osteoarthritis: An Overview of Systematic Review. *PloS one* 12 (12), e0189884. doi:10.1371/journal.pone.0189884

Zeng, C., Wei, J., Persson, M. S. M., Sarmanova, A., Doherty, M., Xie, D., et al. (2018). Relative Efficacy and Safety of Topical Non-steroidal Anti-inflammatory Drugs for Osteoarthritis: a Systematic Review and Network Meta-Analysis of Randomised Controlled Trials and Observational Studies. *Br. J. Sports Med.* 52 (10), 642–650. May. doi:10.1136/bjsports-2017-098043

Zhang, L., Shi, X., Huang, Z., Mao, J., Mei, W., Ding, L., et al. (2020). Network Pharmacology Approach to Uncover the Mechanism Governing the Effect of Radix Achyranthis Bidentatae on Osteoarthritis. *BMC Complement. Med. Ther.* 20 (1), 121. Apr 21. doi:10.1186/s12906-020-02909-4

Zhang, W., Wang, S., Zhang, R., Zhang, Y., Li, X., Lin, Y., et al. (2016). Evidence of Chinese Herbal Medicine Duhuo Jisheng Decoction for Knee Osteoarthritis: a Systematic Review of Randomised Clinical Trials. *BMJ open* 6 (1), e008973. Jan 4. doi:10.1136/bmjopen-2015-008973

Zhang, Z., Huang, C., Jiang, Q., Zheng, Y., Liu, Y., Liu, S., et al. (2020). Guidelines for the Diagnosis and Treatment of Osteoarthritis in China (2019 Edition). *Ann. Transl Med.* 8 (19), 1213. Oct;. doi:10.21037/atm-20-4665

Zhu, N., Hou, J., Ma, G., and Liu, J. (2019). Network Pharmacology Identifies the Mechanisms of Action of Shaoyao Gancao Decoction in the Treatment of Osteoarthritis. *Med. Sci. Monit.* 25, 6051–6073. Aug 14. doi:10.12659/msm.915821

2

Unveiling Active Constituents and Potential Targets Related to the Hematinic Effect of Steamed *Panax notoginseng* Using Network Pharmacology Coupled With Multivariate Data Analyses

Yin Xiong[1,2,3†], Yupiao Hu[1†], Lijuan Chen[1†], Zejun Zhang[1], Yiming Zhang[1], Ming Niu[4*] and Xiuming Cui[1,2,3*]*

[1] Faculty of Life Science and Technology, Kunming University of Science and Technology, Kunming, China, [2] Yunnan Key Laboratory of Panax Notoginseng, Kunming, China, [3] Laboratory of Sustainable Utilization of Panax Notoginseng Resources, State Administration of Traditional Chinese Medicine, Kunming, China, [4] China Military Institute of Chinese Materia Medica, 302 Military Hospital of China, Beijing, China

***Correspondence:**
Yin Xiong
yhsiung@163.com
Ming Niu
nmbright@163.com
Xiuming Cui
sanqi37@vip.sina.com

† These authors have contributed equally to this work

Steamed *Panax notoginseng* (SPN) has been used as a tonic to improve the blood deficiency syndrome (BDS) in the theory of traditional Chinese medicine. Here, we aim to unveil active constituents and potential targets related to the hematinic effect of SPN, which has not been answered before. In the study a constituent-target-disease network was constructed by combining the SPN-specific and anemia-specific target proteins with protein-protein interactions. And the network pharmacology was used to screen out the underlying targets and mechanisms of SPN treating anemia. Also, the multivariate data analyses were performed for the double screening. According to the results, 11 targets related to chemical constituents of SPN were found to be closely associated with the hematinic effect of SPN. Among them, the direct target protein of mitochondrial ferrochelatase (FECH) had the major role through the metabolic pathway. Meanwhile, Rk_3 and 20(*S*)-Rg_3 were predicted to be major constituents related to the hematinic effect of SPN by both multivariate data analyses and network pharmacology. And it was been validated by the pharmacologic tests that Rk_3 and 20(*S*)-Rg_3 could significantly increase the levels of blood routine parameters, FECH and its downstream protein of heme in mice with BDS. The study provides evidences for the mechanism understanding and drug development of SPN for the treatment of anemia.

Keywords: steamed *Panax notoginseng*, hematinic effect, active constituents, mechanism, network pharmacology, multivariate data analyses

---

Abbreviations: APH, acetylphenylhydrazine; BDS, blood deficiency syndrome; CCA, canonical correlation analysis; CTX, cyclophosphamide; FECH, ferrochelatase; FEJ; *Fufang E'jiao Jiang*; Hb, hemoglobin; OMIM, Online Mendelian Inheritance in Man; PLSR, partial least squares regression; PLT, platelet; PN, *Panax notoginseng*; PPI, protein–protein interaction; RBC, red blood cells; SPN, steamed *Panax notoginseng*; TCM, traditional Chinese medicine; TDT, TCM Database@Taiwan; WBC, white blood cells.

INTRODUCTION

Blood deficiency syndrome (BDS) is a common syndrome with high incidence in clinic of traditional Chinese medicine (TCM), which often occurs in patients with anemia. It is characterized by a decreased quantity of red blood cells (RBC) and white blood cells (WBC), usually accompanied by the diminished hemoglobin (Hb) levels or altered RBC morphology (Kassebaum et al., 2014). Patients with BDS are often accompanied with tachycardia, dizziness, shortness of breath, poor ability to exercise, and even loss of consciousness (Janz et al., 2013). The causes giving rise to BDS are similar to anemia, including the reduced erythropoiesis, excessive hemorrhage, and destruction of RBC, of which the last one mainly refers to hemolytic anemia (Tian et al., 2017). Hemolytic anemia can be induced by the administration of acetylphenylhydrazine (APH) and cyclophosphamide (CTX), which is also a classical model for BDS (Zhang et al., 2014). Today, hemolytic anemia is mainly treated with blood transfusion. This treatment is associated with mechanical shearing forces that accelerate red blood cell rupture, and lead to severe clinical complications, including intravascular hemolysis, tissue oxidative stress, and multi-organ dysfunctions (Baek et al., 2012). Therefore, the development of effective therapies or drugs with blood-enriching efficacy is beneficial for the prevention and treatment of the disease.

Panax notoginseng (PN) (Burk.) F. H. Chen, a well known medicinal herb in Asia, has been used to treat blood disorders for thousands of years (Li et al., 2017). In 1944, PN and the relative products were classified as dietary supplements according to the United States Dietary Supplement Health and Education Act (103rd Congress, 1994). Traditionally, PN has been used in both non-steamed and steamed forms. Unlike the non-steamed one treating bleeding and removing blood stasis, the steamed PN (SPN) is used as a tonic to enrich blood and tonify the body, which can improve the BDS by increasing the production of various blood cells in anemic conditions (Ge et al., 2015; Gu et al., 2015). In our previous study (Xiong et al., 2017b), we found that the treatment of SPN could reverse significantly the decrease of levels of WBC, RBC, Hb, and platelet (PLT) of anemic mice induced by APH and CTX, which were inapparent when treated with non-steamed PN. The result was consistent with the report from Zhou et al. (2014). This could be due to the variation in the chemical composition of PN during the steaming process (Wang et al., 2012a). Despite various studies on the processing methods, chemical components and bioeffects of PN (Lau et al., 2009; Sun et al., 2010), much less attention has been paid on its steamed form, let alone the specific active constituents and the underlying mechanisms related to the hematinic effect of SPN, which hinders the development and application of this valuable medicine.

Network pharmacology, as a system biology-based methodology, offers an effective approach to evaluate the pharmacological effects of herbal medicines at the molecular level by predicting the complex interactions of small molecules and proteins in a biological system (Tang et al., 2015; Li et al., 2017). It is considered to be a promising way to unveil properties of herbal medicines and provide valuable insights into current drug discovery and development. Compared with conventional "one target, one drug, one disease" mode, network pharmacology focuses on "multi-targets, multi-constituents treatment to diseases," which coincides with the holistic and systematic concepts of TCM (Li et al., 2015; Quan et al., 2016). It was reported that network pharmacology has been applied to detect new pharmacologic effects of herbal medicines, to uncover the interactions between herbal compounds/formulas and complex syndrome systems, to determine the active constituents and their mechanisms of action (Tao et al., 2013; Sheng et al., 2014). Therefore, to better understand the molecular basis of the enriching-blood effect of SPN, we computationally recognized the active constituents and potential targets of SPN treating anemia by the network pharmacology approach coupled with multivariate data analyses, and experimentally validated the predicted results.

MATERIALS AND METHODS

Computational Prediction of Hematinic Constituents and Targets of SPN Using Network Pharmacology Analyses

Database Construction

Based on the literature research and our previous works on chemical analysis of SPN (Sun et al., 2010; Xiong et al., 2017a,b), 20 compounds were selected, including ginsenosides of F_2 (1), Rb_1 (2), Rb_2 (3), Rb_3 (4), Rc (5), Rd (6), Re (7), Rg_1 (8), Rh_2 (9), Rh_4 (10), Rk_3 (11), 20(*R*)-Rg_2 (12), 20(*S*)-Rg_2 (13), 20(*R*)-Rg_3 (14), 20(*S*)-Rg_3 (15), 20(*R*)-Rh_1 (16), and 20(*S*)-Rh_1 (17); and notoginsenosides of C (18), R_1 (19), and R_2 (20) in SPN. The chemical structures of the composite compounds in SPN were obtained from TCM Database@Taiwan (TDT) or drawn with ChemDraw professional 15.0 (Chen, 2011). The targets of constituents were predicted by the online target prediction software of PharmMapper with a criterion of "fit score" >4[1] (Wang et al., 2017). Gene and protein targets associated with the disease of anemia were collected from the Online Mendelian Inheritance in Man (OMIM) database (Amberger et al., 2015). Database of Interacting Proteins for protein-protein interactions (PPI) was employed to identify the possible interactions of the aforementioned targets. And all protein ID codes were converted to UniProt IDs (Wei et al., 2016).

Network Construction and Analysis

To provide the scientific and reasonable interpretation of the complex relationships between the constituents and targets associated with anemia, network analysis was performed. The chemical constituents, SPN putative targets, and anemia targets were all connected to construct a "constituent-target-disease" network with PPI information. Cytoscape 4.3 (Smoot et al., 2011) was applied to visualize and analyze the network, and calculate the topological features of each node in the network. Only the hub nodes (twofolds above the median "degree" value of all nodes)

[1] http://lilab.ecust.edu.cn/pharmmapper/index.php

with higher values of "betweenness centrality" and "closeness centrality" (above the median value of all nodes) were identified as the candidate SPN targets for anemia.

Targets and Pathways Analyses

To unveil the mechanism of SPN treatment of anemia, DAVID Functional Annotation Bioinformatics Microarray Analysis[2] was performed (Dennis et al., 2003) for the pathway enrichment analysis. The key target in the most significant enriched pathway was verified by performing *in vivo* experiment in the SPN treatment on anemia.

Screening Hematinic Constituents of SPN Based on the Fingerprint-Effect Analyses

Chemicals

The reference standards of ginsenosides 20 (S)-Rg_3 and Rk_3 with a purity $\geq$ 98% were purchased from the National Institutes for the Control of Pharmaceutical and Biological Products (Beijing, China). Methyl alcohol and acetonitrile of HPLC grade were purchased from Sigma-Aldrich, Inc. (St. Louis, MO, United States). Ultrapure water was generated with an UPT-I-20T ultrapure water system (Chengdu Ultrapure Technology, Inc., Chengdu, Sichuan, China). APH was purchased from HuaXia Chemical Reagent Co., Ltd. (Chengdu, China). CTX was purchased from Xiya Chemical Industry Co., Ltd. (Shangdong, China). Mouse ferrochelatase (FECH) enzyme-linked immunoassay kit and heme enzyme-linked immunosorbent assay kit were purchased from Shanghai MLBIO Biotechnology Co., Ltd. (Shanghai, China). All other chemicals used were of analytical grade.

Sample Preparation

The preparation of SPN refers to our previous study (Xiong et al., 2017a). "Samples were obtained from a single batch of PN root in Yunnan, China. Steamed PN samples were prepared by steaming the crushed raw PN in an autoclave (Shanghai, China) for 2, 4, 6, 8, and 10 h at 105, 110, and 120°C, respectively. The steamed powder was then dried in a heating-air drying oven at about 45°C to constant weight, then powdered and sieved through a 40-mesh sieve."

Animals

Animal experimental procedures in the study were strictly conformed to the Guide for the Care and Use of Laboratory Animals and related ethics regulations of Kunming University of Science and Technology. The protocol was approved by the Experimental Animal Welfare and Ethics Committee, Kunming University of Science and Technology. The experimental method refers to our previous study (Xiong et al., 2017a), that "Kunming mice, male and female, weighing 18–22 g, were purchased from TianQin Biotechnology Co., Ltd., Changsha, Hunan [SCXK (Xiang) 2014-0011]. Before the experiments, the mice were given one-week acclimation period in a laboratory at room temperature (20–25°C) and constant humidity (40–70%), and fed with standard rodent chow and tap water freely."

HPLC Analyses

The sample solutions were prepared according to the method in our previous research (Xiong et al., 2017a). "HPLC analyses were done on an Agilent 1260 series system (Agilent Technologies, Santa Clara, CA, United States) consisting of a G1311B Pump, a G4212B diode array detector, and a G1329B autosampler. A Vision HT C_{18} column (250 mm × 4.6 mm, 5 μm) was adopted for the analyses. The mobile phase consisted of A (ultra pure water) and B (acetonitrile). The gradient mode was as follows: 0–20 min, 80% A; 20–45 min, 54% A; 45–55 min, 45% A; 55–60 min, 45% A; 60–65 min, 100% B; 65–70 min, 80% A; 70–90 min, 80% A. The flow rate was set at 1.0 ml/min. The detection wavelength was set at 203 nm. The column temperature was set at 30°C and sample volume was set at 10 μl."

Blood Routine Test

210 km mice, half male and half female, were randomly divided into seven groups, namely the control group, model group, *Fufang E'jiao Jiang* (FEJ) group, and drug groups including raw PN (S1-S3), SPN at 105°C (S4-S8), SPN at 110°C (S9-S13), and SPN at 120°C (S14-S18), 10 mice in each group. The APH and CTX-induced anemia model was applied to evaluate the "blood enriching" function of PN combined with previous methods (He et al., 2015). The anemia model was established by intraperitoneal injected of CTX of 0.07 g/kg for the first 3 days and hypodermic injection of APH of 0.02 g/kg at the fourth day. Mice in the control group were administered with 0.9% normal saline, whereas other groups were administered with FEJ (8 ml/kg), and SPN samples at different steamed conditions (0.9 g/kg), respectively, by gavage for 12 days. Then the blood was collected for the routing analysis, including levels of WBC, RBC, Hb, and PLT after 30 min of the last administration. And the liver tissues were collected for the determination of FECH and heme levels.

Multivariate Data Analyses

Canonical correlation analysis (CCA)

Canonical correlation analysis is a multivariate analysis used to study the correlation between two sets of variables. It is used for the dimension reduction of PCA and to extract the main principal components, and then describes the whole linear relationship of two sets of variables by the relevance of two principal components (Shi et al., 2016). In our study, CCA was used to analyze the relevance between the peak area values from the HPLC fingerprints and blood parameters data.

Partial least squares regression (PLSR)

Partial least squares regression is performed to find the inner relationship between the independent variables (X) and dependent variables (Y), which are simultaneously modeled by taking into account X variance, and the covariance between X and Y (Martens and Naes, 1991). In our study, the X matrix is composed of the enhanced fingerprints, and the Y vector is constructed with the reference values of hematinic effect obtained by measuring the levels of WBC, RBC, Hb, and PLT. Then, X and

[2]https://david.ncifcrf.gov/

Y are decomposed in a product of another two matrices of scores and loadings; as described by the following equations:

$$X = TP^T + E \quad (1)$$

$$Y = UQ^T + F \quad (2)$$

Where TP^T approximates to the chromatographic data and UQ^T to the true Y values; notice that the relationship between T and U scores is a summary of the relationship between X and Y. The terms E and F from the equations are error matrices. Hence, the PLS algorithm attempts to find latent variables that maximize the amount of variation explained in X that is relevant for predicting Y; i.e., capture variance and achieve correlation (Sundberg, 2008).

Experimental Validation for the Predicted Results

Validation for the Screened Active Constituents

Peaks in the HPLC profile predicted to be responsible for the hematinic activity of SPN were then identified by reference standards, of which the activities were finally verified by pharmacologic evaluation using the methods described in the section of "Blood routine test." 90 km mice, half male and half female, were randomly divided into seven groups, namely the control group, model group, FEJ group, and drug groups [including low, moderate, and high-dose ginsenoside 20(*S*)-Rg_3 group; and low, moderate, and high-dose ginsenoside Rk_3 group], 10 mice in each group. Mice in the control group were intraperitoneal injected with 0.9% normal saline, whereas other groups were intraperitoneal injected with FEJ (8 ml/kg), 20(*S*)-Rg_3 (2.5, 5, and 10 mg/kg, respectively), and Rk_3 (2.5, 5, and 10 mg/kg, respectively), respectively.

Validation for the Predicted Targets and Its Downstream Protein

The livers of mice from different groups were removed to detect the levels of FECH and heme. The livers of different groups of mice were homogenized with a homogenizer and centrifuged for 20 min to collect the supernatant. Mouse FECH enzyme-linked immunosorbent assay kit and mouse heme enzyme-linked immunosorbent assay kit were used to detect the levels of FECH and heme in the supernatant.

Statistical Analyses

All data were expressed as means ± SD. SPSS 21.0 software (Statistical Program for Social Sciences, SPSS Inc., United States) was applied to carry out the two-tailed unpaired *t*-test. Umetrics SIMCA-P 11.5 software (Sartorius Stedim Biotech, Sweden) was applied for PLSR analysis. CCA was performed using MATLAB 7.0 (Matrix Laboratory, United States). A value of $P < 0.05$ was considered to be significant difference. A value of $P < 0.01$ was considered to be highly significant difference. EC_{50} value was fitted by probit regression with Origin 7.5 software for windows (OriginLab Corporation, United States).

RESULTS

Computational Prediction Using Network Pharmacology Analyses

Constituents and Targets Prediction

On the basis of database construction, 203 putative targets with "fit score" >4 were predicted by PharmMapper for 14 compounds and 90 candidate protein targets associated with anemia therapy were collected by keyword-based searching over the OMIM database, which included 19 common targets out of SPN constituents and anemia. Therefore, ginsenosides 20 (*R*)-Rg_2, 20 (*S*)-Rg_2, Rb_3, Rb_1, F_2, and Rc were eliminated due to their low binding affinity to all the candidate targets.

Network Construction

The "constituent-target-disease" network was constructed and the noteworthy features of the network analyzed could provide some important information for us to understand the "drug–target" interaction mechanism of a certain drug on a specific disease. Our study was focused on the effect of SPN on treating anemia. In **Figure 1**, the network for the constituents and their potential targets was illustrated with color-coded nodes. The intermolecular interactions (constituent-target or target- disease interactions) were indicated as links, i.e., edges between nodes (Tao et al., 2013). The red triangles represented the analyzed constituents of SPN, the blue dots represented the indirect targets of those constituents, the yellow dots represented the targets of anemia, the purple dots represented the interactional proteins of the anemia targets and SPN constituents, and the yellow squares represented the common targets of SPN constituents and anemia. Obviously, the common targets, as the directed targets of SPN on treating anemia, were relatively important for further screening.

Based on the network analysis, three topological parameters of "degree," "betweenness centrality," and "closeness centrality" were chosen to screen the potential anemia targets that SPN might affect. After calculating the values of the three parameters for each significant protein in the PPI network, the median values of "degree," "betweenness centrality," and "closeness centrality" were 1, 0, and 0.2183, respectively. The protein targets of which the "degree" was more than twofolds of the median value, and "betweenness centrality" and "closeness centrality" were higher than the median value, were chosen as the major targets of SPN treating anemia (Wang et al., 2018). As shown in **Table 1**, we finally determined that 11 common protein targets with degree $\geqq 2$, betweenness centrality $\geqq 0$, and closeness centrality $\geqq 0.2183$ for anemia therapy.

Pathway Analysis of SPN Treating Anemia

Kyoto Encyclopedia of Genes and Genomes (KEGG) is a knowledge base for systematic analysis of gene functions in terms of the networks of genes and molecules. The major component of KEGG is the pathway database that consists of graphical diagrams of biochemical pathways including most of the known metabolic pathways and some of the known regulatory pathways (Kanehisa and Goto, 2000). As shown in **Figure 2**, 10 KEGG pathways were enriched by the pathway-enrichment analysis. And there was the maximum quantity of targets involved in the metabolic pathways.

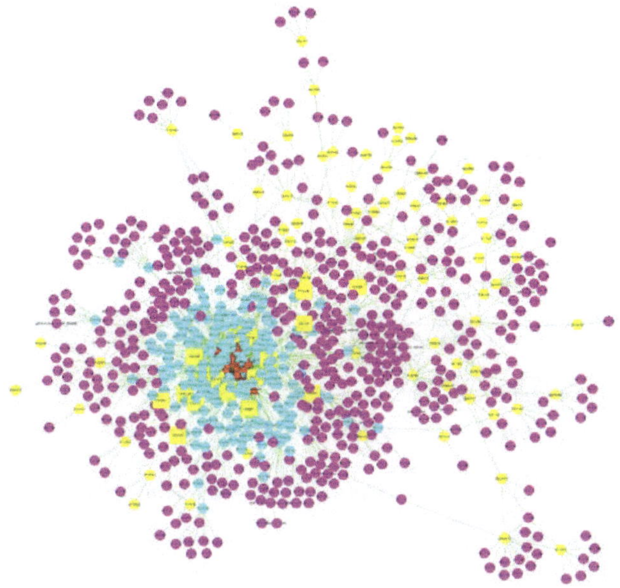

FIGURE 1 | The "constituent–target–disease" network for the treatment of anemia with SPN. The red triangles represented the analyzed constituents of SPN, the blue dots represented the indirect targets of those constituents, the yellow dots represented the targets of anemia, the purple dots represented the interactional proteins of the anemia targets and SPN constituents, and the yellow squares represented the common targets of SPN constituents and anemia. SPN, steamed *Panax notoginseng*.

Based on the analysis of KEGG, these target proteins were P22830 (FECH, mitochondrial), P16442 (histo-blood group ABO system transferase), P00374 (dihydrofolate, reductase), P06744 (glucose-6-phosphate isomerase), P19367 (hexokinase-1), P35228 (nitric oxide synthase, inducible), and P30613 (pyruvate kinase PKLR). Combined with the results in **Table 1**, FECH and histo-blood group ABO system transferase showed higher values of degree than others. And based on the literature research, FECH was reported to be a mitochondrial membrane-associated protein catalyzing the terminal step of heme biosynthesis (Yoon and Cowan, 2004), of which the abnormal synthesis can lead to anemia (Iolascon et al., 2009). Therefore, the protein of FECH and its downstream protein of heme (**Figure 3**) were chosen from the map of metabolic pathways for further verification. Constituents related to the target of FECH included ginsenosides Rh_4 (10), Rk_3 (11), 20(*R*)-Rg_3 (14), 20(*S*)-Rg_3 (15), 20(*R*)-Rh_1 (16), 20(*S*)-Rh_1 (17), and notoginsenoside R_2 (20).

Prediction of Hematinic Constituents of SPN Based on Multivariate Data Analyses

HPLC Analyses

HPLC fingerprints for 18 batches of PN samples were shown in **Figure 4** (Xiong et al., 2017a). "Peaks with good segregation, which also occupied large areas from consecutive peaks, were determined as the common peaks of PN samples. Therefore, fifteen peaks were selected by comparing their ultraviolet spectra and HPLC retention time." The areas of 15 peaks in 18 batches of PN samples were listed in **Supplementary Table S1**. "The peak area was defined as 0 for peaks lacked in chromatograms. The coefficients of variance for almost all common peaks were higher than 46.6%. This is due to the diversity in the levels of constituents contained in samples under different process conditions. The areas of 15 common peaks were used for the following analysis" (Xiong et al., 2017a).

Blood Routine Test

After the administration for 15 days, the quantities of WBC, RBC, Hb and PLT from the peripheral blood of mice were shown in **Figure 5**. Compared with the control group, the levels of WBC, RBC, Hb, and PLT in the model group were significantly decreased ($P < 0.01$), indicating the anemia model was successfully established. Compared with the model group, WBC, RBC, Hb, and PLT levels in the FEJ and all of PN groups were increased at different degrees. Besides, there were more significant differences in the levels of the above four parameters

TABLE 1 | The information of common target proteins and their corresponding active constituents predicted by network pharmacology analyses.

UniProt No.	Protein name	Closeness centrality	Degree	Betweenness centrality	Constituent
P22830	FECH, mitochondrial	0.2810	9	0.0011	(10) (11) (14) (15) (16) (17) (20)
P16442	Histo-blood group ABO system transferase	0.2995	16	0.0041	(3) (6) (7) (9) (10) (11) (14) (15) (17) (18) (19) (20)
P06702	Protein S100-A9	0.2811	8	0.0036	(3) (6) (7) (8) (10) (11) (17) (19)
P60568	Interleukin-2	0.2404	4	0.0056	(3) (14)
P06744	Glucose-6-phosphate isomerase	0.2490	2	0.0001	(20)
P30613	Pyruvate kinase PKLR	0.2747	4	0.0014	(7) (20)
Q06124	Tyrosine-protein phosphatase non-receptor type 11	0.2812	6	0.0078	(6) (10) (11)
P19367	Hexokinase-1	0.2635	2	0.0005	(7)
P00374	Dihydrofolate reductase	0.2677	2	0.0006	(7)
P35228	Nitric oxide synthase, inducible	0.2552	4	0.0114	(7)
P42224	Signal transducer and activator of transcription 1-alpha/beta	0.2188	2	0.0024	(18)

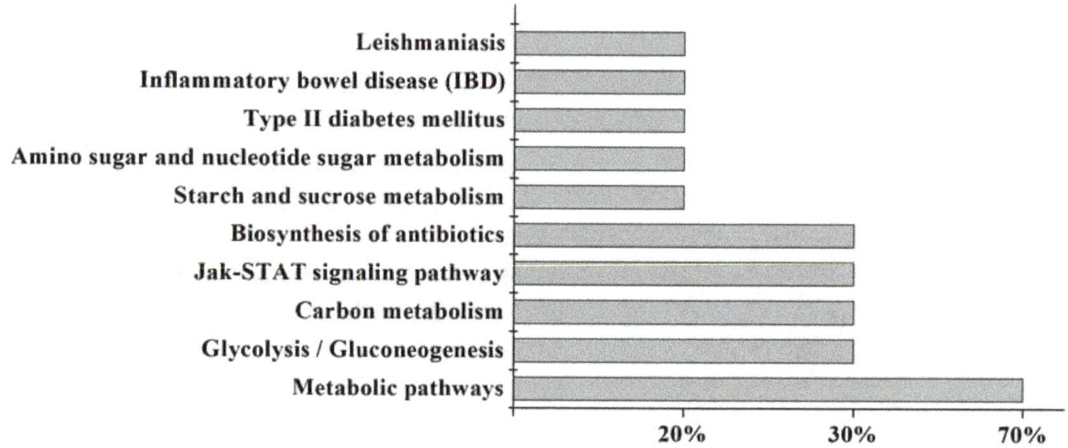

FIGURE 2 | Ten enriched pathways with putative targets. *X*-axis represents the percentage of targets involved in the pathway. *Y*-axis represents the name of putative pathway.

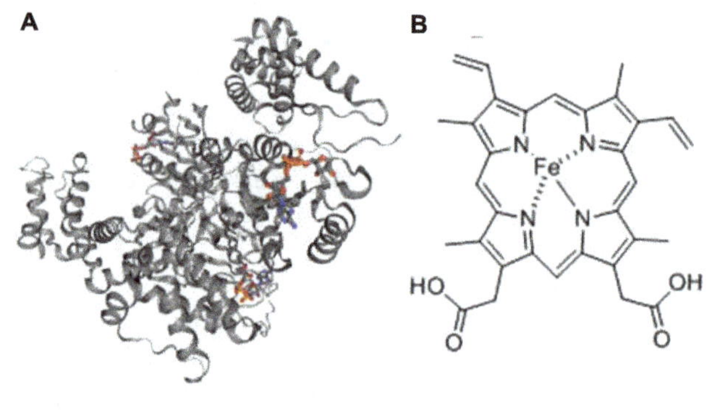

FIGURE 3 | The structures of **(A)** FECH and **(B)** heme. FECH, ferrochelatase.

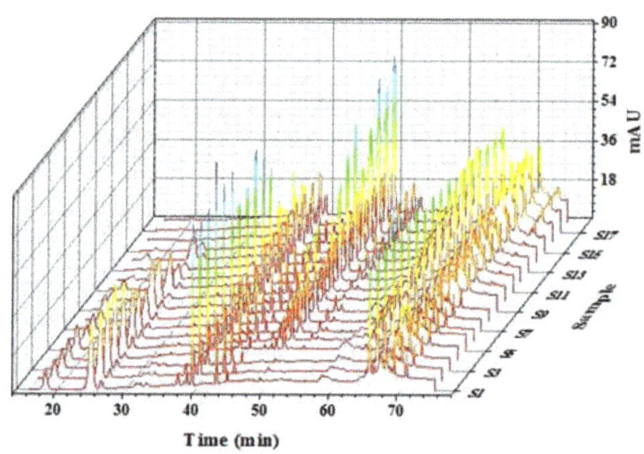

FIGURE 4 | HPLC fingerprints of 18 batches of PN extracts. HPLC analyses were done on a Vision HT C_{18} column (250 mm × 4.6 mm, 5 μm) at 30°C. The mobile phase consisting of A (ultra pure water) and B (acetonitrile) was used at a flow rate of 1.0 ml/min as the following gradient mode: 0–20 min, 80% A; 20–45 min, 54% A; 45–55 min, 45% A; 55–60 min, 45% A; 60–65 min, 100% B; 65–70 min, 80% A; and 70–90 min, 80% A. The detection wavelength was set at 203 nm and the injection column was set at 10 μl. PN, *Panax notoginseng* (Xiong et al., 2017a).

between the model group and SPN groups steamed at higher temperature and longer time, suggesting that SPN steamed at higher temperature and longer time could significantly reverse the decrease of the quantities of WBC, RBC, Hb, and PLT. While for mice treated with raw PN, the level of RBC was significantly increased, whereas there was no significant difference in levels of WBC, Hb, and PLT between raw PN and the model group, indicating that the blood-enriching effect of raw PN was generally weaker than SPN. According the results, SPN was observed to enhance the hematopoietic effect on mice with chemotherapy-induced anemia, which was consistent with the traditional use of SPN (Gu et al., 2015).

Uncovering Active Constituents by Multivariate Data Analyses

CCA

Canonical correlation analysis was used to establish the fingerprint-effect relationships between area values of 15 common peaks in the HPLC data and four blood routine parameters (WBC, RBC, Hb, and PLT). The analysis result was shown in **Table 2**. The correlation coefficients showed that the four parameters were positively correlated with X_4, X_5, X_9, X_{10}, X_{11}, X_{12}, X_{13}, X_{14}, and X_{15}. Besides, eight peaks: X_5, X_9, X_{10}, X_{11}, X_{12}, X_{13}, X_{14}, and X_{15} were highly correlated ($|R| > 0.6$) with the blood parameters. This indicates that the decrease of the quantities of WBC, RBC, Hb, and PLT might be reversed by these compounds.

PLSR

The PLSR models to correlate chromatographic data and hematinic effect of 18 batches of PN samples were constructed. Since the total number of samples (18) was small and the prediction for new samples was not our first concern, no division

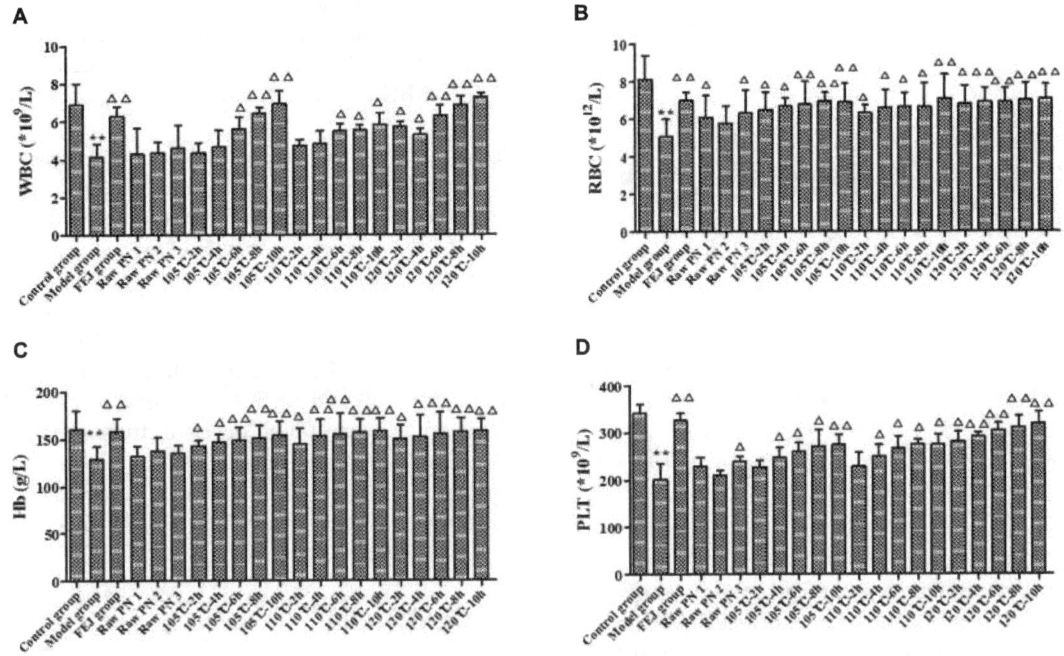

FIGURE 5 | The contents of **(A)** WBC, **(B)** RBC, **(C)** Hb, and **(D)** PLT in the blood of mice after treated with different PN samples. Each value represents means ± SD (n = 10). $^{**}P < 0.01$, compared with the control group; $^{\triangle}$ $P < 0.05$ and $^{\triangle\ \triangle}$ $P < 0.01$, compared with the model group. FEJ, *Fufang E'jiao Jiang*; Hb, hemoglobin; PLT, platelet; PN, *Panax notoginseng*; RBC, red blood cell; SD, standard deviation; WBC, white blood cell.

was made into a calibration set to build a PLSR model and a test set to validate the predictive properties. Our main concern was to focus on the indication of hematinic effect peaks from the modeling results. PLSR models were built from the normalized data matrix X containing the 18 PN fingerprints and the response matrix Y (including Y_1, Y_2, Y_3, and Y_4, which represented WBC, RBC, Hb, and PLT, respectively). For the model, four principle components were achieved, accounting for an explained variance of 86.4% for X variable, 87.1% for Y variable, and a predictive ability (Q^2) of 81.5% (**Supplementary Table S2**), indicating that the obtained model was excellent. As shown in the regression coefficients plot (**Figure 6**), peaks 1, 3, 6, and 8–15 were positively correlated with the quantities of WBC, RBC, Hb, and PLT, whereas peaks 2, 4, 5, and 7 were negatively correlated with the quantities of the four parameters.

Besides, the importance of the X-variables for the model could be summarized by variable importance for the projection (VIP) values (usually with a threshold >1.0). Thus, constituents corresponding to peaks 5, 9, 11, 12, 14, and 15, of which the VIP values were >1.0 (**Table 3**) with high absolute values of coefficients were considered to be highly related to the hematinic effect of different PN samples. Furthermore, false discovery rate (FDR, usually with a threshold ≤0.05) can effectively solve the control of false positive error in multiple comparisons of high-dimensional data, and can significantly improve the efficiency of hypothesis testing (Benjamini and Hochberg, 1995). Therefore, constituents corresponding to peaks 5, 7, 9, 10, and 12, of which the FDR values were ≤ 0.05, indicated that constituents corresponding to peaks 5, 7, 9, 10, and 12 were positively correlated with the hematinic effect. Among them, only peak 10 and 12 had significant correlation with the hematinic effect by P-value correcting ($P < 0.05$).

Identification of active constituents corresponding to predicted peaks

Based on CCA and PLSR results, constituents corresponding to peaks 10 and 12 were predicted to be the major active ones related to the hematinic effect of SPN. By comparing the chromatogram

TABLE 2 | The correlation coefficients between the common characteristic peaks and four blood parameters.

Blood parameters	Common characteristic peaks														
	1	2	3	4	5	6	7	8	9	10	11	12	13	14	15
WBC	−0.689	−0.789	−0.595	0.122	0.5932	−0.590	−0.662	−0.274	0.740	0.782	0.783	0.805	0.738	0.684	0.747
RBC	−0.702	−0.777	−0.601	0.338	0.7276	−0.442	−0.611	−0.181	0.798	0.785	0.782	0.763	0.753	0.644	0.744
Hb	−0.854	−0.845	−0.712	0.156	0.757	−0.653	−0.748	−0.170	0.824	0.867	0.862	0.845	0.790	0.671	0.788
PLT	−0.845	−0.934	−0.776	0.212	0.7195	−0.676	−0.781	−0.479	0.905	0.940	0.939	0.909	0.907	0.886	0.933

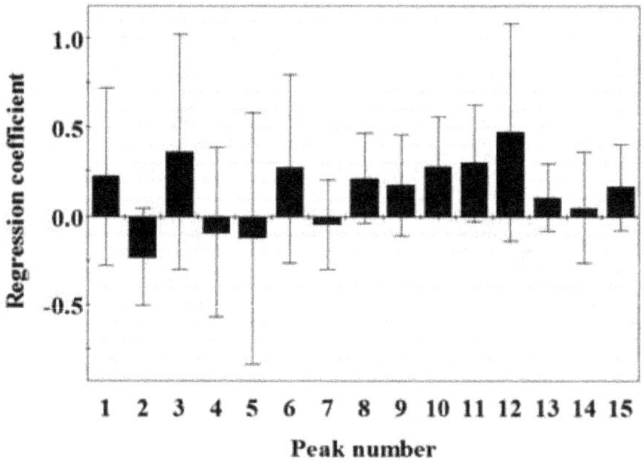

FIGURE 6 | Regression coefficient plots of hematinic effect of 15 peaks in the chromatograms of PN samples. PN, *Panax notoginseng*.

of SPN sample to that of the mixed standard solution (**Figure 7**), peaks 10 and 12 were identified to be ginsenosides Rk_3 and 20(*S*)-Rg_3, respectively, which had the major role in the hematinic effect of SPN.

According to the results of network pharmacology analyses, the two constituents were also predicted to be the active ones. Therefore, ginsenosides Rk_3 and 20(*S*)-Rg_3 were determined to be the target constituents for the further investigation of their hematinic effect.

Experimental Validation for the Predicted Results

Validation for the Screened Active Constituents

After intraperitoneal injected ginsenosides Rk_3 and 20(*S*)-Rg_3 for 15 days, the quantities of WBC, RBC, Hb, and PLT from the peripheral blood of mice were shown in **Figures 8, 9**, respectively. Compared with the control group, the levels of WBC, RBC, Hb, and PLT in the model group were significantly decreased ($P < 0.01$), indicating the anemia model was successfully established. Compared with the model group, the levels of WBC, RBC, Hb, and PLT after treated three doses of ginsenoside Rk_3 were all increased. Meanwhile, the levels of WBC, RBC, and PLT in the high-dose group were significantly increased ($P < 0.05$), suggesting that Rk_3 could reverse the decrease of the quantities of WBC, RBC, Hb, and PLT in a dose-dependent way. For the treatment with ginsenoside 20(*S*)-Rg_3 of three doses, the levels of WBC, RBC, Hb, and PLT were all increased compared with the model group. Besides, the levels of WBC and Hb in the moderate-dose and high-dose groups were significantly increased ($P < 0.05$); and the levels of RBC and PLT in the high-dose group were significantly increased ($P < 0.05$), suggesting that the ginsenoside 20(*S*)-Rg_3 could reverse the decrease of the quantities of WBC, RBC, Hb, and PLT in a dose-dependent way.

Validation for the Predicted Target Proteins

As shown in **Figure 10**, the level of FECH in the model group was significantly decreased compared with the control group ($P < 0.05$), suggesting that the model was well established. Compared with the model group, the levels of FECH and heme were all significantly increased after the administration of different doses of Rk_3 and 20(*S*)-Rg_3 ($P < 0.05$). In general, the levels of FECH and heme in livers of mice treated with the middle-dose Rk_3 and 20(*S*)-Rg_3 were relatively higher than those treated with low and high doses of drugs. The results indicated that ginsenosides Rk_3 and 20(*S*)-Rg_3 had a positive effect on improving the levels of FECH and heme, which was consistent with the predicted results of network pharmacology analyses.

DISCUSSION

Herbal medicines exert their therapeutic effects through the synergistic effects of multiple constituents and targets. PN in raw and steamed forms are historically supposed to be different in the efficacies. Lau et al. (2009) reported that the bleeding time of rats treated with raw PN was shorter than those treated with SPN. Zhou et al. (2014) found that SPN could significantly increase the levels of Hb and WBC, as well as the organ index of mice with BDS induced by CTX, which were unconspicuous when treated with raw PN. Based on our previous studies (Xiong et al., 2017b), there was a significant variation in the chemical composition between the two forms of PN, which leaded to the difference in the pharmacologic effects of raw and steamed PN. As shown in **Figure 3**, the levels of blood routine parameters of mice treated with SPN were significantly increased compared with the model group, which were also obviously higher than those of mice treated with raw PN. The result was consistent with the traditional use of SPN as a tonic to enrich the blood.

Currently, methods for uncovering active constituents of herbal medicines treating diseases mainly rely on retrospective analyses. However, this method depends on large consumption of manpower and material resources, which hinders the development of drugs. To address this issue, we have developed firstly a more comprehensive approach that integrates anemia-SPN networks to effectively discover potential active constituents and targets involved. Technically, the prediction accuracy of the drug targets and the completeness of the databases are important to the method and will affect the creditability of the

TABLE 3 | Variable importance for the projection of PLSR.

Peak	1	2	3	4	5	6	7	8	9	10	11	12	13	14	15
VIP	0.987	0.70	0.56	0.29	1.03	0.37	0.57	0.45	1.121	1.37	1.24	1.41	0.902	1.09	1.23
FDR	0.097	0.085	0.092	0.088	0.041	0.067	0.034	0.068	0.042	0.048	0.072	0.022	0.099	0.061	0.060
P-value	0.091	0.097	0.098	0.558	0.055	0.150 0.0.235	0.185	0.235	0.079	0.011	0.062	0.001	0.086	0.079	0.058

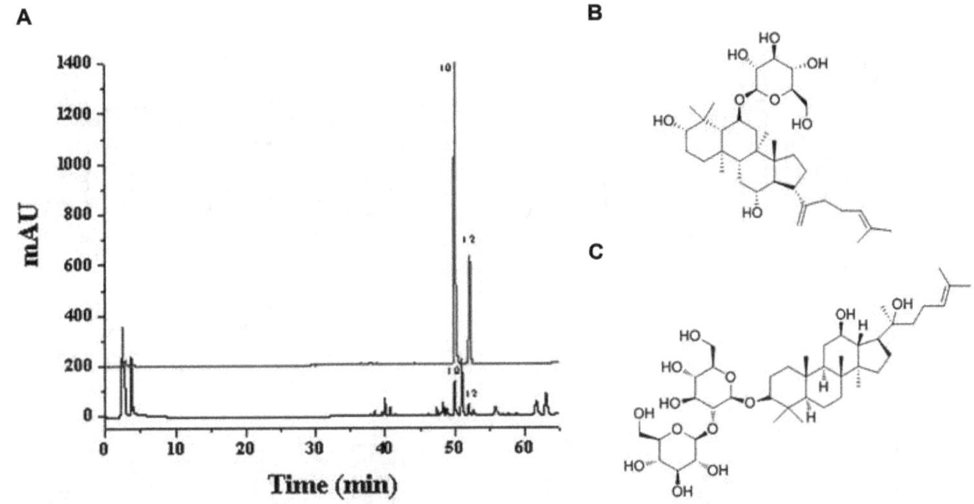

FIGURE 7 | The **(A)** chromatograms of SPN sample (black) and the mix standard solution (red), and structures of **(B)** ginsenosides Rk_3 and **(C)** 20(*S*)-Rg_3. Peak 10 and 12 correspond to ginsenosides Rk_3 and 20(*S*)-Rg_3, respectively. SPN, steamed *Panax notoginseng*.

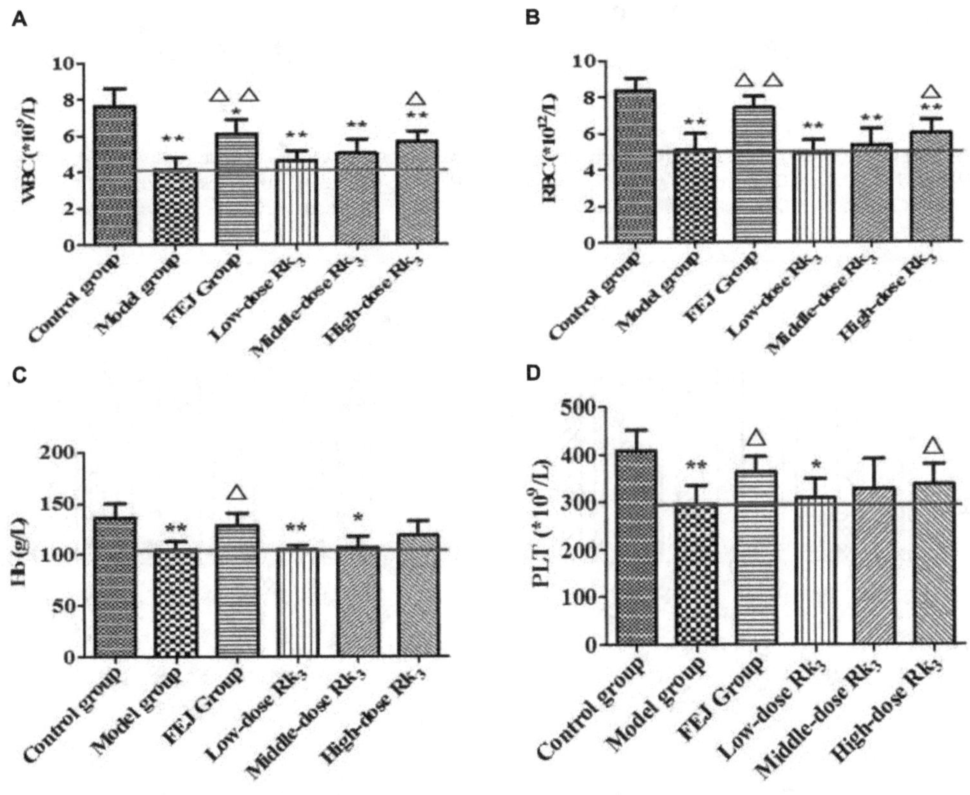

FIGURE 8 | The contents of **(A)** WBC, **(B)** RBC, **(C)** Hb, and **(D)** PLT in the blood of mice after treated with ginsenoside Rk_3. Each value represents means ± SD ($n = 10$). $^*P < 0.05$ and $^{**}P < 0.01$, compared with the control group; $^{\Delta} P < 0.05$ and $^{\Delta\Delta} P < 0.01$, compared with the model group. FEJ, *Fufang E'jiao Jiang*; Hb, hemoglobin; PLT, platelet; RBC, red blood cell; SD, standard deviation; WBC, white blood cell.

final results. Therefore, we tried to reduce the false positive cases, such as threshold filtering with the fit score in the drug target prediction, significance analyzing with hypergeometric distribution approach in disease targets enrichment, and reasonable topologic parameter screening in the analyses of network (Wang et al., 2018). In addition, the combined prediction of multivariate data analyses and verification of pharmacologic tests confirmed the credibility of the model. The

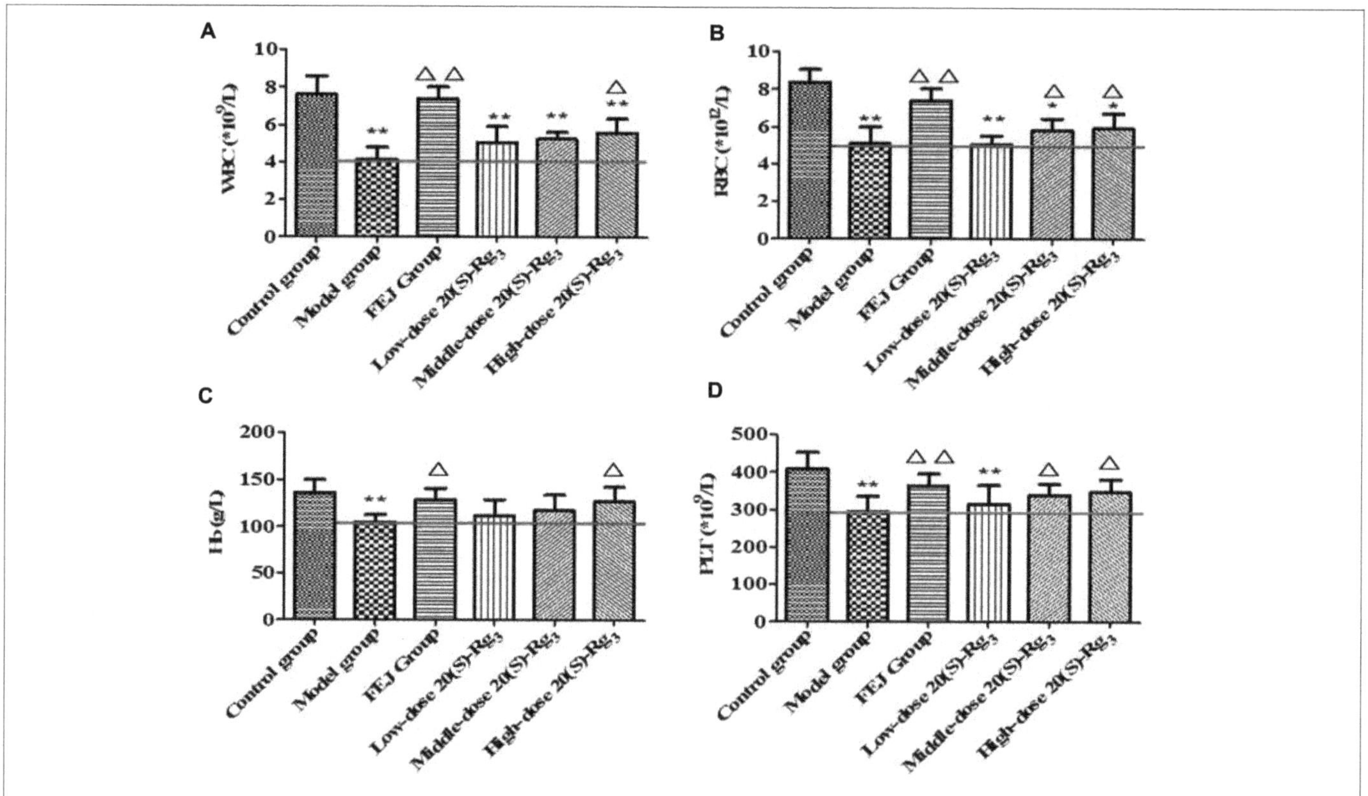

FIGURE 9 | The contents of **(A)** WBC, **(B)** RBC, **(C)** Hb, and **(D)** PLT in the blood of mice after treated with ginsenoside 20(S)-Rg3. Each value represents means ± SD (n = 10). *P < 0.05 and **P < 0.01, compared with the control group; $^{\triangle}$ P < 0.05 and $^{\triangle\triangle}$ P < 0.01, compared with the model group. FEJ, *Fufang E'jiao Jiang*; Hb, hemoglobin; PLT, platelet; RBC, red blood cell; SD, standard deviation; WBC, white blood cell.

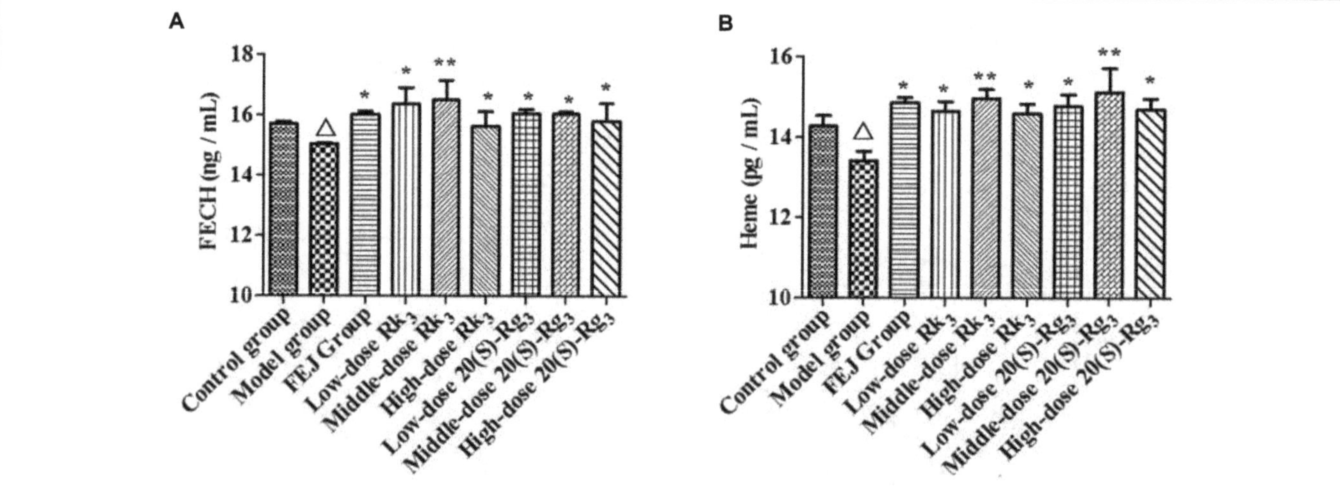

FIGURE 10 | The contents of **(A)** FECH and **(B)** heme in the livers of mice. Each value represents means ± SD (n = 10). $^{\triangle}$ P < 0.05, compared with the control group; *P < 0.05 and **P < 0.01, compared with the model group. FECH, ferrochelatase; FEJ, *Fufang E'jiao Jiang*; SD, standard deviation.

predicted results indicated that 14 constituents of SPN were interacted with 11 targets related to anemia in the network. As shown in **Table 1**, many candidate proteins were targeted by more than one compound. It suggested that these targets might play an important role in the hematopoiesis, the modulation of which could lead to the stimulation of various cytokines in the hematopoietic microenvironment, enhancement of the function of internal free radical scavenging system, facilitation of the absorption and utilization of iron, improvement of the bone marrow hematopoietic microenvironment, *etc.* (Wang et al., 2012b; Liu M. et al., 2014). The common cross-targets shared by multiple constituents implied that SPN might exert the

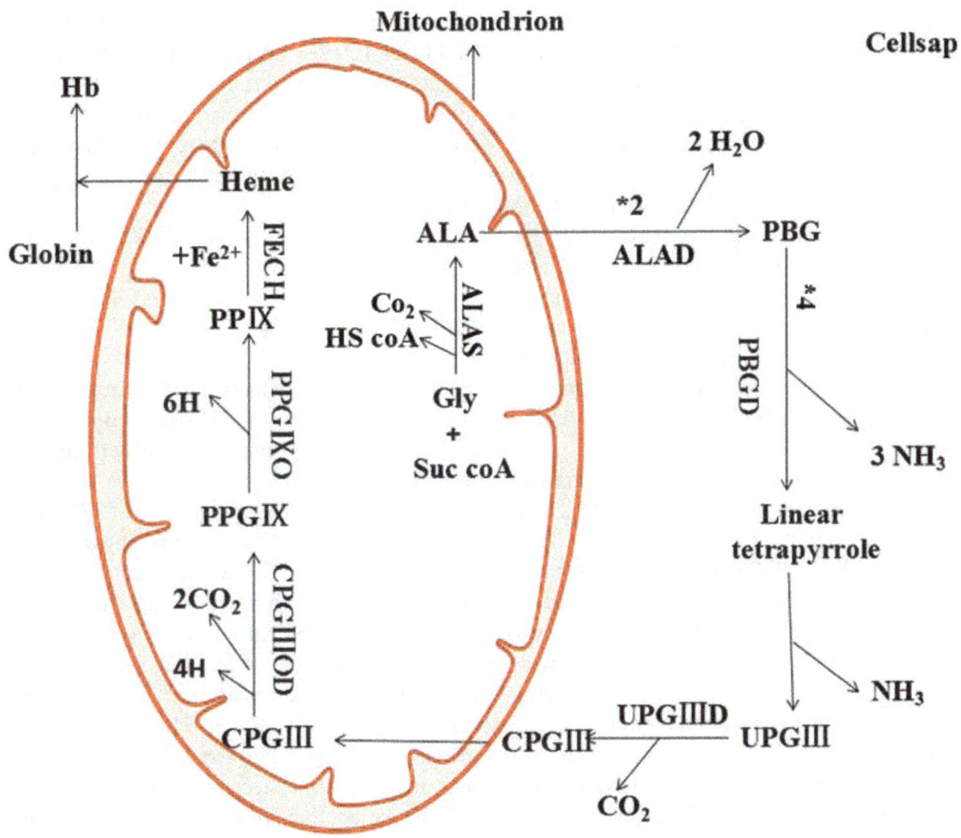

FIGURE 11 | The metabolic pathway of FECH and heme. ALA, δ-aminolevulinic acid; ALAD, δ-aminolevulinic acid dehydrase; ALAS, δ-aminolevulinic acid synthase; CPGIII, coproporphyrinogen III; CPGIIIOD, coproporphyrinogen III oxidized decarboxylase; FECH, ferrochelatase; Gly, glycine; Hb, hemoglobin; PBG, porphobilinogen; PBGD, porphobilinogen deaminase; PPIX, protoporphyrinIX PPGIX, protoporphyrinogenIX; PPGIXO, protoporphyrinogenIX oxidase; Suc-CoA, succinyl–coenzyme A; UPGIX, uroporphyrinogen III; UPG?D, uroporphyrinogen III decarboxylase.

synergistic therapeutic effect on anemia, which was probably more effective than single compound. This suggested that the herbal medicine might act on polypharmacological level, rather than on one specific protein in order to combat complex diseases, such as anemia.

"Degree," "betweenness centrality," and "closeness centrality" are three key topological parameters that characterize the most influential nodes in a network. According to Li et al. (2007), if the "degree" of a node was more than twofolds of the median degree of all nodes in a network, such gene or protein was believed to play a critical role in the network structure, and it could be treated as a hub gene or a hub protein. "Betweenness centrality" was one of the significant indicators of network essentiality because proteins with high betweenness were essential for the functioning of the system by serving as a bridge of communication between several other proteins in the network (Melak and Gakkhar, 2015). And "closeness centrality" was another one of the significant indicators of network essentiality which represented the average length of the shortest paths to access all other proteins in the network. The higher the value, the more central the protein (Zhuang et al., 2015). Therefore, we used the above parameters to determine the importance of active constituents and action targets (the nodes in our network), as well as the extent of their influence on the spread of information through the network (Tang et al., 2015). Among the 11 predicted targets involved in the pathogenic process of anemia, FECH was shown relatively higher values of degree and closeness centrality, and was reported to be closely related to the production of heme. According to **Figure 11**, FECH is the terminal heme synthesis enzyme to catalyze the insertion of the imported iron into protoporphyrin IX to produce heme. Gene mutation in FECH may cause pathological changes like erythropoietic protoporphyria, an autosomal dominant disease which can develop into cholelithiasis and varying degrees of liver diseases (Casanova-González et al., 2010). It was reported that FECH forms an oligomeric complex with Mfrn1 and Abcb10 to synergistically integrate mitochondrial iron importation for heme biosynthesis (Chen et al., 2010). Since heme is an important raw material for hemoglobin synthesis and the increased heme level can resulted in a significant enhancement of human hemoglobin production (Liu L. et al., 2014), the variation of FECH and heme could be investigated to verify the hemopoiesis induced by active constituents of SPN.

From **Table 1**, the majority of compounds were linked with more than one target, indicating that these compounds might play the therapeutic effect by acting on multi-targets. Among the 14 compounds in our network, several of them might be essential. For example, in our previous work (Xiong et al., 2017a), we found the levels of some saponins in PN were increased along with the steaming time and temperature. Among them, ginsenosides Rh_4, Rk_3, 20(*R*)-Rg_3, and 20(*R*)-Rh_1 with higher contents or exclusively existed in SPN showed higher contributions to the activities of SPN. The result was consistent with the prediction in this research, that seven constituents of ginsenosides Rh_4 (10), Rk_3 (11), 20(*R*)-Rg_3 (14), 20(*S*)-Rg_3 (15), 20(*R*)-Rh_1 (16), and 20(*S*)-Rh_1 (17), and notoginsenoside R_2 (20) were predicted to be interacting with the target of FECH for the treatment of anemia. It indicated that the network pharmacology approach had great potential to identify active constituents and alternative targets for the mechanism understanding and drug development of herbal medicines.

To further determine the active constituents, the analysis of fingerprint-effect relationship has been applied to screen characteristic constituents related to the hematinic effect of SPN. Multivariate data analyses such as PLSR and CCA are often used to specify a linear relationship between a set of dependent variables from a large set of independent variables, especially when the sample size is small relative to the dimension of these variables (Garza-Juárez et al., 2011; Wu et al., 2015). According to the results, Rk_3 and 20(*S*)-Rg_3 were predicted to be the major bioactive constituents of SPN treating anemia, which were also included in the prediction of network pharmacology analyses. The two constituents were reported to own various protective effects in previous studies. For example, 20(*S*)-Rg_3 could prevent the progression of renal damage (Kang et al., 2010), protect against benzo[*a*]pyrene-induced genotoxicity in human cells (Poon et al., 2012), and protect against lipopolysaccharide-induced oxidative tissue injury in the liver of rats (Kang et al., 2009). And ginsenoside Rk_3 was shown a protective effect against hypoxia-reoxygenation induced H9c2 cardiomyocytes damage, which was often used as a major ingredient of the compound preparation for ischemic heart diseases (Sun et al., 2013). To validate the predicted results, the effects of Rk_3 and 20(*S*)-Rg_3 on levels of blood routine parameters were investigated based on the BDS model. Compared to the model group, the high-dose Rk_3 and 20(*S*)-Rg_3 could significantly increase the levels of WBC, RBC, and PLT in a dose-dependent way. The high-dose 20(*S*)-Rg_3 also made a significant difference on improving the content of Hb. It indicated that the two constituents had positive effect on improving the BDS of mice, which was consistent with the predicted results of network pharmacology and multivariate data analyses. Besides, the levels of FECH and heme could be increased by the treatment of Rk_3 and 20(*S*)-Rg_3 (**Figure 10**), suggesting that the two constituents exert the hematinic effect by regulating the predicted target and its downstream protein. Meanwhile, we noticed that the high-dose of ginsenosides Rk_3 and 20(*S*)-Rg_3 also inhibited the production of FECH and heme. That might be due to the bidirectional adjustment between FECH and heme that FECH was an integral factor for the biosynthesis of heme, whereas an excessive level of heme could inhibit the production of FECH (Dailey and Fleming, 1983; Wu et al., 2016). These results also indicated that the metabolism of FECH and heme was involved in the development of anemia, of which the stabilization could be regulated by SPN to resist hemolysis. However, further studies are needed to understand the precise nature of these contributing factors.

CONCLUSION

To unveil the bioactive constituents and investigate the action mechanism of SPN for improving BDS, the network pharmacology approach coupled with multivariate data analyses were performed. In this study, we firstly predicted the active constituents and potential targets of SPN related to the treatment of anemia disease. The results showed that ginsenosides Rk_3 and 20(*S*)-Rg_3 were active constituents related to the hematinic effect of SPN, which acted on the targets of FECH and heme to improve the BDS. Although there could be various pathogens causing the incident of anemia and only the hemolytic type was investigated in the research, it also indicated potential areas for further research of SPN as a botanical remedy for the treatment of related diseases. The strategy employed does not only provide new insights for a deeper understanding of the chemical basis and pharmacology of SPN, but also demonstrate an efficient method for potential discovery of drugs originating from herbal medicines. Additional study on the therapeutic effect of SPN on other types of anemia and the involved pathways will be further carried out.

AUTHOR CONTRIBUTIONS

YX wrote this paper and carried out parts of data analyses. YH constructed the network and verified the predicted targets. LC did the multivariate data analyses and parts of pharmacologic tests. ZZ and YZ conducted parts of the pharmacologic tests. MN provided the technical support of network pharmacology. YX and XC supervised the project. All authors read and approved the final manuscript.

FUNDING

This work was supported by National Natural Science Foundation of China (81660661), Kunming University of Science and Technology (KKSY201526065), and Yunnan Applied Basic Research Project (2016FD040).

REFERENCES

103rd Congress (1994). *Dietary Supplement Health and Education Act of 1994, Pub Law 103-417*. Bethesda, MD: National Institutes of Health.

Amberger, J. S., Bocchini, C. A., Schiettecatte, F., Scott, A. F., and Hamosh, A. (2015). OMIM.org: online Mendelian Inheritance in Man (OMIM®), an online catalog of human genes and genetic disorders. *Nucleic Acids Res.* 43, 789–798. doi: 10.1093/nar/gku1205

Baek, J. H., D'Agnillo, F., Vallelian, F., Pereira, C. P., Williams, M. C., Jia, Y., et al. (2012). Hemoglobin-driven pathophysiology is an in vivo consequence of the red blood cell storage lesion that can be attenuated in guinea pigs by haptoglobin therapy. *J. Clin. Invest.* 122, 1444–1458. doi: 10.1172/JCI59770

Benjamini, Y., and Hochberg, Y. (1995). Controlling the false discovery rate: a practical and powerful approach to multiple testing. *J. R. Stat. Soc. B* 57, 289–300. doi: 10.1111/j.2517-6161.1995.tb02031.x

Casanova-González, M. J., Trapero-Marugán, M., Jones, E. A., and Moreno-Otero, R. (2010). Liver disease and erythropoietic protoporphyria:a concise review. *World J. Gastroenterol.* 16, 4526–4531. doi: 10.3748/wjg.v16.i36.4526

Chen, C. Y. (2011). Tcm database@taiwan: the world's largest traditional Chinese medicine database for drug screening in silico. *PLoS One.* 6:e15939. doi: 10.1371/journal.pone.0015939

Chen, W., Dailey, H. A., and Paw, B. H. (2010). Ferrochelatase forms an oligomeric complex with mitoferrin-1 and Abcb10 for erythroid heme biosynthesis. *Blood* 116, 628–630. doi: 10.1182/blood-2009-12-259614

Dailey, H. A., and Fleming, J. E. (1983). Bovine ferrochelatase. Kinetic analysis of inhibition by N-methylprotoporphyrin, manganese, and heme. *J. Biol. Chem.* 258, 11453–11459.

Dennis, G., Sherman, B. T., Hosack, D. A., Yang, J., Gao, W., Lane, H. C., et al. (2003). DAVID: database for annotation, visualization, and integrated discovery. *Genome Biol.* 4:R60.

Garza-Juárez, A., de la Luz Salazar-Cavazos, M., Salazar-Aranda, R., Pérez-Meseguer, J., and de Torres, N. W. (2011). Correlation between chromatographic fingerprint and antioxidant activity of *Turnera diffusa* (Damiana). *Planta Med.* 77, 958–963. doi: 10.1055/s-0030-1250684

Ge, F., Huang, Z., Yu, H., Wang, Y., and Liu, D. (2015). Transformation of *Panax notoginseng* saponins by steaming and *Trichoderma longibrachiatum*. *Pharm. Biotechnol. Eq.* 30, 165–172. doi: 10.1080/13102818.2015.1102611

Gu, C., Lv, J., Zhang, X., Qiao, Y., Yan, H., Li, Y., et al. (2015). Triterpenoids with promoting effects on the differentiation cells from the steamed roots of Panax notoginseng. *J. Nat. Prod.* 78, 1829–1840. doi: 10.1021/acs.jnatprod.5b00027

He, Y., Sang, W., Yang, G., Zou, J., Yang, X., Ji, Q., et al. (2015). Study on the effect of bloodenriching and mechanism of steamed notoginseng powder based on the theory of "prepared notoginseng can enrich the Blood and Qi while the raw one do the opposite". *World Chin. Med.* 10, 647–651.

Iolascon, A., De, F. L., and Beaumont, C. (2009). Molecular basis of inherited microcytic anemia due to defects in iron acquisition or heme synthesis. *Haematologica* 94, 395–408. doi: 10.3324/haematol.13619

Janz, T. G., Johnson, R. L., and Rubenstein, S. D. (2013). Anemia in the emergency department: evaluation and treatment. *J. Emerg. Med.* 15, 1–15; quiz 15–16.

Kanehisa, M., and Goto, S. (2000). KEGG: kyoto encyclopedia of genes and genomes. *Nucleic Acids Res.* 27, 29–34. doi: 10.1093/nar/27.1.29

Kang, K. S., Kim, H. Y., Yamabe, N., Park, J. H., and Yokozawa, T. (2009). Preventive effect of 20(S)-ginsenoside Rg3 against lipopolysaccharide-induced hepatic and renal injury in rats. *Free Radic. Res.* 41, 1181–1188. doi: 10.1080/10715760701581740

Kang, K. S., Yamabe, N., Kim, H. Y., Park, J. H., and Yokozawa, T. (2010). Effects of heat-processed ginseng and its active component ginsenoside 20 (S)-Rg3 on the progression of renal damage and dysfunction in type 2 diabetic Otsuka Long-Evans Tokushima Fatty rats. *Biol. Pharm. Bull.* 33, 1077–1081. doi: 10.1248/bpb.33.1077

Kassebaum, N. J., Jasrasaria, R., Naghavi, M., Wulf, S. K., Johns, N., Lozano, R., et al. (2014). A systematic analysis of global anemia burden from 1990 to 2010. *Blood* 123, 615–624. doi: 10.1182/blood-2013-06-508325

Lau, A. J., Toh, D. F., Chua, T. K., Pang, Y. K., Woo, S. O., and Koh, H. L. (2009). Antiplatelet and anticoagulant effects of Panax notoginseng: comparison of raw and steamed *Panax notoginseng* with *Panax ginseng* and *Panax quinquefolium*. *J. Ethnopharmacol.* 125, 380–386. doi: 10.1016/j.jep.2009.07.038

Li, J., Zhao, P., Li, Y., Tian, Y., and Wang, Y. (2015). Systems pharmacology-based dissection of mechanisms of chinese medicinal formula Bufei Yishen as an effective treatment for chronic obstructive pulmonary disease. *Sci. Rep.* 5, 15290. doi: 10.1038/srep15290

Li, S., Zhang, Z. Q., Wu, L. J., Zhang, X. G., Li, Y. D., and Wang, Y. Y. (2007). Understanding ZHENG in traditional Chinese medicine in the context of neuro-endocrine-immune network. *IET Syst. Biol.* 1, 51–60. doi: 10.1049/iet-syb:20060032

Li, W., Yuan, G., Pan, Y., Wang, C., and Chen, H. (2017). Network pharmacology studies on the bioactive compounds and action mechanisms of natural products for the treatment of diabetes mellitus: a review. *Front. Pharmacol.* 8:74. doi: 10.3389/fphar.2017.00074

Liu, L., Martínez, J. L., Liu, Z., Petranovic, D., and Nielsen, J. (2014). Balanced globin protein expression and heme biosynthesis improve production of human hemoglobin in *Saccharomyces cerevisiae*. *Metab. Eng.* 21, 9–16. doi: 10.1016/j.ymben.2013.10.010

Liu, M., Tan, H., Zhang, X., Liu, Z., Cheng, Y., Wang, D. L., et al. (2014). Hematopoietic effects and mechanisms of Fufang E'jiao Jiang on radiotherapy and chemotherapy-induced myelosuppressed mice. *J. Ethnopharmacol.* 152, 575–584. doi: 10.1016/j.jep.2014.02.012

Martens, H. E., and Naes, T. (1991). Multivariate calibration. *Biometrics* 47, 1203–1205.

Melak, T., and Gakkhar, S. (2015). Comparative genome and network centrality analysis to identify drug targets of mycobacterium tuberculosis h37rv. *Biomed. Res. Int.* 2015:212061. doi: 10.1155/2015/212061

Poon, P. Y., Kwok, H. H., Yue, P. Y., Yang, M. S., Mak, N. K., Wong, C. K., et al. (2012). Cytoprotective effect of 20 (S)-Rg3 on benzo[a]pyrene-induced DNA damage. *Drug Metab. Dispos.* 40, 120–129. doi: 10.1124/dmd.111.039503

Quan, Q. R., Li, H. Y., Cao, M. B., Bal, X. J., Fan, S. Y., Wang, B., et al. (2016). Identification of the anti-tumor activity and mechanisms of nuciferine through a network pharmacology approach. *Acta Pharmacol. Sin.* 37, 963–972. doi: 10.1038/aps.2016.53

Sheng, S. J., Wang, J. X., Wang, L. R., Liu, H., Li, P. B., Liu, M. H., et al. (2014). Network pharmacology analyses of the antithrombotic pharmacological mechanism of Fufang Xueshuantong Capsule with experimental support using disseminated intravascular coagulation rats. *J. Ethnopharmacol.* 154, 735–744. doi: 10.1016/j.jep.2014.04.048

Shi, Z., Liu, Z., Liu, C., Wu, M., Su, H., Ma, X., et al. (2016). Spectrum-effect relationships between chemical fingerprints and antibacterial effects of Lonicerae japonicae Flos and Lonicerae Flos base on UPLC and microcalorimetry. *Front. Pharmacol.* 7:12. doi: 10.3389/fphar.2016.00012

Smoot, M. E., Ono, K., Ruscheinski, J., Wang, P. L., and Ideker, T. (2011). Cytoscape 2.8: new features for data integration and network visualization. *Bioinformatics* 27, 431–432. doi: 10.1093/bioinformatics/btq675

Sun, J., Sun, G., Meng, X., Wang, H., Wang, M., Qin, M., et al. (2013). Ginsenoside Rk3 prevents hypoxia-reoxygenation induced apoptosis in H9c2 cardiomyocytes via AKT and MAPK pathway. *Evid Based Compl. Alt.* 2013:690190. doi: 10.1155/2013/690190

Sun, S., Wang, C. Z., Tong, R., Li, X. L., Fishbein, A., Wang, Q., et al. (2010). Effects of steaming the root of *Panax notoginseng*, on chemical composition and anticancer activities. *Food Chem.* 118, 307–314. doi: 10.1016/j.foodchem.2009.04.122

Sundberg, R. (2008). Applied chemometrics for scientists. *J. Am. Stat. Assoc.* 103, 1317–1318. doi: 10.1198/jasa.2008.s244

Tang, F., Tang, Q. F., Tian, Y. X., Qin, F., Yao, H., and Tan, X. M. (2015). Network pharmacology-based prediction of the active ingredients and potential targets of Mahuang Fuzi Xixin decoction for application to allergic rhinitis. *J. Ethnopharmacol.* 176, 402–412. doi: 10.1016/j.jep.2015.10.040

Tao, W., Xu, X., Wang, X., Li, B., Wang, Y., Li, Y., et al. (2013). Network pharmacology-based prediction of the active ingredients and potential targets of Chinese herbal Radix Curcumae formula for application to cardiovascular disease. *J. Ethnopharmacol.* 145, 1–10. doi: 10.1016/j.jep.2012.09.051

Tian, J. S., Zhang, X., Liu, H., Xiang, H., Xing, J., Zhang, L. Z., et al. (2017). The hematinic effect of Colla corii asini (Ejiao) using 1 H-NMR metabolomics coupled with correlation analysis in APH-induced anemic rats. *RSC Adv.* 7, 8952–8962. doi: 10.1039/C6RA26899D

Wang, D., Liao, P., Zhu, H., Chen, K., Min, X., Zhang, Y., et al. (2012a). The processing of *Panax notoginseng* and the transformation of its saponin components. *Food Chem.* 132, 1808–1813. doi: 10.1016/j.foodchem.2011.12.010

Wang, D., Liu, M., Cao, J., Cheng, Y., Zhuo, C., Xu, H., et al. (2012b). Effect of Colla corii asini (E'jiao) on D-galactose induced aging mice. *Biol. Pharm. Bull.* 35, 2128–2132. doi: 10.1248/bpb.b12-00238

Wang, J., Cui, H., Wang, R., Zhang, C., Niu, M., Bai, Z., et al. (2018). A systems pharmacology-oriented discovery of a new therapeutic use of the TCM formula Liuweiwuling for liver failure. *Sci. Rep.* 8:5645. doi: 10.1038/s41598-018-21515-6

Wang, X., Shen, Y., Wang, S., Li, S., Zhang, W., Liu, X., et al. (2017). Pharmmapper 2017 update: a web server for potential drug target identification with a comprehensive target pharmacophore database. *Nucleic Acids Res.* 45, W356–W360. doi: 10.1093/nar/gkx374

Wei, S., Niu, M., Wang, J., Wang, J., Su, H., Luo, S., et al. (2016). A network pharmacology approach to discover active compounds and action mechanisms of San-Cao Granule for treatment of liver fibrosis. *Drug Des. Dev. Ther.* 10, 733–743. doi: 10.2147/DDDT.S96964

Wu, J., Wen, S., Zhou, Y., Chao, H., and Shen, Y. (2016). Human ferrochelatase: insights for the mechanism of ferrous iron approaching into protoporphyrin IX by QM/MM and QTCP free energy studies. *J. Chem. Inf. Model.* 56, 2421–2433. doi: 10.1021/acs.jcim.6b00216

Wu, X. D., Chen, H. G., Zhou, X., Huang, Y., Hu, E. M., Jiang, Z. M., et al. (2015). Studies on chromatographic fingerprint and fingerprinting profile-efficacy relationship of *Saxifraga stolonifera* Meerb. *Molecules* 20, 22781–22798. doi: 10.3390/molecules201219882

Xiong, Y., Chen, L., Hu, Y., and Cui, X. (2017a). Uncovering active constituents responsible for different activities of raw and steamed Panax notoginseng roots. *Front. Pharmacol.* 8:745. doi: 10.3389/fphar.2017.00745

Xiong, Y., Chen, L., Man, J., Hu, Y., and Cui, X. (2017b). Chemical and bioactive comparison of *Panax notoginseng* root and rhizome in raw and steamed forms. *J. Gins. Res.* (in press). doi: 10.1016/j.jgr.2017.11.004

Yoon, T., and Cowan, J. A. (2004). Frataxin-mediated iron delivery to ferrochelatase in the final step of heme biosynthesis. *J. Biol. Chem.* 279, 25943–25946. doi: 10.1074/jbc.C400107200

Zhang, H., Wang, H. F., Liu, Y., Huang, L. J., Wang, Z. F., and Li, Y. (2014). The haematopoietic effect of *Panax japonicus* on blood deficiency model mice. *J. Ethnopharmacol.* 154, 818–824. doi: 10.1016/j.jep.2014.05.008

Zhou, X. H., Long, L. L., Li, C. M., Zhao, R. H., Zhang, R. P., and Mao, X. J. (2014). Raw versus steamed *Panax notoginseng* in pharmacological effects. *Glob. Tradit. Chin. Med.* 7, 420–426.

Zhuang, D. Y., Jiang, L. I., He, Q. Q., Zhou, P., and Yue, T. (2015). Identification of hub subnetwork based on topological features of genes in breast cancer. *Int. J. Mol. Med.* 35, 664–674. doi: 10.3892/ijmm.2014.2057

3

In Silico Study of Anti-Insomnia Mechanism for Suanzaoren Prescription

Jian Gao[1], Qiming Wang[1], Yuwei Huang[1], Kailin Tang[1], Xue Yang[2] and Zhiwei Cao[1]**

[1] Shanghai 10th People's Hospital, School of Life Sciences and Technology, Tongji University, Shanghai, China,
[2] Department of Traditional Chinese Medicine, Yangpu Hospital, School of Medicine, TongJi University, Shanghai, China

***Correspondence:**
Xue Yang
yxkxl@163.com
Zhiwei Cao
zwcao@tongji.edu.cn

Insomnia is a common and widespread sleeping disorder caused by various risk factors. Though beneficial, conventional treatments of insomnia have significant limitations. As an alternative treatment, Chinese herbal formula Suanzaoren prescription (SZRP), composed of Suanzaoren [seeds of *Ziziphus jujuba* var. *spinosa* (Bunge) Hu ex H.F.Chow] and four additional herbs, has been reported with significant anti-insomnia effects. Yet the anti-insomnia mechanism of the herb formulae remains unknown. In this study, we attempted to extrapolate the holistic anti-insomnia mechanism of SZRP through herbal targeting and network pharmacology. The results indicated that the ingredients of Suanzaoren can target multi-neurotransmitter receptors at synapse interface, which was reported to be associated with sedative and hypnotic effects, while the four additional herbs can hit multiple pathways downstream of membrane neurotransmitters. Furthermore, the four additional herbs showed highly cooperative targeting patterns in the paralleled and cross-talked pathways related to inflammatory regulation and endocrine system, which may contribute to the additional relief of insomnia caused by inflammation, anxiety, or endocrine disorder. The interesting complementary mechanism we found among the herbal groups of SZRP may provide an example to study Chinese herbal formula and offers clues to future design of anti-insomnia strategy.

Keywords: network pharmacology, suanzaoren prescription, insomnia, bioinformatics, systematic analysis

INTRODUCTION

Insomnia is a common sleep disorder in which people have difficulty falling asleep or staying asleep (Punnoose et al., 2012). It can sap quality of life and even cause damage to health. Short-term insomnia can cause daytime sleeping and low energy (Lande and Gragnani, 2010), while long-term insomnia may lead to serious problems including driving accident, anxiety, chronic pain, cardiovascular disease, and heart failure (Taylor et al., 2007). According to its etiology, insomnia can be classified as primary or secondary (National Heart, 2016). Primary insomnia is not directly associated with any other health conditions or problems, and its pathogenesis remains unclear. On the contrary, secondary insomnia is related to those obvious triggers, and it is generally caused by the following reasons: 1) emotional disorder including psychological stress, depression, and anxiety; 2) health conditions of chronic pain, such as arthritis, headache, and other inflammations; 3) hormone disorder including menstruation, menopause, and hyperglycemia (Pepin et al., 2014; Santoro et al., 2015); and 4) some medicines and substances.

Anti-insomnia treatment often includes lifestyle change, cognitive-behavioral therapy, and prescription medicines (Buysse, 2013). Nonpharmacologic treatments are usually recommended as the first-line treatment (Trauer et al., 2015), while pharmacologic treatments including benzodiazepines and benzodiazepine-like medications are applied as additional treatment if nonpharmacologic treatments fail (Asnis et al., 2015). Though pharmacologic treatments can be effective, patients may not tolerate their side effects such as rebound withdrawal effects, disruption in sleep architecture, grogginess, memory impairment, and undesired behaviors during sleep (Tiller et al., 2003; Wilt et al., 2016). In addition to those drugs mentioned above, antidepressants, antipsychotics, and antihistamines may also be applied for sedative effect. Yet they are usually not recommended in the absence of corresponding disease symptoms. Due to the present limited treatment, a substantial number of patients worldwide have started to seek their sleeping aids in herbal medicine as an alternative approach (Chen et al., 2009; Frass et al., 2012). It has been reported that Chinese herbal formulae "Xiao Yao Wan," "liquorice, wheat, and jujube soup," "Tian Wang Bu Xin Dan," and "Suanzaoren prescription (SZRP)" are clinically effective against insomnia (Chen et al., 2011; Liu et al., 2015; Ko et al., 2016); among them, SZRP is the most widely used and well documented for refractory insomnia. It was first recorded in *Shennong Bencao Jing*, which is the earliest authoritative monograph on pharmacy in China (Gu, 2007). In addition to the clinical practice, high-quality randomized controlled trials have confirmed its efficacy and safety (Wang et al., 2010; Wang et al., 2013; Yuan et al., 2013). Moreover, a meta-analysis study covering 1,454 patients showed that both SZRP monotherapy and combinational treatment can improve sleep quality significantly with minimal side effects (Zhou et al., 2018).

SZRP contains the main herb seeds of *Ziziphus jujuba* var. *spinosa* (Bunge) Hu ex H.F.Chow (Suanzaoren) and four additional herbs: *Anemarrhena asphodeloides* Bunge (Zhimu), *Wolfiporia extensa* (Peck) Ginns (Fuling), *Ligusticum sinense* Oliv. (Chuanxiong), and *Glycyrrhiza uralensis* Fisch. (Zhigancao). According to the TCM theory and Chinese Pharmacopeia (China, 2015), Suanzaore is the *Emperor* (*Jun*), Zhimu and Fuling are the *Ministers* (*Chen*), Chuanxiong is the *Adjuvant* (*Zuo*), and Zhigancao is the *Courier* (*Shi*) (WHO, 2007). The functions of herb are usually believed to be multiple because of the vast chemical diversity. Previous literatures have reported that Suanzaoren is anti-insomnia (Shergis et al., 2017), Zhimu is laxative and anti-inflammatory (Park et al., 2018; Ji et al., 2019; Li et al., 2019), Fuling is diuretic (Zhao et al., 2012), and Chuanxiong is anti-migraine (Shan et al., 2018). However, current studies about the pharmacological mechanism of SZRP are mainly focused on the main herb Suanzaoren. Photochemical analysis indicated that Suanzaoren contains flavonoids, saponins, and triterpenes. Jujuboside A, sanjoinine A, and flavonoids in Suanzaoren were reported to have sedative and hypnotic effects. Further study showed that jujuboside A affected GABAergic and serotonergic system in rat through glutamate-mediated excitatory signal pathway (Cao et al., 2010). The hydrolysis product of jujuboside A, jujubogenin, was predicted to have high potential of blood–brain barrier penetration ability (Chen et al., 2008). In addition, sanjoinine A was found to be able to prolong sleeping time through increasing chloride influx and GABA synthesis (Zhang et al., 2003). In addition, the flavonoid 6-hydroxyflavone in Suanzaoren showed GABA agonistic action by binding to GABAA receptors (Ren et al., 2010). These aforementioned studies provide a glimpse of the partial mechanism of anti-insomnia effects of Suanzaoren herb. The holistic mechanism of SZRP formulae remains unclear. What is the mechanism of additional herbs in treating insomnia? How can they help to improve the therapeutic effects of the main herb? No systematic studies have been published so far. In this work, first, we conducted a global analysis of all known targets of herbal ingredients for five herbs of SZRP to elucidate the overall anti-insomnia mechanisms of SZRP, and then we analyzed the targeting network patterns herb by herb for better understanding of their potential roles in TCM formulae.

METHODS

Dataset

The information of herbal ingredients and targets was collected from online TCM databases Traditional Chinese Medicine Systems Pharmacology (Ru et al., 2014), Herb Ingredients' Targets (HIT) (Ye et al., 2011), and Natural Product Activity & Species Source Database (NPASS) (Zeng et al., 2018). The following key words were used to search in these databases: *Ziziphus jujuba* var. *spinosa* (Bunge) Hu ex H.F.Chow OR Suanzaoren; *Anemarrhena asphodeloides* Bunge OR Zhimu; *Wolfiporia extensa* (Peck) Ginns OR Fuling; *Ligusticum sinense* Oliv. OR Chuanxiong; and *Glycyrrhiza uralensis* Fisch. OR Zhigancao. Therapeutic targets were collected from Therapeutic Targets Database (TTD) (Li et al., 2018). The validated information of plants was collected from Kew Royal Botanic Garden (https://mpns.science.kew.org/mpns-portal/) and The Plant List (http://www.theplantlist.org).

Functional Annotation and Enrichment Analysis

Statistical analysis of KEGG function enrichment of the target profile was performed by Metascape (Tripathi et al., 2015) (http://metascape.org). The pathways significantly enriched were selected (p-value < 0.01). Then only terms with both −Log (p-value) > 5 and more than 5% targets falling into the category were retained. The retained terms were mapped into bubble graph by "pyplot" of matplotlib. Finally, bubble graphs of each herb were combined and labeled with Adobe Photoshop software (Adobe, San Jose, California).

Network Construction for SZRP

To better elaborate the holistic mechanism of SZRP, three subnetworks were compiled by following the procedures: 1) All targets of SZRP were submitted to an online tool KEGG Search Pathway (https://www.genome.jp/kegg/tool/map_pathway1.html). 2) All result maps of KEGG were downloaded and integrated. 3) Maps related to "nervous," "immune," or "endocrine" were reserved. 4) For each label of "nervous," "immune," and "endocrine," multiple pathways were integrated and overlapped according to cross-talk targets in these maps. Detailed information such as targets names and integrated pathways are shown in **Table S3**. 5) Subnetworks were drawn with Adobe Illustrator software, where intermediate genes were hidden for better display.

RESULTS

Overall Ingredients and Targets of SZRP

To understand the potential anti-insomnia mechanism of SZRP holistically, known targets for herbal ingredient in the formula were collected and analyzed. Five medicinal species were validated by botanical documentation (**Figure 1**). *Z. jujube*, *A. asphodeloides*, *L. sinense*, and *G. uralensis* were validated by Kew Database and TPL. *W. extensa* was reported as an edible fungus (Esteban, 2009; Wei et al., 2016). Through database searching, 497 unique targets were collected for five herbs in SZRP (**Table 1**); 24% of proteins (119) were reported as therapeutic targets in TTD (Li et al., 2018). Three known therapeutic targets of anti-insomnia drugs were covered by SZRP targets including gamma-aminobutyric acid type A receptor (GABAR), 5-hydroxytryptamine receptor (HTR), and histamine receptor (HRH). All information of targets is shown in **Table S1**. The distribution of targets of five herbs is shown in **Figure 2**. Eighty known targets were retrieved for Suanzaoren, among which 26 were shared by all five herbs. In terms of target abundance, *A. asphodeloides* retrieved the most targets, while *L. sinense* had the most abundant unique targets.

TABLE 1 | Number of ingredients and known targets for each herb in SZRP.

Species name	TCM name	Ingredients	Targets
Ziziphus jujuba var. *spinosa* (Bunge) Hu ex H.F.Chow	Suanzaoren	35	80
Anemarrhena asphodeloides Bunge	Zhimu	82	228
Wolfiporia extensa (Peck) Ginns	Fuling	58	184
Ligusticum sinense Oliv.	Chuanxiong	292	296
Glycyrrhiza uralensis Fisch.	Zhigancao	272	201
Total (SZRP)		**711**	**497**

Functional Analysis of Separated SZRP

To investigate the functional relationship among the five individual herbs of SZRP, targets of each herb were mapped to KEGG for functional enrichment analysis. The top 5 functional pathways for each herb in SZRP are listed in **Table 2**. It can be seen that apart from the main herb, the top enriched pathway profiles were highly similar for the four additional herbs. In **Table S2**, the overall pathway enrichment of total formulae is shown with their targets combined. Aside from cellular processes, metabolism, and signal transduction terms, organismal systems of nervous, endocrine, immune infections (NEIs) were significantly enriched. As our aim is to interpolate the potential anti-insomnia mechanism, we tentatively focused on organismal systems of NEIs, which are known to closely relate with insomnia pathology (Santoro et al., 2015; Xiang et al., 2019). To display the functional similarity and difference among herbal groups of SZRP, significant pathway terms of KEGG were mapped into a bubble graph in **Figure 3**.

The big and higher bubbles in **Figure 3** represent those highly significantly enriched pathway terms. It can be seen that the main

TCM Name	Suanzaoren	Zhimu	Fuling	Chuanxiong	Zhigancao
Species Name	*Ziziphus jujuba* var. *spinosa* (Bunge) Hu ex H.F.Chow	*Anemarrhena asphodeloides* Bunge	*Wolfiporia extensa* (Peck) Ginns	*Ligusticum sinense* Oliv.	*Glycyrrhiza uralensis* Fisch.
Botanical Documentation	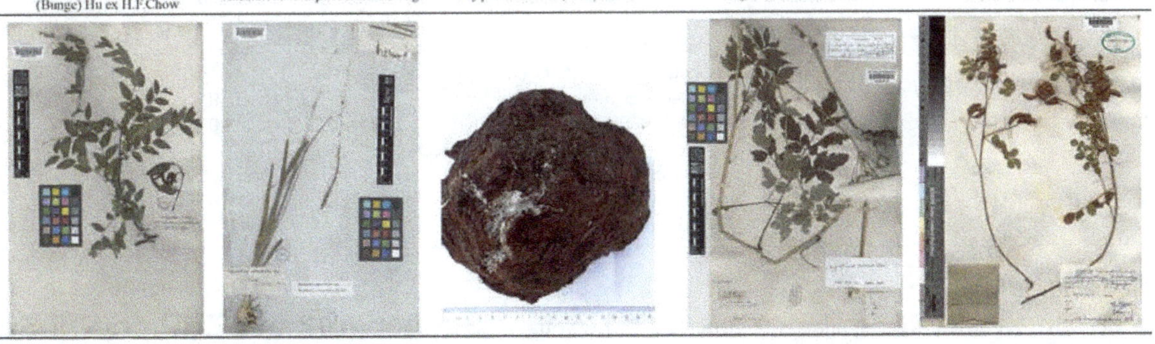				
Validated Source	Kew Royal Botanic Gardens K000723006 The Plant List kew-2891502	Kew Royal Botanic Gardens K000794610 The Plant List kew-299155	Esteban, C. I., 2009 Wei et al., 2016	Kew Royal Botanic Gardens K000685139 The Plant List kew-2343931	Kew Royal Botanic Gardens K000118170 The Plant List ild-32406
Location	China	China	Yingshan County Hubei Province China	Hubei Province China	Kazakstan
Used Parts	Seeds	Rhizomes	Sclerotium	Rhizomes	Roots and Rhizomes

FIGURE 1 | The validated information of five herbs in SZRP, including botanical documentation (voucher specimen deposited in herbarium), location (the collection location of voucher specimen), and used part (used part of medicinal species).

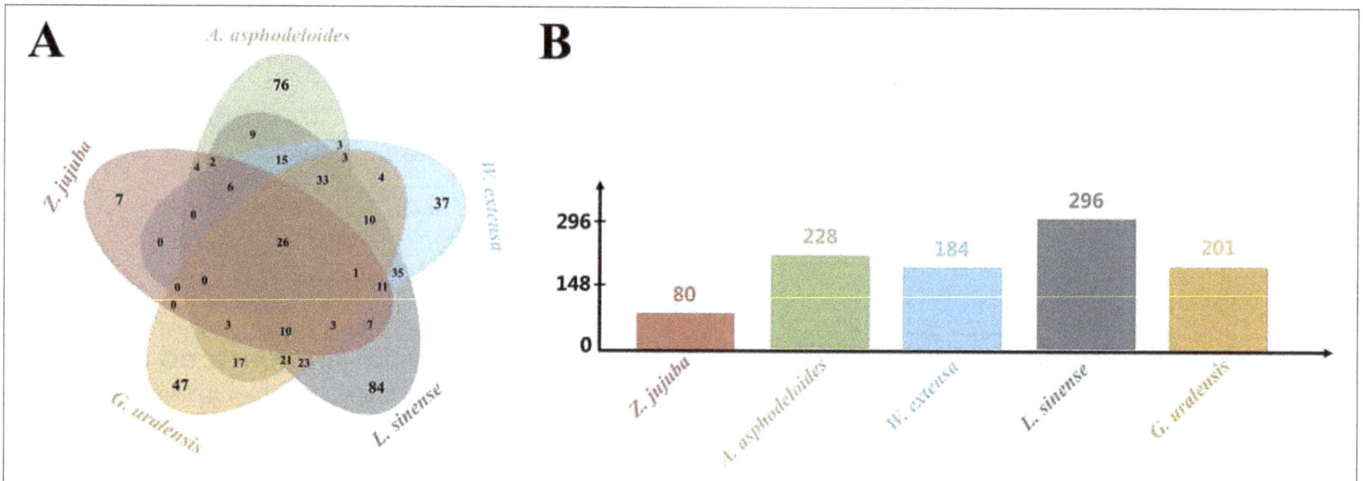

FIGURE 2 | The target distribution of five herbs. **(A)** Unique and overlapping target of five herbs. **(B)** The number of targets for different herbs.

TABLE 2 | Top five pathways enriched by targets of each herb in SZRP.

Species name	Herbal group	Pathway name	KEGG ID	Ratio (%)	–Log(*p*-value)
Ziziphus jujuba var. *spinosa* (Bunge) Hu ex H.F.Chow	*Emperor* (*Jun*)	Serotonergic synapse	hsa04726	12.5	11.09
		Dopaminergic synapse	hsa04728	10	7.7
		Amphetamine addiction	hsa05031	7.5	6.82
		Adrenergic signaling in cardiomyocytes	hsa04261	8.75	6.09
		Cocaine addiction	hsa05030	6.25	6.08
Anemarrhena asphodeloides Bunge	*Minister* (*Chen*)	Fluid shear stress and atherosclerosis	hsa05418	8.81	16.73
		AGE-RAGE signaling pathway	hsa04933	6.17	11.88
		Influenza A	hsa05164	7.49	11.67
		Ovarian steroidogenesis	hsa04913	4.85	11.65
		Adipocytokine signaling pathway	hsa04920	5.29	11.36
Wolfiporia extensa (Peck) Ginns	*Minister* (*Chen*)	Hepatitis B	hsa05161	13.66	25.55
		Influenza A	hsa05164	13.11	22.1
		AGE-RAGE signaling pathway	hsa04933	9.84	18.85
		Chagas disease (American trypanosomiasis)	hsa05142	9.84	18.6
		Hepatitis C	hsa05160	10.38	17.93
Ligusticum sinense Oliv.	*Adjuvant* (*Zuo*)	AGE-RAGE signaling pathway	hsa04933	9.18	27.63
		Hepatitis B	hsa05161	9.86	25.51
		Fluid shear stress and atherosclerosis	hsa05418	8.84	21.77
		Chagas disease (American trypanosomiasis)	hsa05142	7.14	18.79
		Prolactin signaling pathway	hsa04917	6.12	18.05
Glycyrrhiza uralensis Fisch.	*Courier* (*Shi*)	AGE-RAGE signaling pathway	hsa04933	14	33.98
		Fluid shear stress and atherosclerosis	hsa05418	15	32.19
		Th17 cell differentiation	hsa04659	11.5	24.88
		IL-17 signaling pathway	hsa04657	11	24.81
		Hepatitis B	hsa05161	11.5	21.73

herb of SZRP significantly regulates the function of nervous system, such as dopaminergic and serotonergic synapse pathways, suggesting that the *Emperor* (*Jun*) herb may enable hypnotic effects through modulating excitement in nervous system. In contrast, four additional herbs concentrated more significantly on the endocrine system, immunology system, and infections, offering complementary effects against insomnia. Specifically, the *Minister* (*Chen*) herb significantly targets virus infection pathways and immune cell pathways, while the *Adjuvant* (*Zuo*) and *Courier* (*Shi*) herbs affected signaling regulation of oxidative stress (AGE–RAGE) and hormone secretion (Prolactin).

Subnetwork of SZRP on NEI System

For further investigation, subnetworks were constructed based on enriched pathways for multi-neurotransmitter regulation, inflammatory regulation, and endocrine regulation (**Figures 4** and **5**). Each target in the pathways was labeled according to the different targeting patterns of the four herbal groups.

Figure 4 shows the targeting patterns of SZRP herbs in a multi-neurotransmitter regulation network. These targets can be roughly divided into three classes: 1) interacted directly with multi-neurotransmitter receptors and downstream pathways; 2) related to the synthesis, secretion, and recycling

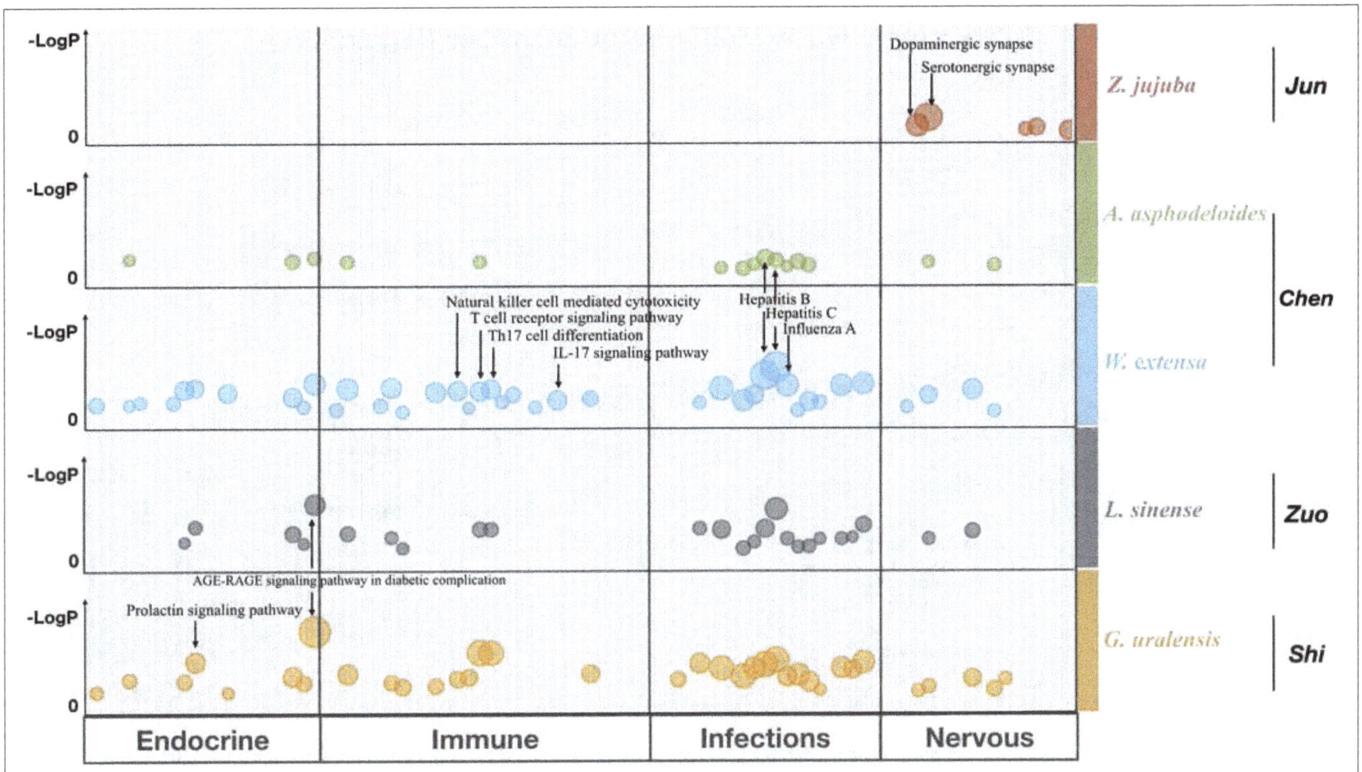

FIGURE 3 | Bubble graph for significantly enriched pathway terms from KEGG by Metascape. Each bubble represents one KEGG pathway term. The size of the bubble correlates with the relative ratio of targets hitting each pathway over the total targets, with larger bubbles indicating the more enriched terms. The LogP shows the statistical significance of *p*-values, with larger and higher numbers indicating the more significant ones. And only those functional terms were retained with both –Log(*p*-value) > 5 and enrichment ratio > 5%. The detailed statistical data are shown in **Table S2**.

of neurotransmitters; and 3) related to the sedative or hypnotic effects, such as opioid receptor (OPR) and adenosine receptor (ADORA). Of interest is that all herbal groups can target transporter proteins of dopamine and serotonin in the pre-synaptic membrane. When being examined from the perspective of herbal groups, the *Emperor* (*Jun*) herb significantly targeted on interfacial neurotransmitter receptors (**Figure 4**). The four additional herbs not only targeted those receptors but also targeted those in downstream, such as Raf, Akt, PKC, and CaM. Specifically speaking, the *Courier* (*Shi*) herb mainly regulated major downstream targets of multi-neurotransmitter regulation pathway. The synapse formation, axonal outgrowth, synaptic plasticity, and neuroprotection medicated by targets nAChR, DR, and HTR may be beneficial to maintain circadian rhythm; in addition, targets of SZRP such as GABRA, ADORA, and HRH have been reported to participate in sleep induction (Huang et al., 2014; Wisden et al., 2017).

Besides, SZRP can regulate immune-related inflammatory pathways and their upstream targets (**Figure 5**). The *Emperor* (*Jun*) herb mainly influenced COX2, while the four additional herbs took part in the regulation of inflammatory factors such as IL-1, IL-2, IL-6, IL-8, and IL-10. And the *Courier* (*Shi*) herb covered the largest area of inflammation pathways. Two compounds from the *Adjuvant* (*Zuo*) herb *L. sinense* have been reported to inhibit inflammation through downregulating IL-1 and IL-8 (Diodovich et al., 2003; Medeiros et al., 2007) and upregulating IL-10 (Sarkar et al., 2006). Inflammation and chronic pain are widely reported with insomnia (Cheatle et al., 2016), while inhibition of inflammation and chronic pain was shown to improve sleep quality (Trenkwalder et al., 2017; Wells et al., 2017).

Endocrine disorder associated with premenstrual and menopausal syndromes in women shows outstanding effects on secondary insomnia (Santoro et al., 2015). **Figure 5** shows the targeting patterns of SZRP herbs in endocrine regulation pathways. These targets were related to the regulation of blood sugar, blood pressure, and hormone system. All herbal groups mainly exerted a wide range of hormonal regulating effect by targeting the key receptors such as estrogen receptor (ER), progesterone receptor (PR), and adrenergic receptor (ADR). The whole formula played holistic and complementary roles in blood pressure and hormone regulation, while other herbal groups of *Minister* (*Chen*), *Adjuvant* (*Zuo*), and *Courier* (*Shi*) showed unique effects on blood sugar regulation by targeting insulin (INS), insulin receptor (INSR), and glucagon-like peptide 1 receptor (GLP-1R). Menstruation- and menopause-related insomnia is often caused by endocrine disorder (Santoro et al., 2015); moreover, hyperglycemia and hypertension are the high-risk factors of insomnia.

To understand the mechanistic relationship within TCM formulae, SZRP was disassembled into individual herbal groups. The *Emperor* (*Jun*) herb was found to mainly target receptors in synapse membrane, which might relieve the primary insomnia. The *Minister* (*Chen*) herbs can target not only the nervous system

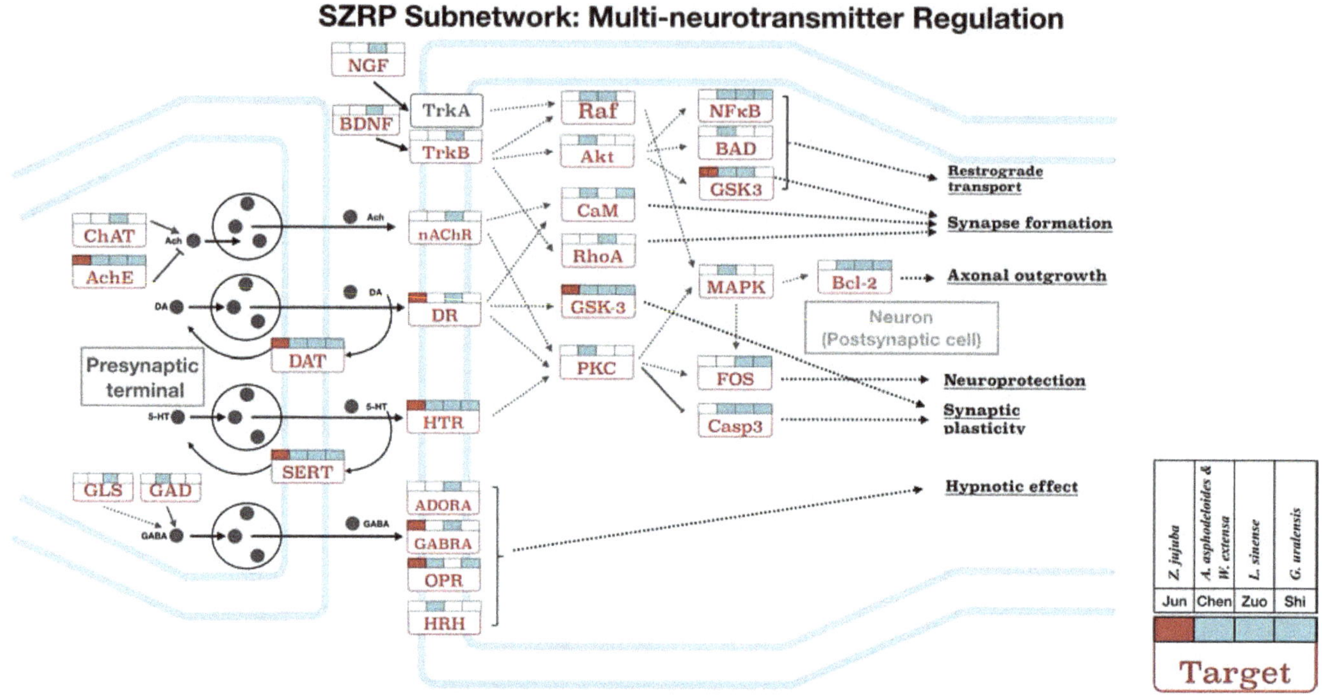

FIGURE 4 | The targeting subnetwork showing multi-neurotransmitter regulation at both pre-synapse and post-synapse for SZRP. Target names are shown in rectangles, and their full gene names can be found in **Table S3**. The gray dots illustrate neurotransmitter/hormone. The colored flags above each target show the targeting pattern from four herbal groups of SZRP, where the *Emperor*'s (*Jun*) targets are labeled in red. The solid arrows in the figure mean directed actions, and dashed arrows represent intermediate genes abbreviated for better illustration.

helping the *Emperor* (*Jun*) herb but also inflammation and endocrine pathways, providing potential assistance to secondary insomnia. Zhimu has been reported to act on HRH, an effective target for sedative effect (Krystal et al., 2013). Among the herbs, only the Adjuvant (Zuo) herb can upregulate IL-10, the well-known anti-inflammatory cytokine (Ouyang et al., 2011; Iyer and Cheng, 2012). It is noted that no unique function has been found for the *Courier* (*Shi*) herb in the network we constructed. Its function may be relates to the pharmacokinetics. Previous study showed that the *Courier* (*Shi*) herb was able to facilitate the adsorption of Suanzaoren (Shen et al., 2012; Bi et al., 2014). These results agree with the TCM theory that *Jun*, *Chen*, *Zuo*, and *Shi* perform their own functions and cooperate with each other (Fan et al., 2006). In summary, the holistic mechanism of SZRP was first studied in a systematic way by network pharmacology.

DISCUSSION

In this study, the anti-insomnia mechanism of SZRP was first studied in a distinctive way by networking pharmacology. As a prevalent sleeping disorder, insomnia can be induced by various risk factors. Our research found that multiple pathways were involved in the anti-insomnia effects of SZRP. Five herbs in SZRP seem to play different roles in a complimentary way. The ingredients of the main herb mainly targeted multi-neurotransmitter proteins at the pre-synapse and post-synapse interface exerting sedative and hypnotic effects. This effect was likely enhanced by additional herbs through holistically regulating the nervous system related to insomnia symptoms. On top of that, the additional herbs were suggested to intensely regulate the immune system, particularly inflammation cytokines, which were often reported as an important influential factor for insomnia (Quartana et al., 2015; Irwin et al., 2016; Fernandez-Mendoza et al., 2017). Moreover, the whole formula can target the endocrine system to balance the hormone, blood pressure, and blood sugar, enhancing the sedative and hypnotic effects of the main herb.

By decomposing the formula, the *Emperor* (*Jun*) herb, *Z. jujuba*, was found to target synapse membrane, which may fight the main symptom of insomnia. The *Minister* (*Chen*) herbs, *A. asphodeloides* and *W. extensa*, not only can regulate the nervous system helping *Jun* herb in relieving the main symptom but also can densely target inflammation and endocrine pathways treating the likely pathological causes or secondary symptoms. *A. asphodeloides* is reported to act on HRH, which is an effective sedative target (Krystal et al., 2013). Interestingly, only the *Adjuvant* (*Zuo*) herb can uniquely upregulate IL-10, the well-known inflammation-inhibiting factor (Ouyang et al., 2011; Iyer and Cheng, 2012) that seems to counteract the inflammation-inhibiting effects of other herbal groups. It is noted that no unique function has been found for the *Courier* (*Shi*) herb *G. uralensis* from current MOA networking. We suggest that its possible role in ADME processes cannot be detected in the current analysis (Shen et al., 2012; Bi et al., 2014). The most interesting is to see the targeting patterns in the subnetworks among the herbal groups, such as targeting multi-points of the same pathway, parallel

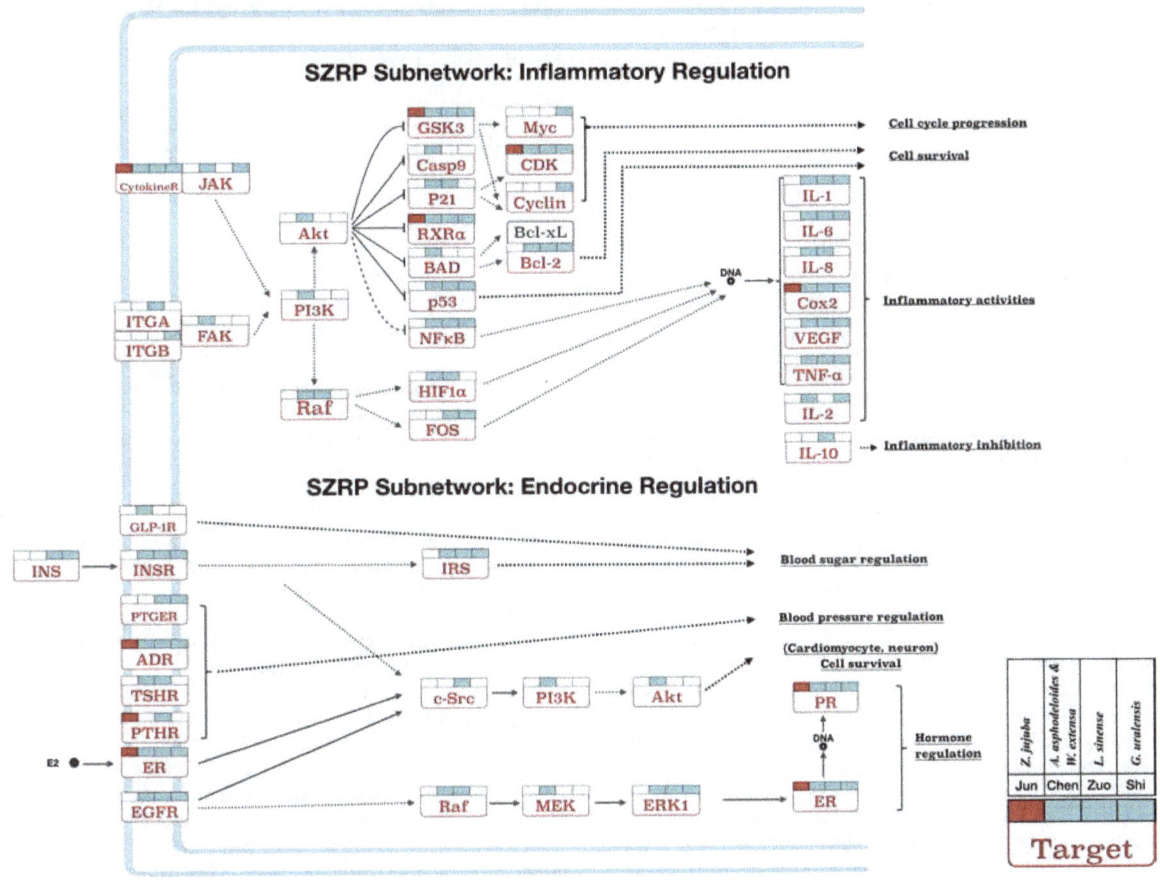

FIGURE 5 | The pathway of inflammatory and endocrine regulation effect in SZRP. Target names are shown in rectangles, and their full gene names can be found in **Table S3**. All labels are same as **Figure 4**.

pathways, and cross-talked pathways. These patterns have been reported to have beneficial synergistic effects (Jia et al., 2009) and have been applied to design synergistic drug combinations for cancer (Sun et al., 2015).

Meanwhile, the above results seem to support the TCM theory that the *Emperor* (*Jun*) herb often deals with the main symptoms of a disorder, while the *Minister* (*Chen*) assists the *Emperor* (*Jun*) herb to fight the main symptoms and also to remove those accompanying symptoms and signs. The *Adjuvant* (*Zuo*) herbs usually coordinate the effects of the *Emperor* (*Jun*) and *Minister* (*Chen*) herbs by counteracting their toxic or side effects, and the *Courier* (*Shi*) herb helps to deliver or guide the other herbs in the prescription to the target organs (Fan et al., 2006). As such, the future design of anti-insomnia drugs may cover not only the nervous system but also the endocrine and immune systems holistically for better clinical efficacy.

Herbal medicines are usually believed to be multi-functional because of their vast chemical diversity. In this work, we only focused on the widely reported anti-insomnia effects of SZRP. This does not exclude the possibility of additional functions of the formulae. In the pathway enrichment analysis, cancer, cardiovascular disease, signal transformation, and lipid metabolism were also detected for the whole formulae, inferring potential functions to be discovered. In fact, one is often involved with multiple functions and labeled with many different pathways. For instance, NFKB1 was labeled by 67 pathways in KEGG, suggesting its important role as a cross-talk gene. In our case, the ratio of NEI targets chosen for anti-insomnia analysis is about 51.7% of total unique targets.

It is realized that our study aims to explain the global mechanism of traditional formula by decomposing the herbal formula. The current conclusion may be limited by the data quality and quantity, as well as clinical evidence. To avoid noise induction, we started with a widely acknowledged formula as an example, and their targets with literature support, instead of predicting targets. In the future, more efforts should be devoted to mutual interactions between herbal constituents and the dosage effects. Therefore, we here recommend our method of TCM formula with clear clinical effects and validated targets at the current stage.

AUTHOR CONTRIBUTIONS

JG wrote the manuscript and contributed to the overall design. QW, YH, and JG analyzed and interpreted the results. YH, KT, and QW modified the manuscript. XY and ZC supervised the project. All authors read, critically reviewed, and approved the final manuscript.

FUNDING

This work was supported in part by the National Key R&D Program of China (2017YFC1700200 and 2017YFC0908400) and the National Natural Science Foundation of China (31671379).

SUPPLEMENTARY MATERIAL

TABLE S1 | 497 targets of 5 herbs in SZRP.

TABLE S2 | Top 50 pathways of functional enrichment analysis.

TABLE S3 | Original information of targets in Figure 4-5.

REFERENCES

Asnis, G. M., Thomas, M., and Henderson, M. A. (2015). Pharmacotherapy treatment options for insomnia: a primer for clinicians. *Int. J. Mol. Sci.* 17 (1), 50. doi: 10.3390/ijms17010050

Bi, X., Gong, M., and Di, L. (2014). Review on prescription compatibility of shaoyao gancao decoction and reflection on pharmacokinetic compatibility mechanism of traditional Chinese medicine prescription based on *in vivo* drug interaction of main efficacious components. *Evid. Based Complement. Alternat. Med.* 2014, 208129. doi: 10.1155/2014/208129

Buysse, D. J. (2013). Insomnia. *JAMA* 309 (7), 706–716. doi: 10.1001/jama.2013.193

Cao, J. X., Zhang, Q. Y., Cui, S. Y., Cui, X. Y., Zhang, J., Zhang, Y. H., et al. (2010). Hypnotic effect of jujubosides from Semen Ziziphi Spinosae. *J. Ethnopharmacol.* 130 (1), 163–166. doi: 10.1016/j.jep.2010.03.023

Cheatle, M. D., Foster, S., Pinkett, A., Lesneski, M., Qu, D., and Dhingra, L. (2016). Assessing and managing sleep disturbance in patients with chronic pain. *Anesthesiol. Clin.* 34 (2), 379–393. doi: 10.1016/j.anclin.2016.01.007

Chen, C. Y., Chen, Y. F., and Tsai, H. Y. (2008). What is the effective component in suanzaoren decoction for curing insomnia? Discovery by virtual screening and molecular dynamic simulation. *J. Biomol. Struct. Dyn.* 26 (1), 57–64. doi: 10.1080/07391102.2008.10507223

Chen, F. P., Jong, M. S., Chen, Y. C., Kung, Y. Y., Chen, T. J., Chen, F. J., et al. (2011). Prescriptions of Chinese Herbal medicines for insomnia in Taiwan during 2002. *Evid. Based Complement. Alternat. Med.* 2011, 236341. doi: 10.1093/ecam/nep018

Chen, L. C., Chen, I. C., Wang, B. R., and Shao, C. H. (2009). Drug-use pattern of Chinese herbal medicines in insomnia: a 4-year survey in Taiwan. *J. Clin. Pharm. Ther.* 34 (5), 555–560. doi: 10.1111/j.1365-2710.2009.01038.x

Diodovich, C., Malerba, I., Bowe, G., Acquati, F., Bianchi, M. G., Taramelli, R., et al. (2003). Naphthalene exposure: effects on gene expression and proliferation in human cord blood cells. *J. Biochem. Mol. Toxicol.* 17 (5), 286–294. doi: 10.1002/jbt.10091

Esteban, C. I. (2009). Medicinal interest of *Poria cocos* (= *Wolfiporia extensa*). *Rev. Iberoam. Micol.* 26 (2), 103–107. doi: 10.1016/S1130-1406(09)70019-1

Fan, T. P., Yeh, J. C., Leung, K. W., Yue, P. Y., and Wong, R. N. (2006). Angiogenesis: from plants to blood vessels. *Trends Pharmacol. Sci.* 27 (6), 297–309. doi: 10.1016/j.tips.2006.04.006

Fernandez-Mendoza, J., Baker, J. H., Vgontzas, A. N., Gaines, J., Liao, D., and Bixler, E. O. (2017). Insomnia symptoms with objective short sleep duration are associated with systemic inflammation in adolescents. *Brain Behav. Immun.* 61, 110–116. doi: 10.1016/j.bbi.2016.12.026

Frass, M., Strassl, R. P., Friehs, H., Mullner, M., Kundi, M., and Kaye, A. D. (2012). Use and acceptance of complementary and alternative medicine among the general population and medical personnel: a systematic review. *Ochsner J.* 12 (1), 45–56. doi: 10.1043/1524-5012-12.1.45

Gu, G. (2007). *Shennong's classic of materia medica, annotated by PJ Yang*. Beijing: Academy Press.

Huang, Z. L., Zhang, Z., and Qu, W. M. (2014). Roles of adenosine and its receptors in sleep-wake regulation. *Int. Rev. Neurobiol.* 119, 349–371. doi: 10.1016/B978-0-12-801022-8.00014-3

Irwin, M. R., Olmstead, R., and Carroll, J. E. (2016). Sleep disturbance, sleep duration, and inflammation: a systematic review and meta-analysis of cohort studies and experimental sleep deprivation. *Biol. Psychiatry* 80 (1), 40–52. doi: 10.1016/j.biopsych.2015.05.014

Iyer, S. S., and Cheng, G. (2012). Role of interleukin 10 transcriptional regulation in inflammation and autoimmune disease. *Crit. Rev. Immunol.* 32 (1), 23–63. doi: 10.1615/CritRevImmunol.v32.i1.30

Ji, K. Y., Kim, K. M., Kim, Y. H., Im, A. R., Lee, J. Y., Park, B., et al. (2019). The enhancing immune response and anti-inflammatory effects of *Anemarrhena asphodeloides* extract in RAW 264.7 cells. *Phytomedicine* 59, 152789. doi: 10.1016/j.phymed.2018.12.012

Jia, J., Zhu, F., Ma, X., Cao, Z., Cao, Z. W., Li, Y., et al. (2009). Mechanisms of drug combinations: interaction and network perspectives. *Nat. Rev. Drug Discov.* 8 (2), 111–128. doi: 10.1038/nrd2683

Ko, C. H., Koon, C. M., Yu, S. L., Lee, K. Y., Lau, C. B., Chan, E. H., et al. (2016). Hypnotic effects of a novel anti-insomnia formula on *Drosophila* insomnia model. *Chin. J. Integr. Med.* 22 (5), 335–343. doi: 10.1007/s11655-014-1625-1

Krystal, A. D., Richelson, E., and Roth, T. (2013). Review of the histamine system and the clinical effects of H1 antagonists: basis for a new model for understanding the effects of insomnia medications. *Sleep Med. Rev.* 17 (4), 263–272. doi: 10.1016/j.smrv.2012.08.001

Lande, R. G., and Gragnani, C. (2010). Nonpharmacologic approaches to the management of insomnia. *J. Am. Osteopath. Assoc.* 110 (12), 695–701

Liu, L., Liu, C., Wang, Y., Wang, P., Li, Y., and Li, B. (2015). Herbal medicine for anxiety, depression and insomnia. *Curr. Neuropharmacol.* 13 (4), 481–493. doi: 10.2174/1570159X1304150831122734

Li, X., Liu, Y., Guan, W., Xia, Y., Zhou, Y., Yang, B., et al. (2019). Physicochemical properties and laxative effects of polysaccharides from Anemarrhena asphodeloides Bge. in loperamide-induced rats. *J. Ethnopharmacol.* 240, 111961. doi: 10.1016/j.jep.2019.111961

Li, Y. H., Yu, C. Y., Li, X. X., Zhang, P., Tang, J., Yang, Q., et al. (2018). Therapeutic target database update 2018: enriched resource for facilitating bench-to-clinic research of targeted therapeutics. *Nucleic Acids Res.* 46 (D1), D1121–D1127. doi: 10.1093/nar/gkx1076

Medeiros, R., Passos, G. F., Vitor, C. E., Koepp, J., Mazzuco, T. L., Pianowski, L. F., et al. (2007). Effect of two active compounds obtained from the essential oil of *Cordia verbenacea* on the acute inflammatory responses elicited by LPS in the rat paw. *Br. J. Pharmacol.* 151 (5), 618–627. doi: 10.1038/sj.bjp.0707270

National Heart, L.a.B.I. (2016). *What is insomnia* [Online]. Available: https://www.nhlbi.nih.gov/health-topics/insomnia [Accessed].

Ouyang, W., Rutz, S., Crellin, N. K., Valdez, P. A., and Hymowitz, S. G. (2011). Regulation and functions of the IL-10 family of cytokines in inflammation and disease. *Annu. Rev. Immunol.* 29, 71–109. doi: 10.1146/annurev-immunol-031210-101312

Park, B. K., So, K. S., Ko, H. J., Kim, H. J., Kwon, K. S., Kwon, Y. S., et al. (2018). Therapeutic potential of the rhizomes of *Anemarrhena asphodeloides* and timosaponin A-III in an animal model of lipopolysaccharide-induced lung inflammation. *Biomol. Ther. (Seoul)* 26 (6), 553–559. doi: 10.4062/biomolther.2017.249

Pepin, J. L., Borel, A. L., Tamisier, R., Baguet, J. P., Levy, P., and Dauvilliers, Y. (2014). Hypertension and sleep: overview of a tight relationship. *Sleep Med. Rev.* 18 (6), 509–519. doi: 10.1016/j.smrv.2014.03.003

Punnoose, A. R., Golub, R. M., and Burke, A. E. (2012). JAMA patient page. Insomnia. *JAMA* 307 (24), 2653. doi: 10.1001/jama.2012.6219

Quartana, P. J., Finan, P. H., Page, G. G., and Smith, M. T. (2015). Effects of insomnia disorder and knee osteoarthritis on resting and pain-evoked inflammatory markers. *Brain Behav. Immun.* 47, 228–237. doi: 10.1016/j.bbi.2014.12.010

Ren, L., Wang, F., Xu, Z., Chan, W. M., Zhao, C., and Xue, H. (2010). GABAA receptor subtype selectivity underlying anxiolytic effect of 6-hydroxyflavone. *Biochem. Pharmacol.* 79 (9), 1337–1344. doi: 10.1016/j.bcp.2009.12.024

Ru, J., Li, P., Wang, J., Zhou, W., Li, B., Huang, C., et al. (2014). TCMSP: a database of systems pharmacology for drug discovery from herbal medicines. *J. Cheminform.* 6, 13. doi: 10.1186/1758-2946-6-13

Santoro, N., Epperson, C. N., and Mathews, S. B. (2015). Menopausal symptoms and their management. *Endocrinol. Metab. Clin. North Am.* 44 (3), 497–515. doi: 10.1016/j.ecl.2015.05.001

Sarkar, S., Khan, M. F., Kaphalia, B. S., and Ansari, G. A. (2006). Methyl palmitate inhibits lipopolysaccharide-stimulated phagocytic activity of rat peritoneal macrophages. *J. Biochem. Mol. Toxicol.* 20 (6), 302–308. doi: 10.1002/jbt.20150

Shan, C. S., Xu, Q. Q., Shi, Y. H., Wang, Y., He, Z. X., and Zheng, G. Q. (2018). Chuanxiong formulae for migraine: a systematic review and meta-analysis of high-quality randomized controlled trials. *Front. Pharmacol.* 9, 589. doi: 10.3389/fphar.2018.00589

Shen, L., Hu, R. W., Lin, X., Cong, W. J., Hong, Y. L., Feng, Y., et al. (2012). Pharmacokinetics of characteristic effective ingredients from individual and combination Shaoyao and Gancao treatment in rats using HPLC fingerprinting. *Eur. J. Drug Metab. Pharmacokinet.* 37 (2), 133–140. doi: 10.1007/s13318-011-0052-y

Shergis, J. L., Ni, X., Sarris, J., Zhang, A. L., Guo, X., Xue, C. C., et al. (2017). *Ziziphus spinosa* seeds for insomnia: a review of chemistry and psychopharmacology. *Phytomedicine* 34, 38–43. doi: 10.1016/j.phymed.2017.07.004

Sun, Y., Sheng, Z., Ma, C., Tang, K., Zhu, R., Wu, Z., et al. (2015). Combining genomic and network characteristics for extended capability in predicting synergistic drugs for cancer. *Nat. Commun.* 6, 8481. doi: 10.1038/ncomms9481

Taylor, D. J., Mallory, L. J., Lichstein, K. L., Durrence, H. H., Riedel, B. W., and Bush, A. J. (2007). Comorbidity of chronic insomnia with medical problems. *Sleep* 30 (2), 213–218. doi: 10.1093/sleep/30.2.213

Tiller, J. W. (2003). The management of insomnia: an update. Available: https://www.nps.org.au/australian-prescriber/articles/the-management-of-insomnia-an-update

Trauer, J. M., Qian, M. Y., Doyle, J. S., Rajaratnam, S. M., and Cunnington, D. (2015). Cognitive behavioral therapy for chronic insomnia: a systematic review and meta-analysis. *Ann. Intern. Med.* 163 (3), 191–204. doi: 10.7326/M14-2841

Trenkwalder, C., Zieglgansberger, W., Ahmedzai, S. H., and Hogl, B. (2017). Pain, opioids, and sleep: implications for restless legs syndrome treatment. *Sleep Med.* 31, 78–85. doi: 10.1016/j.sleep.2016.09.017

Tripathi, S., Pohl, M. O., Zhou, Y., Rodriguez-Frandsen, A., Wang, G., Stein, D. A., et al. (2015). Meta- and orthogonal integration of influenza "OMICs" data defines a role for UBR4 in virus budding. *Cell Host Microbe* 18 (6), 723–735. doi: 10.1016/j.chom.2015.11.002

Wang, S., Liu, J., Ma, G., Lan, H., and Zhao, Z. (2013). Clinical study of Zaorenanshen tablet treating insomnia. *Hebei J. Tradit. Chin. Med.* 35 (8), 1217–1219. doi: 10.3969/j.issn.1002-2619.2013.08.058

Wang, Z., He, M., and Jiang, J. (2010). Sanqi Granule the treatment of insomnia of deficiency heart blood and stagnant heat type randomized double-blind clinical curative effect observation. *Liaoning J. Tradit. Chin. Med.* 37 (12), 2289–2292.

Wei, W., Shu, S., Zhu, W., Xiong, Y., and Peng, F. (2016). The kinome of edible and medicinal fungus *Wolfiporia cocos*. *Front. Microbiol.* 7, 1495. doi: 10.3389/fmicb.2016.01495

Wells, A. M., Ridener, E., Bourbonais, C. A., Kim, W., Pantazopoulos, H., Carroll, F. I., et al. (2017). Effects of chronic social defeat stress on sleep and circadian rhythms are mitigated by kappa-opioid receptor antagonism. *J. Neurosci.* 37 (32), 7656–7668. doi: 10.1523/JNEUROSCI.0885-17.2017

WHO (2007). *WHO international standard terminologies on traditional medicine in the Western Pacific Region.*

Wilt, T. J., MacDonald, R., Brasure, M., Olson, C. M., Carlyle, M., Fuchs, E., et al. (2016). Pharmacologic treatment of insomnia disorder: an evidence report for a clinical practice guideline by the American College of Physicians. *Ann. Intern. Med.* 165 (2), 103–112. doi: 10.7326/M15-1781

Wisden, W., Yu, X., and Franks, N. P. (2017). "GABA Receptors and the pharmacology of sleep" in *Handbook of Experimental Pharmacology*. Berlin, Heidelberg: Springer, 1–26.

Xiang, B., Liu, K., Yu, M., Liang, X., Huang, C., Zhang, J., et al. (2019). Systematic genetic analyses of GWAS data reveal an association between the immune system and insomnia. *Mol. Genet. Genomic Med.* 7 (7), e00742. doi: 10.1002/ mgg3.742

Ye, H., Ye, L., Kang, H., Zhang, D., Tao, L., Tang, K., et al. (2011). HIT: linking herbal active ingredients to targets. *Nucleic Acids Res.* 39 (Database issue), D1055–D1059. doi: 10.1093/nar/gkq1165

Yuan, C., Chen, Y., and Li, J. (2013). Adjuvant treatment of insomnia of liver-yin deficiency pattern by Mei'an grannule: a randomized double-blind and placebo-controlled trial. *Shanghai J. Tradit. Chin. Med.* 47 (5), 57–71. doi: 10.16305/j.1007-1334.2013.05.027

Zeng, X., Zhang, P., He, W., Qin, C., Chen, S., Tao, L., et al. (2018). NPASS: natural product activity and species source database for natural product research, discovery and tool development. *Nucleic Acids Res.* 46 (D1), D1217–D1222. doi: 10.1093/nar/gkx1026

Zhang, M., Ning, G., Shou, C., Lu, Y., Hong, D., and Zheng, X. (2003). Inhibitory effect of jujuboside A on glutamate-mediated excitatory signal pathway in hippocampus. *Planta Med.* 69 (8), 692–695. doi: 10.1055/s-2003-42786

Zhao, Y. Y., Feng, Y. L., Du, X., Xi, Z. H., Cheng, X. L., and Wei, F. (2012). Diuretic activity of the ethanol and aqueous extracts of the surface layer of *Poria cocos* in rat. *J. Ethnopharmacol.* 144 (3), 775–778. doi: 10.1016/j.jep.2012.09.033

Zhou, Q. H., Zhou, X. L., Xu, M. B., Jin, T. Y., Rong, P. Q., Zheng, G. Q., et al. (2018). Suanzaoren formulae for insomnia: updated clinical evidence and possible mechanisms. *Front. Pharmacol.* 9, 76. doi: 10.3389/fphar.2018.00076

4

Antidepressant Mechanism of Traditional Chinese Medicine Formula Xiaoyaosan in CUMS-Induced Depressed Mouse Model via RIPK1-RIPK3-MLKL Mediated Necroptosis Based on Network Pharmacology Analysis

Zhi-Yi Yan[1,2†], Hai-Yan Jiao[1†], Jian-Bei Chen[1], Kai-Wen Zhang[1], Xi-Hong Wang[1], You-Ming Jiang[1], Yue-Yun Liu[1], Zhe Xue[1], Qing-Yu Ma[3], Xiao-Juan Li[3]* and Jia-Xu Chen[1,3]**

[1]School of Traditional Chinese Medicine, Beijing University of Chinese Medicine, Beijing, China, [2]Dongfang Hospital Affiliated to Beijing University of Chinese Medicine, Beijing, China, [3]Formula-pattern Research Center, School of Traditional Chinese Medicine, Jinan University, Guangzhou, China

***Correspondence:**
Qing-Yu Ma
tmaqingyu@jnu.edu.cn
Xiao-Juan Li
lixiaojuan@jnu.edu.cn
Jia-Xu Chen
chenjiaxu@hotmail.com*

†These authors contributed equally to this work

Background: Depression is a stress-related disorder that seriously threatens people's physical and mental health. Xiaoyaosan is a classical traditional Chinese medicine formula, which has been used to treat mental depression since ancient times. More and more notice has been given to the relationship between the occurrence of necroptosis and the pathogenesis of mental disorders.

Objective: The purpose of present study is to explore the potential mechanism of Xiaoyaosan for the treatment of depression using network pharmacology and experimental research, and identify the potential targets of necroptosis underlying the antidepressant mechanism of Xiaoyaosan.

Methods: The mice model of depression was induced by chronic unpredictable mild stress (CUMS) for 6 weeks. Adult C57BL/6 mice were randomly divided into five groups, including control group, chronic unpredictable mild stress group, Xiaoyaosan treatment

---

Abbreviations: ADME, absorption, distribution, metabolism and enhancement; ANOVA, one-way analysis of variance; BDNF, brain-derived neurotrophic factor; CTD, Comparative Toxicogenomic database; CUMS, chronic unpredictable mild stress; CNS, central nervous system; DL, drug likeness; DMSO, dimethyl sulphoxide; DAMPs, damage-associated molecular pattern molecules; ECL, enhanced chemiluminescence; ETCM, Encyclopedia of Traditional Chinese Medicine; FS, forced swimming; H&E, hematoxylin and eosin; HPA, hypothalamic pituitary adrenal; HRP, horseradish peroxidase; HERB, High-throughput Experiment- and Reference-guided database of Traditional Chinese Medicine; IF, immunofluorescence; IHC, immunohistochemical; LSD, least significant difference; MOD, mean optical density; MFI, mean fluorescence intensity; MLKL, mixed lineage kinase domain-like; Nec-1, necrostatin-1; NSF, novelty-suppressed feeding; OB, bioavailability; OMIM, Online Mendelian Inheritance in Man; PFA, paraformaldehyde; PPI, protein–protein interaction; PVDF, polyvinylidene fluoride; RIPK, receptor interacting protein kinas; SAC, sacrificed; SP, sucrose preference; SPF, specific-pathogen free; SEM, standard error of mean; SSRIs, selective serotonin reuptake inhibitors; TCM, traditional Chinese medicine; TCMSP, TCM Systems Pharmacology database and Analysis Platform; TBST, tris buffered saline tween; TLR, toll-like receptor; TNF, tumor necrosis factor; TTD, Therapeutic Target database; UPLC-MS/MS, ultra-performance chromatography-electrospray tandem mass spectrometr; UniProt, universal Protein Resource; WB, western blot; WHO, World Health Organization.

group, necrostatin-1 (Nec-1) group and solvent group. Drug intervention performed from 4th to 6th week of modeling. The mice in Xiaoyaosan treatment group received Xiaoyaosan by intragastric administration (0.254 g/kg/d), and mice in CUMS group received 0.5 ml physiological saline. Meanwhile, the mice in Nec-1 group were injected intraperitoneally (i.p.) with Nec-1 (10 mg/kg/d), and the equivalent volume of DMSO/PBS (8.3%) was injected into solvent group mice. The behavior tests such as sucrose preference test, forced swimming test and novelty-suppressed feeding test were measured to evaluate depressive-like behaviors of model mice. Then, the active ingredients in Xiaoyaosan and the related targets of depression and necroptosis were compiled through appropriate databases, while the "botanical drugs-active ingredients-target genes" network was constructed by network pharmacology analysis. The expressions of RIPK1, RIPK3, MLKL, *p*-MLKL were detected as critical target genes of necroptosis and the potential therapeutic target compounds of Xiaoyaosan. Furthermore, the levels of neuroinflammation and microglial activation of hippocampus were measured by detecting the expressions of IL-1β, Lipocalin-2 and IBA1, and the hematoxylin and eosin (H&E) stained was used to observe the morphology in hippocampus sections.

Results: After 6-weeks of modeling, the behavioral data showed that mice in CUMS group and solvent group had obvious depressive-like behaviors, and the medication of Xiaoyaosan or Nec-1 could improve these behavioral changes. A total of 96 active ingredients in Xiaoyaosan which could regulate the 23 key target genes were selected from databases. Xiaoyaosan could alleviate the core target genes in necroptosis and improve the hippocampal function and neuroinflammation in depressed mice.

Conclusion: The activation of necroptosis existed in the hippocampus of CUMS-induced mice, which was closely related to the pathogenesis of depression. The antidepressant mechanism of Xiaoyaosan included the regulation of multiple targets in necroptosis. It also suggested that necroptosis could be a new potential target for the treatment of depression.

Keywords: xiaoyaosan, chronic unpredictable mild stress, depression, necroptosis, neuroinflammation, microglial activation

INTRODUCTION

Depression is a common clinical mental disorder characterized by constant down in spirits and cognitive impairment, and the prevalence of which is increasing year by year with the lifetime prevalence as high as 10–15% (Moussavi et al., 2007; Chiriță et al., 2015). According to the latest statistics of the World Health Organization (WHO) in 2019, more than 350 million people worldwide suffer from depression, which has covered all age groups and increased by more than 18% from 2005 to 2015. It is also a major factor contributing to the increase in global burden of disease and medical expenses.

The classic Chinese formula Xiaoyaosan, originated from the book *Prescriptions of the Bureau of Taiping People's Welfare Pharmacy* in Song Dynasty of China, is one of the effective traditional Chinese compound recipes in treating psycho-emotional related symptoms and diseases (Zhang et al., 2019). According to the recent clinical and basic studies, Xiaoyaosan has a multi-target regulating effect which is reflected in the treatment of depression-related diseases (Li et al., 2015; Jiao et al., 2019; Xiong et al., 2019; Liu et al., 2020; Zhou et al., 2021). In the pathogenesis study of depression, it is found that psychological and physical stressors can activate the immune system, lead to inflammation, and then participate in the development of depression (Iwata et al., 2013). Overproduction of pro-inflammatory cytokines is a key factor in the interaction between immune system and central nervous system (CNS) (Dowlati et al., 2010). Microglia is innate immune-related glial cell in CNS, which is the most widely-investigated in stress-related neuroinflammation (Sawada et al., 2014). Meanwhile, many studies have confirmed that inhibition of necroptosis can provide neuroprotective effect, so necroptosis is also a potential target for the treatment of CNS-related diseases (Liu et al., 2015). Xiaoyaosan has also been shown to play a therapeutic role by improving inflammation and regulating the function of hippocampal microglia (Li et al., 2017; Jiao et al., 2021).

Necroptosis is an active cell death process characterized by cell necrosis and inflammation. Studies have confirmed that

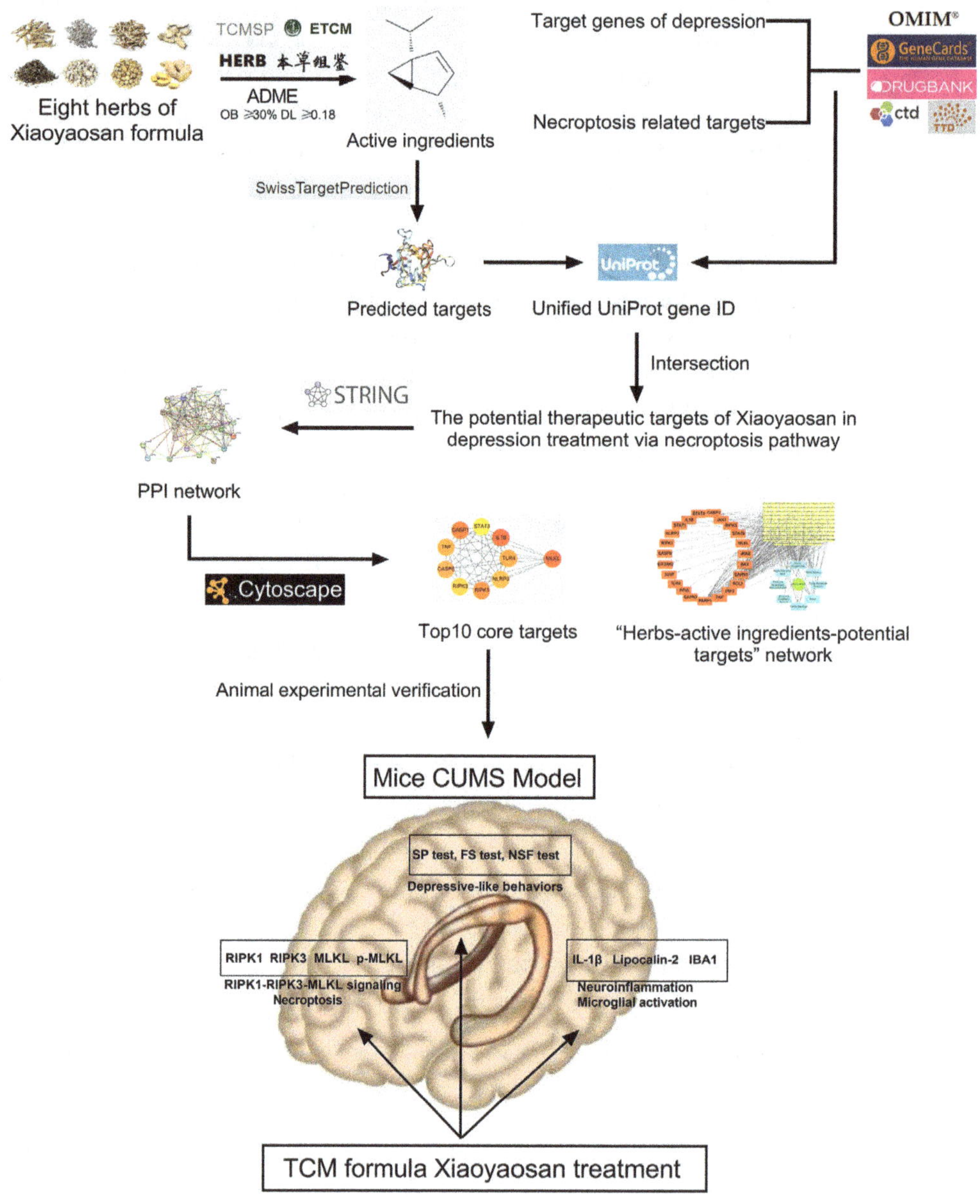

FIGURE 1 | Flow chart of network pharmacological analysis and experimental study of Xiaoyaosan for depression treatment through necroptosis pathway.

necroptosis has a unique signal transduction pathway, which is closely related to the function of receptor interacting protein kinase 1 (RIPK1) and RIPK3(Galluzzi et al., 2009). Necroptosis is often accompanied by significant inflammatory response, characterized by a large number of inflammatory cell infiltration and activation of inflammatory pathways (Newton and Manning, 2016). The formation of a RIPK1–RIPK3–mixed lineage kinase domain-like (MLKL) complex leads to the initiation of necroptosis, while the phosphorylation of MLKL protein by RIPK3 eventually leads to necroptosis by destroying plasma membrane and cytolysis (Cho et al., 2009; Shan et al., 2018). Moreover, inflammatory response is triggered by the release of intracellular contents from necrotic cells, and inflammatory factors further promote cell death, which forms a circulatory circuit (Pasparakis et al., 2015). Here, Necrostatin-1 (Nec-1) as an effective, selective and permeable necroptosis inhibitor, can effectively block the active sites of RIPK1 and RIPK3, thus inhibit the necroptosis pathway by controlling the phosphorylation (Degterev et al., 2008). Therefore, the detection of RIPK1, RIPK3 and MLKL can verify the occurrence of necroptosis, and the effective measurement to regulate necroptosis may alleviate the inflammatory response of the lesion regions, thereby slowing down the pathological changes of the corresponding diseases (Schwabe and Luedde, 2018).

Under the guidance of the overall concept of traditional Chinese medicine (TCM) and the thought of syndrome differentiation and treatment, TCM formula is a treatment method with specific therapeutic efficacy based on the principles of drug properties, drug properties and compatibility, which contains profound and complex scientific connotation (Wang et al., 2008). However, due to the lack of quantifiable and objective data support, it is very difficult to clarify the mechanism of TCM formula, which has become an important reason why TCM formula is difficult to be accepted by the international community (Luo et al., 2020). Network pharmacology, a new discipline to reveal the mechanism of diseases and the pharmacodynamic mechanism of drugs from the perspective of biological network, is well meet the concept of holism in TCM, while the core element of network pharmacology –"network target, multi-components" theory was also proposed by TCM researchers (Li and Zhang, 2013). Nowadays, network pharmacology has become an important breakthrough in the cross-innovation of information science and medical science, and has been widely used in the research of traditional Chinese medicine (Li et al., 2014; Guo et al., 2021; Sheng et al., 2021). Thus far, studies have shown that necroptosis plays an important role in neuroinflammation and central nervous system related diseases (Chen et al., 2021; Thadathil et al., 2021), and the role of necroptosis remains largely unexamined in the depression-related CNS mechanism. Also, the antidepressant effect of Xiaoyaosan has still not yet been comprehensively studied. Therefore, this study utilized network pharmacology approach to explore the therapeutic effects of Xiaoyaosan on depression via necroptosis pathway, then the antidepressant mechanism was observed *in vivo* using CUMS mice. **Figure 1** showed the flow chart of the study.

METHODS

Preparation of Traditional Chinese Medicine

TCM formula Xiaoyaosan consists of the following eight Chinese botanical drugs: Bupleurum chinense DC (Description: Apiaceae), Angelica sinensis (Oliv.) Diels (Description: Apiaceae), Paeonia lactiflora Pall (Description: Paeoniaceae), Poria cocos (Schw.) Wolf (Description: Polyporaceae), Atractylodes macrocephala Koidz (Description: Compositae), Glycyrrhiza uralensis Fisch (Description: Leguminosea), Zingiber officinale Rosc (Description: Zingiberaceae), and Mentha haplocalyx Briq (Description: Lamiaceae) at a ratio of 5:5:5:5:5:4:5:1. The prepared drug in pieces of Xiaoyaosan were purchased from Beijing Tongrentang (Bozhou) Pieces Co. Ltd., Bozhou, China, while the ultra-performance chromatography-electrospray tandem mass spectrometry (UPLC-MS/MS) was used to identify the samples of these decoction pieces (Ding et al., 2017; Yuan et al., 2020). The Xiaoyaosan dry powder (J2447) used in experimental studies was prepared by Jiuzhitang Co. Ltd, Changsha, China, in accord with the process recorded in the Chinese Pharmacopoeia 2015 Edition (Pan et al., 2019; Zhu et al., 2019). 2.36 g of crude drug yielded One Gram the finished dry powder administered experimentally.

Network Pharmacology Approach

The active ingredients and potential targets of TCM formula Xiaoyaosan for application to depression were investigated based on network pharmacology. The active ingredients in Xiaoyaosan were screened according to absorption, distribution, metabolism and enhancement (ADME) of drugs, while the bioavailability (OB) and drug likeness (DL) were used as screening parameters (Vugmeyster et al., 2012). According to ADME (OB ≥ 30% and DL ≥ 0.18), the active ingredients of Xiaoyaosan were collected from traditional Chinese medicine databases including the TCM Systems Pharmacology database and Analysis Platform (TCMSP, https://tcmsp-e.com/) (Ru et al., 2014), the Encyclopedia of Traditional Chinese Medicine (ETCM, http://www.tcmip.cn/ETCM/) (Zhang et al., 2019) and the High-throughput Experiment- and Reference-guided database of Traditional Chinese Medicine (HERB, http://herb.ac.cn/) (Fang et al., 2021), then SwissTargetPrediction database (http://www.swisstargetprediction.ch/) (Daina et al., 2019) was used to predict the targets of active ingredients in Xiaoyaosan, the reliability screening of predicted targets was also carried out (Probability ≥30%).

The related genes with depression and necroptosis pathway were collected from GeneCards database (https://www.genecards.org/) (Stelzer et al., 2016), Online Mendelian Inheritance in Man (OMIM, https://omim.org/) (Amberger et al., 2015), Comparative Toxicogenomic database (CTD, http://ctdbase.org/) (Davis et al., 2020), Therapeutic Target database (TTD, http://db.idrblab.net/ttd/) (Wang et al., 2020), and DrugBank database (http://www.drugbank.ca/) (Wishart et al., 2018), using "Depression", "Depressive disorder" or "Necroptosis" as the search term. Then, the gene symbols of the ingredients in Xiaoyaosan, depression and necroptosis pathway were searched in the universal Protein Resource (UniProt, https://www.UniProt.org/) to get the unified UniProt gene ID.

The potential therapeutic targets of Xiaoyaosan in depression treatment via necroptosis pathway were obtained by overlapping the predicted targets of the ingredients in Xiaoyaosan and the target genes of depression and necroptosis pathway. Furthermore, the STRING database (https://string-db.org/) (Szklarczyk et al., 2019) was used to generate the protein–protein interaction (PPI) network of potential target genes of Xiaoyaosan with the species limited to human (Homo sapiens) and the interaction score ≥0.4. Then, the Cytoscape software (version 3.7.2, http://www.cytoscape.org/, Boston, MA, United States) was used to construct the "botanical drugs-active ingredients-potential targets" network, and identify the core target genes from the results of PPI network with the cytoHubba plugin (Guo et al., 2021).

Animals

The study was approved by the Institutional Animal Care and Use Committee of Beijing University of Chinese Medicine (BUCM-4-2018120401-4053). Experimental protocols applied in our study were performed in agreement with the existing current animal welfare guidelines. Specific-pathogen free (SPF) male C57BL/6 mice aged 8-week-old (SYXK (Jing) 2016-0006, Beijing Vital River Laboratory Animal

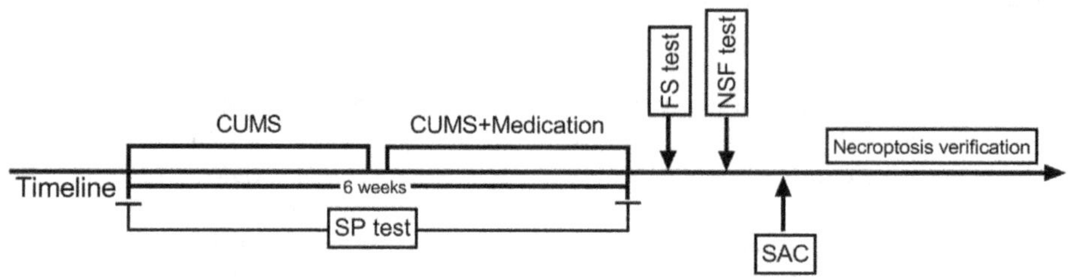

FIGURE 2 | Schedule of the experimental design.

Technology Limited Company, Beijing, China) were housed separately in a standard animal feeding room (room temperature: 22 ± 2°C; relative humidity: 30–40%; light condition: a 12 h/12 h dark/light cycle) and fed standard rodent diet. Animals were adapted to their new environment for 7 days before CUMS procedure.

CUMS Model and Medication Process

A total of 75 mice were randomly assigned to five groups (n = 15), including control group (no stress + physiological saline), CUMS group (CUMS + physiological saline), solvent group [CUMS + dimethyl sulphoxide (DMSO)/phosphate buffered saline (PBS)], Nec-1 group (CUMS + Nec-1), and Xiaoyaosan treatment group (CUMS + Xiaoyaosan). The CUMS modeling was performed as previously reported (Yan et al., 2019). Briefly, animals except the control group mice were subjected to the following stressors for six consecutive weeks: food deprivation for 24 h; water deprivation for 24 h; empty cages for 11 h; crowded cages for 24 h; restraint stress for 3 h; exposed to wet and soiled cages for 24 h; and 4°C cold water swimming for 5 min. The schedule of the study was showed in **Figure 2**.

Drug intervention lasted for 3 weeks, starting from the 4th week of modeling. The dosage of Xiaoyaosan and the duration of administration were confirmed according to the previous publications (Ding et al., 2017; Liu Y. et al., 2019). The Xiaoyaosan dry powder was dissolved in distilled water, then the mice in Xiaoyaosan treatment group received Xiaoyaosan by intragastric administration (0.254 g/kg/d), meanwhile mice in the CUMS group received 0.5 ml physiological saline (Yan et al., 2018). The concentration and volume of the gavage administration were adjusted once a week according to the changes in the body weight of the mice. Nec-1 (product number: RH82010-10mg, CAS number: 4311-88-0, BIORuler, Danbury, CT, United States) was dissolved in DMSO/PBS (1 mg in 125 μL of DMSO diluted with 1,375 μL of 0.1 M PBS). The Nec-1 group were injected intraperitoneally (i.p.) with Nec-1 (10 mg/kg) daily for 3 weeks, and the equivalent volume of DMSO/PBS (8.3%) was injected into solvent group mice (Dara et al., 2016).

The SP test was performed every week during the modeling process. The scheme lasted for successive 6 weeks, and the 3-weeks's daily medication of Xiaoyaosan or Nec-1 was conducted. After the modeling, the FS test, and NSF test were carried out, then the mice were sacrificed for further detection.

Behavioral Assessment

To evaluate the depressive behaviors of model animals, the sucrose preference (SP) test, forced swimming (FS) test and novelty-suppressed feeding (NSF) test were conducted as previous described with minor modifications (Barfield et al., 2013; Liao et al., 2018).

The SP test was performed every week during the modeling process. In brief, each mouse in this study was given two bottles filled with deionized water and 1% sucrose solution after 24-h fasting and water deprivation, then the consumption of sucrose solution and deionized water in 1 h was recorded, respectively. The sucrose preference rate was presented as the percentage of the 1% sucrose solution consumed out of the total amount of liquid consumed, which represented the parameter of hedonic behavior.

The FS test and NSF test were conducted after the 6-weeks modeling to further assess the depressed behaviors in mice. In the FS test, each mouse was placed in a clear glass aquarium (24 cm height and 19 cm diameter) containing approximately 6 cm of water (24 ± 1°C) for 5 min, and the whole time was recorded using a high definition camera. The mouse was accepted and considered to be immobile when it stopped swimming and kept afloat on the water which reflected the despair of animals after they failed to cope with the attempt, the immobility time was recorded in our study. The NSF test was performed in a white plastic box (25 × 25 × 20 cm) with a single food pellet of regular chow placed in the center. After 24 h of food deprivation, the mouse was placed in a corner of the box, the latency to chew the food pellet was recorded, followed by the measurement of the food consumption in the subsequent 5 min.

Preparation of Tissue Samples

After 6 weeks of modeling, mice sacrificed by decapitation after behavioral tests. The hippocampal tissues of five mice in each group were collected for western blot analysis, the RNA preservation solution (Biotech, #2714) was used to preserve the hippocampi of five mice in each group for quantitative RT-PCR assay. The whole brains of the remaining mice in each group were fixed in 4% paraformaldehyde (PFA) solution (4% PFA, 2.5% glutaraldehyde, and 0.1 M PBS) and prepared for tissue slicing.

Quantitative RT-PCR Analysis

Total RNA of hippocampus was extracted using Trizol® reagent (Applied Biosystems, Waltham, MA, United States), then the quality and concentration of total RNA were determined by 1%

TABLE 1 | Primer sequences used in the quantitative RT-PCR analysis.

Gene	–	Sequences
IBA1	Forward	5′-TGGCTCCGAGGAGACGTTCAG-3′
	Reverse	5′-GGACCAGTTGGCCTCTTGTGTTC-3′
IL-1β	Forward	5′-TCGCAGCAGCACATCAACAAGAG-3′
	Reverse	5′-TGCTCATGTCCTCATCCTGGAAGG-3′
Lipocalin-2	Forward	5′-CGCTACTGGATCAGAACATTTG-3′
	Reverse	5′-CTTGCACATTGTAGCTCTGTAC-3′

agarose gel electrophoresis and Q3000 micro-volume spectrophotometer (Quawell Technology, San Jose, CA, United States). The RevertAid First Strand cDNA Synthesis Kit (Termo Fisher Scientifc, Waltham, MA, United States) was used to transfer total RNA into cDNA. **Table 1** showed the sequences for primers used in our study which were designed based on published mRNA sequences in NCBI and synthesized by Sangon Biotech Co., Ltd, Shanghai, China. HPRT1 (BBI LifeScience, Amherst, MA, United States) was selected as the housekeeping gene in the experiment through reference genes selection method by geNorm, NormFinder, and BestKeeper software (Dongliang et al., 2011). The quantitative RT-PCR (qRT-PCR) reaction system was prepared by SYBR® Green PCR Master Mix (Applied Biosystems) in a final volume of 25 μL, then performed on Multicolor Real-time PCR Detection System (Bio-Rad, Hercules, CA, United States) with the following thermal cycling conditions: preincubation at 94 °C for 3 min, followed by 40 cycles of denaturation at 94°C for 30 s, annealing at 55°C for 30 s, and extending at 72°C for 30 s. The signals were normalized to HPRT1 and the relative expression of mRNA in each sample was calculated by $2^{-\Delta\Delta Ct}$ method.

Western Blot Analysis

Protein levels of IBA1, IL-1β, Lipocalin-2, RIPK1, RIPK3, MLKL, and *p*-MLKL were measured by western blot analysis. The total protein of hippocampal tissues was extracted using RIPA Lysis buffer (Biomiga, Santiago, CA, United States). The proteins were loaded onto 12% SDS-PAGE gels at 30 μg per lane, and then transferred onto polyvinylidene fluoride (PVDF) membranes. The 5% non-fat dry milk in 0.05% tris buffered saline tween (TBST) was used to block the membranes, and the membranes were incubated with primary antibodies at 4 °C overnight (IBA1, 1:1,000 dilution, ab178847, Abcam, San Francisco, CA, United States; IL-1β, ab9722, 1:1,000 dilution, Abcam; Lipocalin-2, ab216462, 1:100 dilution, Abcam; RIPK1, 1:1,000 dilution, ab72139, Abcam; RIPK3, 1:1,000 dilution, ab56164, Abcam; phosphorylated MLKL (*p*-MLKL), 1:1,000 dilution, ab196436, Abcam; MLKL, 1:2000 dilution, orb32399, Biorbyt, Cambridge, UK; β-actin, 1:5,000 dilution, #5125, Cell Signal, Danvers, MA, United States). Then, the membranes were incubated with horseradish peroxidase- (HRP-) conjugated secondary antibody [Goat Anti-Rabbit IgG H&L (HRP), 1: 10,000 dilution, ab205718, Abcam; Goat Anti-Mouse IgG H&L (HRP), 1:10,000 dilution, ab205719, Abcam] for 1 h at room temperature. The enhanced chemiluminescence (ECL) detection reagent (Thermo Fisher Scientific) was used to develop the membranes for 1 min, and the Tanon-5200 system (Tanon, Shanghai, China) was used to visualize the protein bands. The optical density of protein bands was quantified by Tanon Gis software (Tanon).

Histopathological Examination, Immunohistochemistry and Immunofluorescence

The brain samples fixed in 4% PFA solution were used to prepared paraffin-embedded tissue sections which included hippocampal CA1 and CA3 regions based on the stereotaxic atlases of the mouse brain (Konsman, 2003). The sections were stained with hematoxylin-eosin (H&E) to observe the cellular morphology and infiltration of inflammatory cells. A four-point severity scale (0, normal; 1, mild; 2, moderate; 3, severe) was used to score the H&E stained sections by an experienced pathologist in a blinded manner.

Immunohistochemical (IHC) staining was used to observe the levels of IBA1 and *p*-MLKL in hippocampus followed the previous described procedures (Yan et al., 2018). After dewaxing, dehydration and antigen retrieval, the brain sections were incubated with 3% H_2O_2 solution at room temperature for 10 min. Next, sections were incubated with primary antibodies (IBA1, 1:8,000 dilution, ab178847, Abcam; *p*-MLKL, 1:250 dilution, ab196436, Abcam) overnight at 4 °C. Then sections were incubated with secondary antibodies, and the diaminobezidin 3, 3 (DAB) solution (Invitrogen, Carlsbad, CA, United States) was used for coloration. For quantitative analysis, the original immunohistochemical images were collected with an image analyzer (MIAS99, Fubo-Tech Co., Beijing, China) with a color video camera (TK-C1381, JVC, Beijing, China) and BX50 microscope (Olympus Co., Tokyo, Japan), and the positive staining of hippocampal CA1 and CA3 regions at high power magnification (×400) was assessed by mean optical density (MOD) using Image-pro Plus software (version 6.0, Rockville, MD, United States).

Immunofluorescence (IF) staining was used to observe the expression of *p*-MLKL as previous described (Qu et al., 2017). The brain sections were incubated with 0.5% TritonX-100 solution at room temperature for 10 min. Next, sections were incubated with primary antibody (*p*-MLKL, 1:100 dilution, ab196436, Abcam) overnight at 4°C. Then sections were incubated with fluorescent-conjugated goat anti-rabbit IgG, follow by the Thioflavin T and DAPI staining. The fluorescence signal of sections was observed and photographed under an Olympus BX53 fluorescence microscope (Olympus Co., Tokyo, Japan), and the mean fluorescence intensity (MFI) was analyzed using Image-pro Plus software.

Statistical Analysis

In this study, all data were analyzed using SPSS software (version 20.0, Chicago, IL, United States) and expressed as means ± SEM. The statistical analyses were performed by one-way analysis of variance (ANOVA) with least significant difference (LSD) post hoc multiple comparisons when equal variances were assumed, Dunnett's T3 test was used when the data had a normal

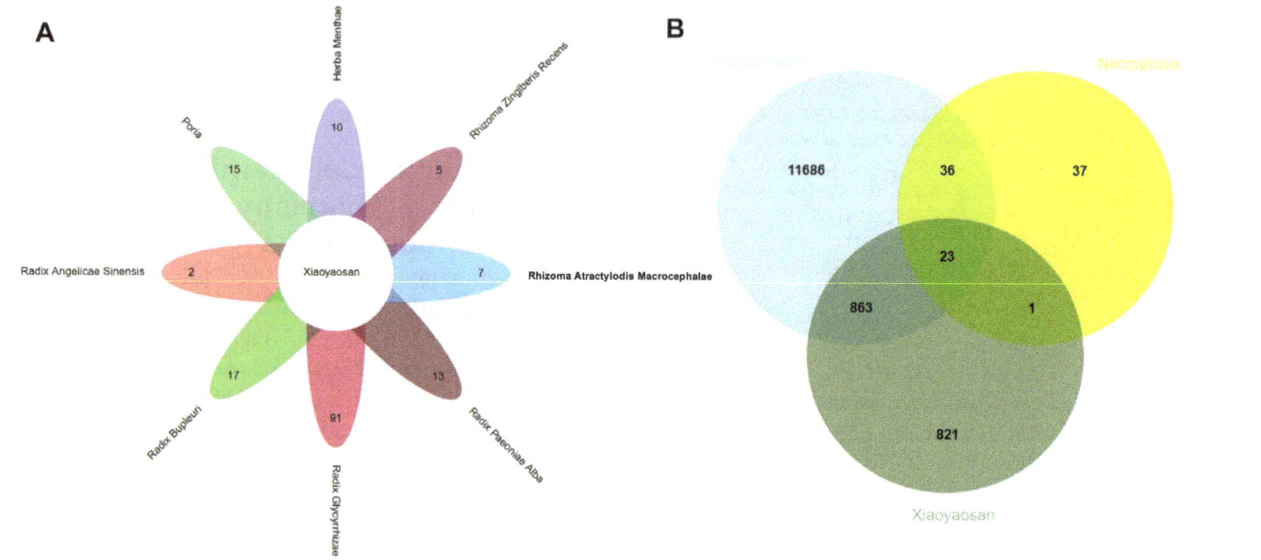

FIGURE 3 | Wynn maps for the active ingredients of Xiaoyaosan and potential treatment targets **(A)** Based on the ADME parameters (OB ≥ 30% and DL ≥ 0.18), there were 17 ingredients in *Radix Bupleuri*, two ingredients in *Radix Angelicae Sinensis*, 13 ingredients in *Radix Paeoniae Alba*, 15 ingredients in *Poria*, seven ingredients in *Rhizoma Atractylodis Macrocephalae*, 91 ingredients in *Radix Glycyrrhizae*, five ingredients in *Rhizoma Zingiberis Recens* and 10 ingredients in *Herba Menthae* **(B)** A total of 1708 predicted targets of TCM formula Xiaoyaosan, 12,608 therapeutic targets for depression and 97 necroptosis related targets were intersected, and there were 23 potential treatment target genes.

distribution but the variances are not homogeneous. A p-value of 0.05 was considered statistically significant.

RESULTS

Active Ingredients of Xiaoyaosan Regulated Necroptosis in Depression

The network pharmacology method was used to initial investigate whether the active components of Xiaoyaosan could improve necroptosis pathway in depression.

As showed in **Figure 3**, a total of 148 active ingredients in the eight botanical drugs of Xiaoyaosan were collected based on the ADME parameters (OB ≥ 30% and DL ≥ 0.18), and we obtained 23 potential treatment targets (BAX, BCL2, CAPN1, CAPN2, CASP1, CASP8, EIF2AK2, IL1B, JAK1, JAK2, JAK3, MLKL, NLRP3, PARP1, PPIA, RIPK1, RIPK3, STAT1, STAT3, STAT6, TLR4, TNF, XIAP) that might be associated with the antidepressant mechanism of Xiaoyaosan through necroptosis pathway by taking the intersection of 1708 putative targets of the active ingredients in Xiaoyaosan, 12,608 therapeutic targets for depression and 97 necroptosis related targets.

Figure 4A showed the "botanical drugs-active ingredients-potential targets" network, eight botanical drugs of TCM formula Xiaoyaosan had 96 active ingredients which could regulate the 23 key target genes. Therefore, based on the network pharmacological analysis we can speculate that traditional Chinese formula Xiaoyaosan could regulate the necroptosis pathway in depression. **Figure 4B** showed the PPI network of potential target genes of Xiaoyaosan and the sub-network of the top 10 core targets which was picked up using the cytoHubba plugin in Cytoscape software. As showed in **Table 2**, the hub nodes of sub-network were ranked by maximal clique centrality (MCC) method, and MLKL, IL1B, CASP8, CASP1, RIPK1, TLR4, NLRP3, RIPK3, TNF, STAT3 were the top 10 potential treatment targets of Xiaoyaosan.

Depressive-like Behaviors of CUMS Mice

We performed the sucrose preference (SP) test, forced swimming (FS) test and novelty-suppressed feeding (NSF) test to observe the effects of Xiaoyaosan on depressive-like behaviors. As shown in **Figure 5A**, the baseline sucrose preference rate of control group, CUMS group, solvent group, Nec-1 group and Xiaoyaosan group had no significant differences. However, after CUMS modeling, the mice in CUMS group had a significant drop in sucrose preference rate compared with the control group mice ($p < 0.01$), while the Nec-1 group and Xiaoyaosan treatment group had no differences with the stress groups. Then, the CUMS progress continued for another 3 weeks with medication procedure, the mice in CUMS group and solvent group still had a low sucrose preference rate ($p < 0.01$), while the sucrose preference rate of Nec-1 group and Xiaoyaosan treatment group mice was significant increased (both $p < 0.01$). The CUMS group and solvent group mice exhibited significantly longer immobility time in the FS test ($p < 0.01$), and Xiaoyaosan or Nec-1 ameliorated this depressive-like behavior in comparison with the CUMS group and solvent group (both $p < 0.01$) (**Figure 5B**). For the NSF test, it was shown that mice in CUMS group had a significant longer latency to chew the food pellet compared with the control mice ($p < 0.01$) (**Figure 5C**), and the food consumption significantly decreased ($p < 0.01$) (**Figure 5D**). There was no significant difference between the

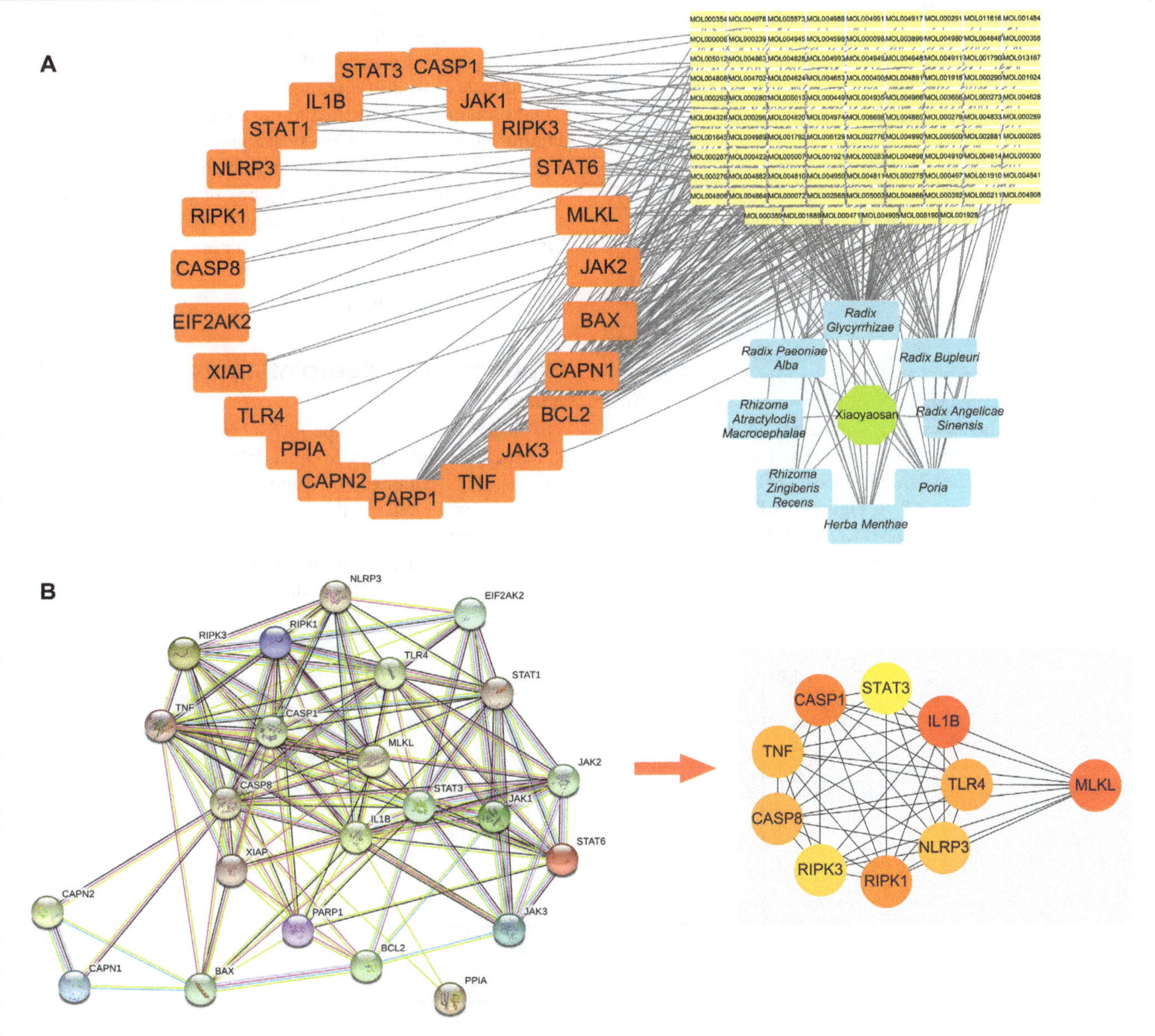

FIGURE 4 | "Botanical drugs-active ingredients-potential targets" network and PPI network of potential target genes of Xiaoyaosan **(A)** The "Botanical drugs-active ingredients-potential targets" network: These eight botanical drugs of TCM formula Xiaoyaosan had 96 active ingredients which could regulate the 23 key target genes according to the network pharmacological analysis **(B)** PPI network of the 23 key target genes: The sub-network of the top 10 core targets was picked up from the PPI network of potential target genes of Xiaoyaosan using the cytoHubba plugin in Cytoscape software.

solvent group and the CUMS group. Xiaoyaosan or Nec-1 could reverse these changes in the NSF test (both $p < 0.05$).

Necroptosis in the Hippocampus of CUMS Mice

In order to explore the possible mechanism of necroptosis in the mouse model of depression, the expressions of RIPK1, RIPK3, MLKL, *p*-MLKL were detected by western blot assay. As shown in **Figure 6**, the levels of RIPK1, RIPK3, MLKL and *p*-MLKL significant up-regulated in the hippocampi of CUMS-exposed mice compared to the control group ($p < 0.01$). Compared with the solvent group, these necroptosis biomarkers in Nec-1 group were significant down-regulated (both $p < 0.01$). Also, the effects of Xiaoyaosan were similar to Nec-1, which could mitigate the stress-induced elevation of RIPK1, RIPK3, MLKL and *p*-MLKL levels, as shown in the comparison between Xiaoyaosan treatment group and CUMS group ($p < 0.05$ or $p < 0.01$).

To further verified the process of necroptosis in CUMS-induced mice, the IHC and IF staining methods were used to observe the distribution of *p*-MLKL in hippocampus. **Figure 7** exhibited the representative micrographs of IHC and IF staining for *p*-MLKL in the CA1 and CA3 regions of hippocampus, and the results were set out in **Figure 8**. The MOD of *p*-MLKL in both

TABLE 2 | The Top 10 core target genes in PPI network ranked by MCC method.

Rank	Name	Score
1	MLKL	147,962
2	IL1B	142,802
3	CASP8	137,046
4	CASP1	131,880
5	RIPK1	131,040
6	TLR4	92,280
7	NLRP3	85,680
8	RIPK3	80,640
8	TNF	80,640
10	STAT3	67,446

CA1 and CA3 regions of CUMS group mice was significantly increased when compared with the control group ($p < 0.05, p < 0.01$, respectively), and there was no significant difference between solvent group and CUMS group. Then the treatment of Nec-1 or Xiaoyaosan reversed the CUMS-induced *p*-MLKL changes in the CA1 and CA3 ($p < 0.05$ or $p < 0.01$, **Figures 8A,B**). Compared with the control group, the MFI of *p*-MLKL of CUMS group mice was significantly increased, and CUMS group had no significant difference with solvent group. Similarly to IHC staining results, the *p*-MLKL MFI was decreased in Nec-1 and Xiaoyaosan group mice ($p < 0.05, p < 0.01$, **Figures 8C,D**). The outcomes of thioflavine T staining showed that the MFI of thioflavine T labelled amyloid-like polymers was also increased in the CA1 and CA3 regions of CUMS group mice compared to the control group (both $p < 0.01$, **Figures 8E,F**). In the end, the IF staining results revealed that high levels of the *p*-MLKL colocalized with thioflavin T staining was detected in the CA1 and CA3 regions of CUMS group mice, in contrast with the low colocalization in control group ($p < 0.01$, **Figures 8G,H**). The low levels of colocalization were observed in the CA1 and CA3 regions of mice in Xiaoyaosan group and Nec-1 group as well ($p < 0.05$, $p < 0.01$).

Hippocampal Neuroinflammation of CUMS Mice

The H&E staining was performed in order to evaluate the inflammatory infiltrates in mice hippocampal CA1 and CA3 regions. As exhibited in **Figure 9A**, a large number of inflammatory cell infiltration was observed in the hippocampus of the mice in chronically stressed groups treated with vehicle (physiological saline and solvent group). The histological scores of the hippocampus in each group

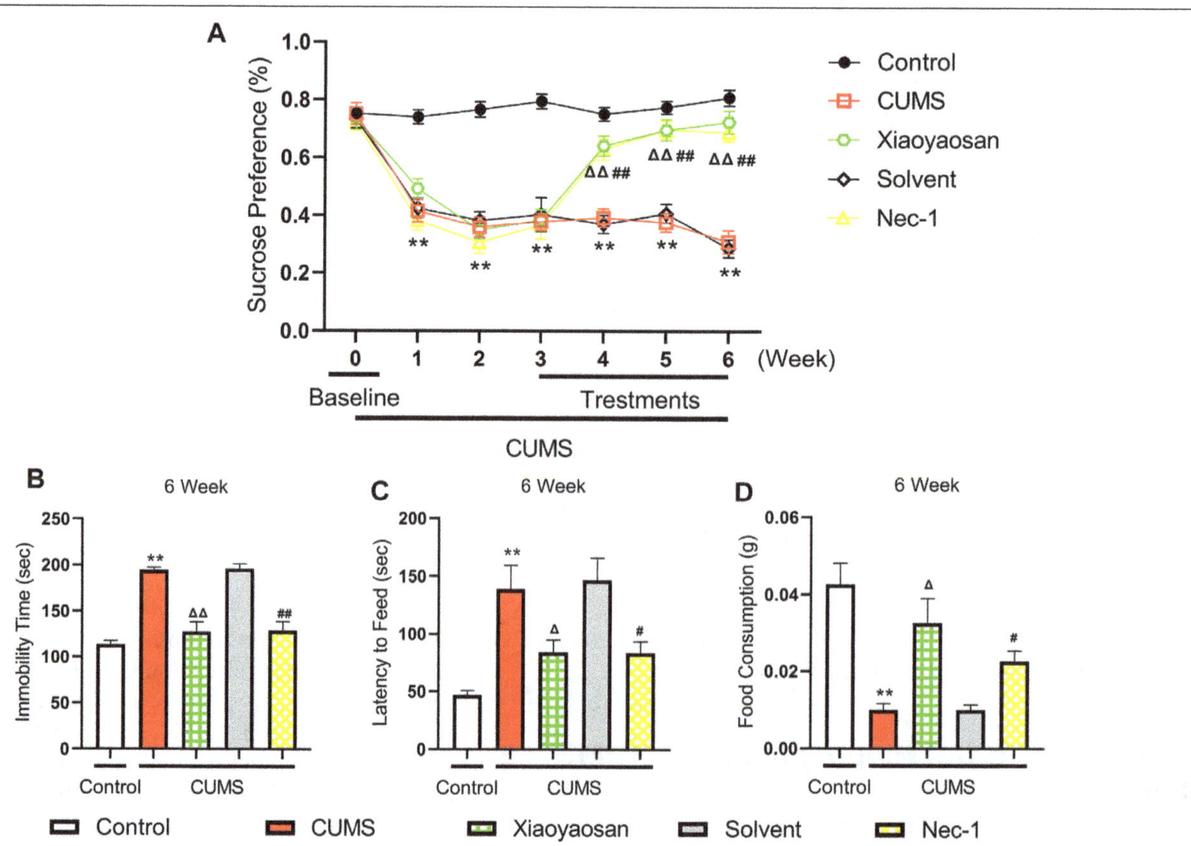

FIGURE 5 | Changes in the Depressive-like behaviors of CUMS mice **(A)** Changes of sucrose preference rate during the CUMS modeling period (n = 15) **(B)** FS test results after the 6-weeks modeling (n = 15) **(C)** The results of latency to feed in NSF test after the 6-weeks modeling (n = 15) **(D)** The results of food consumption in NSF test after the 6-weeks modeling (n = 15). Data were expressed as means ± SEM, **$p < 0.01$ versus control group; Δ$p < 0.05$, ΔΔ$p < 0.01$ versus CUMS group; #$p < 0.05$, ##$p < 0.01$ versus solvent group.

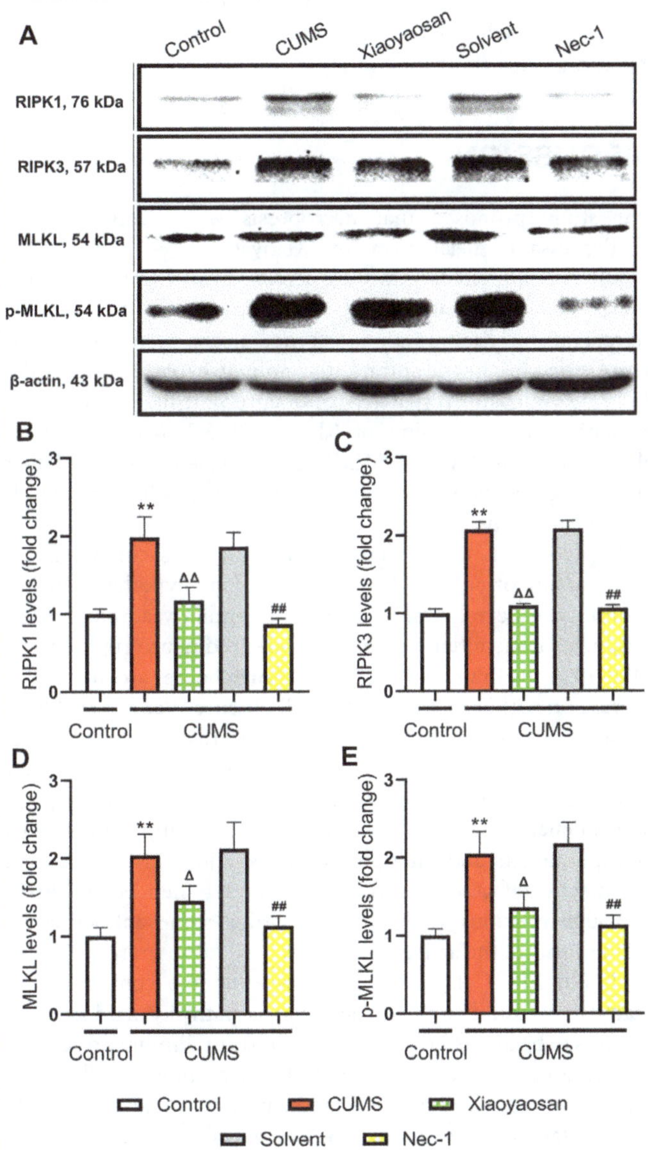

FIGURE 6 | Changes of necroptosis biomarkers in the hippocampi of CUMS mice **(A)** Representative micrographs of WB for necroptosis biomarkers **(B)** The expression of RIPK1 in the hippocampus of experimental mice (n = 5) **(C)** The expression of RIPK3 in the hippocampus of experimental mice (n = 5) **(D)** The expression of MLKL in the hippocampus of experimental mice (n = 5) **(E)** The expression of *p*-MLKL in the hippocampus of experimental mice (n = 5). Data were expressed as means ± SEM, $^{**}p < 0.01$ versus control group; $\Delta p < 0.05$, $\Delta\Delta p < 0.01$ versus CUMS group; $^{\#\#}p < 0.01$ versus solvent group.

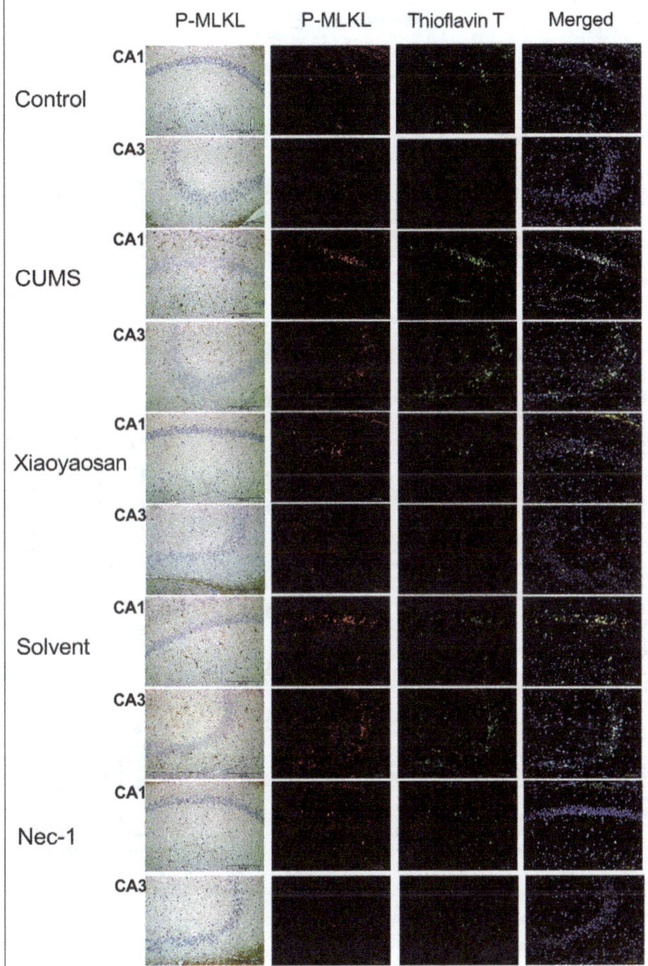

FIGURE 7 | Representative micrographs of IHC and IF staining for *p*-MLKL (scale bar = 200 μm, ×400 magnification) in the CA1 and CA3 regions.

were judged, it was found that the scores of CUMS group and solvent group in CA1 and CA3 regions were significantly higher than that of control group (both $p < 0.01$), Xiaoyaosan or Nec-1 treatment notably mitigated CUMS-induced inflammatory infiltrates (both $p < 0.05$) (**Figures 9B,C**). The expression levels of IL-1β and Lipocalin-2 were measured by qRT-PCR and western blot. The results indicated that the 6-weeks CUMS significant up-regulated the mRNA and protein levels of IL-1β in the hippocampus of CUMS-exposed mice (both $p < 0.01$), and the mice in the Xiaoyaosan treatment group and Nec-1 group showed a significant increase in IL-1β expression compared with the CUMS group mice (both $p < 0.01$) (**Figures 10A,C**). The CUMS modeling also increased the Lipocalin-2 level ($p < 0.01$), whereas the administration of Xiaoyaosan and Nec-1 noticeably inhibited the expressions of Lipocalin-2 (both $p < 0.01$) (**Figures 10B,D**).

Hippocampal Microglial Activation of CUMS Mice

To initial test the level of microglial activation in the hippocampi of CUMS-exposed mice, the expression of IBA1 was detected. **Figure 11A** presented the representative micrographs of IHC staining for IBA1 in the CA1 and CA3 regions of hippocampus. As showed in **Figures 11B,C**, the MOD of IBA1 in CA1 and CA3 of CUMS mice was significantly increased when compared to the control group (both $p < 0.05$), whereas the expression of IBA1 in

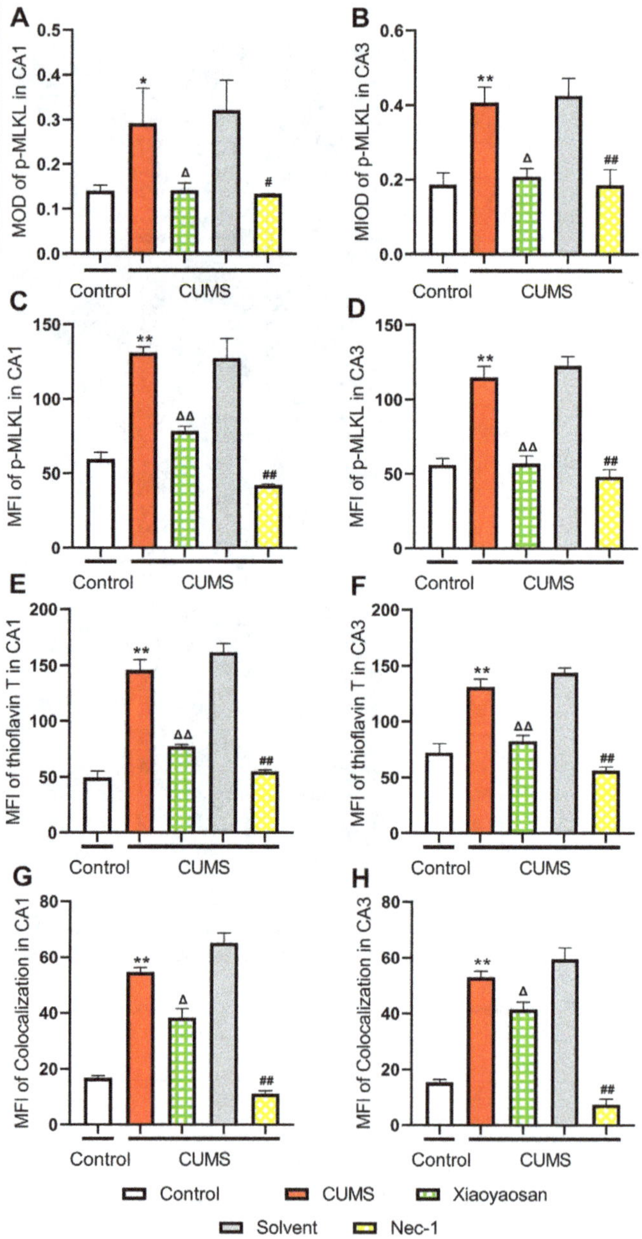

FIGURE 8 | Expression of *p*-MLKL in CA1 and CA3 regions of the hippocampus **(A)** The MOD level of *p*-MLKL in the CA1 region (n = 5) **(B)** The MOD level of *p*-MLKL in the CA3 region (n = 5) **(C)** The MFI level of *p*-MLKL in the CA1 region (n = 5) **(D)** The MFI level of *p*-MLKL in the CA3 region (n = 5) **(E)** The MFI level of thioflavine T staining in the CA1 region (n = 5) **(F)** The MFI level of thioflavine T staining in the CA3 region (n = 5) **(G)** The MFI level of *p*-MLKL colocalized with thioflavin T staining in the CA1 region (n = 5) **(H)** The MFI level of *p*-MLKL colocalized with thioflavin T staining in the CA3 region (n = 5). Data were expressed as means ± SEM, *$p < 0.05$, **$p < 0.01$ versus control group; Δ $p < 0.05$, ΔΔ $p < 0.01$ versus CUMS group; #$p < 0.05$, ##$p < 0.01$ versus solvent group.

CA1 and CA3 was noticeably reduced by the interference of Nec-1 and Xiaoyaosan ($p < 0.05$, $p < 0.01$). As showed in **Figures 11D,E**, the qRT-PCR and western blot data also demonstrated the high level of IBA1 in the hippocampus of the chronically stressed mice (both $p < 0.01$), and the treatment with Nec-1 or Xiaoyaosan significantly reduced the expression of IBA1 as compared to stressed groups (both $p < 0.01$).

DISCUSSION

Our study proposed that necroptosis was involved in the antidepressant mechanism of Xiaoyaosan. A total of 23 potential treatment targets were screened out through network pharmacological analysis that might be related to the active ingredients of Xiaoyaosan intervened necroptosis pathway in depression. In the meantime, the animal experiment revealed that Xiaoyaosan displayed antidepressant-like effects via regulating the expression of RIPK1, RIPK3, MLKL, and the phosphorylation level of MLKL of depressed mice, and then improving the neuroinflammation and microglia function in the hippocampus.

Depression is a prevalent and persistent psychiatric illness affecting millions of people worldwide. Many hypotheses such as inflammatory cytokines, hypothalamic pituitary adrenal (HPA) axis, neurotransmitter system, brain-derived neurotrophic factor (BDNF) in the brain and endogenous metabolites are involved in depression pathogenesis, but it is still obscure (Peng et al., 2015). Today, there is still lack of precise and effective diagnostic or therapeutic methods for depression. Xiaoyaosan is a common TCM formula for treating syndrome of stagnation of liver qi and spleen deficiency with the characteristics of multiple ingredients, multiple targets and multiple pathways, and it also has a good therapeutic effect on depressive diseases (Chen et al., 2020). Although previous studies have revealed some antidepressant mechanisms of the active ingredients of Xiaoyaosan (Liu X. et al., 2021; Liu XJ. et al., 2021), while whether the components of Xiaoyaosan could improve necroptosis pathway in depression remains to be discussed. The present study preliminary disclosure that Xiaoyaosan could regulate the necroptosis pathway in depression via its 96 active ingredients that could regulate the 23 key target genes based on the network pharmacological analysis. Through PPI network analysis of these 23 target genes, we confirmed that MLKL, IL1B, CASP8, CASP1, RIPK1, TLR4, NLRP3, RIPK3, TNF, STAT3 as the potential target genes of Xiaoyaosan in the treatment of depression, among which the MCC score of MLKL was the highest. Mounting evidence suggested that necroptosis depended on RIPK1/RIPK3/MLKL activities, RIPK1 and RIPK3 upregulated upon activation of death receptors, triggered a signaling cascade involving phosphorylation of MLKL which contributes to the change of plasm membrane permeability, then resulting in cellular necrosis (Liu C. et al., 2021; Marunouchi et al., 2021; Yu et al., 2021). Therefore, the expressions of RIPK1, RIPK3, MLKL were evaluated as biomarkers of necroptosis in the study.

Stress was closely related to neurological disorders, and the sustained psychosocial stress is one of the main causes of depression. Chronic or repeated stress can cause neuronal disturbances, which was similar to changes observed in the brain during depression (de Kloet and Joëls, 2005). Animal model of depression was an important method to explore the

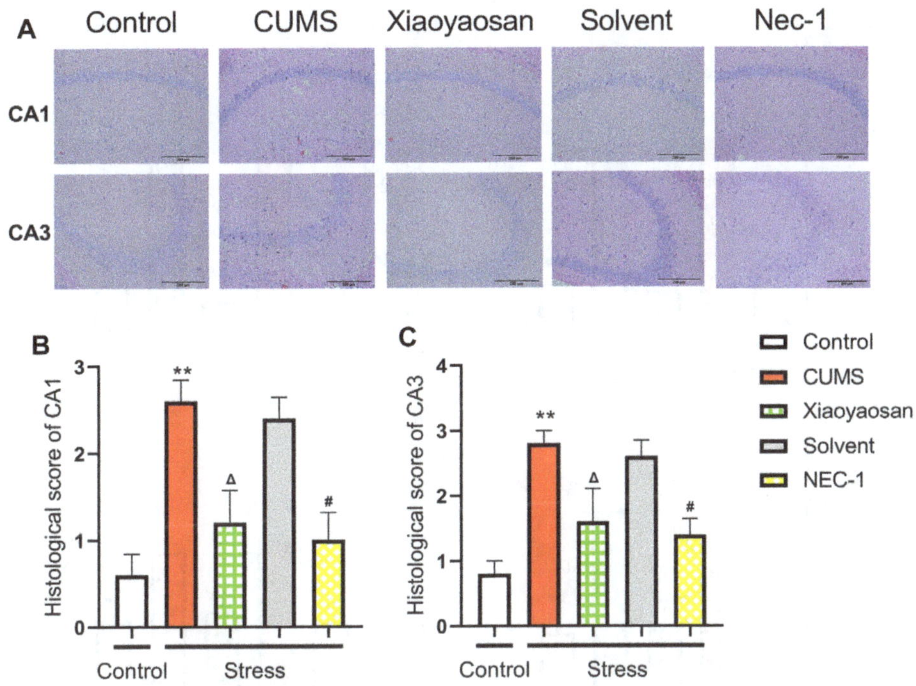

FIGURE 9 | The histological changes in CA1 and CA3 regions of the hippocampi in CUMS mice **(A)** Representative micrographs of H&E staining (scale bar = 200 μm, ×400 magnification) in the CA1 and CA3 regions **(B)** The histological scores in the CA1 region (n = 5) **(C)** The histological scores in the CA1 region (n = 5). Data were expressed as means ± SEM, $^{**}p < 0.01$ versus control group; $\Delta\ p < 0.05$ versus CUMS group; $\#p < 0.05$ versus Solvent group.

dysregulatory mechanisms of depression and the regulatory mechanisms by which antidepressant treatments alleviate the various depressive symptoms (Frazer and Morilak, 2005). The depression model by CUMS method was widely recognized and applied for mechanism research and drug selection. Also, some studies showed that the depressive behaviors induced by CUMS was similar to the clinical manifestations of depression induced by long-term exposure to multiple stresses (D'Aquila et al., 1994; Papp et al., 1996). Here, we found that after 6 weeks of CUMS, mice were observed to exhibit significant depressive symptoms through behavioral evaluation, which was consistent with other studies (Cao et al., 2013). This study used classical evaluation methods to observe depressive behavior in CUMS-induced mice, including SP test, FS test and NSF test. The performance of anhedonia was manifested by lack of interest in reward stimulus, which was a manifestation of affective disorders including depression, while SP test was a method to evaluate the degree of pleasure loss in rodents (Weiss, 1997). FS test was a kind of negative stress experiment that animals could not escape from hostile environment and produce hopeless behaviors, the immobility time was used as an important index to evaluate depressive behaviors (Bächli et al., 2008). So, it was widely used in the exploration of the pathogenesis of stress and the pharmacological study of potential antidepressants. The NSF test observed the contradiction between the fear of new environment and the great need for things, the food consumption and latency of feed could represent the degree of depression and anxiety in animals (Shalom et al., 2006). The results showed that there were obvious behavioral changes in the CUMS model group, including decreased sucrose preference rate, prolonged immobility time, longer latency of feed and decreased appetite. Thus, it could be proved that the 6-weeks modeling successfully established depressive-like changes in mice. In the meantime, we found that the treatment of Xiaoyaosan could significantly improve the depressive-like behavioral changes in mice which was consistent with the results of previous studies, indicating that Xiaoyaosan exhibited good antidepressant performances (Wang et al., 2018; Liu X. et al., 2019).

The mechanism of cell death had always been one of the focuses of biomedical research, and it was common believed that cell death patterns included apoptosis, necrosis and autophagy at present. Apoptosis and autophagy required the synthesis of new proteins and energy supplies, which was an active process of cell self-regulation, also known as programmed death (M Stacey and Wei-Xing, 2006). Cell necrosis was previously considered to be a passive disordered process that occurred under overwhelming physical and chemical damage from the outside world, and therefore could not be regulated (Vandenabeele et al., 2008). With the in-depth study of the mechanism of cell death, it was found that cell necrosis was also a programmed death process with notable necrosis features, then it was redefined as necroptosis (Degterev et al., 2005). Necroptosis was mainly initiated by the members of tumor necrosis factor (TNF) receptor family and toll-like receptor (TLR) family, which phosphorylated MLKL by transmitting death signals through RIPK1 and RIPK3(Galluzzi and Kroemer, 2008). Thus, as the executor of cell death, phosphorylation of MLKL eventually led to cell necrosis. The necrotic cells released their contents as damage-

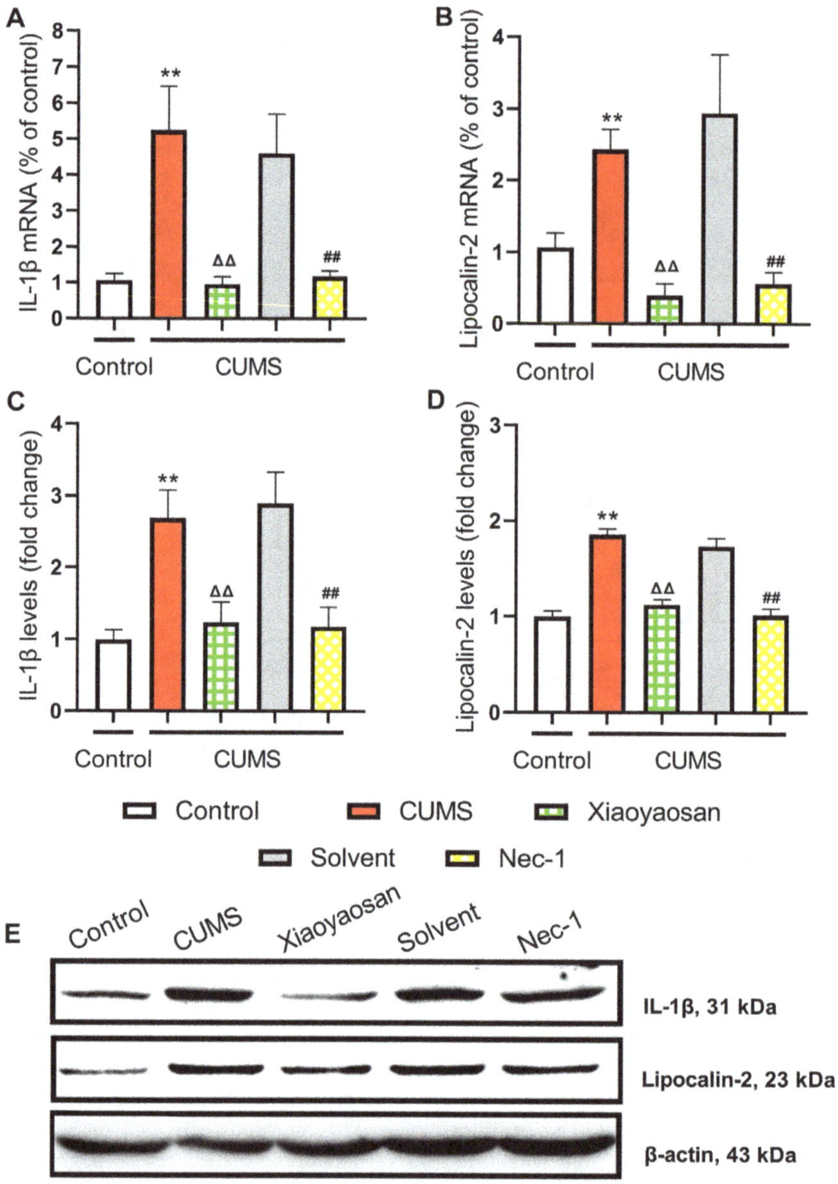

FIGURE 10 | The levels of IL-1β and Lipocalin-2 in the hippocampus of CUMS mice **(A)** The mRNA results of IL-1β (n = 5) **(B)** The mRNA results of Lipocalin-2 (n = 5) **(C)** The protein results of IL-1β (n = 5) **(D)** The protein results of Lipocalin-2 (n = 5) **(E)** Representative micrographs of WB for IL-1β and Lipocalin-2. Data were expressed as means ± SEM, $^{**}p < 0.01$ versus control group; ΔΔ $p < 0.01$ versus CUMS group; $^{\#\#}p < 0.01$ versus Solvent group.

associated molecular pattern molecules (DAMPs) to stimulate inflammation in peripheral cells, then activated immune responses of the body (Sonenshine and Macaluso, 2017). Therefore, the role of necroptosis in the neurological diseases involved a variety of biological mechanisms related to neuroinflammation (Liu et al., 2014; Bian et al., 2017; Shao et al., 2018). Nec-1 could inhibit necroptosis and reduce inflammation, which was beneficial to the improvement of pathological damage (Takahashi et al., 2012). The increased inflammation was associated with stress-related affective disorders (Stein et al., 2018), while the activations of immune system and inflammatory cytokines might be involved in the pathogenesis of some patients with depression (Haapakoski et al., 2016). The involvement of chronic low-grade inflammatory response, compensatory anti-inflammatory reflex system, and cellular mediated immunity might be the key factors leading to depression (Maes, 1995). Also, higher level of inflammation was associated with increased risk of depression (Pasco et al., 2010). The treatment of antidepressants, especially selective serotonin reuptake inhibitors (SSRIs), could significantly reduce the production of pro-inflammatory cytokines and inflammatory markers, such as IL-1β, IL-6 and TNF-α, and increase the production of anti-inflammatory cytokines, such as IL-10 (Berk et al., 2013). Accordingly, anti-inflammatory

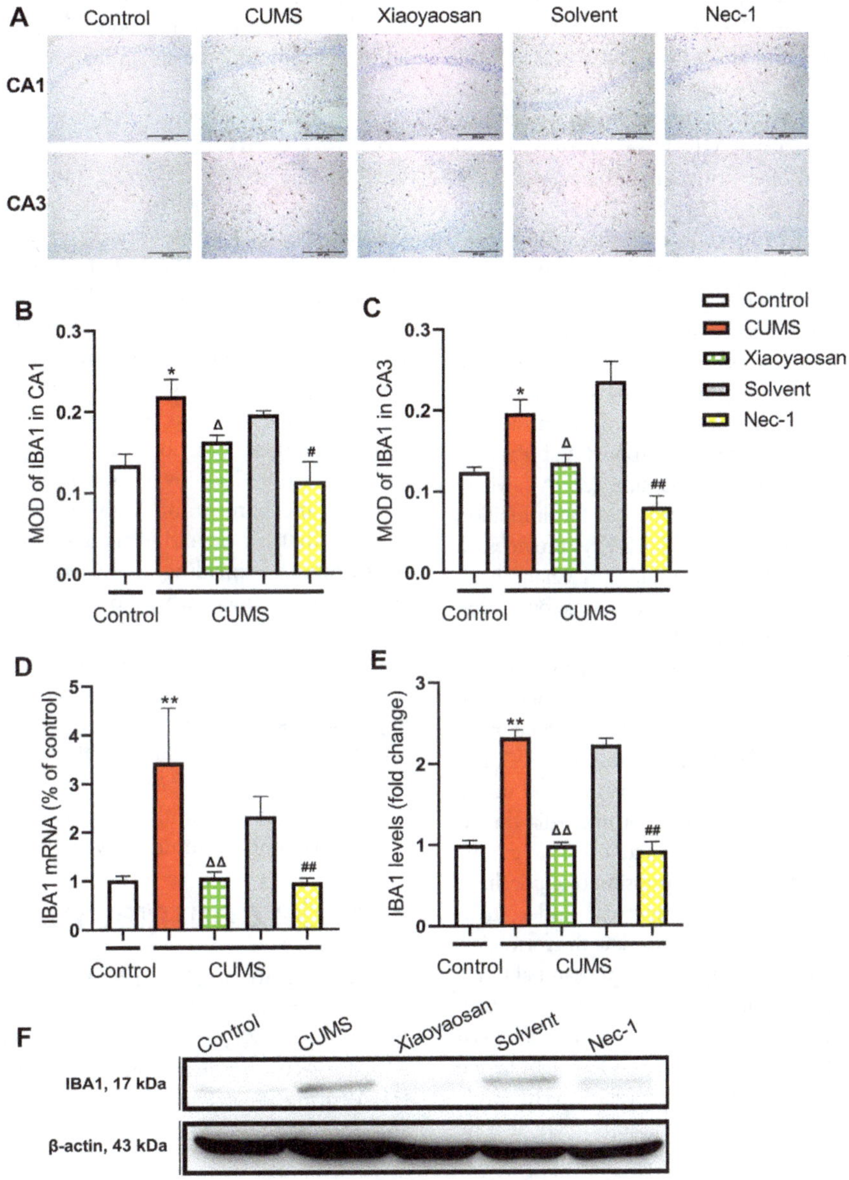

FIGURE 11 | Expression of IBA1 in CA1 and CA3 regions of the hippocampi in CUMS mice **(A)** Representative micrographs of immunohistochemical staining for IBA1 (scale bar = 200 μm, ×400 magnification) in the CA1 and CA3 regions **(B)** The MOD level of IBA1 in the CA1 region (n = 5) **(C)** The MOD level of IBA1 in the CA3 region (n = 5) **(D)** The mRNA results of IBA1 (n = 5) **(E)** The protein results of IBA1 (n = 5). Data were expressed as means ± SEM, $^*p < 0.05$, $^{**}p < 0.01$ versus control group; $\Delta\ p < 0.05$, $\Delta\Delta\ p < 0.01$ versus CUMS group; $\#p < 0.05$, $\#\#p < 0.01$ versus Solvent group.

could be an effective strategy for the treatment of depression and had great research value (Müller and Schwarz, 2010; Hayley, 2011).

Our results explained that the necroptosis inhibitor Nec-1 could improve depressive-like behaviors in mice, which suggested that the necroptosis pathway might be associated with the pathogenesis of depression. Hippocampus, as the most learning and memory function-related brain area, was also the main target of stress injury (Christie, 2015). Studies have found that inflammation of hippocampus and overactivation of microglia were important central mechanisms of depression (Streit et al., 2004; Xu et al., 2015), and the regulation of necroptosis on CNS function was also closely related to the occurrence of neuroinflammation (Antunes et al., 2019). Therefore, in order to further investigate the results of network pharmacology, and further explore the relationship between the pathogenesis of depression and necroptosis, we detected the expressions of RIPK1, RIPK3, MLKL and *p*-MLKL in hippocampus of CUMS-induced mice to confirm the level of necroptosis. It was observed that RIPK1, RIPK3 and MLKL in hippocampus of model mice were significantly up-regulated, and the phosphorylation level of MLKL was also increased, meanwhile, Nec-1 played a significant role in regulating the expressions of the above indicators. Phosphorylated MLKL was the most precise protein, which could definitely indicate the necroptosis activated via RIPK-mediated MLKL signaling (Rodriguez et al., 2016). In other words, the phosphorylation of MLKL at ser345 was crucial for the recruitment of MLKL and the activation of necroptosis pathway (Rodriguez et al., 2016). We also found high level of the *p*-MLKL colocalized with thioflavin T staining in the hippocampus of CUMS group mice, indicating that MLKL was phosphorylated in the presence of amyloid-like polymers, characteristic of necrosome complexes (Li et al., 2012; Liu et al., 2017).

Finally, our results displayed a large number of inflammatory cells infiltrated into the hippocampus of CUMS-exposed mice and revealed that the expressions of IL-1β, Lipocalin-2 and IBA1 were significantly increased, which proved that the existence of neuroinflammation and excessive activation of microglia were associated with the necroptosis pathway. Necroptosis can be specifically blocked by small molecule compound Nec-1, but not by specific inhibitors of apoptosis and autophagy, such as z-vad. fmk (N-benzyloxycarbonyl Val ala ASP (o-me) fluoromethylketone) and 3-methyladenine (3 mA). Many studies on different perspectives have revealed that the inhibition of necroptosis mediated by RIPK1/RIPK3/MLKL provides a protective effect against inflammation (Moriwaki and Chan, 2016 Duan et al., 2020; Kumari et al., 2021). Therefore, it was found that Nec-1 could also suppress neuroinflammation and activation of microglia in hippocampus. It was reported that Lipocalin-2 was an inflammatory-related protein closely correlated to hippocampal structure and function, and it might be a key regulator of emotional behaviors and cognitive function (Ferreira et al., 2013). Lipocalin-2 secreted by microglia and astrocytes participated in the activation of microglia, then excessive activation of microglia caused neuroinflammation and injured the structure and function of neurons (Kim et al., 2017). Normally, there was low expression of Lipocalin-2 in hippocampus, but it might continuously increase under stress stimulation, which was related to its ability to regulate the formation and maturation of dendritic spines of neurons in hippocampal CA1-CA3 regions (Mucha et al., 2011). Moreover, the activation of MLKL during necroptosis triggered the release of IL-1β, IL-6 and TNF(Wu et al., 2013). The inflammatory cytokines such as IL-1β might be the key substance regulating the expression of Lipocalin-2 (Hu et al., 2015). At this point we could conclude that necroptosis might activate the Lipocalin-2 involved inflammatory pathway, induce the neuroinflammation and microglial over-activation, and then participate in the functional changes of hippocampus leading to depressive-like behaviors in depressed mice. Grounded on rigorous science, the TCM formula Xiaoyaosan was an antidepressant therapy conceptually based on a multiple component, multiple targeting principle. As showed in this study, Xiaoyaosan might mediate the RIPK1-RIPK3-MLKL signaling and its subsequent inflammatory pathway, regulate the inflammatory-related mediator Lipocalin-2, and then improve the function of hippocampal microglia to exert antidepressant and anti-inflammatory effect.

CONCLUSION

According to the network pharmacological study, the active ingredients of Xiaoyaosan may exert the antidepressant effect via 23 necroptosis related potential targets. Then, the animal experiment found that the RIPK1-RIPK3-MLKL signaling was triggered in the stress-induced depression in mice. These findings were consistent with the cytokine hypothesis of depression that postulated stress may activate the necroptosis pathway in hippocampus, leading to neuroinflammation and microglial activation, then contribute to the development of depressive-like behaviors. Moreover, our findings further illustrated the possible mechanism of Xiaoyaosan with explicit experiment results that it could regulate the necroptosis mediated inflammatory signaling pathway to alleviated the depressive symptoms of mice, which provided an experimental basis for the clinical application of Xiaoyaosan in the treatment of depression. For future research, whether necroptosis can be used as a new potential pathway for the treatment of depression still needs to be confirmed with RIPK or MLKL knockout mice, and the functional impact of necroptosis in depression with the specific role of the active components of Xiaoyaosan on neuroinflammation could be further explored by more novel and accurate network pharmacological analysis.

AUTHOR CONTRIBUTIONS

Conceptualization, ZY, HJ and JC; Data curation, ZY and HJ; Formal analysis, ZY and HJ; Funding acquisition, JC; Investigation, ZY, JC, KZ and XW; Methodology, HJ, JC and XW; Project administration, ZY and KZ; Visualization, ZY and HJ; Writing — original draft, ZY and HJ; Writing — review andamp; editing, YJ, YL, ZX, QM, XL and JC.

FUNDING

This research was supported by grants from National Natural Science Foundation of China (No. 81630104, 81973748), and Huang Zhendong Research Fund for Traditional Chinese Medicine of Jinan University (No. 201911).

REFERENCES

Amberger, J. S., Bocchini, C. A., Schiettecatte, F., Scott, A. F., and Hamosh, A. (2015). OMIM.org: Online Mendelian Inheritance in Man (OMIM®), an Online Catalog of Human Genes and Genetic Disorders. *Nucleic Acids Res.* 43, D789–D798. doi:10.1093/nar/gku1205

Antunes, D. P. E., Rodrigues, O. S., Dias, A. J. S. o. J., and Pereira, R. C. M. (2019). Loss of Microglial Parkin Inhibits Necroptosis and Contributes to Neuroinflammation. *Mol. Neurobiol.*, 1–15. doi:10.1007/s12035-018-1264-9

Bächli, H., Steiner, M. A., Habersetzer, U., and Wotjak, C. T. (2008). Increased Water Temperature Renders Single-Housed C57BL/6J Mice Susceptible to Antidepressant Treatment in the Forced Swim Test. *Behav. Brain Res.* 187 (1), 67–71. doi:10.1016/j.bbr.2007.08.029

Barfield, E. T., Moser, V. A., Hand, A., and Grisel, J. E. (2013). β-Endorphin Modulates the Effect of Stress on Novelty-Suppressed Feeding. *Front. Behav. Neurosci.* 7 (6), 19. doi:10.3389/fnbeh.2013.00019

Berk, M., Williams, L. J., Jacka, F. N., O'Neil, A., Pasco, J. A., Moylan, S., et al. (2013). So Depression Is an Inflammatory Disease, but Where Does the Inflammation Come From? *BMC Med.* 11 (1), 200. doi:10.1186/1741-7015-11-200

Bian, P., Zheng, X., Wei, L., Ye, C., Fan, H., Cai, Y., et al. (2017). MLKL Mediated Necroptosis Accelerates JEV-Induced Neuroinflammation in Mice. *Front. Microbiol.* 8, 303. doi:10.3389/fmicb.2017.00303

Cao, X., Li, L. P., Wang, Q., Wu, Q., Hu, H. H., Zhang, M., et al. (2013). Astrocyte-Derived ATP Modulates Depressive-Like Behaviors. *Nat. Med.* 19 (1), 773–777. doi:10.1038/nm.3162

Chen, C., Yin, Q., Tian, J., Gao, X., Qin, X., Du, G., et al. (2020). Studies on the Potential Link Between Antidepressant Effect of Xiaoyao San and its Pharmacological Activity of Hepatoprotection Based on Multi-Platform Metabolomics. *J. Ethnopharmacol.* 249, 112432. doi:10.1016/j.jep.2019.112432

Chen, Y., Gong, K., Guo, L., Zhang, B., Chen, S., Li, Z., et al. (2021). Downregulation of Phosphoglycerate Mutase 5 Improves Microglial Inflammasome Activation after Traumatic Brain Injury. *Cell Death Discov.* 7 (1), 290. doi:10.1038/s41420-021-00686-8

Chiriţă, A. L., Gheorman, V., Bondari, D., and Rogoveanu, I. (2015). Current Understanding of the Neurobiology of Major Depressive Disorder. *Rom. J. Morphol. Embryol.* 56 (2 Suppl. l), 651–658.

Cho, Y. S., Challa, S., Moquin, D., Genga, R., Ray, T. D., Guildford, M., et al. (2009). Phosphorylation-Driven Assembly of the RIP1-RIP3 Complex Regulates Programmed Necrosis and Virus-Induced Inflammation. *Cell.* 137 (6), 1112–1123. doi:10.1016/j.cell.2009.05.037

Christie, B. R. (2015). Long-Term Depression (LTD) in the hippocampus. *Hippocampus.* 6 (1), 1–2.

D'Aquila, P. S., Brain, P., and Willner, P. (1994). Effects of Chronic Mild Stress on Performance in Behavioural Tests Relevant to Anxiety and Depression. *Physiol. Behav.* 56 (5), 861–867. doi:10.1016/0031-9384(94)90316-6

Daina, A., Michielin, O., and Zoete, V. (2019). SwissTargetPrediction: Updated Data and New Features for Efficient Prediction of Protein Targets of Small Molecules. *Nucleic Acids Res.* 47 (W1), W357–w364. doi:10.1093/nar/gkz382

Dara, L., Johnson, H., Suda, J., Win, S., Gaarde, W., Han, D., et al. (2016). Receptor Interacting Protein Kinase 1 Mediates Murine Acetaminophen Toxicity Independent of the Necrosome and Not Through Necroptosis. *Hepatology.* 62 (6), 1847–1857. doi:10.1002/hep.27939

Davis, A. P., Grondin, C. J., Johnson, R. J., Sciaky, D., Wiegers, J., Wiegers, T. C., et al. (2020). Comparative Toxicogenomics Database (CTD): Update 2021. *Nucleic Acids Res.* 49, D1138–D1143. doi:10.1093/nar/gkaa891

de Kloet, E. R., and Joëls, F. (2005). Jo?lsStress and the Brain: From Adaptation to Disease. *Nat. Rev. Neurosci.* 6 (6), 463–475. doi:10.1038/nrn1683

Degterev, A., Hitomi, J., Germscheid, M., Ch'En, I. L., Korkina, O., Teng, X., et al. (2008). Identification of RIP1 Kinase as a Specific Cellular Target of Necrostatins. *Nat. Chem. Biol.* 4 (5), 313–321. doi:10.1038/nchembio.83

Degterev, A., Huang, Z., Boyce, M., Li, Y., Jagtap, P., Mizushima, N., et al. (2005). Chemical Inhibitor of Nonapoptotic Cell Death With Therapeutic Potential for Ischemic Brain Injury. *Nat. Chem. Biol.* 1 (2), 112–119. doi:10.1038/nchembio711

Ding, X. F., Li, Y. H., Chen, J. X., Sun, L. J., Jiao, H. Y., Wang, X. X., et al. (2017). Involvement of the Glutamate/Glutamine Cycle and Glutamate Transporter GLT-1 in Antidepressant-like Effects of Xiao Yao San on Chronically Stressed Mice. *BMC Complement. Altern. Med.* 17 (1), 326. doi:10.1186/s12906-017-1830-0

Dongliang, C., Xiaoping, P., Peng, X., Farwell, M. A., and Baohong, Z. (2011). Evaluation and Identification of Reliable Reference Genes for Pharmacogenomics, Toxicogenomics, and Small RNA Expression Analysis. *J. Cell Physiol.* 226 (10), 2469–2477. doi:10.1002/jcp.22725

Dowlati, Y., Herrmann, N., Swardfager, W., Liu, H., Sham, L., Reim, E. K., et al. (2010). A Meta-Analysis of Cytokines in Major Depression. *Biol. Psychiatry.* 67 (5), 446–457. doi:10.1016/j.biopsych.2009.09.033

Duan, X., Liu, X., Liu, N., Huang, Y., Jin, Z., Zhang, S., et al. (2020). Inhibition of Keratinocyte Necroptosis Mediated by RIPK1/RIPK3/MLKL Provides a Protective Effect against Psoriatic Inflammation. *Cell Death Dis.* 11 (2), 134. doi:10.1038/s41419-020-2328-0

Fang, S., Dong, L., Liu, L., Guo, J., Zhao, L., Zhang, J., et al. (2021). HERB: a High-Throughput Experiment- and Reference-Guided Database of Traditional Chinese Medicine. *Nucleic Acids Res.* 49 (D1), D1197–d1206. doi:10.1093/nar/gkaa1063

Ferreira, A. C., Pinto, V., Dá Mesquita, S., Novais, A., Sousa, J. C., Correia-Neves, M., et al. (2013). Lipocalin-2 Is Involved in Emotional Behaviors and Cognitive Function. *Front Cell Neurosci.* 7 (31), 122. doi:10.3389/fncel.2013.00122

Frazer, A., and Morilak, D. A. (2005). What Should Animal Models of Depression Model? *Neurosci. Biobehav Rev.* 29 (4), 515–523. doi:10.1016/j.neubiorev.2005.03.006

Galluzzi, L., Kepp, O., and Kroemer, G. (2009). RIP Kinases Initiate Programmed Necrosis. *J. Mol. Cell Biol.* 1 (1), 8–10. doi:10.1093/jmcb/mjp007

Galluzzi, L., and Kroemer, G. (2008). Necroptosis: A Specialized Pathway of Programmed Necrosis. *Cell.* 135 (7), 1161–1163. doi:10.1016/j.cell.2008.12.004

Guo, X., Wu, Y., Zhang, C., Wu, L., Qin, L., and Liu, T. (2021). Network Pharmacology Analysis of ZiShenWan for Diabetic Nephropathy and Experimental Verification of its Anti-Inflammatory Mechanism. *Drug Des. Devel Ther.* 15, 1577–1594. doi:10.2147/dddt.s297683

Haapakoski, R., Ebmeier, K. P., Alenius, H., and Kivimäki, M. (2016). Innate and Adaptive Immunity in the Development of Depression: An Update on Current Knowledge and Technological Advances. *Prog. Neuropsychopharmacol. Biol. Psychiatry.* 66, 63–72. doi:10.1016/j.pnpbp.2015.11.012

Hayley, S. (2011). Toward an Anti-inflammatory Strategy for Depression. *Front. Behav. Neurosci.* 5 (19), 19. doi:10.3389/fnbeh.2011.00019

Hu, Y., Xue, J., Yang, Y., Zhou, X., Qin, C., Zheng, M., et al. (2015). Lipocalin 2 Upregulation Protects Hepatocytes from IL1-β-Induced Stress. *Cell Physiol Biochem.* 36 (2), 753–762. doi:10.1159/000430135

Iwata, M., Ota, K. T., and Duman, R. S. (2013). The Inflammasome: Pathways Linking Psychological Stress, Depression, and Systemic Illnesses. *Brain Behav. Immun.* 31 (7), 105–114. doi:10.1016/j.bbi.2012.12.008

Jiao, H., Yan, Z., Ma, Q., Li, X., Jiang, Y., Liu, Y., et al. (2019). Influence of Xiaoyaosan on Depressive-Like Behaviors in Chronic Stress-Depressed Rats Through Regulating Tryptophan Metabolism in Hippocampus. *Neuropsychiatr. Dis. Treat.* 15, 21–31. doi:10.2147/ndt.S185295

Jiao, H., Yang, H., Yan, Z., Chen, J., Xu, M., Jiang, Y., et al. (2021). Traditional Chinese Formula Xiaoyaosan Alleviates Depressive-Like Behavior in CUMS Mice by Regulating PEBP1-GPX4-Mediated Ferroptosis in the Hippocampus. *Neuropsychiatr. Dis. Treat.* 17, 1001–1019. doi:10.2147/ndt.s302443

Kim, J. H., Ko, P. W., Lee, H. W., Jeong, J. Y., Lee, M. G., Kim, J. H., et al. (2017). Astrocyte-Derived Lipocalin-2 Mediates Hippocampal Damage and Cognitive Deficits in Experimental Models of Vascular Dementia. *Glia.* 65 (9), 1471–1490. doi:10.1002/glia.23174

Konsman, J.-P. (2003). The Mouse Brain in Stereotaxic Coordinates. *Psychoneuroendocrinology.* 28 (6), 827–828. doi:10.1016/s0306-4530(03)00088-x

Kumari, S., Van, T. M., Preukschat, D., Schuenke, H., Basic, M., Bleich, A., et al. (2021). NF-κB Inhibition in Keratinocytes Causes RIPK1-Mediated Necroptosis and Skin Inflammation. *Life Sci. Alliance.* 4 (6). doi:10.26508/lsa.202000956

Li, H., Zhao, L., Zhang, B., Jiang, Y., Wang, X., Guo, Y., et al. (2014). A Network Pharmacology Approach to Determine Active Compounds and Action Mechanisms of Ge-Gen-Qin-Lian Decoction for Treatment of Type 2 Diabetes. *Evid. Based Complement. Alternat Med.* 2014, 495840. doi:10.1155/2014/495840

Li, J., McQuade, T., Siemer, A. B., Napetschnig, J., Moriwaki, K., Hsiao, Y. S., et al. (2012). The RIP1/RIP3 Necrosome Forms a Functional Amyloid Signaling Complex Required for Programmed Necrosis. *Cell.* 150 (2), 339–350. doi:10.1016/j.cell.2012.06.019

Li, P., Tang, X. D., Cai, Z. X., Qiu, J. J., Lin, X. L., Zhu, T., et al. (2015). CNP Signal Pathway Up-Regulated in Rectum of Depressed Rats and the Interventional Effect of Xiaoyaosan. *World J. Gastroenterol.* 21 (5), 1518–1530. doi:10.3748/wjg.v21.i5.1518

Li, S., and Zhang, B. (2013). Traditional Chinese Medicine Network Pharmacology: Theory, Methodology and Application. *Chin. J. Nat. Med.* 11 (2), 110–120. doi:10.1016/s1875-5364(13)60037-0

Li, X. J., Ma, Q. Y., Jiang, Y. M., Bai, X. H., Yan, Z. Y., Liu, Q., et al. (2017). Xiaoyaosan Exerts Anxiolytic-Like Effects by Down-Regulating the TNF-A/jak2-STAT3 Pathway in the Rat hippocampus. *Sci. Rep.* 7 (1), 353. doi:10.1038/s41598-017-00496-y

Liao, D., Xiang, D., Dang, R., Xu, P., Wang, J., Han, W., et al. (2018). Neuroprotective Effects of Dl-3-N-Butylphthalide Against Doxorubicin-Induced Neuroinflammation, Oxidative Stress, Endoplasmic Reticulum Stress, and Behavioral Changes. *Oxid Med. Cell Longev.* 2018, 9125601–9125613. doi:10.1155/2018/9125601

Liu, C., Chen, Y., Cui, W., Cao, Y., Zhao, L., Wang, H., et al. (2021a). Inhibition of Neuronal Necroptosis Mediated by RIP1/RIP3/MLKL Provides Neuroprotective Effects on Kaolin-Induced Hydrocephalus in Mice. *Cell Prolif.* 54, e13108. doi:10.1111/cpr.13108

Liu, X., Wei, F., Liu, H., Zhao, S., Du, G., and Qin, X. (2021b). Integrating Hippocampal Metabolomics and Network Pharmacology Deciphers the Antidepressant Mechanisms of Xiaoyaosan. *J. Ethnopharmacol.* 268, 113549. doi:10.1016/j.jep.2020.113549

Liu, X. J., Wang, Y. Z., Wei, F. X., Lv, M., Qu, P., Chen, S. J., et al. (2021c). The Synergistic Anti-Depression Effects of Different Efficacy Groups of Xiaoyaosan as Demonstrated by the Integration of Network Pharmacology and Serum Metabolomics. *J. Pharm. Biomed. Anal.* 197, 113949. doi:10.1016/j.jpba.2021.113949

Liu, S., Liu, H., Johnston, A., Hanna-Addams, S., Reynoso, E., Xiang, Y., et al. (2017). MLKL Forms Disulfide Bond-Dependent Amyloid-like Polymers to Induce Necroptosis. *Proc. Natl. Acad. Sci. U S A.* 114 (36), E7450–e7459. doi:10.1073/pnas.1707531114

Liu, S., Wang, X., Li, Y., Xu, L., Yu, X., Ge, L., et al. (2014). Necroptosis Mediates TNF-Induced Toxicity of Hippocampal Neurons. *Biomed. Res. Int.* 2014 (11), 290182. doi:10.1155/2014/290182

Liu, T., Bao, Y. H., Wang, Y., and Jiang, J. Y. (2015). The Role of Necroptosis in Neurosurgical Diseases. *Braz. J. Med. Biol. Res.* 48 (4), 292–298. doi:10.1590/1414-431X20144310

Liu, X., Liu, C., Tian, J., Gao, X., Li, K., Du, G., et al. (2020). Plasma Metabolomics of Depressed Patients and Treatment With Xiaoyaosan Based on Mass Spectrometry Technique. *J. Ethnopharmacol.* 246, 112219. doi:10.1016/j.jep.2019.112219

Liu, X., Zheng, X., Du, G., Li, Z., and Qin, X. (2019a). Brain Metabonomics Study of the Antidepressant-Like Effect of Xiaoyaosan on the CUMS-Depression Rats by 1H NMR Analysis. *J. Ethnopharmacol* 235, 141–154. doi:10.1016/j.jep.2019.01.018

Liu, Y., Ding, X. F., Wang, X. X., Zou, X. J., Li, X. J., Liu, Y. Y., et al. (2019b). Xiaoyaosan Exerts Antidepressant-Like Effects by Regulating the Functions of Astrocytes and EAATs in the Prefrontal Cortex of Mice. *BMC Complement. Altern. Med.* 19 (1), 215. doi:10.1186/s12906-019-2613-6

Luo, T. T., Lu, Y., Yan, S. K., Xiao, X., Rong, X. L., and Guo, J. (2020). Network Pharmacology in Research of Chinese Medicine Formula: Methodology, Application and Prospective. *Chin. J. Integr. Med.* 26 (1), 72–80. doi:10.1007/s11655-019-3064-0

Maes, M. (1995). Evidence for an Immune Response in Major Depression: A Review and Hypothesis. *Prog. Neuropsychopharmacol. Biol. Psychiatry.* 19 (1), 11–38. doi:10.1016/0278-5846(94)00101-m

Marunouchi, T., Ito, T., Onda, S., Kyo, L., Takahashi, K., Uchida, M., et al. (2021). Effects of 17-AAG on the RIP1/RIP3/MLKL Pathway During the Development of Heart Failure Following Myocardial Infarction in Rats. *J. Pharmacol. Sci.* 147 (2), 192–199. doi:10.1016/j.jphs.2021.06.009

Moriwaki, K., and Chan, F. K. (2016). Necroptosis-Independent Signaling by the RIP Kinases in Inflammation. *Cell Mol Life Sci.* 73 (11-12), 2325–2334. doi:10.1007/s00018-016-2203-4

Moussavi, S., Chatterji, S., Verdes, E., Tandon, A., Patel, V., and Ustun, B. (2007). Depression, Chronic Diseases, and Decrements in Health: Results From the World Health Surveys. *Lancet.* 370 (9590), 851–858. doi:10.1016/s0140-6736(07)61415-9

Mucha, M., Skrzypiec, A. E., Schiavon, E., Attwood, B. K., Kucerova, E., and Pawlak, R. (2011). Lipocalin-2 Controls Neuronal Excitability and Anxiety by Regulating Dendritic Spine Formation and Maturation. *Proc. Natl. Acad. Sci. U S A.* 108 (45), 18436–18441. doi:10.1073/pnas.1107936108

Müller, N., and Schwarz, M. J. (2010). S03-03 - Antiinflammatory Treatment Approaches in Major Depression. *Eur. Psychiatry.* 25 (10), 120. doi:10.1016/s0924-9338(10)70120-6

Newton, K., and Manning, G. (2016). Necroptosis and Inflammation. *Annu. Rev. Biochem.* 85 (1), 743–763. doi:10.1146/annurev-biochem-060815-014830

Pan, Q., Wu, J., Liu, Y., Li, X., and Chen, J. (2019). Involvement of Hepatic SHIP2 and PI3K/Akt Signalling in the Regulation of Plasma Insulin by Xiaoyaosan in Chronic Immobilization-Stressed Rats. *Molecules.* 24 (3), 480. doi:10.3390/molecules24030480

Papp, M., Moryl, E., and Willner, P. (1996). Pharmacological Validation of the Chronic Mild Stress Model of Depression. *Eur. J. Pharmacol.* 296 (2), 129–136. doi:10.1016/0014-2999(95)00697-4

Pasco, J. A., Nicholson, G. C., Williams, L. J., Jacka, F. N., Henry, M. J., Kotowicz, M. A., et al. (2010). Association of High-Sensitivity C-Reactive Protein With De Novo Major Depression. *Br. J. Psychiatry.* 197 (5), 372–377. doi:10.1192/bjp.bp.109.076430

Pasparakis, M., and Vandenabeele, P. (2015). Necroptosis and its Role in Inflammation. *Nature.* 517 (7534), 311–320. doi:10.1038/nature14191

Peng, G. J., Tian, J. S., Gao, X. X., Zhou, Y. Z., and Qin, X. M. (2015). Research on the Pathological Mechanism and Drug Treatment Mechanism of Depression. *Curr. Neuropharmacol.* 13 (4), 514–523. doi:10.2174/1570159x1304150831120428

Qu, Y., Tang, J., Wang, H., Li, S., Zhao, F., Zhang, L., et al. (2017). RIPK3 Interactions With MLKL and CaMKII Mediate Oligodendrocytes Death in the Developing Brain. *Cell Death Dis.* 8 (2), e2629. doi:10.1038/cddis.2017.54

Rodriguez, D. A., Weinlich, R., Brown, S., Guy, C., Fitzgerald, P., Dillon, C. P., et al. (2016). Characterization of RIPK3-Mediated Phosphorylation of the Activation Loop of MLKL during Necroptosis. *Cell Death Differ.* 23 (1), 76–88. doi:10.1038/cdd.2015.70

Ru, J., Li, P., Wang, J., Zhou, W., Li, B., Huang, C., et al. (2014). TCMSP: a Database of Systems Pharmacology for Drug Discovery From Herbal Medicines. *J. Cheminform.* 6, 13. doi:10.1186/1758-2946-6-13

Sawada, A., Niiyama, Y., Ataka, K., Nagaishi, K., Yamakage, M., and Fujimiya, M. (2014). Suppression of Bone Marrow-Derived Microglia in the Amygdala Improves Anxiety-Like Behavior Induced by Chronic Partial Sciatic Nerve Ligation in Mice. *Pain.* 155 (9), 1762–1772. doi:10.1016/j.pain.2014.05.031

Schwabe, R. F., and Luedde, T. (2018). Apoptosis and Necroptosis in the Liver: a Matter of Life and Death. *Nat. Rev. Gastroenterol. Hepatol.* 15 (12), 738–752. doi:10.1038/s41575-018-0065-y

Shalom, G., Lifschytz, T., Lerer, B., and Newman, M. E. (2006). Effects of T3 and Fluoxetine in the Novelty-Suppressed Feeding Test Model of Depression and Anxiety: Gender Differences. *Eur. Neuropsychopharmacol.* 16 (06), S48–S49. doi:10.1016/s0924-977x(06)80058-1

Shan, B., Pan, H., Najafov, A., and Yuan, J. (2018). Necroptosis in Development and Diseases. *Genes Dev.* 32 (5-6), 327–340. doi:10.1101/gad.312561.118

Shao, L., Liu, X., Zhu, S., Liu, C., Gao, Y., and Xu, X. (2018). The Role of Smurf1 in Neuronal Necroptosis after Lipopolysaccharide-Induced Neuroinflammation. *Cell Mol Neurobiol.* 38 (4), 809–816. doi:10.1007/s10571-017-0553-6

Sheng, Q., Du, R., Ma, C., Zhou, Y., Shen, X., Hou, X., et al. (2021). NMPA-Approved Traditional Chinese Medicine-Pingwei Pill: New Indication for Colistin Recovery Against MCR-Positive Bacteria Infection. *Chin. Med.* 16 (1), 106. doi:10.1186/s13020-021-00518-y

Sonenshine, D. E., and Macaluso, R. K. (2017). Microbial Invasion vs. Tick Immune Regulation. *Front. Cell Infect. Microbiol.* 7, 390. doi:10.3389/fcimb.2017.00390

Stacey, R., and Wei-Xing, Z. (2006). Chemotherapeutic Approaches for Targeting Cell Death Pathways. *Oncologist.* 11 (4), 342–357. doi:10.1634/theoncologist.11-4-342

Stein, D. J., Naudé, P. J., and Berk, M. (2018). Stress, Depression, and Inflammation: Molecular and Microglial Mechanisms. *Biol. Psychiatry.* 83 (1), 5. doi:10.1016/j.biopsych.2017.10.025

Stelzer, G., Rosen, N., Plaschkes, I., Zimmerman, S., Twik, M., Fishilevich, S., et al. (2016). The GeneCards Suite: From Gene Data Mining to Disease Genome Sequence Analyses. *Curr. Protoc. Bioinformatics.* 54, 131–3031. doi:10.1002/cpbi.5

Streit, W. J., Mrak, R. E., and Griffin, W. S. T. (2004). Microglia and Neuroinflammation: a Pathological Perspective. *J. Neuroinflammation.* 1 (1), 14. doi:10.1186/1742-2094-1-14

Szklarczyk, D., Gable, A. L., Lyon, D., Junge, A., Wyder, S., Huerta-Cepas, J., et al. (2019). STRING V11: Protein-Protein Association Networks With Increased Coverage, Supporting Functional Discovery in Genome-Wide Experimental Datasets. *Nucleic Acids Res.* 47 (D1), D607–d613. doi:10.1093/nar/gky1131

Takahashi, N., Duprez, L., Grootjans, S., Cauwels, A., Nerinckx, W., DuHadaway, J. B., et al. (2012). Necrostatin-1 Analogues: Critical Issues on the Specificity, Activity and *In Vivo* Use in Experimental Disease Models. *Cell Death Dis.* 3 (11), e437. doi:10.1038/cddis.2012.176

Thadathil, N., Nicklas, E. H., Mohammed, S., Lewis, T. L., Jr., Richardson, A., and Deepa, S. S. (2021). Necroptosis Increases With Age in the Brain and Contributes to Age-Related Neuroinflammation. *Geroscience.* doi:10.1007/s11357-021-00448-5

Vandenabeele, P., Declercq, W., and Berghe, T. V. (2008). Necrotic Cell Death and 'Necrostatins': Now We Can Control Cellular Explosion. *Trends Biochem. Sci.* 33 (8), 352–355. doi:10.1016/j.tibs.2008.05.007

Vugmeyster, Y., Harrold, J., and Xu, X. (2012). Absorption, Distribution, Metabolism, and Excretion (ADME) Studies of Biotherapeutics for Autoimmune and Inflammatory Conditions. *Aaps J.* 14 (4), 714–727. doi:10.1208/s12248-012-9385-y

Wang, L., Zhou, G. B., Liu, P., Song, J. H., Liang, Y., Yan, X. J., et al. (2008). Dissection of Mechanisms of Chinese Medicinal Formula Realgar-Indigo Naturalis as an Effective Treatment for Promyelocytic Leukemia. *Proc. Natl. Acad. Sci. U S A.* 105 (12), 4826–4831. doi:10.1073/pnas.0712365105

Wang, M., Huang, W., Gao, T., Zhao, X., and Lv, Z. (2018). Effects of Xiao Yao San on Interferon-Alpha-Induced Depression in Mice. *Brain Res. Bull.* 139, 197–202. doi:10.1016/j.brainresbull.2017.12.001

Wang, Y., Zhang, S., Li, F., Zhou, Y., Zhang, Y., Wang, Z., et al. (2020). Therapeutic Target Database 2020: Enriched Resource for Facilitating Research and Early Development of Targeted Therapeutics. *Nucleic Acids Res.* 48 (D1), D1031–d1041. doi:10.1093/nar/gkz981

Weiss, J. M. (1997). Does Decreased Sucrose Intake Indicate Loss of Preference in CMS Model? *Psychopharmacology.* 134 (4), 368–370. doi:10.1007/s002130050472

Wishart, D. S., Feunang, Y. D., Guo, A. C., Lo, E. J., Marcu, A., Grant, J. R., et al. (2018). DrugBank 5.0: a Major Update to the DrugBank Database for 2018. *Nucleic Acids Res.* 46 (D1), D1074–d1082. doi:10.1093/nar/gkx1037

Wu, J., Huang, Z., Ren, J., Zhang, Z., He, P., Li, Y., et al. (2013). Mlkl Knockout Mice Demonstrate the Indispensable Role of Mlkl in Necroptosis. *Cell Res.* 23 (8), 994–1006. doi:10.1038/cr.2013.91

Xiong, X., Wang, P., Duan, L., Liu, W., Chu, F., Li, S., et al. (2019). Efficacy and Safety of Chinese Herbal Medicine Xiao Yao San in Hypertension: A Systematic Review and Meta-Analysis. *Phytomedicine.* 61, 152849. doi:10.1016/j.phymed.2019.152849

Xu, Y., Sheng, H., Tang, Z., Lu, J., and Ni, X. (2015). Inflammation and Increased Ido in hippocampus Contribute to Depression-Like Behavior Induced by Estrogen Deficiency. *Behav. Brain Res.* 288, 71–78. doi:10.1016/j.bbr.2015.04.017

Yan, Z., Jiao, H., Ding, X., Ma, Q., and Chen, J. (2018). Xiaoyaosan Improves Depressive-Like Behaviors in Mice Through Regulating Apelin-APJ System in Hypothalamus. *Molecules.* 23 (5), 1073. doi:10.3390/molecules23051073

Yan, Z. Y., Li, X. J., Ding, X. F., Liu, Y. Y., and Chen, J. X. (2019). Evaluating the Anti-sepression Effect of Xiaoyaosan on Chronically-Stressed Mice. *J. Vis. Exp.* 143. doi:10.3791/58276

Yu, Z., Jiang, N., Su, W., and Zhuo, Y. (2021). Necroptosis: A Novel Pathway in Neuroinflammation. *Front. Pharmacol.* 12, 701564. doi:10.3389/fphar.2021.701564

Yuan, N., Gong, L., Tang, K., He, L., Hao, W., Li, X., et al. (2020). An Integrated Pharmacology-Based Analysis for Antidepressant Mechanism of Chinese Herbal Formula Xiao-Yao-San. *Front. Pharmacol.* 11, 284. doi:10.3389/fphar.2020.00284

Zhang, B. B., Liu, Y. M., Hu, A. L., Xu, S. F., Fan, L. D., Cheng, M. L., et al. (2019). HgS and Zuotai Differ From HgCl(2) and Methyl Mercury in Intestinal Hg Absorption, Transporter Expression and Gut Microbiome in Mice. *Toxicol. Appl. Pharmacol.* 379, 114615. doi:10.1016/j.taap.2019.114615

Zhou, X. M., Liu, C. Y., Liu, Y. Y., Ma, Q. Y., Zhao, X., Jiang, Y. M., et al. (2021). Xiaoyaosan Alleviates Hippocampal Glutamate-Induced Toxicity in the CUMS Rats via NR2B and PI3K/Akt Signaling Pathway. *Front. Pharmacol.* 12, 586788. doi:10.3389/fphar.2021.586788

Zhu, H. Z., Liang, Y. D., Ma, Q. Y., Hao, W. Z., Li, X. J., Wu, M. S., et al. (2019). Xiaoyaosan Improves Depressive-Like Behavior in Rats with Chronic Immobilization Stress through Modulation of the Gut Microbiota. *Biomed. Pharmacother.* 112, 108621. doi:10.1016/j.biopha.2019.108621

5

Closing the Gap Between Therapeutic Use and Mode of Action in Remedial Herbs

*Joaquim Olivés[1] and Jordi Mestres[1,2]**

[1] Research Group on Systems Pharmacology, Research Programme on Biomedical Informatics (GRIB), IMIM Hospital del Mar Medical Research Institute, Barcelona, Spain, [2] Department of Experimental and Health Sciences, University Pompeu Fabra, Barcelona, Spain

***Correspondence:**
Jordi Mestres
jmestres@imim.es

The ancient tradition of taking parts of a plant or preparing plant extracts for treating certain discomforts and maladies has long been lacking a scientific rationale to support its preparation and still widespread use in several parts of the world. In an attempt to address this challenge, we collected and integrated data connecting metabolites, plants, diseases, and proteins. A mechanistic hypothesis is generated when a metabolite is known to be present in a given plant, that plant is known to be used to treat a certain disease, that disease is known to be linked to the function of a given protein, and that protein is finally known or predicted to interact with the original metabolite. The construction of plant–protein networks from mutually connected metabolites and diseases facilitated the identification of plausible mechanisms of action for plants being used to treat analgesia, hypercholesterolemia, diarrhea, catarrh, and cough. Additional concrete examples using both experimentally known and computationally predicted, and subsequently experimentally confirmed, metabolite–protein interactions to close the connection circle between metabolites, plants, diseases, and proteins offered further proof of concept for the validity and scope of the approach to generate mode of action hypotheses for some of the therapeutic uses of remedial herbs.

Keywords: ethnopharmacology, traditional medicine, network pharmacology, mechanism of action, phytochemicals, endogenous metabolites, plant metabolomics

INTRODUCTION

Plant leaves, roots, barks, and extracts have been used since the dawn of human history to treat various discomforts and maladies. The healing properties of remedial herbs were most likely identified through a long and serendipitous learning process that once acquired was carefully passed through generations. Still today, traditional medicines represent a well-established therapeutic alternative to synthetic drugs in vast parts of the world (Tao et al., 2014). However, there is still a profound lack of understanding about the specific chemical ingredient(s) and the exact mechanism(s) of action by which medicinal plants exert their therapeutic effect.

In recent years, global efforts to generate, collect, store, and make publicly available data connecting plants with their endogenous metabolites (phytoconstituents), interacting proteins, and disease indications have set the ground to develop novel systems approaches to unveiling the mode of action of remedial herbs (Liu et al., 2013; Lagunin et al., 2014; Chen et al., 2017). This is schematically illustrated in **Figure 1**. A number of publicly available well annotated databases on medicinal plants

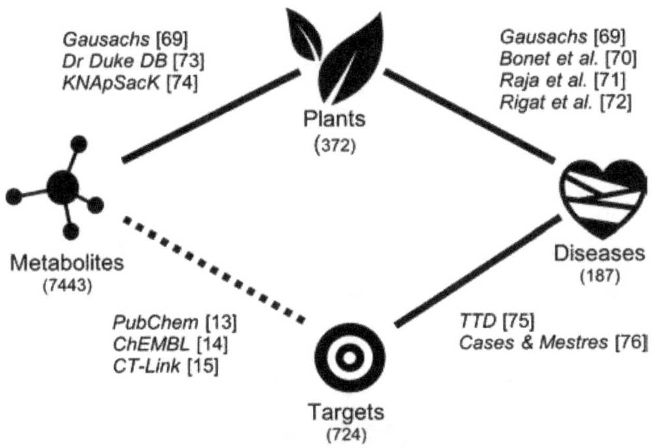

FIGURE 1 | Scheme showing the data sources and the process of closing the gap between the therapeutic use of plants and the protein targets predicted for the endogenous plant metabolites.

in use in different regions of the planet exist already (Chen, 2011; James et al., 2013; Ntie-Kang et al., 2013; Tota et al., 2013; Pathania et al., 2015; Mohanraj et al., 2018). Once data connecting the different aspects of ethnopharmacological relevance are known, the circle is closed and mechanistic hypotheses emerge naturally. The problem arises when gaps of data exist and the circles cannot be closed. In this respect, most current ethnomedicinal studies still focus on which parts of the plant are used to treat common ailments (Chassagne et al., 2016). Initiatives to identify and isolate some of the chemical structures present in those parts of therapeutic interest are expensive and inefficient. This notwithstanding, at least 50,000 endogenous plant metabolites have been already identified (Hounsome et al., 2008).

However, *in vitro* affinity data between plant metabolites and human proteins are scarce to find in public repositories (Bolton et al., 2008; Gaulton et al., 2012). Therefore, more efforts are needed in this direction to close the gap between therapeutic use and mode of action in remedial herbs (represented as a dotted line in **Figure 1**). One option is to process large libraries of isolated small molecules from plants through *in vitro* high-throughput screening assays to identify affinities for therapeutically relevant proteins. This is a highly tedious and expensive endeavor if one wants to be comprehensive. Alternatively, modern state-of-the-art computational methods to predict the affinity of small molecules across thousands of proteins can be used to prioritize any further *in vitro* testing of selected small molecules on particular proteins (Vidal et al., 2011; Garcia-Serna et al., 2015). Applications on predicting the targets of natural medicines are increasingly being reported (Keum et al., 2016; Fang et al., 2017; Sawada et al., 2018; Yi et al., 2018).

The last step involves connecting those confirmed interacting proteins with the actual disease for which the plant is prescribed. This task is now facilitated by the recent construction of databases connecting human genes with diseases (Piñero et al., 2017). The aim of this work is to collect and integrate all pieces of data and processes that allow for automatically generating mechanistic hypotheses for the known therapeutic uses of plants.

RESULTS AND DISCUSSION

Among the 372 medicinal plants present in our integrated database, *Sambucus nigra* (black elder) is the plant associated with the highest number of therapeutic uses (31). It is recommended for bronchitis, migraine, diarrhea, nausea, hyperuricemia, and influenza, to name just a few. Genus *Sambucus* belongs to the Caprifoliaceae family of flowering plants, whose leaves, flowers, and berries are traditionally used worldwide for a wide variety of medicinal applications (Dulf et al., 2013; Mahmoudi et al., 2014). Following *Sambucus nigra* in the list of plants with widest therapeutic use are *Allium sativum* (24), *Rosmarinus officinalis* (22), *Mentha spicata* (21), *Urtica dioica* (21), *Salvia officinalis* (21), and *Thymus vulgaris* (21), all of them found easily in many parts of the world and used as food and/or spice.

If we focus on cardiovascular diseases, a total of 171 plants were found to be associated with 46 different therapeutic uses. For illustrative purposes, the network of plants linked to cardiovascular diseases is shown in **Figure 2**. Among those, *Ginkgo biloba* is the plant with the most cardiovascular uses (with 14), followed by *Camellia sinensis* (with 8) and *Allium cepa, Crataegus monogyna, Olea europea, Urtica doica*, and *Vitis vinifera* (with 7). Among diseases, hypertension, hypercholesterolemia, hyperglycemia, and haemorrhoids are clearly the cardiovascular aspects being most addressed by remedial herbs.

Ginkgo biloba and *Camellia sinensis* are indigenous plants from Asia (Cybulska-Heinrich et al., 2012; Moore et al., 2009). The extracts of the leaves and nuts from *Ginkgo biloba* have been used for hundreds of years to treat a wide variety of disorders, such as asthma, vertigo, tinnitus, as well as general circulatory problems (Cybulska-Heinrich et al., 2012). *Camellia sinensis* is a plant from which green tea can be produced. This beverage has a long traditional use as social drink but also as medicine in the treatment and prevention of disorders, dysfunctions, or diseases in humans and other animals (Batista et al., 2009; Moore et al., 2009). *Aesculus hippocastanum* (horse chestnut) is native to the countries of the Balkan Peninsula, but it is cultivated worldwide for its beauty. Historically, seed extracts from this plant have been used as a treatment for many ailments (Anonymous, 2009). *Crataegus monogyna* (hawthorn) is known as a traditional medicinal plant in many countries, growing in shrub communities and decidious thin forests (Öztürk and Tunçel, 2011). *Vitis vinifera* (grapevine) is an indigenous plant from southern and Western Asia, but it is cultivated today in all temperature regions of the world (Nassiri-Asl and Hosseinzadeh, 2009). Finally, *Allium cepa* (onion) is one of the most important vegetables worldwide and is extensively cultivated. It is an herbaceous bulbous plant that has a long tradition of being beneficial against inflammation, general cardiovascular diseases, and cancer (Slimestad et al., 2007).

Regarding knowledge on the chemical composition of plants, *Camellia sinensis* (green tea) is the plant with the highest number of chemical structures identified (710), followed by *Zea mays* (677) and *Panax ginseng* (601). Other chemically well characterized plants are *Citrus sinensis* (orange tree), *Apium graveolens* (celery), and *Daucus carota* (carrot), with 589, 533, and 507 known

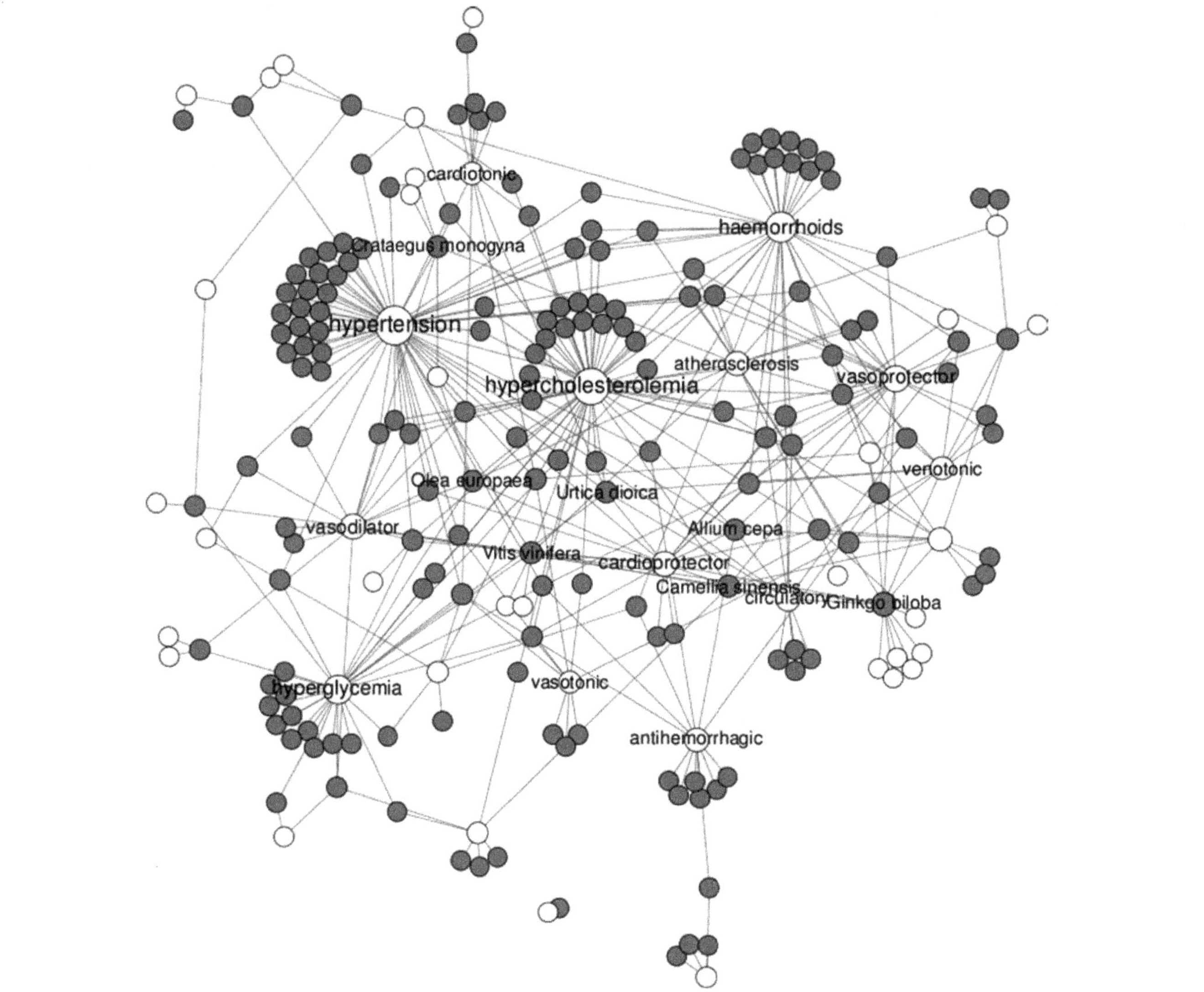

FIGURE 2 | Network of remedial herbs (gray circles) linked to therapeutic uses in cardiovascular diseases (white circles).

molecules, respectively. In contrast, many plants in the database have only one or very few endogenous metabolites identified, such as *Rhamnus alaternus* (Mediterranean blackthorn), *Lonicera etrusca* (honeysuckle), or *Hernaria glabra* (herniaria).

A detailed analysis of all the links between plants, metabolites, targets, and diseases in our integrated database (**Figure 1**) identified a total of 31,808 mechanistic hypotheses. At this stage, a mechanistic hypothesis is generated if a given plant known to have some therapeutic use contains at least one endogenous metabolite that is either known or predicted to interact with a human protein associated with its original therapeutic use. It ought to be stressed here that the concentration of any plant metabolite in a herbal preparation is very low and that, by any means, the results presented below imply that the metabolite assigned to the mechanistic hypothesis is the sole responsible of the therapeutic action of the plant but it will somehow contribute it. In this respect, a total of 893 mechanistic hypotheses for its different therapeutic uses could be generated for *Glycine max* (soybean). Among the plants with the highest number of mechanistic hypotheses generated, we found *Ginkgo biloba* (793), *Camellia sinensis* (781), *Citrus limon* (578), and *Vitis vinifera* (563). Out of the total number of 31,808 mechanistic hypotheses generated, 14,308 involved known interactions between endogenous metabolites and protein targets, whereas the remaining 17,500 hypotheses emerged from predicted interactions (see *Materials and Methods*).

Retrospective Validation

Among the molecules involved in the mechanistic hypotheses generated with known metabolite–protein interactions, we identified some well-known single active principles, such as atropine, morphine, and digitoxin, as well as a mixture of active principles, such as the one composed of quercetin, luteolin, and apigenin (**Figure 3**).

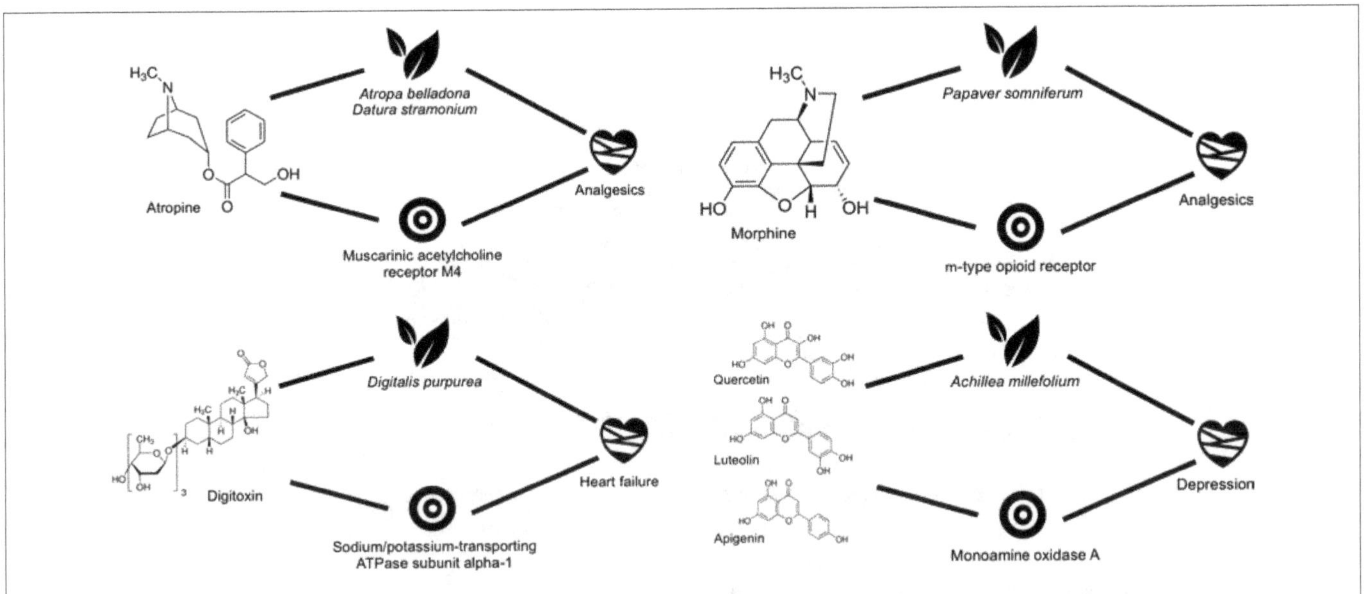

FIGURE 3 | Scheme showing some of the closed circles confirmed retrospectively for some of the plants being used in cardiovascular diseases.

Atropine is found mainly in *Atropa belladonna* and *Datura stramonium* (Kurzbaum et al., 2001; Caksen et al., 2003), both used commonly for their analgesic action (Duttaroy et al., 2002; Overington et al., 2006). This molecule is known to be active against the muscarinic acetylcholine receptor M4, a therapeutic target associated with some analgesics. Therefore, we have all links described in **Figure 1** confirmed and thus forming a mechanistic hypothesis for the analgesic action of these plants (Soni et al., 2012; Owais et al., 2014).

Another widely recognized molecule for its analgesic activity is morphine. It is found in *Papaver somniferum* (opium poppy), and it was the first active alkaloid extracted from this plant (Jurna, 2003). Opium has been used in traditional medicinal as sedative and analgesic (Calixto et al., 2001). According to all links established in our database, morphine would be directly identified as a candidate to contribute to the analgesic action of opium through its interaction with μ-type opioid receptor (Choi et al., 2006; Yamada et al., 2006), a receptor well known for its association with analgesia (Inturrisi, 2002).

Digitoxin is a glycoside with known activity against the sodium/potassium-transporting ATPase subunit α-1, a protein associated with heart failure (Müller-Ehmsen et al., 2002; Hauck et al., 2009). Digitoxin is found in *Digitalis purpurea* (Chen et al., 2001), a plant used in traditional medicine for treating precisely this particular disease. Digitoxin has not only been proven to interact with the sodium/potassium-transporting ATPase subunit α-1, but it has also been shown to be indeed effective in heart failure (Belz et al., 2001).

Finally, we selected an example in which three compounds, namely, quercetin, luteolin, and apigenin, all confirmed endogenous metabolites of *Achillea millefolium* (yarrow), a plant used traditionally for treating depression, are known to have biologically relevant affinities for monoamine oxidase A (Lemmens-Gruber et al., 2006; Han et al., 2007; Benetis et al., 2008; Bandaruk et al., 2014), which, in turn, is one of the target proteins for depression (Thase et al., 1995).

A more systematic analysis of all the mechanistic hypotheses that could be derived directly from known data and associations revealed that, among all disease categories, the circulatory, respiratory, and musculoskeletal systems collectively represented over 47% of all mechanistic hypotheses generated. The plant–protein networks derived for some specific diseases within these categories are shown in **Figure 4**.

In the analgesia network (**Figure 4**, top), one can observe that plants have multiple connections with a diverse range of proteins. This reflects the fact that some of the endogenous metabolites found in those plants have biologically relevant affinities for many of those proteins. Among them, aldose reductase (Young et al., 1983), muscarinic acetylcholine receptors (Duttaroy et al., 2002), and opioid receptors (Inturrisi, 2002) are the ones being most targeted by metabolites from these plants. Altogether, the formation of this complex network is indicative of a variety of plausible mechanisms of action relevant to analgesia, although one cannot exclude the possibility that the proteins involved in this analgesia network are closely related by cross-pharmacology, that is, they interact with similar ligands (Keiser et al., 2007; Briansó et al., 2011).

In contrast, the catarrh and cough networks (**Figure 4**, bottom) show that plants indicated for these therapeutic uses have endogenous metabolites targeting very much the same proteins. For catarrh, all plants contain some chemical entity that is active on the dopamine D1B, D2, and D3 receptors, all of them well known to be associated with respiratory diseases (Birrell et al., 2002). For cough, all plants contain at least one chemical entity with affinity for the μ and δ opioid receptors (Kotzer et al., 2000).

In between these two limit situations, the plant–protein networks obtained for hypercholesterolemia and diarrhea (**Figure 4**, middle) are consistent with different plants linked to these therapeutic uses acting through a small number of different mechanistic hypotheses. In this respect, most plants used for treating hypercholesterolemia

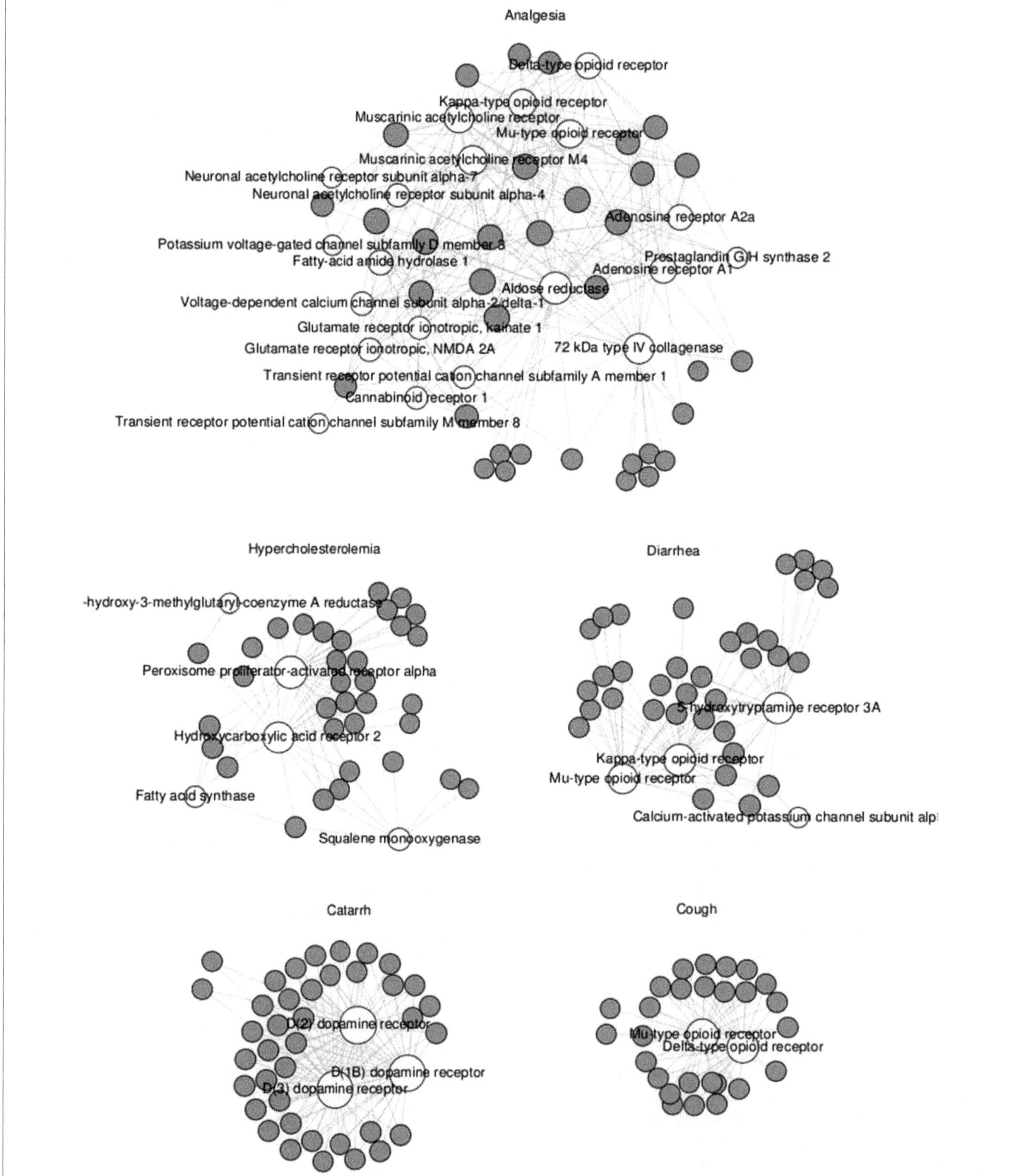

FIGURE 4 | Network of remedial herbs (gray circles) linked to proteins (white circles) associated with various maladies, namely, analgesia, hypercholesterolemia, diarrhea, catarrh, and cough.

seem to contain some chemical ingredient biologically active on the peroxisome proliferator-activated receptor α (56) and the hydroxycarboxylic receptor 2 (Karpe and Frayn, 2004). However, other plants may be exerting their therapeutic effect through interactions with some enzymes also associated with hypercholesterolemia, such as fatty acid synthase (Marseille-Tremblay et al., 2007) and squalene monooxygenase (Belter et al., 2011). Likewise, plants used for treating diarrhea contain chemical entities that have affinities for the μ and κ opioid receptors (Callahan, 2002), the 5-hydroxytryptamine 3A receptor channel (Sikander et al., 2009), and/or the calcium-activated potassium channel subunit α-1 (Deng et al., 2015). Even though many plants are targeting all of them, others seem to target only one or two.

It is important to highlight at this stage that the use of known data only is prone to the effects of completeness, and thus, several links may actually be missing in the networks discussed. In fact, looking at the distribution of the affinity values for those known interactions, we observe that in many cases these interacting chemicals are found also in plants that are not used for treating the disease associated with the interacting protein. Some of the reasons why these plants have not been used for these illnesses could be, for example, that the compound concentration is not enough in the plant or the plant really has this therapeutic action but it is simply not used for it. The same plant may have different uses in different parts of the world. Last but not least, it could well be that the action of some of these compounds requires the presence of some bioenhancer (Dudhatra et al., 2012), the therapeutic action being ultimately the result of multiple compounds acting synergistically. Overall, from the initial number of 372 plants associated with at least one therapeutic use, only 193 contain known data for all necessary links to derive a mechanistic hypothesis. Accordingly, the following section illustrates the use of high-confidence predictions as a means to enlarge the coverage of plants for which mechanistic hypotheses can be derived.

Prospective Evaluation

Before embarking into the analysis of some of the mechanistic hypotheses emerging from predicted interactions, we validated the expected accuracy of those predictions for which known data was available. Overall, a good correlation was found between known and predicted affinity values for the same molecule–protein interactions. The median of the difference in affinities was 0.332, with 25% and 75% quartiles being at −0.1 and 0.7 with respect to the median, respectively, with a standard deviation of 0.794. Then, for those predicted interactions only, we focused on those providing a balance between potency of the predicted affinity and novelty of the prediction, as regarded by the similarity to the closest molecule for which the affinity for the same protein is known already. Among those, we prioritised the confirmation of the proposed mechanistic hypotheses for two single compounds, namely, rybosylzeatin and isorhamnetin, and one compound mixture, composed of cyanidin, delphinidin, and malvidin. The results are compiled in **Figure 5**.

Ribosylzeatin is an endogenous metabolite present in *Ginkgo biloba* (gingko), *Glycine max* (soybean), and *Vitis vinifera* (grapevine). This small molecule was predicted to have low micromolar affinity for the adenosine A1 and A3 receptors and *in vitro* testing performed subsequently confirmed 57% and 65% binding, respectively, at 10mM concentration. Accordingly, a mechanistic hypothesis could be derived suggesting that the interaction of ribosylzeatin with the adenosine A1 and A3 receptors may be contributing to the beneficial effects of those plants in the treatment of a number of cardiovascular diseases where these receptors are known to play a role, namely, cardiac dysrhythmias, supraventricular tachycardia, acute ischaemic heart disease, and mycocardial ischemia (Kiesman et al., 2009; Fishman et al., 2012). In this respect, soybean is known as an important source of proteins in diet, widely used as herbal medicine for the treatment of several cardiovascular diseases. Also, the cardioprotector properties of grapevine have been exploited in folk medicine since

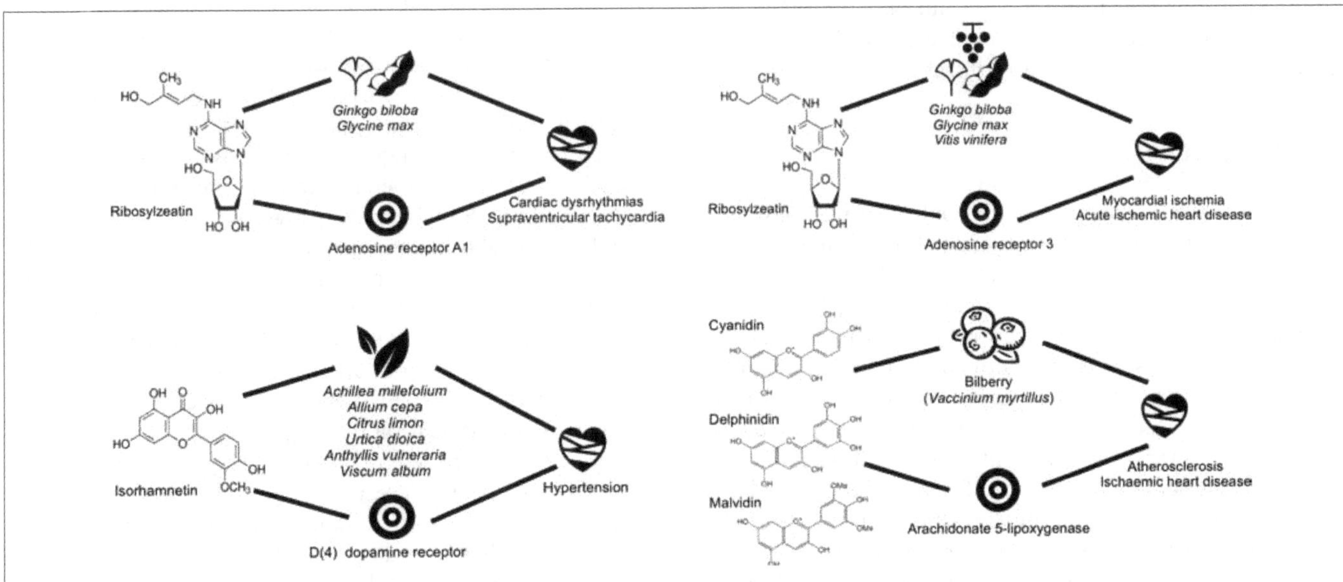

FIGURE 5 | Scheme showing some of the closed circles confirmed prospectively for some of the plants being used in cardiovascular diseases.

ancient times. In particular, the therapeutic action of grapevine against ventricular tachycardia was recently demonstrated in rats (Zhao et al., 2010). However, in this study, the authors used a proanthocyanidin grape seed extract. On the basis of the hypothesis generated here, we would suggest that ribosylzeatin is one of the active ingredients in grapevine participating in this therapeutic effect in synergy with other proanthocyanidins.

Isorhamnetin is a phytochemical present in multiple plants used for the treatment of hypertension. A low micromolar affinity between isorhamnetin and the dopamine D4 receptor was predicted. Upon *in vitro* testing, the experimental value obtained was only 28% binding. Despite this rather low affinity value, we could suggest that this compound may well be contributing to some extent to the effect on hypertension of the plants in which it is present. In fact, a similar chemical present in most of those plants listed and suggested to be partly responsible for their therapeutic action on hypertension is quercetin, reported to have also a low experimental affinity value of 5 μM against the same dopamine D4 receptor.

Finally, very much along the same lines reported above for the hypotheses generated from known metabolite–protein interactions, we were also keen on having a prospective mixture example. Accordingly, we predicted activity of cyanidin, delphinidin, and malvidin, all present in *Vaccinium myrtillus* (bilberry), on the arachidonate 5-lipoxygenase (ALOX5). *In vitro* testing of its mixture confirmed a 41% inhibition. This result provides a mechanistic hypothesis for the therapeutic use of bilberry for atherosclerosis and ischemic heart disease. It has been already suggested that quercetin is partially responsible for the therapeutic action of this plant due to its affinity for the ALOX5. We could add now delphinidin, cyanidin, and malvidin to the list of potential chemical effectors of this plant. Indeed, bilberry fruit contains high concentration of several anthocyanidins (Cassinese et al., 2007; Chu et al., 2011). In fact, other anthocyanidins present in bilberry, such as peonidin and petunidin, were also predicted to be active against this protein. So all these compounds may actually contribute synergistically to the therapeutic effect attributed to bilberry for the treatment of atherosclerosis and ischemic heart disease.

CONCLUSIONS

An effort to integrate data linking metabolites, plants, diseases, and proteins has been shown to be useful to generate mechanistic hypotheses for some of the therapeutic uses of remedial herbs. In this respect, the use of predicted interactions largely increases our ability to generate mechanistic hypotheses for plants for which known data is scarce. This notwithstanding, one ought to admit that many computationally derived hypotheses may either be false positives or not truly contribute to the therapeutic effect exhibited by the medicinal plant. Unfortunately, it is impossible to pursue experimental confirmation of all hypotheses generated and offer general statistics of this limitation. Nonetheless, the examples presented offer clear potential for the use of this type of systems approaches to contribute to finding a scientific rationale for traditional medicines. There is much more to learn about nature and its use for therapeutic purposes, and more research in this direction is certainly necessary.

MATERIALS AND METHODS

Linking plants to diseases. A very first version of the database was created containing the therapeutic use of plants in traditional Catalan medicine (Gausachs, 2008). Plants were stored using their scientific name in Latin, whereas therapeutic uses were mapped to their corresponding disease identifier in ICD-10 (International Classification of Diseases Version 10). This initial database was complemented with additional therapeutic uses found for those plants in other public sources (Raja et al., 1997; Rigat et al., 2007; James et al., 2013). Data from the different sources was integrated using Latin names for plants and ICD-10 identifiers for diseases from 18 categories. In total, 372 medicinal plants associated with 187 therapeutic uses were collected at this stage (**Supplementary Material**).

Linking plants to metabolites. The endogenous metabolites identified at present for every single plant in the database were extracted from three different sources, namely, Dr Duke Phytochemical and Ethnobotanical Database (U.S. Department of Agriculture, Agricultural Research Service., 1992-2016), the KNApSAcK database (Nakamura et al., 2014), and Gausachs' work on Catalan remedial herbs (Gausachs, 2008). Among those, only KNApSacK contains chemical structures linked to chemical names. Structures for the chemical names available only in the other two sources were extracted from PubChem (Bolton et al., 2008). The final set of chemical structures from all sources was unified and stored using InChI Keys. In the end, a total of 7,443 unique chemical structures present in 322 of those 372 medicinal plants could be gathered and added to the database (**Supplementary Material**).

Linking proteins to diseases. Next, a list of both known and explored human proteins associated with diseases was extracted from the Therapeutic Target Database (Zhu et al., 2012). These data was complemented with curated protein–disease links, with focus on cardiovascular diseases, available in the literature (Cases and Mestres, 2009). The final list of proteins was stored and unified using their UniProt identifiers (The UniProt Consortium, 2015). A final number of 724 unique proteins known to be relevant for 166 out of the initial 187 therapeutic uses were ultimately entered into the database (**Supplementary Material**).

Linking metabolites to proteins. Finally, affinity data (pK_i, pK_d, pIC_{50}, pEC_{50}) between chemical structures and proteins was extracted from various public sources (Roth et al., 2004; Bolton et al., 2008; Gaulton et al., 2012; Gilson et al., 2016; Southan et al., 2016). Up to 3,171 known interactions between 705 phytoconstituents and 228 proteins were identified and collected into the database at this stage. In addition, since affinity data are well recognised to be suffering from completeness issues (Mestres et al., 2008; Cases and Mestres, 2009), known interactions between molecules and proteins were complemented with high-confidence predictions obtained using ligand-based computational models implemented in the CT-link software (Vidal et al., 2011; Garcia-Serna et al., 2015). Accordingly, 16,897 additional interactions predicted between 2,796 molecules, present in 297 plants, and 313 proteins were generated. However, the vast majority of the interactions predicted were assigned relatively low confidence scores (CScore). If only high confidence predictions (CScore $\geq$ 0.7) are considered, a total of 1,555 predicted interactions remain. In the end, affinity data for a total of 4,726 interactions between 1,157 endogenous metabolites and 320 therapeutically relevant proteins were assembled and stored in the database (**Supplementary Material**).

Predicting metabolite–protein interactions. All metabolite two-dimensional structures were processed with the CT-link software to obtain predicted affinities for a list of over 2,000 protein targets (Vidal et al., 2011; Garcia-Serna et al., 2015). Predictions are based on six independent ligand-based approaches that include similarity-based methods, pharmacophore clusters, quantitative structure–activity relationships, machine learning techniques, and cross-pharmacology relationships (Vidal et al., 2011). Ligand-based target models were constructed from small molecules for which *in vitro* affinity data was publicly available (Bolton et al., 2008; Gaulton et al., 2012). Each prediction is assigned a confidence score (CScore) that depends on the number and type of methods as well as on the affinity range of the prediction (see **Supplementary Material**). In the last decade, predictions from CT-link have been validated both retrospectively (Vidal and Mestres, 2010; Flachner et al., 2012; Spitzmüller and Mestres, 2013) and prospectively (Areias et al., 2010; Mestres et al., 2011; Antolin et al., 2012; Montolio et al., 2012; Antolin and Mestres, 2015; van Voorhuis et al., 2016; Ellis et al., 2019) in a wide range of applications and therapeutic areas.

Experimental *in vitro* assays. For the prospective validation, two molecules and one herbal extract were selected for testing with *in vitro* assays at Cerep (CEREP Inc). Ribosylzeatin was tested in binding assays to confirm the predicted interactions with adenosine A1 and A3 receptors. Cellular assays were used to confirm the predicted interactions between isorhamnetin and the dopamine D4 receptor, as well as between a compound mixture (containing cyanidin, delphinidin, and malvidin) and 5-lipoxygenase.

For the binding assay, ribosylzeatin was tested twice at a test concentration of 10 μM. The reference agonist ligands used to calculate the compound activity were CPA for the adenosine A1 receptor and IB-MECA for the adenosine A3 receptor, which have IC_{50} values of 0.75 nM and 0.31 nM, respectively. The adenosine A1 receptor assay was performed in the presence of 1 nM of 3H.CCPA. After 60 min of incubation with shaking, bound radioactivity was separated from free by vacuum filtration and determined by scintillation counting. A similar procedure was followed for the adenosine A3 receptor assay. In this case, it was performed in the presence of 0.15 nM of 125I.AB-MECA. It was incubated with shaking during 120 min. After that, bound radioactivity was filtered and measured with scintillation counting. For these binding assays the results are expressed as a percent of measured specific binding relative to control specific binding.

For the dopamine D4 receptor assay, isorhamnetin was tested at a concentration of 10 μM. The reference agonist ligand was dopamine, with an EC_{50} value of 28 nM. D4.4 was incubated for 10 min at 37°C and, after that, cAMP was detected and measured with HTRF. Results are expressed as a percentage of measured response relative to control response.

Finally, for the testing of the compound mixture of cyanidin, delphinidin, and malvidin in the 5-lipoxygenase enzyme assay, the reference compound used was NDGA, which has an IC_{50} of 910 nM. 5-Lipoxygenase was incubated 20 min with shaking and 25 μM arachidonic acid as substrate. Thereafter, rhodamine 123 was measured using fluorimetry. Results are expressed as a percentage of measured specific binding relative to control specific binding.

Compounds showing an inhibition or stimulation higher than 50% were considered to be active for the proteins tested, whereas interactions showing activity values between 25% and 50% were considered to be indicative of at least weak to moderate effects.

AUTHOR CONTRIBUTIONS

JM conceived and designed the study. JO acquired the data for the analysis. JO and JM analyzed and interpreted the data, discussed the results, and wrote the manuscript.

FUNDING

This research was supported by the Spanish Ministerio de Ciencia Innovación y Universidades (project SAF2017-83614-R).

SUPPLEMENTARY MATERIAL

SUPPLEMENTARY TABLE 1 | Collected data connecting diseases and plants, plants and metabolites, metabolites and proteins, and proteins and diseases. Also provided are the different subsets used to construct the plant-disease and plant-protein networks of Figures 2 and 4, respectively.

REFERENCES

Anonymous. (2009). *Aesculus hippocastanum* (Horse chestnut). *Altern. Med. Rev.* 14 (3), 278–283.

Antolin, A. A., and Mestres, J. (2015). Distant polypharmacology among MLP chemical probes. *ACS Chem. Biol.* 10 (2), 395–400. doi: 10.1021/cb500393m

Antolin, A. A., Jalencas, X., Yélamos, J., and Mestres, J. (2012). Identification of pim kinases as novel targets for PJ34 with confounding effects in PARP biology. *ACS Chem. Biol.* 7 (12), 1962–1967. doi: 10.1021/cb300317y

Areias, F. M., Brea, J., Gregori-Puigjané, E., Zaki, M. E. A., Carvalho, M. A., Domínguez, E., et al. (2010). In silico directed chemical probing of the adenosine receptor family. *Bioorg. Med. Chem.* 18 (9), 3043–3052. doi: 10.1016/j.bmc.2010.03.048

Bandaruk, Y., Mukai, R., and Terao, J. (2014). Cellular uptake of quercetin and luteolin and their effects on monoamine oxidase-A in human neuroblastoma SH-SY5Y cells. *Toxicol. Rep.* 1, 639–649. doi: 10.1016/j.toxrep.2014.08.016

Batista, G. de A. P., da Cunha, C. L. P., Scartezini, M., von der Heyde, R., Bitencourt, M. G., et al. (2009). Prospective double-blind crossover study of Camellia sinensis (green tea) in dyslipidemias. *Arq. Bras. Cardiol.* 93 (2), 128–134. doi: 10.1590/S0066-782X2009000800010

Belter, A., Skupinska, M., Giel-Pietraszuk, M., Grabarkiewicz, T., Rychlewski, L., and Barciszewski, J. (2011). Squalene monooxygenase – a target for hypercholesterolemic therapy. *Biol. Chem.* 392 (12), 1053–1075. doi: 10.1515/BC.2011.195

Belz, G. G., Breithaupt-Grogler, K., and Osowski, U. (2001). Treatment of congestive heart failure – current status of use of digitoxin. *Eur. J. Clin. Invest.* 31 Suppl 2, 10–17. doi: 10.1046/j.1365-2362.2001.0310s2010.x

Benetis, R., Radusiene, J., and Janulis, V. (2008). Variability of phenolic compounds in flowers of Achillea millefolium wild populations in Lithuania. *Med. Kaunas Lith.* 44 (10), 775–781. doi: 10.3390/medicina44100097

Birrell, M. A., Crispino, N., Hele, D. J., Patel, H. J., Yacoub, M. H., Barnes, P. J., et al. (2002). Effect of dopamine receptor agonists on sensory nerve activity: possible therapeutic targets for the treatment of asthma and COPD. *Br. J. Pharmacol.* 136 (4), 620–628. doi: 10.1038/sj.bjp.0704758

Bolton, E. E., Wang, Y., Thiessen, P. A., and Bryant, S. H. (2008). PubChem: integrated platform of small molecules and biological activities. *Annual Rep. Comput. Chem.* 4, 217–241. doi: 10.1016/S1574-1400(08)00012-1

Bonet, M. A., Parada, M., Selga, A., and Vallès, J. (1999). Studies on pharmaceutical ethnobotany in the regions of l'Alt Empordà and Les Guilleries (Catalonia, Iberian Peninsula). *J. Ethnopharmacol.* 68 (1–3), 145–168. doi: 10.1016/S0378-8741(99)00083-5

Briansó, F., Carrascosa, M. C., Oprea, T. I., and Mestres, J. (2011). Cross-pharmacology analysis of G protein-coupled receptors. *Curr. Top. Med. Chem.* 11 (15), 1956–1963. doi: 10.2174/156802611796391285

Caksen, H., Odabaş, D., Akbayram, S., Cesur, Y., Arslan, S., Uner, A., et al. (2003). Deadly nightshade (*Atropa belladonna*) intoxication: an analysis of 49 children. *Hum. Exp. Toxicol.* 22 (12), 665–668. doi: 10.1191/0960327103ht404oa

Calixto, J. B., Scheidt, C., Otuki, M., and Santos, A. R. (2001). Biological activity of plant extracts. *Expert Opin. Emerg. Drugs* 6 (2), 261–279. doi: 10.1517/14728214.6.2.261

Callahan, M. J. (2002). Irritable bowel syndrome neuropharmacology. A review of approved and investigational compounds. *J. Clin. Gastroenterol.* 35 (1 Suppl), 58–67. doi: 10.1097/00004836-200207001-00011

Cases, M., and Mestres, J. (2009). A chemogenomic approach to drug discovery: focus on cardiovascular diseases. *Drug Discov. Today* 14 (9–10), 479–485. doi: 10.1016/j.drudis.2009.02.010

Cassinese, C., de Combarieu, E., Falzoni, M., Fuzzati, N., Pace, R., and Sardone, N. (2007). New liquid chromatography method with ultraviolet detection for analysis of anthocyanins and anthocyanidins in Vaccinium myrtillus fruit dry extracts and commercial preparations. *J. AOAC Int.* 90 (4), 911–919.

CEREP Inc. http://www.cerep.fr/.

Chassagne, F., Hul, S., Deharo, E., and Bourdy, G. (2016). Natural remedies used by Bunong people in Mondulkiri province (Northeast Cambodia) with special reference to the treatment of 11 most common ailments. *J. Ethnopharmacol.* 191, 41–70. doi: 10.1016/j.jep.2016.06.003

Chen, C. Y.-C. (2011). TCM Database@Taiwan: the world's largest traditional Chinese medicine database for drug screening *in silico*. *PLoS ONE* 6 (1), e15939. doi: 10.1371/journal.pone.0015939

Chen, J. J., Wang, P. S., Chien, E. J., and Wang, S. W. (2001). Direct inhibitory effect of digitalis on progesterone release from rat granulosa cells. *Br. J. Pharmacol.* 132 (8), 1761–1768. doi: 10.1038/sj.bjp.0703974

Chen, Y., de Bruyn Kops, C., and Kirchmair, J. (2017). Data resources for the computer-guided discovery of bioactive natural products. *J. Chem. Inf. Model.* 57 (9), 2099–2111. doi: 10.1021/acs.jcim.7b00341

Choi, H. S., Kim, C. S., Hwang, C. K., Song, K. Y., Wang, W., Qiu, Y., et al. (2006). The opioid ligand binding of human mu-opioid receptor is modulated by novel splice variants of the receptor. *Biochem. Biophys. Res. Commun.* 343 (4), 1132–1140. doi: 10.1016/j.bbrc.2006.03.084

Chu, W., Cheung, S. C. M., Lau, R. A. W., and Benzie, I. F. F. (2011). "Bilberry (Vaccinium myrtillus L.)," in *Herbal Medicine: Biomolecular and Clinical Aspects* (Boca Raton (FL): CRC Press/Taylor & Francis). chapter 4. doi: 10.1201/b10787-5

Cybulska-Heinrich, A. K., Mozaffarieh, M., and Flammer, J. (2012). Ginkgo bilobal: an adjuvant therapy for progressive normal and high tension glaucoma. *Mol. Vis.* 18, 390–402.

Deng, Y., Han, X., Tang, S., Xiao, W., Tan, Z., Zhou, C., et al. (2015). Magnolol and honokiol regulate the calcium-activated potassium channels signaling pathway in Enterotoxigenic Escherichia coli-induced diarrhea mice. *Eur. J. Pharmacol.* 755, 66–73. doi: 10.1016/j.ejphar.2015.03.002

Dudhatra, G. B., Mody, S. K., Awale, M. M., Patel, H. B., Modi, C. M., Kumar, A., et al. (2012). A comprehensive review on pharmacotherapeutics of herbal bioenhancers. *Sci. World J.* 637953. doi: 10.1100/2012/637953

Dulf, F. V., Oroian, I., Vodnar, D. C., Socaciu, C., and Pintea, A. (2013). Lipid clases and fatty acid regiodistribution in triacylglycerols of seed oils of two Sambucus species (S. nigra L. and S. ebulus L.). *Molecules* 18 (10), 11768–11782. doi: 10.3390/molecules181011768

Duttaroy, A., Gomeza, J., Gan, J.-W., Siddiqui, N., Basile, A. S., Harman, W. D., et al. (2002). Evaluation of muscarinic agonist-induced analgesia in muscarinic acetylcholine receptor knockout mice. *Mol. Pharmacol.* 62 (5), 1084–1093. doi: 10.1124/mol.62.5.1084

Ellis, C. R., Racz, R., Kruhlak, N. L., Kim, M. T., Hawkins, E. G., Strauss, D. G., et al. (2019). Assessing the structural and pharmacological similarity of newly identified drugs of abuse to controlled substances using public health assessment via structural evaluation. *Clin. Pharmacol. Ther.* 106 (1), 116–122. doi: 10.1002/cpt.1418

Fang, J., Wu, Z., Cai, C., Wang, Q., Tang, Y., and Cheng, F. (2017). Quantitative and systems pharmacology. 1. *In silico* prediction of drug-target interactions of natural products enables new targeted cancer therapy. *J. Chem. Inf. Model.* 57 (11), 2657–2671. doi: 10.1021/acs.jcim.7b00216

Fishman, P., Bar-Yehuda, S., Liang, B. T., and Jacobson, K. A. (2012). Pharmacological and therapeutic effects of A3 adenosine receptor antagonists. *Drug Discov. Today* 17 (7–8), 359–366. doi: 10.1016/j.drudis.2011.10.007

Flachner, B., Lörincz, Z., Carotti, A., Nicolotti, O., Kuchipudi, P., Remez, N., et al. (2012). A chemocentric approach to the identification of cancer targets. *PLoS ONE* 7 (4), e35582. doi: 10.1371/journal.pone.0035582

Garcia-Serna, R., Vidal, D., Remez, N., and Mestres, J. (2015). Large-scale predictive drug safety: from structural alerts to biological mechanisms. *Chem. Res. Toxicol.* 28 (10), 1875–1887. doi: 10.1021/acs.chemrestox.5b00260

Gaulton, A., Bellis, L. J., Bento, A. P., Chambers, J., Davies, M., Hersey, A., et al. (2012). ChEMBL: a large-scale bioactivity database for drug discovery. *Nucleic Acids Res.* 40 (Database issue), D1100–D1107. doi: 10.1093/nar/gkr777

Gausachs, R. (2008). *Les Herbes Remeieres* Vol. 2. Barcelona: Rafael Dalmau.

Gilson, M. K., Liu, T., Baitaluk, M., Nicola, G., Hwang, L., and Chong, J. (2016). BindingDB in 2015: a public database for medicinal chemistry, computational chemistry and systems pharmacology. *Nucleic Acids Res.* 44 (D1), D1045–D1053. doi: 10.1093/nar/gkv1072

Han, X. H., Hong, S. S., Hwang, J. S., Lee, M. K., Hwang, B. Y., and Ro, J. S. (2007). Monoamine oxidase inhibitory components from *Cayratia japonica*. *Arch. Pharm. Res.* 30 (1), 13–17. doi: 10.1007/BF02977772

Hauck, C., Potter, T., Bartz, M., Wittwer, T., Wahlers, T., Mehlhorn, U., et al. (2009). Isoform specificity of cardiac glycosides binding to human Na+,K+-ATPase alpha1beta1, alpha2beta1 and alpha3beta1. *Eur. J. Pharmacol.* 622 (1–3), 7–14. doi: 10.1016/j.ejphar.2009.08.039

Hounsome, N., Hounsome, B., Tomos, D., and Edwards-Jones, G. (2008). Plant metabolites and nutritional quality of vegetables. *J. Food Sci.* 73 (4), 48–65. doi: 10.1111/j.1750-3841.2008.00716.x

Inturrisi, C. E. (2002). Clinical pharmacology of opioids for pain. *Clin. J. Pain* 18 (4 Suppl), S3–S13. doi: 10.1097/00002508-200207001-00002

James, P., Mathai, V. A., Shajikumar, S., Pereppadan, P. A., Sudha, P., Keshavachandran, R., et al. (2013). DIACAN: integrated database for antidiabetic and anticancer medicinal plants. *Bioinformation* 9 (18), 941–943. doi: 10.6026/97320630009941

Jurna, I. (2003). Sertürner und Morphin – eine historische Vignette. *Schmerz* 17, 280–283. doi: 10.1007/s00482-003-0220-3

Karpe, F., and Frayn, K. N. (2004). The nicotinic acid receptor – a new mechanism for an old drug. *Lancet* 363 (9424), 1892–1894. doi: 10.1016/S0140-6736(04)16359-9

Keiser, M. J., Roth, B. L., Armbruster, B. N., Ernsberger, P., Irwin, J. J., and Shoichet, B. K. (2007). Relating protein pharmacology by ligand chemistry. *Nat. Biotechnol.* 25 (2), 197–206. doi: 10.1038/nbt1284

Keum, J., Yoo, S., Lee, D., and Nam, H. (2016). Prediction of compound-target interactions of natural products using large-scale drug and protein information. *BMC Bioinformatics* 17 (Suppl 6), 219. doi: 10.1186/s12859-016-1081-y

Kiesman, W. F., Elzein, E., and Zablocki, J. (2009). A1 adenosine receptor antagonists, agonists, and allosteric enhancer. *Handb. Exp. Pharmacol.* 193, 25–58. doi: 10.1007/978-3-540-89615-9_2

Kotzer, C. J., Hay, D. W., Dondio, G., Giardina, G., Petrillo, P., and Underwood, D. C. (2000). The antitussive activity of delta-opioid receptor stimulation in guinea pigs. *J. Pharmacol. Exp. Ther.* 292 (2), 803–809.

Kurzbaum, A., Simsolo, C., Kvasha, L., and Blum, A. (2001). Toxic delirium due to *Datura stramonium*. *Isr. Med. Assoc. J.* 3 (7), 538–539.

Lagunin, A. A., Goel, R. K., Gawande, D. Y., Pahwa, P., Gloriozova, T. A., Dmitriev, A. V., et al. (2014). Chemo- and bioinformatics resources for in silico drug discovery from medicinal plants beyond their traditional use: a critical review. *Nat. Prod. Rev.* 31 (11), 1585–1611. doi: 10.1039/C4NP00068D

Lemmens-Gruber, R., Marchart, E., Rawnduzi, P., Engel, N., Benedek, B., and Kopp, B. (2006). Investigation of the spasmolytic activity of the flavonoid fraction of *Achillea millefolium* s.l. on isolated guinea-pig ilea. *Arzneimittelforschung* 56 (8), 582–588. doi: 10.1055/s-0031-1296755

Liu, H., Wang, J., Zhou, W., Wang, Y., and Yang, L. (2013). Systems approaches and polypharmacology for drug discovery from herbal medicines: an example using licorise. *J. Ethnopharmacol.* 146 (3), 773–793. doi: 10.1016/j.jep.2013.02.004

Mahmoudi, M., Ebrahimzadeh, M. A., Dooshan, A., Arimi, A., Ghasemi, N., and Fathiazad, F. (2014). Antidepressant activities of *Sambucus ebulus* and *Sambucus nigra*. *Eur. Rev. Med. Pharmacol. Sci.* 18 (22), 3350–3353.

Marseille-Tremblay, C., Gravel, A., Lafond, J., and Mounier, C. (2007). Effect of an enriched cholesterol diet during gestation on fatty acid synthase, HMG-CoA reductase and SREBP-1/2 expressions in rabbits. *Life Sci.* 81 (9), 772–778. doi: 10.1016/j.lfs.2007.07.016

Mestres, J., Gregori-Puigjané, E., Valverde, S., and Solé, R. V. (2008). Data completeness – the Achilles heel of drug-target networks. *Nat. Biotechnol.* 26 (9), 983–984. doi: 10.1038/nbt0908-983

Mestres, J., Seifert, S. A., and Oprea, T. I. (2011). Linking pharmacology to clinical reports: cyclobenzaprine and its possible association with serotonin syndrome. *Clin. Pharmacol. Ther.* 90 (5), 662–665. doi: 10.1038/clpt.2011.177

Mohanraj, K., Karthikeyan, B. S., Vivek-Ananth, R. P., Chand, R. P. B., Aparna, S. R., Mangalapandi, P., et al. (2018). IMPPAT: a curated database of Indian medicinal plants, phytochemistry and therapeutics. *Sci. Rep.* 8 (1), 4329. doi: 10.1038/s41598-018-22631-z

Montolio, M., Gregori-Puigjané, E., Pineda, D., Mestres, J., and Navarro, P. (2012). Identification of small molecule inhibitors of amyloid b-induced neuronal apoptosis acting through the imidazoline I(2) receptor. *J. Med. Chem.* 55 (22), 9838–9846. doi: 10.1021/jm301055g

Moore, R. J., Jackson, K. G., and Minihane, A. M. (2009). Green tea (Camellia sinensis) catechins and vascular function. *Br. J. Nutr.* 102 (12), 1790–1802. doi: 10.1017/S0007114509991218

Müller-Ehmsen, J., McDonough, A. A., Farley, R. A., and Schwinger, R. H. G. (2002). Sodium pump isoform expression in heart failure: implication for treatment. *Basic Res. Cardiol.* 97 Suppl 1, 25–30. doi: 10.1007/s003950200025

Nakamura, Y., Afendi, F. M., Parvin, A. K., Ono, N., Tanaka, K., Hirai, A., et al. (2014). KNApSAcK metabolite activity database for retrieving the relationships between metabolites and biological activities. *Plant Cell Physiol.* 55 (1), e7. doi: 10.1093/pcp/pct176

Nassiri-Asl, M., and Hosseinzadeh, H. (2009). Review of the pharmacological effects of *Vitis vinifera* (grape) and its bioactive compounds. *Phytother. Res.* 23 (9), 1197–1204. doi: 10.1002/ptr.2761

Ntie-Kang, F., Zofou, D., Babiaka, S. B., Meudom, R., Scharfe, M., Lifongo, L. L., et al. (2013). AfroDb: a select highly potent and diverse natural product library from African medicinal plants. *PLoS ONE* 8 (10), e78085. doi: 10.1371/journal.pone.0078085

Overington, J. P., Al-Lazikani, B., and Hopkins, A. L. (2006). How many drug targets are there? *Nat. Rev. Drug Discov.* 5 (12), 993–996. doi: 10.1038/nrd2199

Owais, F., Anwar, S., Saeed, F., Muhammad, S., Ishtiaque, S., and Mohiuddin, O. (2014). Analgesic, anti-inflammatory and neuropharmacological effects of Atropa belladonna. *Pak. J. Pharm. Sci.* 27 (6 Spec No.), 2183–2187.

Öztürk, N., and Tunçel, M. (2011). Assessment of phenolic acid content and in vitro antiradical characteristics of hawthorn. *J. Med. Food* 14 (6), 664–669. doi: 10.1089/jmf.2010.0063

Pathania, S., Ramakrishnan, S. M., and Bagler, G. (2015). Phytochemica: a platform to explore phytochemicals of medicinal plants. *Database* bav075. doi: 10.1093/database/bav075

Piñero, J., Bravo, A., Queralt-Rosinach, N., Gutiérrez-Sacristán, A., Deu-Pons, J., Centeno, E., et al. (2017). DisGeNET: a comprehensive platform integrating information on human disease-associated genes and variants. *Nucleic Acids Res.* 45 (D1), D833–D839. doi: 10.1093/nar/gkw943

Raja, D., Blanché, C., and Vallès, J. (1997). Contribution to the knowledge of the pharmaceutical ethnobotany of La Segarra region (Catalonia, Iberian Peninsula). *J. Ethnopharmacol.* 57 (3), 149–160. doi: 10.1016/S0378-8741(97)00059-7

Rigat, M., Bonet, M. A., Garcia, S., Garnatje, T., and Vallès, J. (2007). Studies on pharmaceutical ethnobotany in the high river Ter valley (Pyrenees, Catalonia, Iberian Peninsula). *J. Ethnopharmacol.* 113 (2), 267–277. doi: 10.1016/j.jep.2007.06.004

Rimando, A. M., Nagmani, R., Feller, D. R., and Yokoyama, W. (2005). Pterostilbene, a new agonist for the peroxisome proliferator-activated receptor alpha-isoform, lowers plasma lipoproteins and cholesterol in hypercholesterolemic hamsters. *J. Agric. Food Chem.* 53 (9), 3403–3407. doi: 10.1021/jf0580364

Roth, B. L., Sheffler, D. J., and Kroeze, W. K. (2004). Magic shotguns versus magic bullets: selectively non-selective drugs for mood disorders and schizophrenia. *Nat. Rev. Drug Discov.* 3 (4), 353–359. doi: 10.1038/nrd1346

Sawada, R., Iwata, M., Umezaki, M., Usui, Y., Kobayahi, T., Kubono, T., et al. (2018). KampoDB, database of predicted targets and functional annotations of natural medicines. *Sci. Rep.* 8 (1), 11216. doi: 10.1038/s41598-018-29516-1

Sikander, A., Rana, S. V., and Prasad, K. K. (2009). Role of serotonin in gastrointestinal motility and irritable bowel syndrome. *Clin. Chim. Acta* 403 (1–2), 47–55. doi: 10.1016/j.cca.2009.01.028

Slimestad, R., Fossen, T., and Vågen, I. M. (2007). Onions: a source of unique dietary flavonoids. *J. Agric. Food Chem.* 55 (25), 10067–10080. doi: 10.1021/jf0712503

Soni, P., Siddiqui, A. A., Dwivedi, J., and Soni, V. (2012). Pharmacological properties of Datura stramonium L. as a potential medicinal tree: an overview. *Asian Pac. J. Trop. Biomed.* 2 (12), 1002–1008. doi: 10.1016/S2221-1691(13)60014-3

Southan, C., Sharman, J. L., Benson, H. E., Faccenda, E., Pawson, A. J., Alexander, S. P. H., et al. (2016). The IUPHAR/BPS Guide to PHARMACOLOGY in 2016: towards curated quantitative interactions between 1300 protein targets and 6000 ligands. *Nucleic Acids Res.* 44 (D1), D1054–D1068. doi: 10.1093/nar/gkv1037

Spitzmüller, A., and Mestres, J. (2013). Prediction of the P. Falciparum target space relevant to malaria drug discovery. *PLoS Comput. Biol.* 9 (10), e1003257. doi: 10.1371/journal.pcbi.1003257

Tao, L., Zhu, F., Qin, C., Zhang, C., Xu, F., Tan, C. Y., et al. (2014). Nature's contribution to today's pharmacopeia. *Nat. Biotechnol.* 32 (10), 979–980. doi: 10.1038/nbt.3034

Thase, M. E., Trivedi, M. H., and Rush, A. J. (1995). MAOIs in the contemporary treatment of depression. *Neuropsychopharmacology* 12 (3), 185–219. doi: 10.1016/0893-133X(94)00058-8

The UniProt Consortium (2015). UniProt: a hub for protein information. *Nucleic Acids Res.* 43 (Database issue), D204–D212. doi: 10.1093/nar/gku989

Tota, K., Rayabarapu, N., Moosa, S., Talla, V., Bhyravbhatla, B., and Rao, S. (2013). InDiaMed: a comprehensive database of Indian medicinal plants for diabetes. *Bioinformation* 9 (7), 378–380. doi: 10.6026/97320630009378

U.S. Department of Agriculture, Agricultural Research Service. (1992). *Dr. Duke's Phytochemical and Ethnobotanical Databases* [Internet version] Boca Raton, Fla: CRC Press, 183. doi: 10.15482/USDA.ADC/1239279

van Voorhuis, W. C., Adams, J. H., Adelfio, R., Ahyong, V., Akabas, M.H., Alano, P., et al. (2016). Open source drug discovery with the Malaria Box compound collection for neglected diseases and beyond. *PLoS Pathogens* 12 (7), e1005763. doi: 10.1371/journal.ppat.1005763

Vidal, D., and Mestres, J. (2010). In silico receptorome screening of antipsychotic drugs. *Mol. Inform.* 29 (6–7), 543–551. doi: 10.1002/minf.201000055

Vidal, D., Garcia-Serna, R., and Mestres, J. (2011). Ligand-based approaches to in silico pharmacology. *Methods Mol. Biol.* 672, 489–502. doi: 10.1007/978-1-60761-839-3_19

Yamada, H., Shimoyama, N., Sora, I., Uhl, G. R., Fukuda, Y., Moriya, H., et al. (2006). Morphine can produce analgesia *via* spinal kappa opioid receptors in the absence of mu opioid receptors. *Brain Res.* 1083 (1), 61–69. doi: 10.1016/j.brainres.2006.01.095

Yi, F., Li, L., Xu, L.-J., Meng, H., Dong, Y.-M., Liu, H.-B., et al. (2018). *In silico* approach in reveal traditional medicine plants pharmacological material basis. *Chin. Med.* 13, 33. doi: 10.1186/s13020-018-0190-0

Young, R. J., Ewing, D. J., and Clarke, B. F. (1983). A controlled trial of sorbinil, an aldose reductase inhibitor, in chronic painful diabetic neuropathy. *Diabetes* 32 (10), 938–942. doi: 10.2337/diabetes.32.10.938

Zhao, J., Jiang, P., and Zhang, W. (2010). Molecular networks for the study of TCM pharmacology. *Brief. Bioinform.* 11 (4), 417–430. doi: 10.1093/bib/bbp063

Zhu, F., Shi, Z., Qin, C., Tao, L., Liu, X., Xu, F., et al. (2012). Therapeutic target database update 2012: a resource for facilitating target-oriented drug discovery. *Nucleic Acids Res.* 40 (Database issue), D1128–D1136 doi: 10.1093/nar/gkr797

6

Si-Miao-Yong-An Decoction for Diabetic Retinopathy: A Combined Network Pharmacological and In Vivo Approach

Ao Du, Yumin Xie, Hao Ouyang, Bin Lu, Wangya Jia, Hong Xu and Lili Ji**

The MOE Key Laboratory for Standardization of Chinese Medicines, Shanghai Key Laboratory of Compound Chinese Medicines and The SATCM Key Laboratory for New Resources and Quality Evaluation of Chinese Medicines, Institute of Chinese Materia Medica, Shanghai University of Traditional Chinese Medicine, Shanghai, China

***Correspondence:**
Hong Xu
xuhongtcm@163.com
Lili Ji
lichenyue1307@126.com

Si-Miao-Yong-An decoction (SMYAD), a traditional Chinese medicine formula, is mainly used to clear away heat and detoxify and to promote blood circulation and relieve pain. Diabetic retinopathy (DR) is the most common type of microvascular complication caused by diabetes. This study is designed to examine the protective effect of SMYAD against DR and further to reveal the engaged mechanism *via* integrating network pharmacology and *in vivo* experimental evidence. Streptozotocin (STZ) was intraperitoneally injected into mice to induce diabetes. The dysfunction of the blood retina barrier (BRB) was observed by conducting Evan's blue leakage assay, detecting tight junction (TJ) protein expression and counting the number of acellular capillaries in retinas. Our results showed that SMYAD alleviated BRB breakdown *in vivo*. Network pharmacology results demonstrated that regulating inflammation, immune responses, and angiogenesis might be associated with the efficacy of SMYAD in alleviating DR, in which the tumor necrosis factor (TNF) and hypoxia inducible factor 1 (HIF1) signal pathways were involved. Next, immunofluorescence staining results showed that SMYAD decreased microglia activation in retinas and reduced the enhanced adhesion of leukocytes into retinal vessels. SMYAD reduced the elevated serum TNFα content and retinal TNFα expression. SMYAD abrogated the activation of nuclear factor κB (NFκB) and HIF1α and consequently decreased the enhanced expression of some pro-inflammatory molecules and vascular endothelial growth factor (VEGF) in retinas. These results indicate that SMYAD attenuated DR development through suppressing retinal inflammation and angiogenesis *via* abrogating NFκB-TNFα and HIF1α-VEGF signal pathways.

Keywords: Si-Miao-Yong-An decoction, Diabetic retinopathy, network pharmacology, inflammation, angiogenesis

INTRODUCTION

Diabetic retinopathy (DR), a common microvascular complication caused by diabetes, has become the most serious eye disease leading to the adult blindness in the world (Antonetti et al., 2012; Gardlik and Fusekova, 2015). From 2015 to 2019, the prevalence rate of diabetic macular edema (DME) and DR was 27.0% in the world, among which the early period non-proliferative DR (NPDR) accounted for 25.2%, the later period proliferative DR (PDR) was 1.4%, and DME was 4.6% (Thomas et al., 2019). In China, the pooled prevalence rates in people with diabetes between 1990 and 2007 were 18.45, 15.06, and 0.99% for DR, NPDR, and PDR, respectively (Song et al., 2018). Therefore, more attention shall be paid to DR prevention.

At present, DR therapy is mainly based on drug treatment, laser photocoagulation treatment, and pars plana vitrectomy. Laser photocoagulation is an invasive treatment, which can cause postoperative visual field defects, decreased contrast sensitivity, and some other adverse reactions including central dark spots or para-central dark spots (Oellers and Mahmoud, 2016). These side effects greatly limited the clinical application of laser photocoagulation. The vascular endothelial growth factor (VEGF) antagonist, intravitreally injected when applied, is the most common drug used for DR treatment (Bandello et al., 2013). However, the application of the VEGF antagonist only is incapable of curing DR completely. Moreover, it has some side effects such as causing fibrovascular constriction and the sustained elevation of intraocular pressure (Singh and Kim, 2012; Bandello et al., 2013). Therefore, more drugs with better efficacy and fewer side effects need to be found in the future.

According to the theory of traditional Chinese medicine, the pathogenesis of DR was mainly due to the poor blood circulation and stasis caused by Yin deficiency and fire vigour that burned blood vessels. Recently, many traditional Chinese medicines (TCMs) and their active ingredients have been reported to improve DR. These TCMs include *Lonicera japonica* Thunb., *Salvia miltiorrhiza* Bge., *Lycium barbarum* L., *Andrographis paniculata* (Burm.f.) Nees, *Panax notoginseng* (Burkill) F.H.Chen, *Dendrobium officinale* Kimura and Migo, etc., and they all have functions like eliminating heat, improving blood circulation, nourishing Yin, and dissolving blood stasis (Behl and Kotwani, 2017; Vasant More et al., 2017; Xu et al., 2018).

Si-Miao-Yong-An decoction (SMYAD), first recorded in "*YanFangXinBian*" (Qing Dynasty), is composed of *Scrophularia ningpoensis* Hemsl. (Chinese name Xuan-Shen), *Lonicera japonica* Thunb (Chinese name Jin-Yin-Hua), *Angelica sinensis* (Oliv.), Diels (Chinese name Dang-Gui), and *Glycyrrhiza uralensis* Fisch. ex DC. (Chinese name Gan-Cao). It is traditionally applied externally for treating sore, carbuncle, and ulcer. Recently, SMYAD is generally used for the treatment of peripheral vascular diseases such as thromboangiitis obliterans. Among these four TCMs included in SMYAD, Jin-Yin-hua is good at clearing away heat and detoxifying, Xuan-Shen nourishes Yin and relieves fire, Dang-Gui is good at activating blood and dissipating blood stasis, and Gan-Cao reconciles various drugs. Therefore, SMYAD can be used to clear away heat and detoxify, to improve blood circulation, and to relieve pain, which implies its huge potential in DR treatment. Actually, a previous clinical study has demonstrated that SMYAD improved DR and some other diabetic vascular complications in diabetic patients (Zhang et al., 2012). However, the mechanism participating in the SMYAD-provided protection against DR is still not clear.

The pathogenesis of DR is very complex, which implies that modulating multiple targets is required for its treatment. Network pharmacology is generally used to clarify the relationship between the drug's action and molecular targets (Hopkins, 2008). The therapeutic action of the Chinese medicinal formula may be obtained from the joint action of all compounds in the formula, so its pharmacological activity has multi-effects, multi-pathways, and multi-targets, which is consistent with the core theory and method of network pharmacology (Wang et al., 2021). Recently, network pharmacology is commonly used for the prediction of bioactive ingredients and the clarification of molecular targets in TCM's research work (Li et al., 2014; Jiao et al., 2021; Wang et al., 2021).

The alleviation of SMYAD on DR was evaluated *in vivo*, and then, the potential engaged mechanism was investigated by integrating network pharmacology prediction and further *in vivo* experimental validation in this study.

MATERIALS AND METHODS

Reagents

Scrophularia ningpoensis Hemsl., *Lonicera japonica* Thunb., *Angelica sinensis* (Oliv.) Diels, and *Glycyrrhiza uralensis* Fisch. ex DC. were purchased from Kangqiao Co., Ltd. (Shanghai, China). These four TCMs were authenticated by Professor Hong Xu, and voucher samples were kept in the Institute of Chinese Materia Medica (Shanghai University of Traditional Chinese Medicine). Chlorogenic acid (Jin-Yin-Hua), luteoloside (Jin-Yin-Hua), harpagide (Xuan-Shen), harpagoside (Xuan-Shen), ferulic acid (Dang-Gui), glycyrrhizinic acid (Gan-Cao), and liquiritin (Gan-Cao) (purity≥98%) were bought from Dalian Meilun Biotechnology Co., Ltd. (Dalian, China). The intercellular adhesion molecule 1 (ICAM1) antibody (ABclonal, Shanghai, China), the ionized calcium-binding adapter molecule 1 (Iba1) antibody (GeneTax Inc., Alton Parkway Irvine, CA), nuclear factor κB (NFκB) p65, *ß*-actin, Lamin B1, phosphorylated IκB kinase (p-IKK), the phosphorylated NFκ-B inhibitor (p-IκB), VEGF receptor 2 (VEGFR2), and the phosphorylated VEGFR2 antibodies (Cell Signaling Technology, Danvers, MA) were obtained. Tumor necrosis factor-α (TNFα), claudin1, claudin19, hypoxia inducible factor 1α (HIF1*α*), and vascular cell adhesion protein 1 (VCAM1) antibodies (Santa Cruz, Santa Cruz, CA), Alexa Fluor 568 goat anti-rabbit IgG (BD Biosciences, Franklin Lakes, NJ), and peroxidase-conjugated goat anti-rabbit immunoglobulin G (IgG) (H + L) and anti-mouse IgG (H + L) (Jackson ImmunoResearch, West Grove, PA) were obtained. BCA Protein Assay Kits and NE-PER nuclear and cytoplasmic extraction reagents were bought from Thermo Fisher Scientific (Waltham, MA). Enzyme-linked immunosorbent assay (ELISA) kits were from R and D (Minneapolis, MN). PrimeScript RT Master Mix and SYBR Premix Ex Taq kits (Takara, Shiga, Japan) were obtained. Fluorescein isothiocyanate-coupled concanavalin A (FITC-ConA) was bought from Vector Laboratories (Burlingame, CA). 4',6-Diamidino-2-phenylindole (DAPI) and Trizol were purchased from Life Technology (Carlsbad, CA). Other reagents were bought from Sigma Chemical Co. (St. Louis, MO).

Preparation of SMYAD Powder

The SMYAD powder was prepared as recorded in classic literature reports. The mixed *Scrophularia ningpoensis* Hemsl., *Lonicera japonica* Thunb., *Angelica sinensis* (Oliv.) Diels, and *Glycyrrhiza uralensis* Fisch. ex DC. (The ratio of weight is 3:3:2:1) were heated under reflux for 2 h with 10 times the amount of distilled water. The residue was heated under reflux again under the same condition after the extracts were filtered, and this procedure was repeated three times. The filtered extracts were concentrated and further freeze-dried into fine powder with the final yield of 36.5%.

High-Performance Liquid Chromatography Analysis

High-performance liquid chromatography (HPLC) was performed on a Shiseido C18 column (250 nm × 4.6 mm, 5 μm, 30°C). The wavelength was set at 260 nm. The mobile phase consisted of a mixture of acetonitrile–0.05%H_3PO_4–Et_3N (at 0–5 min, 0.2:99.8, v/v; at 5–15 min, increased from 0.2:99.8 to 3:97, v/v; at 15–30 min, 7:93, v/v; at 30–45 min, 8:92, v/v; at 45–65 min, 6:94, v/v; at 65–67 min, 10:90, v/v; at 67–70 min, 11: 89, v/v; at 75–90 min, 12:88, v/v; at 90–115 min, 17:83, v/v; at 115–130 min, 20:80, v/v; at 130–135 min, 23:77, v/v; at 135–145 min, 30:70, v/v; at 145–175 min, 50:50, v/v) with a flow rate of 1.0 ml/min. Seven reference compounds including chlorogenic acid, luteoloside, harpagide, harpagoside, ferulic acid, glycyrrhizinic acid, and liquiritin were dissolved in methanol. The peak of seven main compounds in SMYAD was identified by comparing the retention time with that of reference compounds. Additionally, the contents of those above seven compounds in SMYAD were detected by using the external standard method.

Experimental Animals

Specific-pathogen-free male C57BL/6 mice (20 ± 2 g) were obtained from the Shanghai Laboratory Animal Center of Chinese Academy of Science (Shanghai, China) and fed under a controlled room temperature (22°C ± 1 °C) and humidity (65 ± 5%) with a 12:12 h light/dark cycle. Mice have free access to food and water and have received humane care according to the institutional animal care guidelines approved by the Experimental Animal Ethical Committee of Shanghai University of Traditional Chinese Medicine (approved number: PZSHUTCM200724021).

Animal Treatment

A total of 45 mice were intraperitoneally injected (ip) with 55 mg/kg BW of streptozotocin (STZ) (Sigma No. S0130) in citric acid solution and 0.1 M trisodium citrate solution pH = 4.4 (vehicle) for 5 consecutive days. Also, other 15 mice in the control group were injected with physiological saline. Seven days later, mice with a blood glucose concentration over 16.7 mmol/L were considered as diabetic mice and included in this study. These diabetic mice were randomly divided as follows: DM, DM + SMYAD (1.5 g/kg), and DM + SMYAD (4.5 g/kg). Each group has 15 mice. One month later, SMYAD (1.5, 4.5 g/kg, intragastric administration) was orally given to mice for 1 consecutive month, and then, mice were sacrificed to collect blood samples and eyes. The body weight was monitored and the blood glucose concentration was determined with a Accu-Check glucometer (Roche Diagnostics, Germany) every 7 days during the whole experimental process.

Evan's Blue Leakage Assay

Blood-retina-barrier (BRB) breakdown was detected according to the published method (Mei et al., 2019; Zhang et al., 2019). Briefly, mice were injected with 2% Evan's blue (10 μl/g, i. p.). Two hours later, retinas were dissected after the Evan's blue dye was completely removed from retinal vessels. Formamide was used to dissolve the retinas, and the absorbance in the extracts was determined at 620 nm. The amount of Evan's blue dye was calculated, and the results were normalized to the dried weight of the retina.

Leukostasis Assay

Leukostasis was detected as previously described (Chen et al., 2019). Briefly, FITC-ConA (120 μl) was intravenously injected into mice. Twenty minutes later, the isolated eyes were fixed in a 4% paraformaldehyde (PFA) solution. Retinas were dissected and flat-mounted for the observation under an inverted microscope (IX81, Olympus, Japan). FITC-ConA + cells adhered to retinal blood vessels were counted.

Hematoxylin-Eosin Staining of Acellular Capillaries in Retinas

The retina was fixed in a 4% PFA solution for 24 h and gently rocked overnight after four times of cleaning with ultrapure water and then digested with 3% trypsin and stained with hematoxylin-eosin (H and E) the next day. The morphology of retinal vessels was pictured by using an inverted microscope.

Network Pharmacology Analysis

Network pharmacology analysis was conducted as described in the guidance (Li et al., 2021).

Target Collection: Active targets of SMYAD were acquired from BATMAN-TCM (http://bionet.ncpsb.org.cn/batman-tcm/) and TCMSP (http://tcmspnw.com/) databases. According to the suggested criterion, compounds were selected if the drug-likeness was ≥0.18 and the oral bioavailability was ≥30%. Additionally, the indicator chemical compounds recorded in Chinese Pharmacopoeia from four Chinese botanical drugs included in SMYAD (Chinese Pharmacopoeia Commission, 2020) with low drug-likeness and oral bioavailability values were also retained in this study.

Protein–Protein Interaction (PPI) Network Construction: Diabetic Retinopathy (ICD-11, 9B71.0Z) therapeutic targets were collected by using GeneCards (www.genecards.org/). Cytoscape 3.6. 1 software was used to construct a drugs–ingredients–targets network. A target-to-target and function-related PPI network was established *via* the STRING database.

KEGG and GO Analysis: DAVID 6.8 was used to analyze the KEGG pathway enrichment and GO function of the proteins involved in the PPI network. The R package of ggplot2 was used for enrichment analysis, and the cutoff value was set as $p < 0.05$.

TABLE 1 | List of primers for real-time PCR.

Target	Primer	Sequence
TNFα	Forward	5′- ATGTCTCAGCCTCTTCTCATTC-3′
	Reverse	5′- GCTTGTCACTCGAATTTTGAGA-3′
ICAM1	Forward	5′- CTGAAAGATGAGCTCGAGAGTG-3′
	Reverse	5′- AAACGAATACACGGTGATGGTA-3′
MCP-1	Forward	5′- CAAGAGTGAATCCACACAACAG -3′
	Reverse	5′- GTAGGAGTCAACTCAGCTTTCT -3′
HIF1α	Forward	5′- GAATGAAGTGCACCCTAACAAG -3′
	Reverse	5′- GAGGAATGGGTTCACAAATCAG -3′
VEGF	Forward	5′- TAGAGTACATCTTCAAGCCGTC -3′
	Reverse	5′- CTTTCTTTGGTCTGCATTCACA -3′
Actin	Forward	5′- TTCGTTGCCGGTCCACACCC -3′
	Reverse	5′- GCTTTGCACATGCCGGAGCC -3′

Immunofluorescence Staining

Retinal Iba1 immunofluorescence staining was conducted according to the published method (Mei et al., 2019; Zhang et al., 2019), but in this study, retinas were incubated with the Alexa fluor 568 goat anti-rabbit IgG (H + L) antibody after incubating with the Iba1 antibody overnight.

qPCR Analysis

Retinal RNA was extracted, cDNA was synthesized, and real-time RT-PCR was conducted as described in kits. The relative expression of target genes was normalized to actin, analyzed by the $2^{-\Delta\Delta Ct}$ method, and calculated as the ratio compared with the control. The primer sequences are shown in **Table 1**.

Western-Blot Analysis

Proteins were extracted, and the protein concentration was determined. The denatured samples were run on SDS-PAGE gels and electrophoretically transferred to PVDF membranes that were further incubated with primary and secondary antibodies. The protein expression was visualized by using a chemiluminescent reagent and quantified by calculating gray densities of the target protein blots with internal controls.

ELISA

Serum contents of TNFα, monocyte chemoattractant protein-1 (MCP-1), interleukin-6 (IL-6), and VEGF were detected by using commercial ELISA kits.

Statistical Analysis

Data are shown as the mean ± standard error of the mean (SEM). The statistical significance of differences between groups is obtained through one-way ANOVA with the LSD post hoc test. $p < 0.05$ is considered to be the significant difference.

RESULTS

Chemical Characterization of SMYAD

Data in **Figures 1A–G** demonstrated the HPLC chromatogram of chlorogenic acid, luteoloside, harpagide, harpagoside, ferulic acid, glycyrrhizinic acid, and liquiritin. **Figures 1H–J** demonstrate the HPLC chromatogram of SMYAD, and the above seven compounds were pointed out in SMYAD. Next, the content of these above seven compounds in SMYAD was determined. After calculations, the content of chlorogenic acid, luteoloside, harpagide, harpagoside, ferulic acid, glycyrrhizinic acid, and liquiritin in SMYAD was 0.882, 0.034, 0.284, 0.103, 0.034, 0.258, and 0.201%, respectively.

SMYAD Alleviated BRB Dysfunction *in vivo*

The increased blood glucose concentration and the reduced body weight of diabetic mice did not change after the administration of SMYAD (1.5, 4.5 g/kg) (data not shown). The elevated Evan's blue dye leakage in retinas from diabetic mice was reduced after the administration of SMYAD (1.5, 4.5 g/kg) (**Figure 2A**). As shown in **Figure 2B**, the decreased expression of retinal claudin1 and claudin19 (two typical tight junctions, TJs) in diabetic mice was enhanced when diabetic mice received SMYAD (4.5 g/kg). Moreover, the decreased number of acellular capillaries marked with black arrows in retinas from diabetic mice was enhanced after the administration of SMYAD (1.5, 4.5 g/kg) (**Figure 2C**).

Network Pharmacology Analysis

A total of 109 active compounds and 398 compound-related targets were acquired from TCMSP and BATMAN-TCM. A DR target network was established to find the relationship between compounds in SMYAD and common targets of DR. As shown in **Figure 3A**, the yellow diamond-shape node in the central area represents the total 398 compounds-related targets, the green circular-shape node on the upper-left corner represents 14 active compounds from Jin-Yin-Hua, the red circular-shape node on the upper-right corner represents five compounds from Xuan-Shen, the purple circular-shape node on the bottom-left corner represents one compound from Dang-Gui, the pink circular-shape node on the bottom-right corner represents 84 compounds from Gan-Cao, and the blue circular-shape node represents five co-owned compounds from Jin-Yin-Hua, Xuan-Shen, Dang-Gui, and Gan-Cao. A total of 3,497 targets involved in DR development were obtained from the GeneCards database. After integrating the targets of compounds from SMYAD and the targets involved in DR development, 198 common matched-targets were found, and the Venn diagram is shown in **Figure 3B**. Next, those above 198 common matched-targets were imported into the STRING database to construct a PPI network. After removing 60 disconnected nodes, there were a total of 138 nodes (representing 138 common matched targets) and 817 edges (representing the interaction between two targets) (**Figure 3C**). After screening according to the degree of these nodes, the core targets are shown in **Figure 3D**. The node became larger and its color changed from yellow to red with the increased degree of the targets. Among these core targets, the first six molecular targets with higher degrees were protein kinase B (AKT1), IL-6, tumor protein p53 (TP53), TNF, mitogen-activated protein kinase 8 (MAPK8), and VEGFA.

These above 198 common matched-targets were further imported into the DAVID database, and a total of 960 GO items and 133 KEGG pathways were obtained. As shown in **Figure 3E**, inflammation (GO: 0006954), immune responses (GO: 0006955), and angiogenesis (GO: 0001525) marked with a red square accounted for a large proportion of biological processes. Moreover, the results of KEGG pathways showed that the TNF signaling pathway (hsa04668)

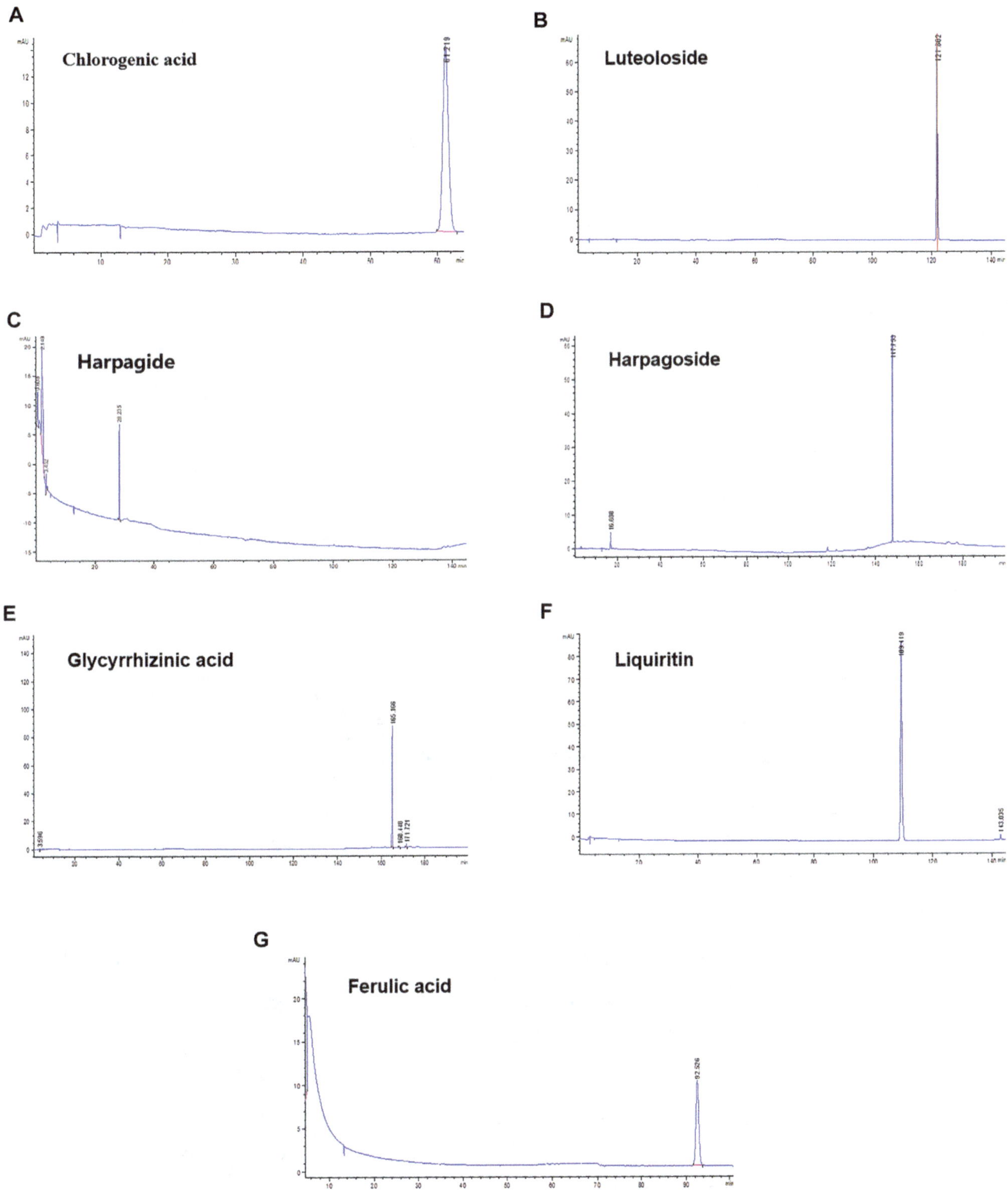

FIGURE 1 | HPLC analysis. HPLC chromatogram of reference compounds including **(A)** chlorogenic acid, **(B)** luteoloside, **(C)** harpagide, **(D)** harpagoside, **(E)** glycyrrhizinic acid, **(F)** liquiritin, and **(G)** ferulic acid. HPLC chromatogram of **(H)** SMYAD and **(I)** SMYAD in arealand **(J)** SMYAD in areaII.

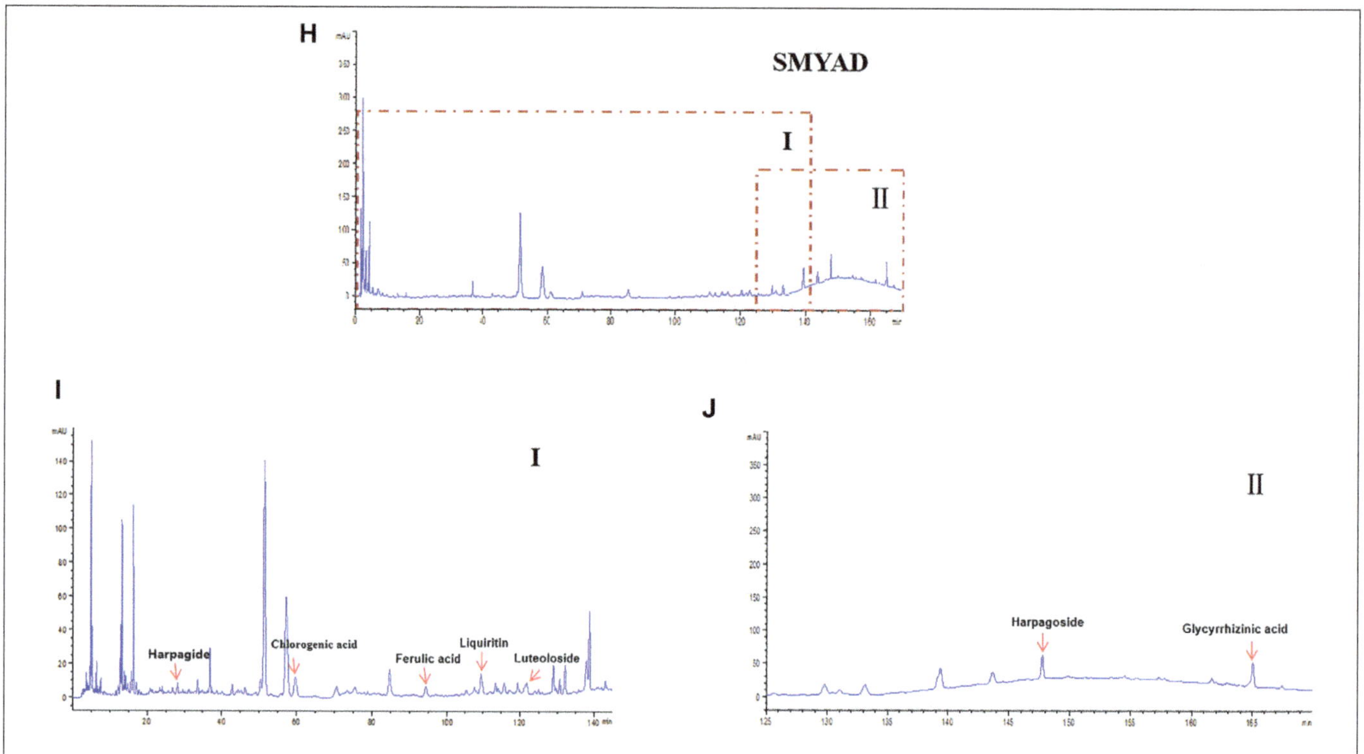

FIGURE 1b | continued

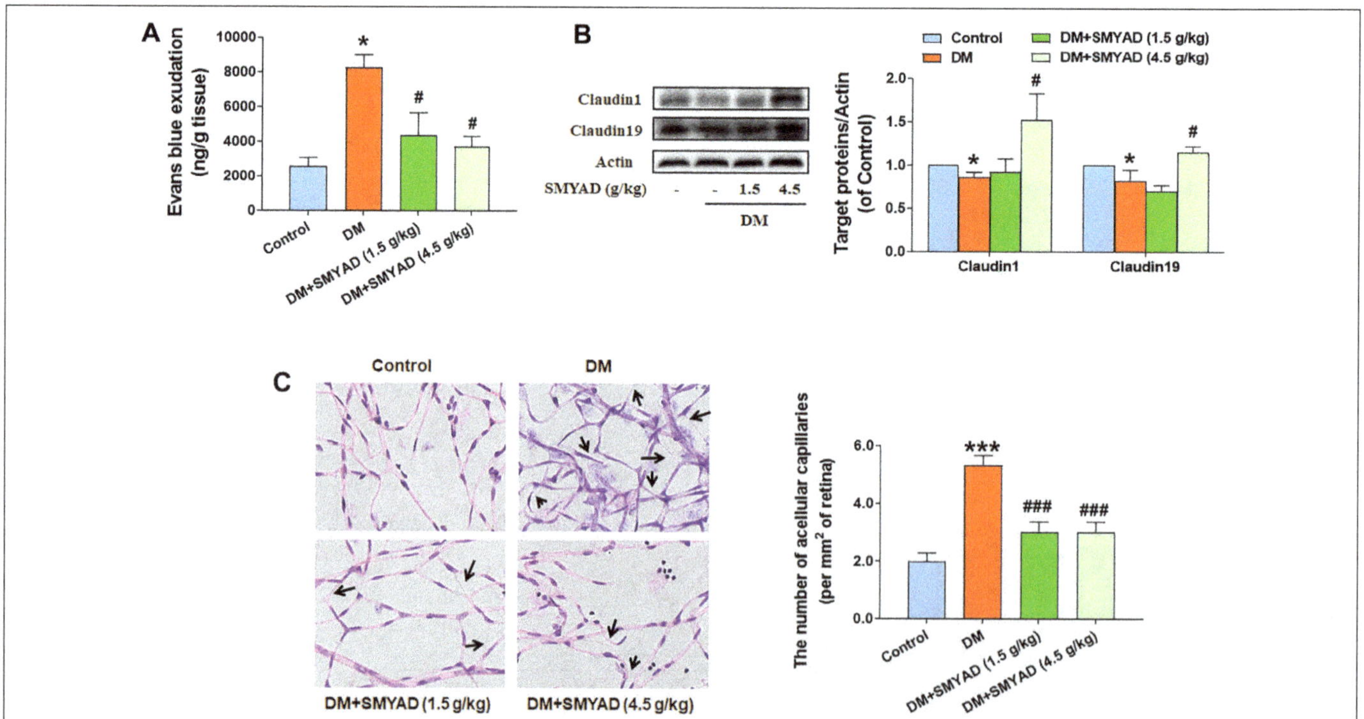

FIGURE 2 | SMYAD alleviated BRB dysfunction *in vivo*. **(A)** Evan's blue leakage assay (n = 4). **(B)** Claudin1 and claudin19 expression in retinas. The quantitative result is shown at right (n = 3). **(C)** Retinal H and E staining. The number of acellular capillaries per field in retinas is shown at right (n = 3). Black arrows indicate acellular capillaries. Data = mean ± SEM. $^{*}p < 0.05$, $^{***}p < 0.001$ vs. control; $^{\#}p < 0.05$, $^{\#\#\#}p < 0.001$ vs. DM.

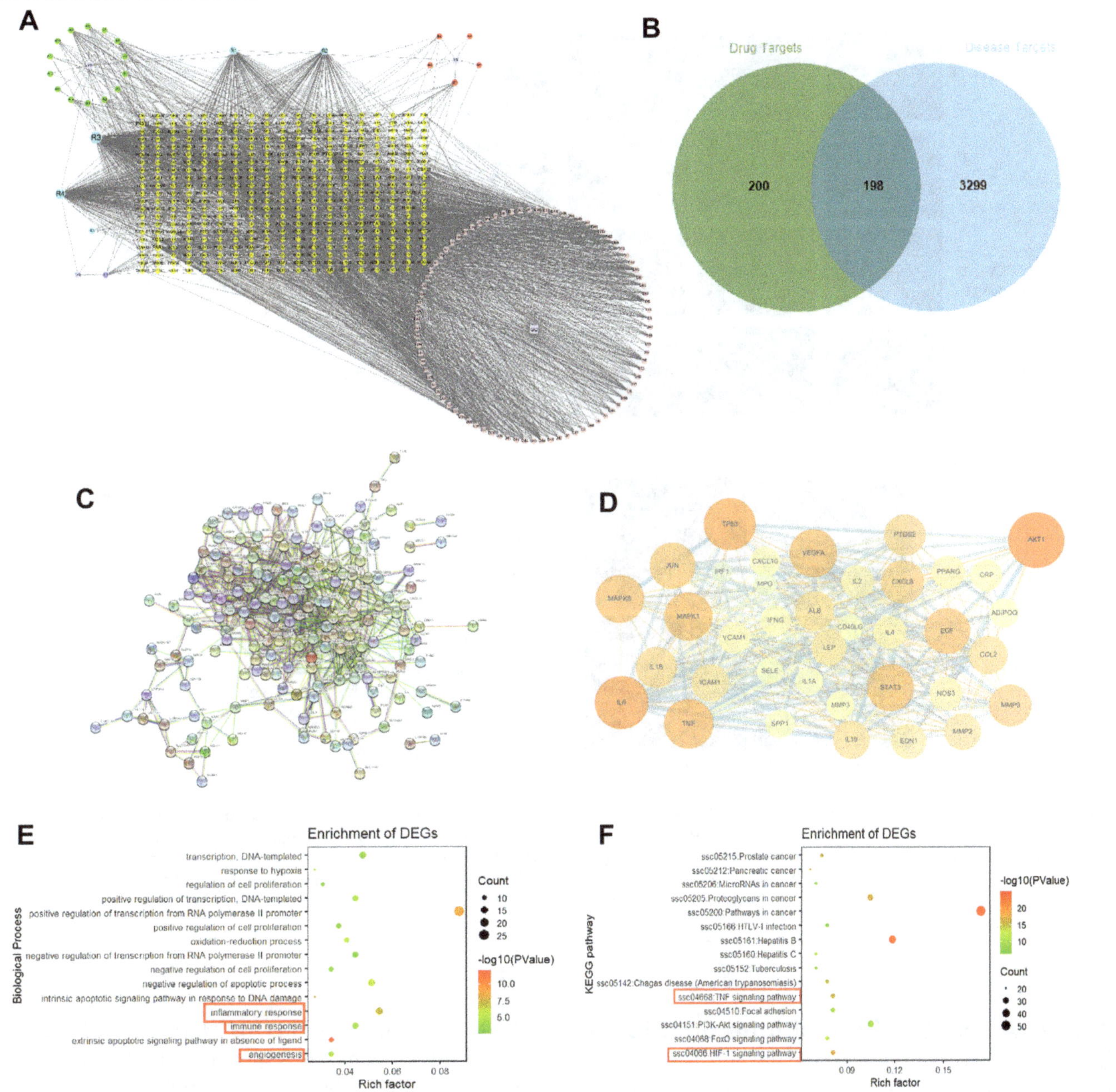

FIGURE 3 | Network pharmacology. **(A)** Drugs–compounds–targets network. The node representing the compound is represented by a multi-color hexagon, and the target point is represented by a yellow diamond. **(B)** Venn diagram. **(C)** PPI network. **(D)** PPI network of core targets extracted from degree centrality. **(E)** GO enrichment analyses. A total of 15 biological process items in descending order of *p*-values in the DAVID database. **(F)** KEGG enrichment analyses.

(critically involved in inflammation and immune responses) and the HIF1 signaling pathway (hsa04066) (critically involved in angiogenesis) marked with a red square were the key signal pathways involved in the SMYAD-provided protection against DR.

Next, we consulted some transcriptome chips conducted in DR research included in GEO Databases (http://www.ncbi.nlm.nih.gov/gds/). The transcriptome chip results from mice at about 6 weeks after STZ injection (GSE111465) showed that the TNF signaling pathway marked with a red square was the most important signaling pathway involved in DR development in mice at 6 weeks after STZ treatment (**Supplementary Figure S1A**). Additionally, the transcriptome chip results from mice at about 12 weeks after STZ injection (GSE19122) showed that the VEGF signaling pathway marked with a red square was the most important signaling pathway involved in DR development in mice at 12 weeks after STZ treatment (**Supplementary Figure S1B**).

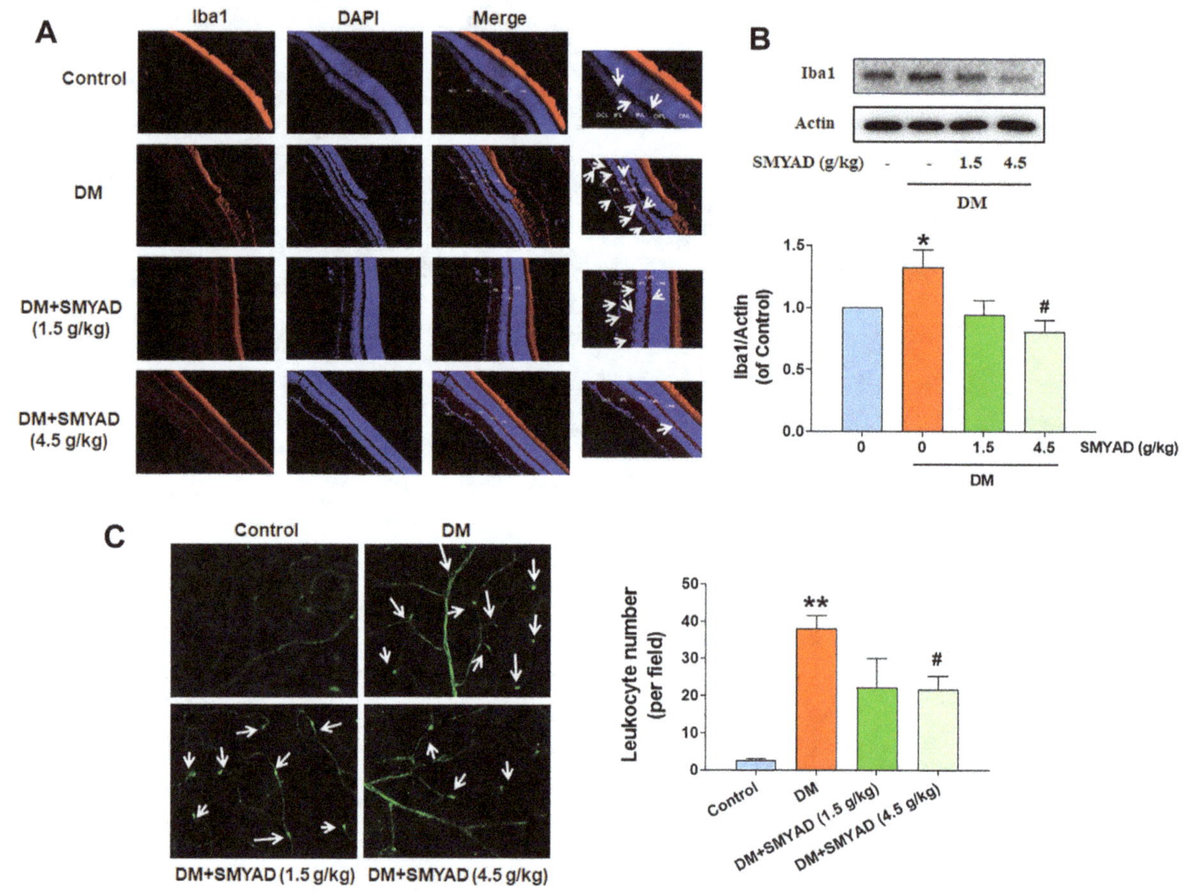

FIGURE 4 | SMYAD alleviated retinal inflammation *in vivo*. **(A)** Representative images of retinal Iba1 immunofluorescence staining (scale bar: 20 mm). Enlarged images are shown at right (scale bar: 5 mm). White arrows indicate microglia. **(B)** SMYAD reduced the enhanced Iba1 expression in retinas. The quantitative result is shown below (n = 3). **(C)** Representative images of retinal FITC-ConA staining. The number of entrapped leukocytes in retinal vessels was calculated and is shown at right (n = 3). **(D)** Serum IL-6 amount (n = 4). **(E)** Serum MCP-1 amount (n = 3). **(F)** Retinal mRNA expression of ICAM1 and MCP-1 (n = 3). **(G)** SMYAD decreased the increased retinal expression of ICAM1 and VCAM1. The quantitative result is shown below (n = 3). Data = mean ± SEM. $^{*}p < 0.05$, $^{**}p < 0.01$ vs. control; $^{\#}p < 0.05$, $^{\#\#}p < 0.01$, $^{\#\#\#}p < 0.001$ vs. DM.

SMYAD Alleviated Retinal Inflammation *in vivo*

Studies have reported that Iba1 is a microglia/macrophage specific marker, which is widely used to label microglia (Kanazawa et al., 2002; Ibrahim et al., 2011). The enhanced number of Iba1-staining microglia (marked with white arrows) in retinas from diabetic mice was decreased after the administration of SMYAD (**Figure 4A**). The elevated retinal Iba1 expression in diabetic mice was decreased when diabetic mice received SMYAD (4.5 g/kg) (**Figure 4B**). The increased number of leukocytes adhered to the retinal capillary (marked with white arrows) from diabetic mice was also decreased after the administration of SMYAD (4.5 g/kg) (**Figure 4C**). Next results showed that the enhanced serum IL-6 and MCP-1 contents in diabetic mice were decreased when diabetic mice received SMYAD (1.5, 4.5 g/kg) (**Figures 4D,E**). The elevated ICAM1 mRNA expression in retinas from diabetic mice was decreased after the administration of SMYAD (4.5 g/kg), and the elevated retinal MCP-1 mRNA expression in diabetic mice was decreased after the administration of SMYAD (1.5, 4.5 g/kg) (**Figure 4F**). Moreover, the elevated protein expression of both ICAM1 and VCAM1 in retinas from diabetic mice was decreased when diabetic mice received SMYAD (4.5 g/kg) (**Figure 4G**).

SMYAD Reduced TNFα Expression and Inhibited NFκB Activation *in vivo*

Data in **Figure 5A** showed that the enhanced serum TNF-α content in diabetic mice was obviously decreased when diabetic mice received SMYAD (1.5, 4.5 g/kg). Meanwhile, the enhanced retinal TNF-α mRNA and protein expression in diabetic mice was also decreased when diabetic mice received SMYAD (4.5 g/kg) (**Figures 5B,C**). Next results showed that SMYAD (4.5 g/kg) abrogated the nuclear accumulation of NFκ-B subunit p65 in retinas from diabetic mice

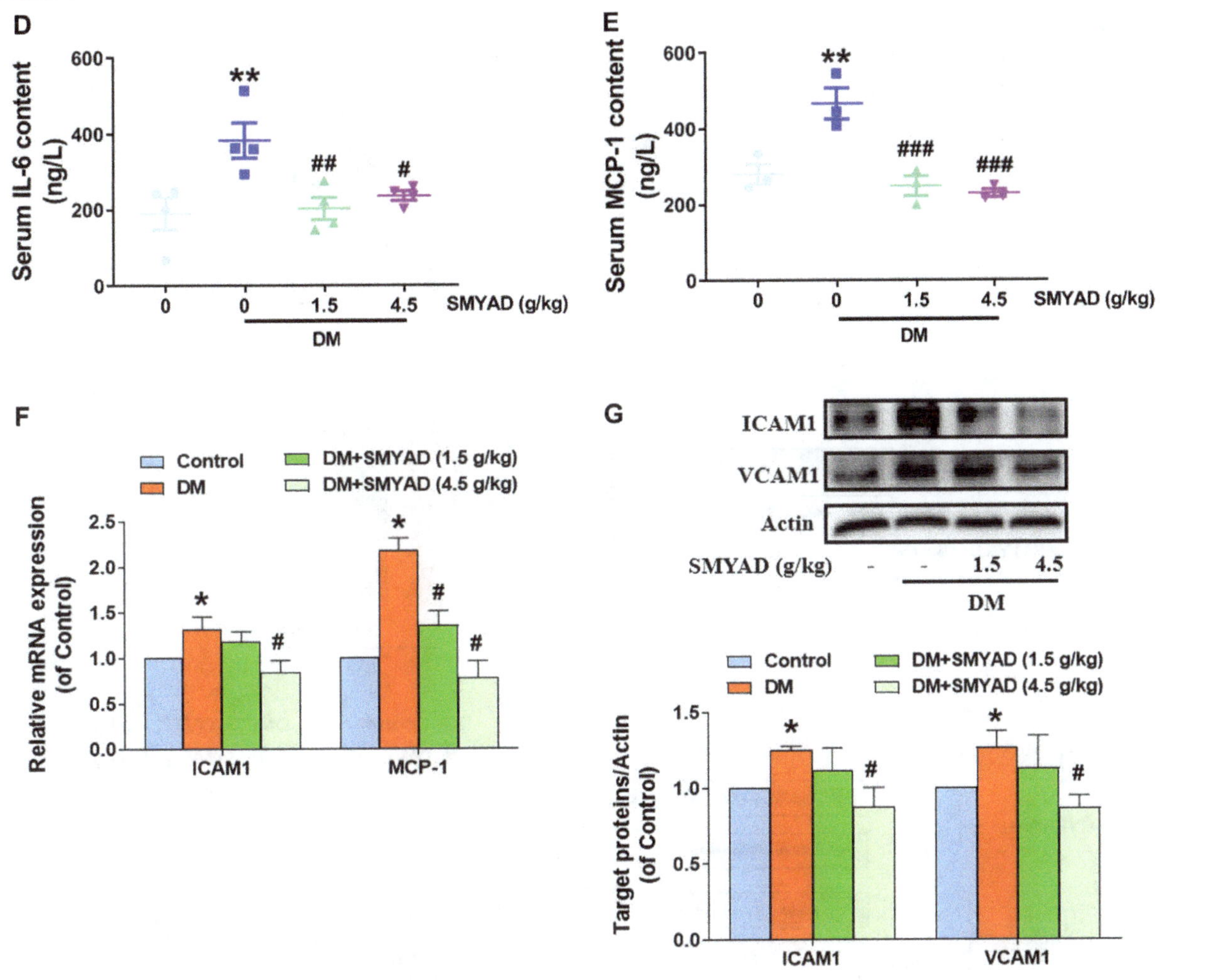

FIGURE 4b | continued

(**Figure 5D**). Moreover, the elevated phosphorylation of IκB and IKK in retinas from diabetic mice was decreased when diabetic mice received SMYAD (1.5, 4.5 g/kg) (**Figure 5E**).

SMYAD Inhibited the HIF1α-VEGF/VEGFR2 Signal Pathway *in vivo*

SMYAD (1.5, 4.5 g/kg) abrogated the nuclear accumulation of HIF1α in retinas from diabetic mice (**Figure 6A**). Data in **Figure 6B** showed that the elevated serum VEGF content in diabetic mice was decreased after the administration of SMYAD (1.5, 4.5 g/kg). The increased retinal VEGF mRNA expression in diabetic mice was decreased when diabetic mice received SMYAD (4.5 g/kg) (**Figure 6C**). The enhanced retinal HIF1α-mRNA expression in diabetic mice was also obviously decreased when diabetic mice received SMYAD (1.5, 4.5 g/kg) (**Figure 6C**). Moreover, the enhanced VEGFR2 phosphorylation in retinas from diabetic mice was decreased when diabetic mice received SMYAD (4.5 g/kg) (**Figure 6D**).

DISCUSSION

The dysfunction of BRB is commonly recognized as the earliest and typical event during DR progression (Zhang et al., 2014). BRB dysfunction is a crucial indicator for reflecting retinal microvascular injury in diabetic patients, which eventually causes severe visual impairment when no prompt intervention is applied (Rudraraju et al., 2020). Claudin1 and claudin19, two important TJs, greatly contributed to maintain the BRB integrity (Erickson et al., 2007). In this study, SMYAD reduced the leakage of Evan's blue dye in retinas. SMYAD also restored the decreased retinal claudin1 and claudin19 expression *in vivo*. These above results indicate that SMYAD ameliorated BRB dysfunction *in vivo*. Acellular capillaries are a kind of microvessels with the blood vessel basal membrane and without endothelial cells. The occurrence of acellular capillaries was commonly used for reflecting the severity of retinopathy (Douglas et al., 2012; Chen et al., 2019). SMYAD decreased the enhanced number of acellular capillaries in retinas from diabetic mice. All these above

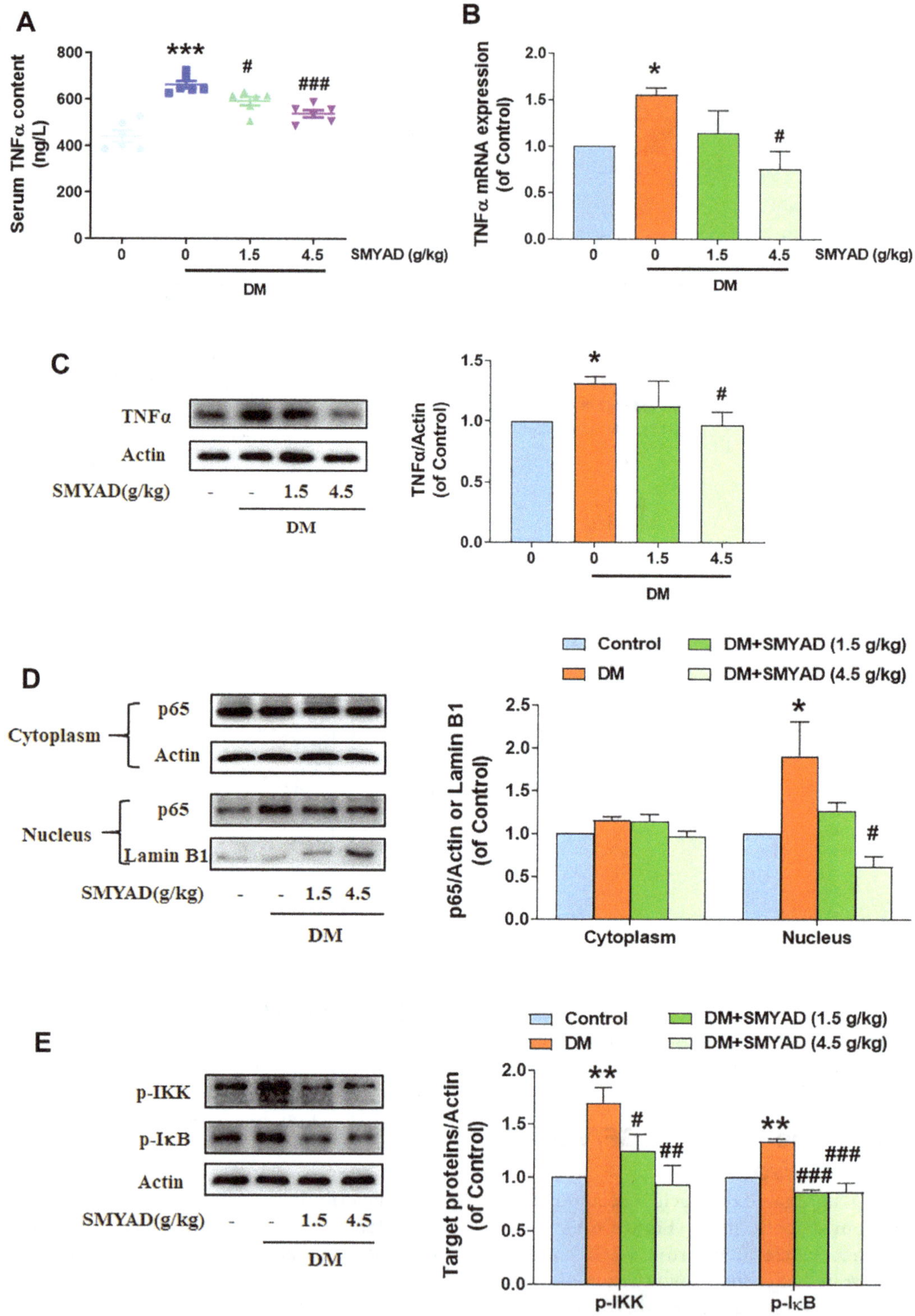

FIGURE 5 | SMYAD reduced TNFα expression and blocked NFκB activation *in vivo*. **(A)** Serum TNFα content (n = 6). **(B)** Retinal mRNA expression of TNFα (n = 3). **(C)** SMYAD reduced the enhanced TNFα expression in retinas. The quantitative result is shown below (n = 3). **(D)** SMYAD abrogated the nuclear accumulation of NFκBp65 in retinas. The quantitative result is shown at right (n = 3). **(E)** SMYAD decreased the enhanced phosphorylation of IκB and IKK. The quantitative result is shown at right (n = 3). Data = mean ± SEM. $^{*}p < 0.05$, $^{**}p < 0.01$, $^{***}p < 0.001$ vs. control; $^{\#}p < 0.05$, $^{\#\#}p < 0.01$, $^{\#\#\#}p < 0.001$ vs. DM.

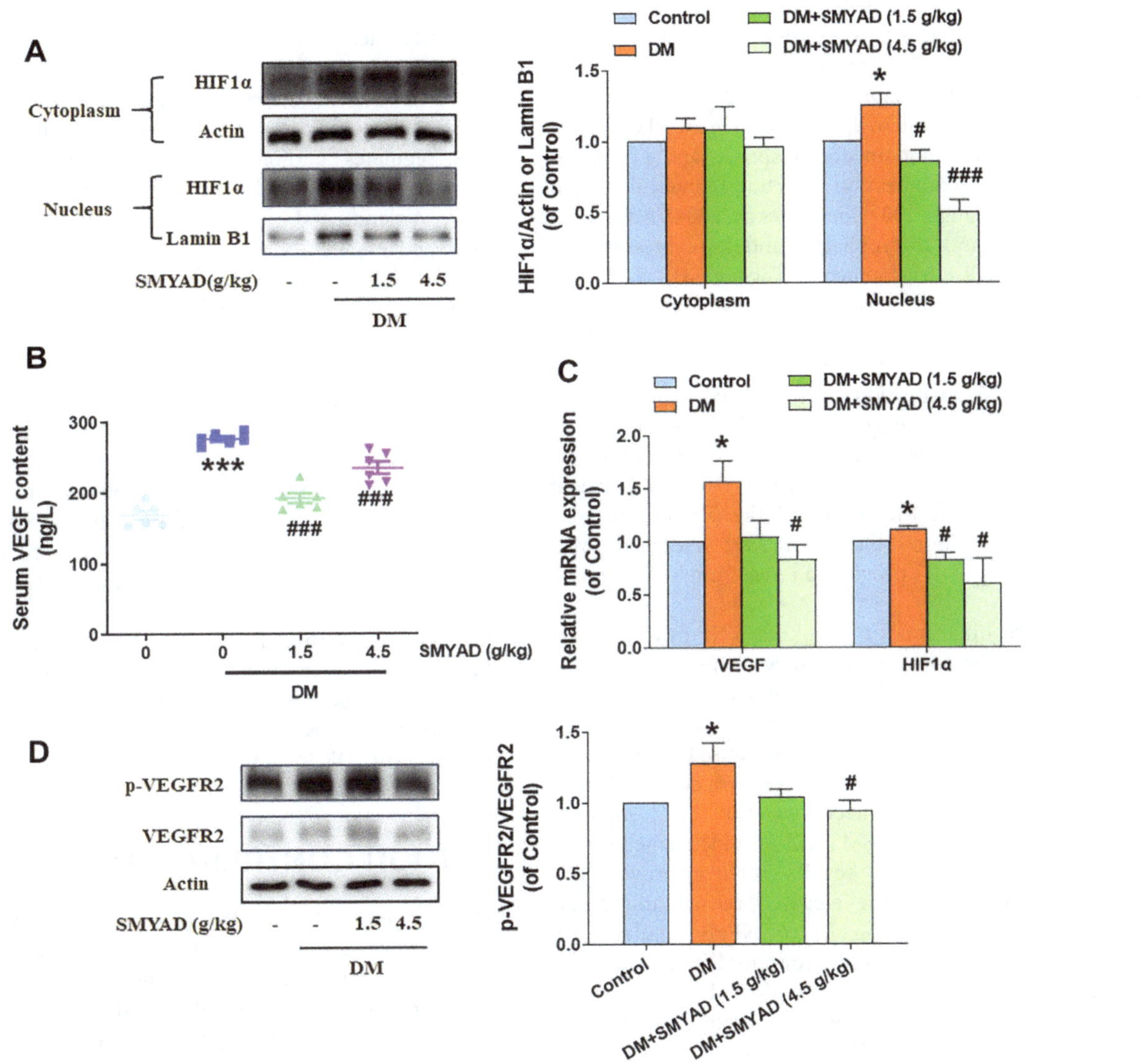

FIGURE 6 | SMYAD inhibited the HIF1α-VEGF/VEGFR2 signal pathway *in vivo*. **(A)** SMYAD reduced nuclear accumulation of HIF1α in retinas. The quantitative result is shown at right (n = 3). **(B)** Serum VEGF content (n = 6). **(C)** HIF1α and VEGF mRNA expression in retinas (n = 3). **(D)** SMYAD decreased the elevated phosphorylation of VEGFR2. The quantitative result is shown at right (n = 3). Data = mean ± SEM. *$p < 0.05$, ***$p < 0.001$ vs. control; #$p < 0.05$, ###$p < 0.001$ vs. DM.

results clearly demonstrated that SMYAD alleviated BRB dysfunction during DR progression.

Next, network pharmacology was performed to find the potential molecular targets involved in the SMYAD-provided alleviation on DR. Among those core molecular targets obtained from network pharmacology, the first six targets with higher degrees were AKT1, IL-6, TP53, TNF, MAPK8, and VEGFA, and they are all reported to regulate inflammation and angiogenesis (Kaštelan et al., 2020; Zhang et al., 2021; Zhou et al., 2021). Moreover, the enrichment results imply the crucial involvement of inflammation, immune responses, and angiogenesis in the SMYAD-provided protection against DR, as well as the potential participation of the TNF signaling pathway and HIF1 signaling pathway. Next, the results from two transcriptome chips conducted in DR research from GEO Databases further validated the previous experimental hints from network pharmacology that TNFα and HIF1α-VEGF signaling pathways participated in the progression of DR. The persistent low-grade inflammation caused by the elevated pro-inflammatory cytokines and other mediators was reported to be closely associated with the injury of retinal vasculature, which will cause BRB breakdown and induce retinal neovascularization during DR progression (Adamis, 2002; Aveleira, et al., 2010; Mesquida, et al., 2019). Therefore, retinal inflammation and neoangiogenesis are crucially involved in the whole course of DR. Our results from network pharmacology indicate that SMYAD may alleviate DR *via* inhibiting TNFα-mediated inflammation and HIF1α-initiated neoangiogenesis in retinas. Meanwhile, these prediction results from network pharmacology were further validated in the next following experiments.

Retinal inflammation initiated by the activated microglia is reported to be associated with DR progression (Baptista et al., 2017; Xu and Chen, 2017). This study showed that SMYAD reduced the enhanced Iba1 expression in retinas, suggesting that SMYAD inhibited retinal microglia activation *in vivo*. Leukostasis is a mild intra-vascular inflammatory response, and it is also an early event during DR progression reflecting retinal ischemia in diabetic patients (Adamis, 2002; Joussen et al., 2004). MCP-1 can recruit monocytes and macrophages, and its expression was elevated during DR development (Taghavi et al., 2019). ICAM1 and VCAM1 can recruit leukocytes to adhere to the endothelium and thus regulate leukostasis (Barouch et al., 2000). We found that SMYAD down-regulated MCP-1, ICAM1, VCAM1, and IL-6 expression and reduced leukostasis in retinas. These results suggest that SMYAD suppressed microglia activation and leukostasis in retina and thus alleviated retinal inflammation during DR development. Moreover, the results further validated the previous network pharmacology prediction that SMYAD alleviated BRB dysfunction during DR progression *via* inhibiting retinal inflammation.

As a main pro-inflammatory cytokine, TNFα was reported to regulate intra-ocular inflammatory responses and DR pathogenesis (Joussen, et al., 2002; Aveleira et al., 2010). TNFα was found to promote the adhesion of leukocytes to the endothelium in the retina and thus caused BRB damage (Joussen et al., 2002; Behl et al., 2008; Aveleira et al., 2010). As predicted in network pharmacology, the TNF signaling pathway participated in the SMYAD-provided amelioration on DR. Next experimental results further proved that SMYAD actually lowered the elevated retinal and serum TNFα contents. Transcription factor NFκB regulates the expression of many pro-inflammatory molecules including TNFα, IL-6, MCP-1, ICAM1, and VCAM1 (Shih et al., 2015). The NFκB signaling pathway is crucial for regulating retinal inflammation during DR progression (Kern, 2007). Our results found that SMYAD suppressed NFκB transcriptional activation and thus contributed to the reduced TNFα amount. All these will contribute to its inhibition on retinal inflammation, which shall be helpful for the alleviation of DR.

Previous network pharmacology results predicted the participation of angiogenesis and the important involvement of the HIF1 signaling pathway in the SMYAD-provided alleviation on DR. The dysfunction of the HIF1α-signaling pathway has already been found to be related with DR progression (Catrina and Zheng, 2021). Our experimental results further evidenced the inhibition of SMYAD on HIF1α activation in retinas *in vivo*. HIF1α can regulate the expression of VEGF, which drives neoangiogenesis *via* binding to its receptors, including VEGFR1, VEGFR2, and VEGFR3, and thus regulates pathological angiogenesis and the elevated vascular permeability during DR development (Witmer et al., 2003; Vriend and Reiter, 2016). SMYAD decreased the enhanced expression of VEGF and phosphorylated VEGFR2 in retinas. These above results suggest that SMYAD reduced retinal angiogenesis through suppressing the HIF1α-VEGF/VEGFR2 signaling cascade.

Our results demonstrated the alleviation of SMYAD on DR *in vivo* for the first time. After integrating the results from network pharmacology and the *in vivo* experimental validation, we found that SMYAD improved DR by inhibiting inflammation and angiogenesis through abrogating the NFκB and HIF1α-VEGF/VEGFR2 signal pathways. However, we must also recognize that the current network pharmacology database cannot yet contain all the signaling molecules involved in DR development, so there may be some other important molecules that have not been found in our study, which needs further deeper investigation in the future. This study provides an experimental basis for the clinical application of SMYAD in patients with DR in the future.

AUTHOR CONTRIBUTIONS

AD, YX, HO, BL, and WJ performed the experiments and analyzed the data. AD drafted the manuscript. HX contributed to the discussion of this study and the revision of this manuscript. LJ conceived and designed this study, wrote and revised the manuscript, conducted the project administration, and acquired the funding grants.

FUNDING

This work was financially supported by the National Natural Science Foundation of China (82074084 and U19A2009) and the leadership in Science and Technology innovation of the third batch of national “Ten Thousand People Plan” for LJ.

REFERENCES

Adamis, A. P. (2002). Is Diabetic Retinopathy an Inflammatory Disease? *Br. J. Ophthalmol.* 86, 363–365. doi:10.1136/bjo.86.4.363

Antonetti, D. A., Klein, R., and Gardner, T. W. (2012). Diabetic Retinopathy. *N. Engl. J. Med.* 366, 1227–1239. doi:10.1056/NEJMra1005073

Aveleira, C. A., Lin, C. M., Abcouwer, S. F., Ambrósio, A. F., and Antonetti, D. A. (2010). TNF-α Signals through PKCζ/NF-Kb to Alter the Tight junction Complex and Increase Retinal Endothelial Cell Permeability. *Diabetes* 59, 2872–2882. doi:10.2337/db09-1606

Bandello, F., Lattanzio, R., Zucchiatti, I., and Del Turco, C. (2013). Pathophysiology and Treatment of Diabetic Retinopathy. *Acta Diabetol.* 50, 1–20. doi:10.1007/s00592-012-0449-3

Baptista, F. I., Aveleira, C. A., Castilho, Á. F., and Ambrósio, A. F. (2017). Elevated Glucose and Interleukin-1β Differentially Affect Retinal Microglial Cell Proliferation. *Mediators Inflamm.* 2017, 4316316. doi:10.1155/2017/4316316

Barouch, F. C., Miyamoto, K., Allport, J. R., Fujita, K., Bursell, S. E., Aiello, L. P., et al. (2000). Integrin-mediated Neutrophil Adhesion and Retinal Leukostasis in Diabetes. *Invest. Ophthalmol. Vis. Sci.* 41, 1153–1158.

Behl, T., and Kotwani, A. (2017). Chinese Herbal Drugs for the Treatment of Diabetic Retinopathy. *J. Pharm. Pharmacol.* 69, 223–235. doi:10.1111/jphp.12683

Behl, Y., Krothapalli, P., Desta, T., DiPiazza, A., Roy, S., and Graves, D. T. (2008). Diabetes-enhanced Tumor Necrosis Factor-Alpha Production Promotes Apoptosis and the Loss of Retinal Microvascular Cells in Type 1 and Type 2 Models of Diabetic Retinopathy. *Am. J. Pathol.* 172, 1411–1418. doi:10.2353/ajpath.2008.071070

Catrina, S. B., and Zheng, X. (2021). Hypoxia and Hypoxia-Inducible Factors in Diabetes and its Complications. *Diabetologia* 64 (4), 709–716. doi:10.1007/s00125-021-05380-z

Chen, M., Obasanmi, G., Armstrong, D., Lavery, N. J., Kissenpfennig, A., Lois, N., et al. (2019). STAT3 Activation in Circulating Myeloid-Derived Cells Contributes to Retinal Microvascular Dysfunction in Diabetes. *J. Neuroinflammation.* 16, 138. doi:10.1186/s12974-019-1533-1

Chinese Pharmacopoeia Commission (2020). *Pharmacopeia of the People's republic of China.* Beijing: The Medicine Science and Technology Press of China. p230, p121, p139, p88.

Douglas, J. Y., Bhatwadekar, A. D., Li Calzi, S., Shaw, L. C., Carnegie, D., Caballero, S., et al. (2012). Bone Marrow-CNS Connections: Implications in the Pathogenesis of Diabetic Retinopathy. *Prog. Retin. Eye Res.* 31, 481–494. doi:10.1016/j.preteyeres.2012.04.005

Erickson, K. K., Sundstrom, J. M., and Antonetti, D. A. (2007). Vascular Permeability in Ocular Disease and the Role of Tight Junctions. *Angiogenesis* 10, 103–117. doi:10.1007/s10456-007-9067-z

Gardlik, R., and Fusekova, I. (2015). Pharmacologic Therapy for Diabetic Retinopathy. *Semin. Ophthalmol.* 30, 252–263. doi:10.3109/08820538.2013.859280

Hopkins, A. L. (2008). Network Pharmacology: the Next Paradigm in Drug Discovery. *Nat. Chem. Biol.* 4, 682–690. doi:10.1038/nchembio.118

Ibrahim, A. S., El-Remessy, A. B., Matragoon, S., Zhang, W., Patel, Y., Khan, S., et al. (2011). Retinal Microglial Activation and Inflammation Induced by Amadori-Glycated Albumin in a Rat Model of Diabetes. *Diabetes* 60, 1122–1133. doi:10.2337/db10-1160

Jiao, X., Jin, X., Ma, Y., Yang, Y., Li, J., Liang, L., et al. (2021). A Comprehensive Application: Molecular Docking and Network Pharmacology for the Prediction of Bioactive Constituents and Elucidation of Mechanisms of Action in Component-Based Chinese Medicine. *Comput. Biol. Chem.* 90, 107402. doi:10.1016/j.compbiolchem.2020.107402

Joussen, A. M., Poulaki, V., Le, M. L., Koizumi, K., Esser, C., Janicki, H., et al. (2004). A central Role for Inflammation in the Pathogenesis of Diabetic Retinopathy. *FASEB J.* 18, 1450–1452. doi:10.1096/fj.03-1476fje

Joussen, A. M., Poulaki, V., Mitsiades, N., Kirchhof, B., Koizumi, K., Döhmen, S., et al. (2002). Nonsteroidal Anti-inflammatory Drugs Prevent Early Diabetic Retinopathy via TNF-Alpha Suppression. *FASEB J.* 16, 438–440. doi:10.1096/fj.01-0707fje

Kanazawa, H., Ohsawa, K., Sasaki, Y., Kohsaka, S., and Imai, Y. (2002). Macrophage/microglia-specific Protein Iba1 Enhances Membrane Ruffling and Rac Activation via Phospholipase C-Gamma -dependent Pathway. *J. Biol. Chem.* 277, 20026–20032. doi:10.1074/jbc.M109218200

Kaštelan, S., Orešković, I., Bišćan, F., Kaštelan, H., and Gverović Antunica, A. (2020). Inflammatory and Angiogenic Biomarkers in Diabetic Retinopathy. *Biochem. Med. (Online)* 30 (3), 030502. doi:10.11613/BM.2020.030502

Kern, T. S. (2007). Contributions of Inflammatory Processes to the Development of the Early Stages of Diabetic Retinopathy. *Exp. Diabetes Res.* 2007, 95103. doi:10.1155/2007/95103

Li, H., Zhao, L., Zhang, B., Jiang, Y., Wang, X., Guo, Y., et al. (2014). A Network Pharmacology Approach to Determine Active Compounds and Action Mechanisms of Ge-Gen-Qin-Lian Decoction for Treatment of Type 2 Diabetes. *Evid. Based Complement. Alternat. Med.* 2014, 495840. doi:10.1155/2014/495840

Li, S., Chen, Y. T., Ding, Q. Y., Dai, J. Y., Duan, X. C., Hu, Y. J., et al. (2021). Network Pharmacology Evaluation Method Guidance-Draft. *World J. Tradit. Chin. Med.* 7 (1), 146–154. doi:10.4103/wjtcm.wjtcm_11_21

Mei, X., Zhang, T., Ouyang, H., Lu, B., Wang, Z., and Ji, L. (2019). Scutellarin Alleviates Blood-Retina-Barrier Oxidative Stress Injury Initiated by Activated Microglia Cells during the Development of Diabetic Retinopathy. *Biochem. Pharmacol.* 159, 82 95. doi:10.1016/j.bcp.2018.11.011

Mesquida, M., Drawnel, F., and Fauser, S. (2019). The Role of Inflammation in Diabetic Eye Disease. *Semin. Immunopathol.* 41, 427–445. doi:10.1007/s00281-019-00750-7

Oellers, P., and Mahmoud, T. H. (2016). Surgery for Proliferative Diabetic Retinopathy: New Tips and Tricks. *J. Ophthalmic Vis. Res.* 11, 93–99. doi:10.4103/2008-322X.180697

Rudraraju, M., Narayanan, S. P., and Somanath, P. R. (2020). Regulation of Blood-Retinal Barrier Cell-Junctions in Diabetic Retinopathy. *Pharmacol. Res.* 161, 105115. doi:10.1016/j.phrs.2020.105115

Shih, R. H., Wang, C. Y., and Yang, C. M. (2015). NF-kappaB Signaling Pathways in Neurological Inflammation: A Mini Review. *Front. Mol. Neurosci.* 8, 77. doi:10.3389/fnmol.2015.00077

Singh, R. S., and Kim, J. E. (2012). Ocular Hypertension Following Intravitreal Anti-vascular Endothelial Growth Factor Agents. *Drugs Aging* 29, 949–956. doi:10.1007/s40266-012-0031-2

Song, P., Yu, J., Chan, K. Y., Theodoratou, E., and Rudan, I. (2018). Prevalence, Risk Factors and burden of Diabetic Retinopathy in China: a Systematic Review and Meta-Analysis. *J. Glob. Health* 8, 010803. doi:10.7189/jogh.08.010803

Taghavi, Y., Hassanshahi, G., Kounis, N. G., Koniari, I., and Khorramdelazad, H. (2019). Monocyte Chemoattractant Protein-1 (MCP-1/CCL2) in Diabetic Retinopathy: Latest Evidence and Clinical Considerations. *J. Cel Commun. Signal* 13, 451–462. doi:10.1007/s12079-018-00500-8

Thomas, R. L., Halim, S., Gurudas, S., Sivaprasad, S., and Owens, D. R. (2019). IDF Diabetes Atlas: A Review of Studies Utilising Retinal Photography on the Global Prevalence of Diabetes Related Retinopathy between 2015 and 2018. *Diabetes Res. Clin. Pract.* 157, 107840. doi:10.1016/j.diabres.2019.107840

Vasant More, S., Kim, I. S., and Choi, D. K. (2017). Recent Update on the Role of Chinese Material Medica and Formulations in Diabetic Retinopathy. *Molecules* 22, 76. doi:10.3390/molecules22010076

Vriend, J., and Reiter, R. J. (2016). Melatonin and the von Hippel-Lindau/HIF-1 oxygen sensing mechanism: A review. *Biochim. Biophys. Acta* 1865, 176–183. doi:10.1016/j.bbcan.2016.02.004

Wang, X., Wang, Z.-Y., Zheng, J.-H., and Li, S. (2021). TCM Network Pharmacology: A New Trend towards Combining Computational, Experimental and Clinical Approaches. *Chin. J. Nat. Med.* 19, 1–11. doi:10.1016/S1875-5364(21)60001-8

Witmer, A. N., Vrensen, G. F., Van Noorden, C. J., and Schlingemann, R. O. (2003). Vascular Endothelial Growth Factors and Angiogenesis in Eye Disease. *Prog. Retin. Eye Res.* 22, 1–29. doi:10.1016/s1350-9462(02)00043-5

Xu, H., and Chen, M. (2017). Diabetic Retinopathy and Dysregulated Innate Immunity. *Vis. Res* 139, 39–46. doi:10.1016/j.visres.2017.04.013

Xu, Z. H., Gao, Y. Y., Zhang, H. T., Ruan, K. F., and Feng, Y. (2018). Progress in Experimental and Clinical Research of the Diabetic Retinopathy Treatment Using Traditional Chinese Medicine. *Am. J. Chin. Med.* 46, 1–27. doi:10.1142/S0192415X1850074X

Zhang, C., Liu, J., Wang, J., Zhang, T., Xu, D., Hu, W., et al. (2021). The Interplay between Tumor Suppressor P53 and Hypoxia Signaling Pathways in Cancer. *Front. Cel Dev. Biol.* 9, 648808. doi:10.3389/fcell.2021.648808

Zhang, C., Wang, H., Nie, J., and Wang, F. (2014). Protective Factors in Diabetic Retinopathy: Focus on Blood-Retinal Barrier. *Discov. Med.* 18, 105–112.

Zhang, R. X., Chen, G. L., and Fang, C. H. (2012). The Application and Mechanism of Simiao Yongan Decoction in Diabetic Complications. *Lishizhen Med. Materia Med. Res.* 23, 2739–2740. doi:10.3969/j.issn.1008-0805.2012.11.033

Zhang, T., Ouyang, H., Mei, X., Lu, B., Yu, Z., Chen, K., et al. (2019). Erianin Alleviates Diabetic Retinopathy by Reducing Retinal Inflammation Initiated by Microglial Cells via Inhibiting Hyperglycemia-Mediated ERK1/2-NF-Kb Signaling Pathway. *FASEB J.* 33, 11776–11790. doi:10.1096/fj.201802614RRR

Zhou, W., Yang, L., Nie, L., and Lin, H. (2021). Unraveling the Molecular Mechanisms Between Inflammation and Tumor Angiogenesis. *Am. J. Cancer Res.* 11 (2), 301–317.

7

Systems Biology Analysis of the Effect and Mechanism of Qi-Jing-Sheng-Bai Granule on Leucopenia in Mice

Saisai Tian[1†], Pengli Huang[2†], Yu Gu[2†], Jian Yang[1], Ran Wu[3], Jing Zhao[2], Ai-Jun Liu[1,4*] and Weidong Zhang[1,2*]*

[1] School of Pharmacy, The Second Military Medical University, Shanghai, China, [2] Institute of Interdisciplinary Complex Research, Shanghai University of Traditional Chinese Medicine, Shanghai, China, [3] Shanghai Tenth People's Hospital, Tongji University, Shanghai, China, [4] Department of Pharmacy, Shanghai Pulmonary Hospital, Shanghai, China

***Correspondence:**
Jing Zhao
zjane_cn@163.com
Ai-Jun Liu
mrliuaijun@163.com
Weidong Zhang
wdzhangy@hotmail.com

† These authors have contributed equally to this work

Qi-Jing-Sheng-Bai granule (QJSB) is a newly developed traditional Chinese medicine (TCM) formula. Clinically, it has been used for the treatment of leucopenia. However, its pharmacological mechanism needs more investigation. In this study, we firstly tested the effects of QJSB on leucopenia using mice induced by cyclophosphamide. Our results suggested that QJSB significantly raised the number of peripheral white blood cells, platelets and nucleated bone marrow cells. Additionally, it markedly enhanced the cell viability and promoted the colony formation of bone marrow mononuclear cells. Furthermore, it reversed the serum cytokines IL-6 and G-CSF disorders. Then, using transcriptomics datasets and metabonomic datasets, we integrated transcriptomics-based network pharmacology and metabolomics technologies to investigate the mechanism of action of QJSB. We found that QJSB regulated a series of biological processes such as hematopoietic cell lineage, homeostasis of number of cells, lymphocyte differentiation, metabolic processes (including lipid, amino acid, and nucleotide metabolism), B cell receptor signaling pathway, T cell activation and NOD-like receptor signaling pathway. In a summary, QJSB has protective effects to leucopenia in mice probably through accelerating cell proliferation and differentiation, regulating metabolism response pathways and modulating immunologic function at a system level.

Keywords: Qi-Jing-Sheng-Bai granule, leucopenia, transcriptomics, metabolomics, network pharmacology

INTRODUCTION

Chemotherapy has been widely used for the treatment of cancers. However, chemotherapy usually induces many adverse effects, including hematologic toxicity and neurotoxicity (Magge and DeAngelis, 2015; Ratti and Tomasello, 2015; Zhou et al., 2018). Among them, hematologic toxicity, like leucopenia, is a very common adverse reaction that can delay the subsequent therapy, induce the risk of cancer metastasis, and even lead to life-threatening events (Xu et al., 2011; Cui et al., 2015). Hence the hematologic indexes, including the white blood cells (WBC), neutrophile granulocytes, blood platelets and monocytes, are important objective indexes for cancer patients after chemotherapy. Studies have shown that granulocyte colony-stimulating factor (G-CSF) and related agents have clinical efficacy. They are recommended to prevent leucopenia (Xu et al., 2011). However, G-CSF only reduces the neutropenia duration for 1–2 days while also increases adverse reactions and the cost of treatment notably (Dygai et al., 2012; Aarts et al., 2013). Traditional Chinese medicine (TCM) formulae have been widely used in China for the treatment of leucopenia (Liu et al., 2014). Formulae usually consist of several types of Chinese medicines. Among them, one herb is the principal component, and the others serve as adjuvant ones to assist the function of the principal component. It is believed that multiple components contained in the formulae could hit multiple targets and exert synergistic effects (Jiang, 2005).

Qi-Jing-Sheng-Bai granule (QJSB) is a modern TCM formula. It is made from extracts of nine Chinese medicines, namely, *Astragalus membranaceus* (Huangqi), *Panax quinquefolium* (Xiyangshen), *Epimedium brevicornum* (Yinyanghuo), *Angelica sinensis* (Danggui), *Polygonatum sibiricum* (Huangjing), *Eclipta pwstmta* (Mohanlian), *Lycium barbarum* (Gouqi), *Psoralea corylifolia* (Buguzhi), and *Spatholobus suberectus* (Jixueteng), as well as one raw material component of Cervi Cornus Colla, at a ratio of 6:2:3:2:2:3:2:2:6:1. Both *A. membranaceus* and Cervi Cornus Colla are principal components. In a clinical study, QJSB has been used for the treatment of leucopenia (Wu et al., 2018). In our previous study, we identified 143 compounds, including 56 flavonoids, 51 saponins, and 36 other compounds, from QJSB (Wu et al., 2018). It has been accepted that the effective ingredients can be detected in serum after medicine administration. After the oral administration of QJSB, 42 compounds, including 24 prototype compounds and 18 metabolites, have been detected in the serum of rats (Wu et al., 2018). Among the 42 compounds, many ingredients have been proven to have bioactivities. For example, ferulic acid improves hematopoietic cell recovery in whole-body gamma irradiated mice and increases levels of granulocyte-colony stimulating factor (G-CSF) (Ma et al., 2011); several flavonoids including formononetin, ononin, calycosin, and calycosin-7-O-β-D-glucoside, induce the expression of erythropoietin in human embryonic kidney fibroblasts via the accumulation of hypoxia-inducible factor-1α (Zheng et al., 2011); quercitrin protects endothelial progenitor cells from oxidative damage via inducing autophagy through extracellular signal-regulated kinase (Zhi et al., 2016); icaritin improves the hematopoietic function in cyclophosphamide-induced myelosuppression mice (Sun et al., 2018). The identification of compounds absorbed into blood revealed the effective substance of QJSB to some extent. However, the therapeutic mechanism of QJSB in leucopenia remains unclear. Thus, the effect on the treatment of leucopenia needs further detailed investigation.

Systems biology studies the pharmacological mechanism of TCM by integrating transcriptomic, proteomic and metabolomic profiles (Su et al., 2011; Meierhofer et al., 2014). Network pharmacology is a new system biology approach, generally describing the association of multiple components with multiple targets and multiple pathways (Ning et al., 2017). Recently, the application of integrated systems biology and network pharmacology is a promising approach for the delineation of effects and mechanisms of TCM formulae.

In this study, we firstly investigated the effect of QJSB on leucopenia using mice induced by cyclophosphamide. We further investigated the therapeutic mechanism of QJSB using the transcriptomics datasets derived from the bone marrow and metabonomic datasets from plasma. Finally, we applied transcriptomics-based network pharmacology and metabolomics technologies to study the mechanism of QJSB for the treatment of leucopenia.

MATERIALS AND METHODS

Chemical Reagents

Cyclophosphamide was purchased from Zaiqi Biotechnology Corporation (Shanghai, China). QJSB granules were kindly provided by Zhendong Pharmaceutical (Shanxi, China).

Animals and Treatments

All animal studies were performed according to the institutional ethical guidelines of animal care and were approved by the Committee on the Ethics of Animal Experiments of the Second Military Medical University, China. Male ICR mice (18–22 g) were obtained from Laboratory Animal Company (Shanghai, China). The mice were acclimated for 2–3 days under conditions of controlled temperature (24 ± 2°C), relative humidity of 60 ± 5%, 12 h light/dark cycle, and *ad libitum* access to standard laboratory food and water. All the mice were randomly allocated into four groups: normal group and 3 leucopenia model groups (cyclophosphamide, 80 mg/kg/day). The model groups were treated with vehicle, leucogen (20 mg/kg/day) and QJSB (3 g/kg/day), respectively. The mice in each group were orally administered with respective medicines for 1 week, and an equivalent volume (0.2 ml/10 g) of 0.9% saline solution was used for normal group and model group. Next, the animals in each group were sacrificed by dislocation of the cervical vertebra and were prepared for subsequent experiments. In each group, the whole blood of 10 mice was used for routine blood examination and bone marrow cells in the femurs were used for the bone marrow nuclear cell count, cell viability assay and colony-forming unit assay. The sera of another 10 mice were used to detect the levels of IL-6 and G-CSF. Bone marrow cells in the femurs of three of these mice were collected for RNA isolation, sequencing and real-time quantitative PCR (RT-qPCR). The plasma of the mice was collected for metabonomic analysis. After 2 weeks of treatment, the mice were sacrificed by dislocation of the cervical vertebra and the whole blood was used for routine blood examination (n = 10).

Leucopenia Model

The leucopenia model was established as follows: for 1 week of treatment, the mice in the model groups were treated with 80 mg/kg/day of cyclophosphamide intraperitoneally for 3 consecutive days (from day 5 to day 7), and the normal group was treated with an equivalent volume (0.1 ml/10 g) of normal saline. For 2 weeks of treatment, the mice were treated with cyclophosphamide (80 mg/kg/day) intraperitoneally for 6 days (3 consecutive days per week), and the normal group was treated with an equivalent volume (0.1 ml/10 g) of normal saline.

Cell Viability Assay

Cell viability was measured using the Cell Counting Kit-8 (CCK8) reagent (Dojindo, Japan). The mice were sacrificed by dislocation of the cervical vertebra and the femurs were immediately collected. Bone marrow was eluted from the shaft by RPMI 1640 medium, and filtered through a 70 micron filter. Bone marrow nuclear cells were dispensed in 96-well culture plates (100 μL/well) at a density of 5×10^5 /mL. Next, the cells were incubated with 10 μl of CCK8 reagent. Finally, the absorbance at 450 nm was measured.

Colony-Forming Units Assay

The mice were sacrificed by dislocation of the cervical vertebra and the femurs were immediately harvested. Next, bone marrow cells were eluted from the shaft by RPMI 1640 medium, and filtered through a 70 micron filter. Thereafter, bone marrow mononuclear cells were obtained by centrifugation in a Ficoll density gradient. The cells were diluted with M3434 methylcellulose medium (StemCell Technologies, Canada) at a density of 3×10^4/mL, dispensed into 6-well culture plates (1 mL/well), and cultured in an atmosphere of 5% CO_2 at 37°C for 12 days. Colonies consisting of 50 cells or more were counted.

The Detection of IL-6 and G-CSF

Whole blood was collected from mice by removing the eyeballs. Blood samples were placed to clot for 2 h at room temperature before centrifuging for 20 min at 2000 × *g*. Serum was collected and stored in aliquots at −80°C for later use. Commercially available sandwich enzyme-linked immunosorbent assay (ELISA) kits (eBiosciences, San Diego, CA, United States) were used for the quantitation of IL-6 and G-CSF. The optical density of each sample at 450 nm was measured. Cytokine levels were quantified using standard curves, and the values were expressed in units of pg/ml.

RNA Isolation, Library Preparation, and Sequencing

The total RNA of bone marrow cells from 12 mice (leucopenia group, $n = 3$, QJSB group, $n = 3$, normal group, $n = 3$, and leucogen group, $n = 3$) were extracted using TRIzol (Invitrogen, Carlsbad, CA, United States) reagent for RNA sequencing and were purified according to the manufacturer's instructions. Strand-specific libraries were prepared using the VAHTS Total RNAseq Library PrepKit for Illumina (Vazyme, China) following the manufacturer's instructions. Using Ribo-Zero rRNA removal beads, ribosomal RNA was removed from total RNA. Following purification, the mRNA was fragmented into small pieces using divalent cations under 94°C for 8 min. The cleaved RNA fragments were copied into first strand cDNA using reverse transcriptase and random primers. This is followed by second strand cDNA synthesis using DNA polymerase I and RNase H. These cDNA fragments then went through an end repair process, the addition of a single "A" base, and then ligation of the adapters. The products were then purified and enriched with PCR to create the final cDNA library. Purified libraries were quantified by Qubit® 2.0 Fluorometer (Life Technologies, United States) and validated by Agilent 2100 bioanalyzer (Agilent Technologies, United States) to confirm the insert size and calculate the mole concentration. Cluster was generated by cBot with the library diluted to 10 pM, followed by sequencing on the Illumina HiSeq 2500 (Illumina, United States).

Data Analysis for Gene Expression

Sequencing raw reads were preprocessed by filtering out rRNA reads, sequencing adapters, short-fragment reads and other low-quality reads using Seqtk. Hisat2 (version 2.0.4) was used to map the cleaned reads to the mouse GRCm38.p4 (mm10) reference genome with two mismatches. Gene expression was evaluated in FPKM (fragments per kilobase per million mapped fragments) from RNAseq data. The formula to calculate FPKM was as follows: FPKM = (number of mapping fragments) $\times 10^3 \times 10^6$/[(length of transcript) × (number of total fragments)]. Differential expression analysis of two groups was performed using the "DESeq2" R package at the cutoff of |log2 fold change| > 0.585 and *P*-value < 0.05 (Love et al., 2013). Then, we constructed a pre-ranked gene list of all differentially expressed genes ordered by the absolute value of log2 fold change and selected the top 300 genes for further analysis.

Pathway Enrichment Analysis and GO Analysis

We firstly used R package "clusterProfiler" to perform pathway enrichment analysis to identify KEGG (Kanehisa and Goto, 2000) (Kyoto Encyclopedia of Genes and Genomes) pathways enriched with the top 300 differentially expressed genes. Significant pathways with *P*-value < 0.05 were selected. Next, GO (Gene Ontology) enrichment analysis was also performed to explore the biological processes of the top 300 differentially expressed genes. At a cutoff of $P < 0.05$.

Evaluation of Drug's Effects by the Network Scores

The background protein-protein interaction (PPI) network was downloaded from the STRING database v10.5[1] and the organism was chosen as "Mus musculus." All genes were standardized by mapping to the Entrez ID for further analysis. In this paper, the top 300 DEGs under the treatment of a drug were regarded as the drug's potential target genes. Similarly, the top 300 DEGs between the model and normal groups were regarded as disease associated genes. We applied the algorithm random walk with restart (RWR) to measure the seed genes' influence on the background network. Specifically, the drug's potential target genes and disease associated genes were used as seed nodes, respectively. Additionally, genes in the background network were scored by RWR. Next, we calculated the Pearson correlation coefficient between the network scores based on each gene set

[1] https://string-db.org/

to estimate the relevance of the drug's potential target genes and disease associated genes. The relevance was estimated as follows:

$$Relevance = cor(Scores_{drug}, Scores_{disease})$$

where *cor* represents the Pearson correlation coefficient and *Scores* represents the genes' network scores. To evaluate the significance of the correlation between the drug's target genes and disease genes, a reference distribution was built. Genes with the same number of drug's target genes were randomly selected from the background network and the correlation coefficient was calculated between the disease genes and random set. We performed 100 repetitions to generate the reference perturbation distribution. The mean and standard deviation of the random correlation coefficients were denoted by $\mu_{Relevance}$ and $\sigma_{Relevance}$, respectively. The Z-score was finally calculated and the absolute value of the Z-score larger than 3 suggests that the drug's effect on the disease was statistically significant.

$$Z_{score} = \frac{|Relevance - \mu_{Relevance}|}{\sigma_{Relevance}}$$

Sample Preparation and LC-MS Conditions for Metabonomic Analysis

Because the endogenous metabolites play an essential role in the physiology of hosts, we explored the host metabolic profiling in the plasma of a subset of 27 subjects by liquid chromatography-mass spectrometry (LC/MS). The detailed method was as follows. Each plasma sample was thawed at 4°C and vortexed for 5 s at room temperature. Next, 100 μL of plasma was transferred into another 1.5 mL tube with 300 μL of methanol and was mixed 45 s in a vortex. Thereafter, the sample was centrifuged for 10 min (12000 rpm, 4°C). Finally, the supernatant was transferred into auto-sampler vials and stored at −80°C for LC-MS analysis. The QC sample was prepared by mixing 10 μL of aliquot from the six above prepared samples, respectively. The QC samples were injected every six samples.

Chromatographic separation was performed on a ACQUITY UPLC® HSS T3 (2.1 × 100 mm, 1.8 μm, Waters, United States) using an ACQUITY Ultra Performance LC system (Waters corp., Milford, MA, United States). The column was maintained at 40°C. The flow rate was set at 0.4 mL/min, and the sample injection was 1 μL. The optimal mobile phase consisted of a linear gradient system of water mixed with 0.1% formic acid (phase A) and acetonitrile (phase B): 0–6.0 min, 5–100% B, 6.0–8.0 min, 100% B; 8.0–9.0 min, 100–90% B; 9.0–14.0 min, 90–80% B; 14.0–14.1 min, 80–5% B; 14.1–19.0 min, 5% B. MS detection was acquired on a Micromass Quadrupole (Q) SYNAPT G2-Si high-resolution mass spectrometer (Waters Corp., Milford, MA, United States) equipped with an electrospray ion (ESI) source. Both positive and negative modes were utilized in the current research. The temperature of the ion source was 120°C. The capillary voltage and cone voltage were 2000 V and 49V, respectively. The desolvation gas temperature and flow were 350°C and 750 L/h, respectively. The cone gas was set at 50 L/h. Data were collected between 50 and 1200 m/z with a 0.2 s scan time and a 0.02 s interscan delay. All analyses were conducted using the lock spray to ensure the accuracy and precision of the mass information for compound identification. Leucine encephalin [$(M+H)^+ = 556.2771$, $(M-H)^- = 554.2615$] was used as the lock spray at a concentration of 1 μg/mL, and the flow rate was set at 5 μL/min. Additionally, mass spectrometry elevated energy (MS^E) collection was applied for compound identification. This technique obtains precursor ion information through low collision energy and full-scan accurate mass fragment information through the ramp of the high collision energy. The collision energy of MS^E was set from 15 to 35 V.

Metabonomic Data Processing and Analysis

The raw plasma LC-MS data were pre-processed using Waters Progenesis QI 2.0 software (Non-linear Dynamics, Newcastle, United Kingdom). Progenesis QI includes the steps of importing data, reviewing alignment, experiment design setup, picking peaks, identifying and reviewing compounds, and performing compound statistical analysis. Then, the data were exported into SICMA 14.1 (Umetric, Umeå, Sweden) for multivariable statistical analysis. The multivariate statistical analysis (MVA) included principal component analysis (PCA), partial least squares discrimination analysis (PLS-DA), and orthogonal partial least square-discriminant (OPLS-DA) models, which were used to observe the classifications for different groups. Thereafter, based on the OPLS-DA plot, the ions were filtered by VIP > 1 (variable importance in the projection) to identify the metabolites contributing to the classifications. Next, ions with P-values < 0.05 were regarded as the differential metabolite ions. Subsequently, the differential metabolites ions with the two filters were structurally identified and interpreted based on the metabonomic associated databases: METLIN[2], HMDB[3], and KEGG[4]. Finally, using the MetaboAnalyst 4.0, we performed pathway analysis for the metabolites contributing to the classifications and identified the most relevant pathways.

RNA Extraction and Real-Time Quantitative PCR

Total RNA was extracted in bone marrow cells from three groups (leucopenia, QJSB and normal groups) mice using the Trizol reagent (Thermo Fisher Scientific) according to the manufacturer's instructions. And cDNA was generated using the High-Capacity cDNA Reverse Transcription Kit (Thermo Fisher Scientific). RT-qPCR was performed using the Stratagene Mx3005P RT-PCR System (Applied Biosystems) and the PowerUp™ SYBR® Green Master Mix (Thermo Fisher Scientific), according to the protocol. Melt curves were analyzed at the end of each assay to confirm the specificity. Fold change was determined using the $2^{-\Delta\Delta CT}$ method normalized with endogenous control GAPDH. The PCR primers used are listed in **Supplementary Table S1**.

[2] https://metlin.scripps.edu/

[3] www.hmdb.ca

[4] https://www.genome.jp/kegg/

Statistical Analysis

GraphPad was used for statistical analysis of the biochemical data. The animals were randomly assigned by using the random permutations table. The data were expressed as the means ± standard deviation (SD). The data were analyzed using by two-tailed Student's *t*-test or one-way analysis of variance (ANOVA). $P < 0.05$ was considered statistically significant. The transcriptomics data were processed by R package with "DESeq2" and "clusterProfiler." SICMA 14.1 (Umetric, Umeå, Sweden) was used for MVA. Cytoscape was used to trace the associated gene–enzyme relationship using KEGG database.

RESULTS

QJSB Increased Peripheral WBCs and Platelets in Leucopenia Model Mice

After treatment with cyclophosphamide, the peripheral WBCs and platelets were significantly decreased. After 1 week of treatment, QJSB increased peripheral WBCs ($P < 0.001$) and platelets ($P < 0.001$) significantly (approximately 2.6-fold and 2.4-fold, respectively) compared with those in model group (**Figures 1A,B**). Administration of QJSB or cyclophosphamide had no significant effect on the other peripheral hemogram parameters such as RBCs and hemoglobin concentration (**Figures 1C,D**). We also got the similar results when the leucopenia model animals were treated by QJSB for 2 weeks (**Figures 1E,F**). For WBC differential counts at 1 week of treatment, cyclophosphamide decreased the percentage of monocytes and increased the percentage of eosinophils. The percentage of eosinophils returned to normal after being administrated with QJSB and leucogen. In addition, an increase was observed in the percentage of basophils in QJSB and leucogen groups (**Figure 2**).

QJSB Increased Bone Marrow Nuclear Cells and Enhanced Cell Viability in Leucopenia Model Mice

The cell number and cell viability of bone marrow nuclear cells were significantly decreased in the cyclophosphamide treatment group ($P < 0.05$). QJSB significantly increased the number of bone marrow nuclear cells, and enhanced the cell viability ($P < 0.001$) (**Figures 3A–C**).

QJSB Promoted Bone Marrow Mononuclear Cells Colony Formation

To determine the effect of QJSB on bone marrow hemopoietic stem/progenitor cells, we performed the methylcellulose semisolid colony-forming units assay. Mononuclear cells were extracted from the bone marrow of ICR mice. Colony formation of bone marrow mononuclear cells was significantly decreased by cyclophosphamide. After 1 week of treatment, the colony number and colony size were both significantly increased by QJSB ($P < 0.001$) (**Figure 3D**).

QJSB Reversed Cytokines Secretion in Serum of Leucopenia Model Mice

The hematopoiesis-related cytokines are important factors for the regulation of hematopoietic function (Alexander, 1998). Both G-CSF and IL-6 in serum were detected. Compared with the normal control group, after cyclophosphamide treatment, the levels of G-CSF and IL-6 in serum were dramatically increased from 100.6 and 5.5 pg/ml to 1143.0 and 89.0 pg/ml, respectively. QJSB significantly reversed the increases of G-CSF (from 1143 to 345 pg/ml, $P < 0.001$) (**Figure 3E**) and IL-6 (from 89.0 to 9.4 pg/ml, $P < 0.001$) (**Figure 3F**) induced by cyclophosphamide.

Differential Expression Genes Identification and Functional Analysis

In order to identify potential molecular mechanisms, high-throughput sequencing was used to identify the affected gene by QJSB in bone tissue. The raw data of fastq format of RNAseq are available through the National Center for Biotechnology Information's Gene Expression Omnibus (GEO[5]), and the GEO series accession number is GSE120707. Then, the top 300 differentially expressed genes between QJSB treatment and model group were identified, which included 172 upregulated and 128 downregulated genes. Comparing the leucopenia groups with the normal groups, the top 300 differentially expressed genes, with 14 upregulated and 286 downregulated genes, were detected. Additionally, comparing the leucogen groups with the leucopenia groups, the top 300 differentially expressed genes, with 177 upregulated and 123 downregulated genes, were also identified. The details of the top 300 differentially expressed genes are listed in **Supplementary Table S2**. To identify potential affected pathways of QJSB, KEGG pathway enrichment analysis was performed using the top 300 differentially expressed genes between QJSB and model group. We found that "hematopoietic cell lineage," "osteoclast differentiation, "B cell receptor signaling pathway, "NOD-like receptor signaling pathway," "arachidonic acid metabolism," and "Ferroptosis" were significantly enriched ($P < 0.05$) (**Figure 4**, left). To further identify the biological processes, we did GO terms enrichment analysis and found the most significantly enriched terms are "homeostasis of number of cells," "cellular response to TGF-β stimulus," "TGF-β receptor signaling pathway," "response to TGF-β," "lymphocyte differentiation," "regulation of immune effector process," and "T cell activation" (**Figure 4**, right). The detail parameters of pathways and GO terms are shown in **Tables 1, 2**. These results indicate that QJSB may influence these pathways and biological process, thus increasing peripheral WBCs and platelets in leucopenia model mice.

RWR-Based Evaluation of QJSB

As mentioned above, the top 300 differentially expressed genes were identified from leucopenia-normal groups, leucogen-leucopenia groups, QJSB-leucopenia groups, respectively. We took the top 300 genes of each set as seeds to apply the RWR

[5]http://www.ncbi.nlm.nih.gov/geo/

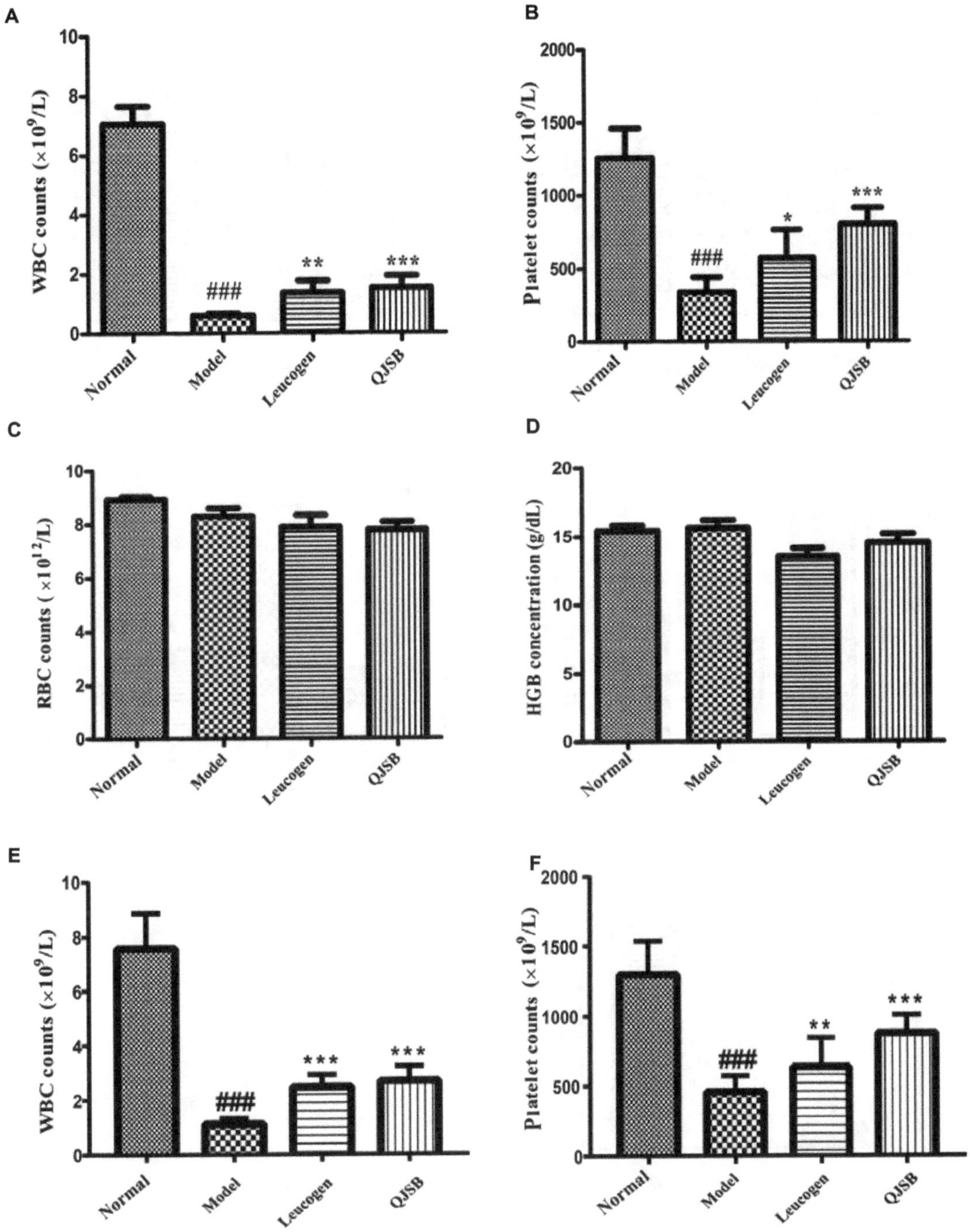

FIGURE 1 | The effect of QJSB on the peripheral WBC **(A)**, platelet **(B)**, RBC **(C)**, and HGB **(D)** parameters in leucopenia mice induced by cyclophosphamide. After 1 week of treatment, QJSB increased peripheral WBCs **(A)** and platelets **(B)** compared with model group, but had no significant effect on the other peripheral hemogram parameters such as RBCs **(C)** and hemoglobin concentration **(D)**. After 2 week of treatment, QJSB also increased peripheral WBCs **(E)** and platelets **(F)**. Data are presented as means ± SD. ###Represent $P < 0.001$ vs. normal group and *, **, and *** represent $P < 0.05$, 0.01, and 0.001 vs. model group, respectively.

algorithm. In total, 153 genes from leucopenia-normal groups were mapped to the background network and set as disease associated genes, while 252 genes from QJSB and 233 genes from leucogen were mapped and set as drug's potential target genes. We calculated the Z-score as described in Materials and Methods. The results are listed in **Table 3**. As shown in **Table 3**, the Z-score for QJSB is 6.156 (larger than 3), and it is 10.823 for leucogen. These results suggest that QJSB and leucogen have significant effects against leucopenia in mice from perspective of network analysis.

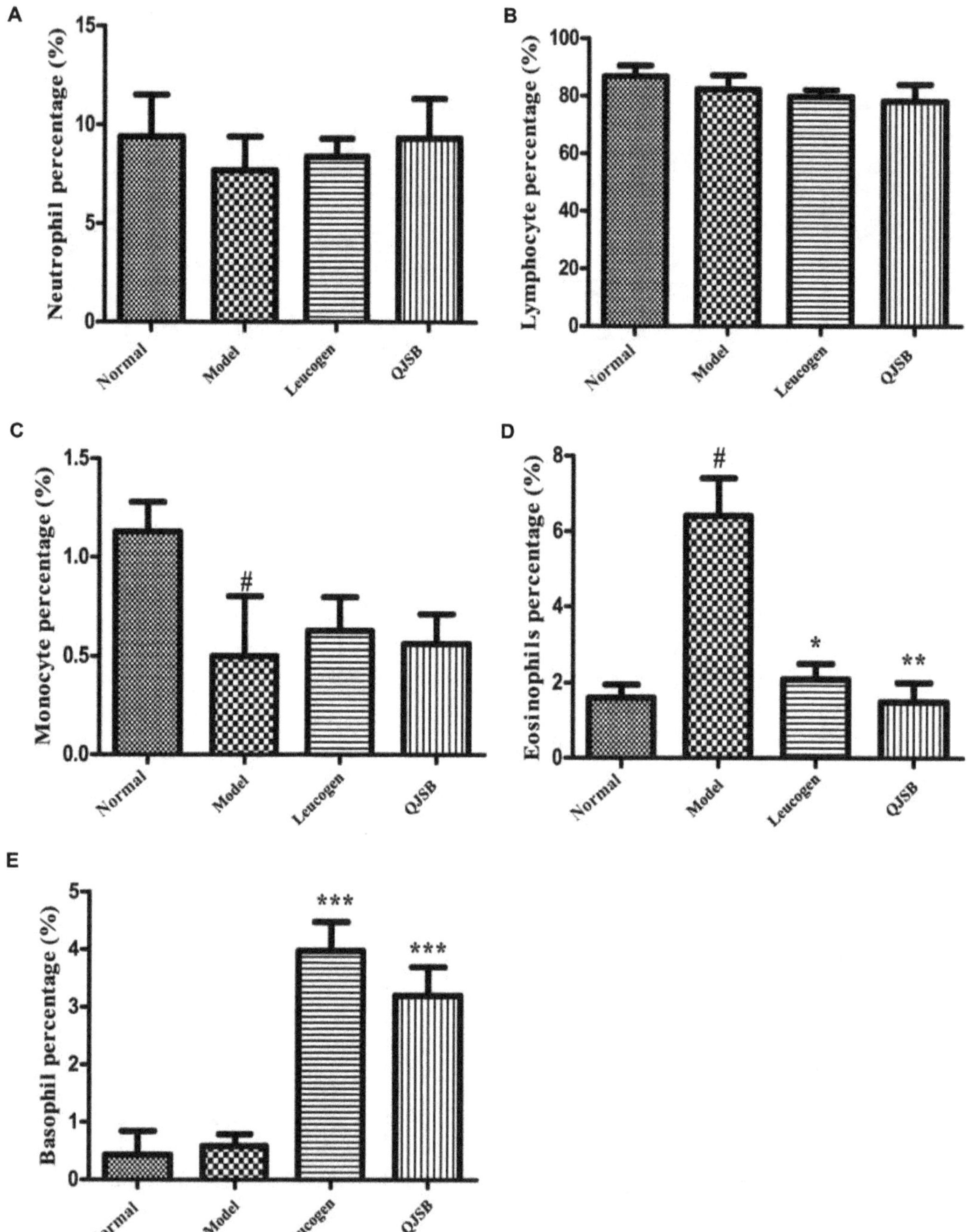

FIGURE 2 | The effect of QJSB on WBC differential counts: neutrophil **(A)**, lymphocyte **(B)**, monocyte **(C)**, eosinophil **(D)**, and basophil **(E)** in leucopenia mice induced by cyclophosphamide. Cyclophosphamide increased the percentage of eosinophils **(D)**, and QJSB returned it to normal. An increase was observed in the percentage of basophils **(E)** in QJSB group. Data are presented as means ± SD. #Represent $P < 0.05$ vs. normal group and *, **, and *** represent $P < 0.05$, 0.01, and 0.001 vs. model group, respectively.

Differential Metabolites Identification and Metabolic Pathway Analysis

The plasma samples were subjected to LC/MS analysis in both the positive ion mode (ESI+) and negative ion mode (ESI−). To discriminate the metabolic profiles among normal, model control and QJSB group, we performed clustering analysis using PCA, and the supervised PLS-DA and OPLS-DA. The plasma sample from different groups tended to separated according to the PCA plots either in ESI+ or ESI-mode (**Figure 5A**). Furthermore, the PLS-DA score scatter plots further evidenced the significant separation among the normal, model and QJSB groups either in

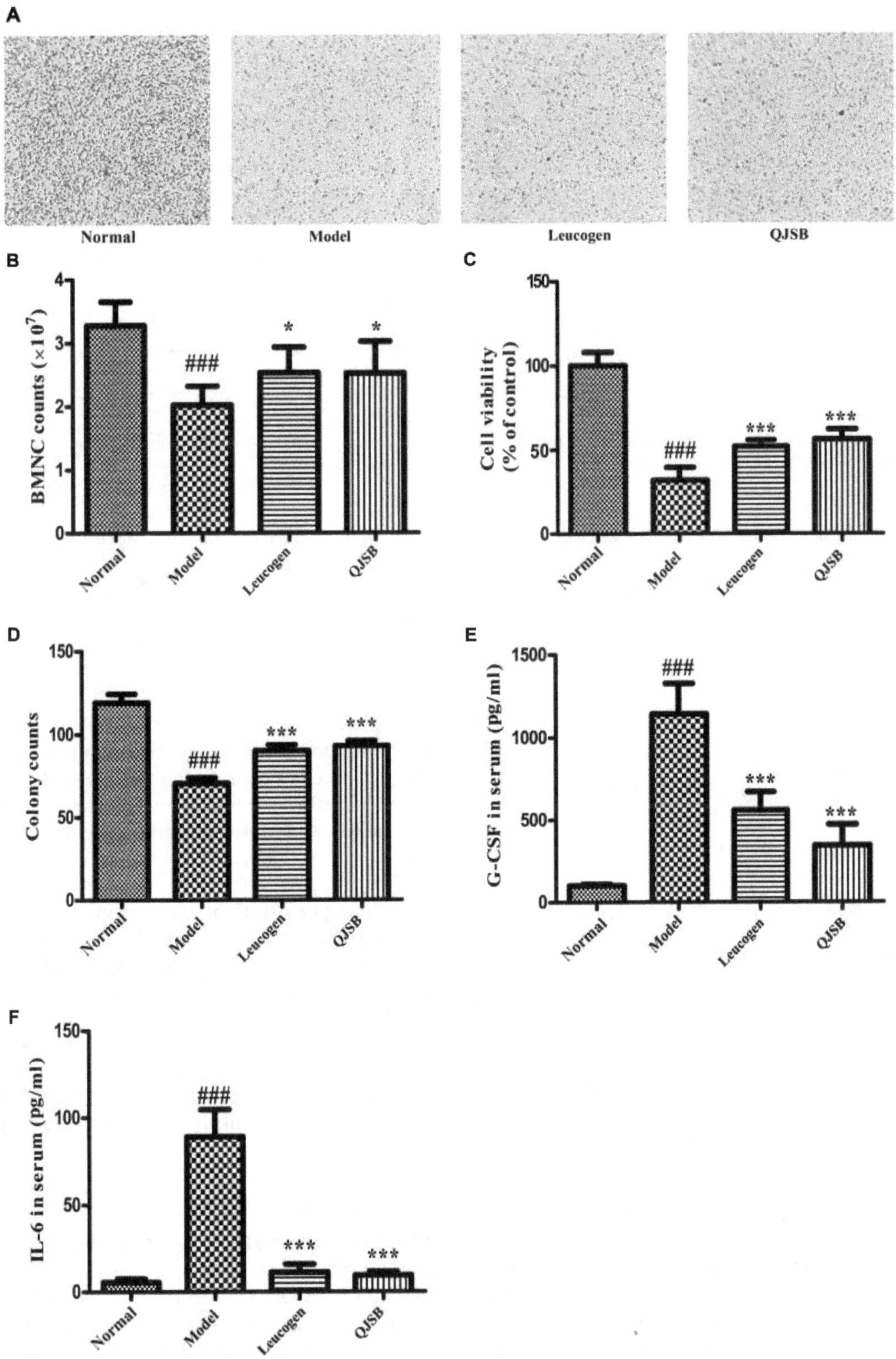

FIGURE 3 | The effect of QJSB on the cell number and cell viability of bone marrow nuclear cells, colony formation of bone marrow mononuclear cells and cytokines secretion. QJSB significantly increased the number of bone marrow nuclear cells **(A,B)**, enhanced the cell viability **(C)** and promoted colony formation of bone marrow mononuclear cells **(D)**. QJSB significantly reversed the increases of G-CSF **(E)** and IL-6 **(F)** induced by cyclophosphamide. Data are presented as means ± SD. ###Represent $P < 0.001$ vs. normal group and * and *** represent $P < 0.05$ and 0.001 vs. model group, respectively.

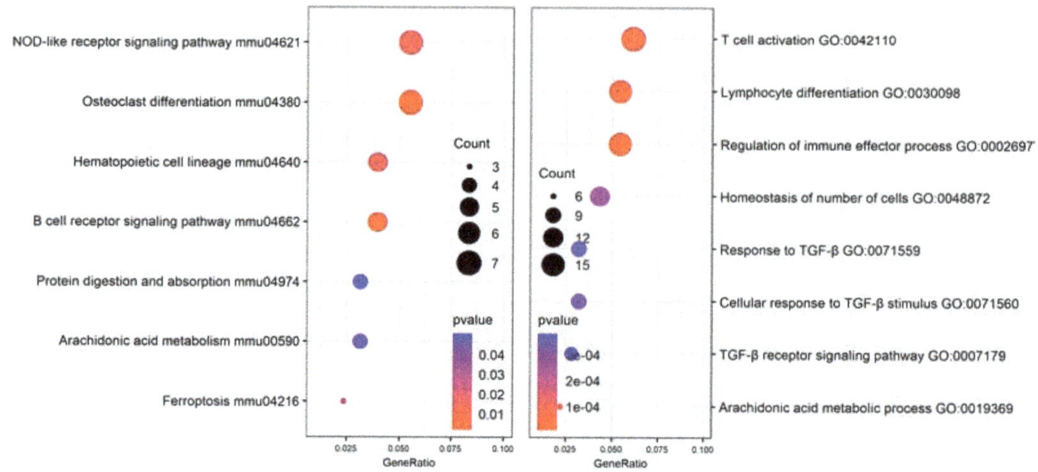

FIGURE 4 | Pathway enrichment analysis and GO analysis. KEGG pathway enrichment analysis for top 300 differentially expressed genes in QJSB-treated mice is shown left. GO analysis for top 300 differentially expressed genes in QJSB-treated mice is shown right.

TABLE 1 | Pathways enrichment analysis of differently expressed genes in bone marrow cells of QJSB-treated mice.

ID	Description	GeneRatio	*P*-value
mmu04380	Osteoclast differentiation	0.0550	0.0035
mmu04662	B cell receptor signaling pathway	0.0390	0.0049
mmu04621	NOD-like receptor signaling pathway	0.0550	0.0148
mmu04640	Hematopoietic cell lineage	0.0390	0.0154
mmu04216	Ferroptosis	0.0240	0.0248
mmu00590	Arachidonic acid metabolism	0.0310	0.0480
mmu04974	Protein digestion and absorption	0.0310	0.0497

TABLE 2 | GO enrichment analysis of differently expressed genes in bone marrow cells of QJSB-treated mice.

ID	Description	GeneRatio	*P*-value
GO:0002697	Regulation of immune effector process	0.0540	0.0000
GO:0030098	Lymphocyte differentiation	0.0540	0.0001
GO:0042110	T cell activation	0.0610	0.0001
GO:0019369	Arachidonic acid metabolic process	0.0220	0.0001
GO:0048872	Homeostasis of number of cells	0.0430	0.0003
GO:0071560	Cellular response to TGF-β stimulus	0.0320	0.0003
GO:0071559	Response to TGF-β	0.0320	0.0004
GO:0007179	TGF-β receptor signaling pathway	0.0280	0.0004

TABLE 3 | The effect scores of QJSB and leucogen on leukopenia.

Drug	QJSB	Leucogen
Overlap	252	233
Revelance	0.1248	0.1590
Z-score	6.1560	10.8230

ESI+ or ESI-mode (**Figure 5B**). To further identify the significant metabolites contributing to the classifications among these three groups, supervised OPLS-DA was adopted between two groups either in the ESI+ or ESI- modes together. The permutations plot was used to assess the OPLS-DA model and the results showed the model was highly significant and non-overfitting (**Supplementary Figure S1**). The quality of the OPLS-DA model was shown in **Supplementary Table S3**. The result suggested that there was the remarkable separation in model vs. normal and model vs. QJSB. There were 51 and 47 metabolites differently regulated in leucopenia (vs. normal) and QJSB treatment (vs. leucopenia model) mice, respectively (**Supplementary Table S4**). Then, in order to identify the key metabolic pathway, we did metabolic pathway enrichment analysis using MetaboAnalyst 4.0 (**Tables 4, 5**). As shown in **Figure 6A**, in leucopenia model (vs. normal), the differential metabolites primarily participate in glycerophospholipid metabolism, primary bile acid biosynthesis phenylalanine, tyrosine and tryptophan biosynthesis and phenylalanine metabolism. These metabolic anomalies were found to be primarily involved in lipid metabolism and amino acid metabolism. After QJSB treatment (vs. leucopenia model), the differential metabolites also were primarily enriched in lipid metabolism (glycerophospholipid metabolism, ether lipid metabolism, and linoleic acid metabolism) and amino acid metabolism (tryptophan metabolism) (**Figure 6B**). The results indicate that QJSB is likely involved in the modulation of the metabolic disorders.

Correlation Networks Construction of Differential Genes and Metabolites

In order to obtain a comprehensive view of the complex mechanisms of QJSB, we combined the transcriptomics-based network pharmacology and metabolomics data to obtain a system-wide view of the therapeutic mechanism of QJSB. Using the Metscape plugin of Cytoscape, we constructed the correlation network between the differential genes and differential metabolites regulated in QJSB-treated mice to analyze their potential relationships. The results suggested that a lot of metabolites and genes were in the same metabolic

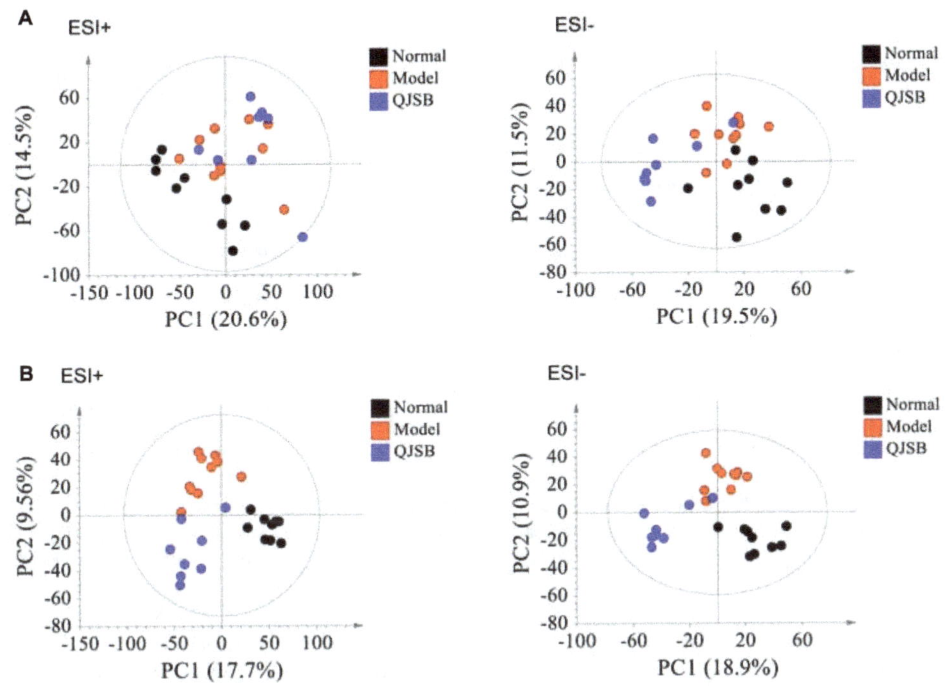

FIGURE 5 | Analysis of metabolic profiles from normal, model and QJSB groups based on UPLC-QTOF-MS. The SIMCA-derived PCA **(A)** and PLS-DA **(B)** score plot among three groups either in ESI+ or ESI− mode, respectively.

TABLE 4 | Pathways enrichment analysis of differential metabolites in bone marrow cells of model mice.

Term	Total	Expected	Hits	Raw *P*-value
Phenylalanine, tyrosine, and tryptophan biosynthesis	4	0.0565	1	0.0553
Glycerophospholipid metabolism	30	0.4234	2	0.0650
D-Glutamine and D-glutamate metabolism	5	0.0706	1	0.0687
Taurine and hypotaurine metabolism	8	0.1129	1	0.1077
Limonene and pinene degradation	8	0.1129	1	0.1077
Phenylalanine metabolism	11	0.1553	1	0.1452
Glycosylphosphatidylinositol (GPI)-anchor biosynthesis	14	0.1976	1	0.1812
Citrate cycle (TCA cycle)	20	0.2823	1	0.2489
Butanoate metabolism	22	0.3105	1	0.2702
Alanine, aspartate, and glutamate metabolism	24	0.3387	1	0.2910
Primary bile acid biosynthesis	46	0.6493	1	0.4855
Purine metabolism	68	0.9598	1	0.6286
Aminoacyl-tRNA biosynthesis	69	0.9739	1	0.6341
Steroid hormone biosynthesis	72	1.0162	1	0.6501

TABLE 5 | Pathways enrichment analysis of differential metabolites in bone marrow cells of QJSB-treated mice.

Term	Total	Expected	Hits	Raw *P*-value
Glycerophospholipid metabolism	30	0.3387	3	0.0040
Synthesis and degradation of ketone bodies	5	0.0565	1	0.0553
Linoleic acid metabolism	6	0.0677	1	0.0660
Alpha-Linolenic acid metabolism	9	0.1016	1	0.0974
Ether lipid metabolism	13	0.1468	1	0.1378
Glycosylphosphatidylinositol (GPI)-anchor biosynthesis	14	0.1581	1	0.1476
Butanoate metabolism	22	0.2484	1	0.2225
Steroid biosynthesis	35	0.3952	1	0.3312
Arachidonic acid metabolism	36	0.4065	1	0.3390
Tryptophan metabolism	40	0.4517	1	0.3691
Purine metabolism	68	0.7678	1	0.5467

pathways, including glycerophospholipid metabolism, linoleate metabolism, squalene and cholesterol biosynthesis, glycine, serine, alanine and threonine metabolism, histidine metabolism, tryptophan metabolism, purine and pyrimidine metabolism, etc. As shown in **Figure 7**, these metabolic pathways mainly were mainly grouped into three classes: lipid metabolism, amino acid metabolism and nucleotide metabolism.

In the lipid metabolic pathways, the levels of metabolites such as phosphatidylcholine (lecithin) and 2-lysolecithin were elevated, and the expression of some genes encoding important metabolic enzymes like Pcyt1a, Phospho1, Cyp4f18, Alox5, and Ggt5 were also augmented by QJSB treatment. Amino acids and nucleotides are essential components of proteins and nucleic acids, respectively, and amino acid metabolism and nucleotide metabolism play an important role in biological synthesis and metabolism of amino acids and nucleotides (Gutteridge

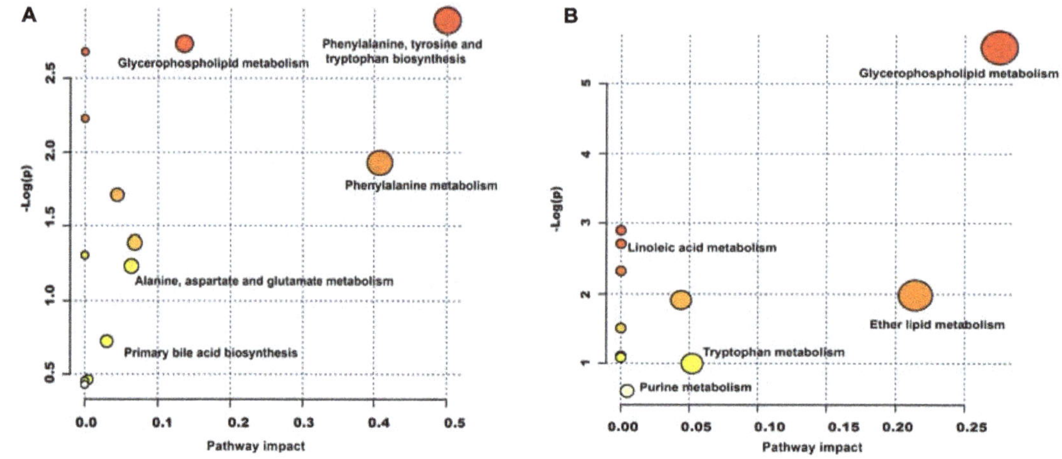

FIGURE 6 | Metabolic pathway analysis of the differential metabolites using the MetaboAnalyst 4.0. **(A)** Representative pathway analysis of the metabolites in leucopenia mice. **(B)** Representative pathway analysis of the metabolites in QJSB-treated mice. All the matched pathways are displayed as circles. The color and size of each circle was based on the *P*-value and pathway impact value, respectively. The smaller *P*-value means the pathway with higher levels of significance.

and Coombs, 1977; Ballantyne, 2001; Bender, 2012). In these metabolic pathways, the level of the metabolite tryptamine and the expression of GGTLA1, HDC, NDST1, and ATP6V1C2 were increased, while the level of the metabolite deoxyadenosine and the expression of ATP6V1G2, ATP2B2, and POLR3H were decreased. These results suggested that QJSB might affect biological synthesis and metabolism of amino acids and nucleotides by regulating amino acid metabolism and nucleotide metabolic pathways.

QJSB Increased the Gene Expression of Ggt5, Cyp4f18, Pcyt1a, Alox5, and Phospho1 in Leucopenia Model Mice

To further investigate the effects of QJSB on the regulation of metabolic pathways, we measured the expression of five genes, Ggt5, Cyp4f18, Pcytla, Alox5, and Phosphol, according to our previous data. They are key genes encoding important metabolic enzymes. RT-qPCR was performed in bone marrow cells from leucopenia model mice induced by cyclophosphamide. Compared to the normal control, the expressions of Ggt5, Cyp4f18, Pcytla, Alox5, and Phosphol were significantly decreased in leucopenia model groups. QJSB significantly increased the mRNA levels of these genes (**Figure 8**, $P < 0.01$). These results are consistent with our data from transcriptomics analysis.

DISCUSSION

Leucopenia is a very common adverse reaction induced by chemotherapy (Xu et al., 2011; Cui et al., 2015). In China, TCM formulae have been widely used to treat leucopenia. Among them, QJSB is a newly developed TCM formula and has been used clinically. In this study, our experiments conclude that QJSB has protective effects against leucopenia. As the theory of pharmachemistry of TCM, more scientists accept the viewpoint that the effective constituents may be detected in serum (Wang, 2006). We have identified 24 prototype compounds in the serum of rats after the oral administration of QJSB (Wu et al., 2018), which revealed the potential active substances of the formula to some extent (**Supplementary Table S5**). The network pharmacology technology is a powerful tool to investigate the therapeutic effects and molecular mechanisms (Zhao et al., 2009; Zhang et al., 2017). We also employed a transcriptomics-based network pharmacology approach to determine that the mechanism was involved in the cell proliferation and differentiation, metabolism response and immunologic function. Functional enrichment analysis was performed to explore the biological processes of the top 300 differentially expressed genes. Usually, the top 300 differentially expressed genes under the treatment of a drug are regarded as the drug's potential target genes, and the top 300 differentially expressed genes between the model and control groups are regarded as disease associated genes. The relevant parameters between the drug's potential target genes and disease associated genes and the Z-score were calculated to evaluate the effect of drugs. A Z-score value greater than 3 often indicates a statistically significant deviation between the actual value and the random ones (Fang et al., 2017). In this study, the Z-score was 6.156. Thus, QJSB might have significant effects against leucopenia disease. Using the transcriptomics-based network pharmacology and metabonomics technology, we propose a model for QJSB multi-pathways treatment mechanism (**Figure 9**). We concluded that QJSB mainly participates in the metabolism response, cell proliferation and differentiation, and the immune response, etc.

The hematopoietic cell lineage is mainly involved in blood cells development progresses from a rare population of hematopoietic stem cells (HSCs). HSCs can undergo either self-renewal or differentiation into multilineage committed progenitor cells: common lymphoid progenitors (CLPs) or common myeloid progenitors (CMPs), and successively become more restricted in their differentiation capacity. They

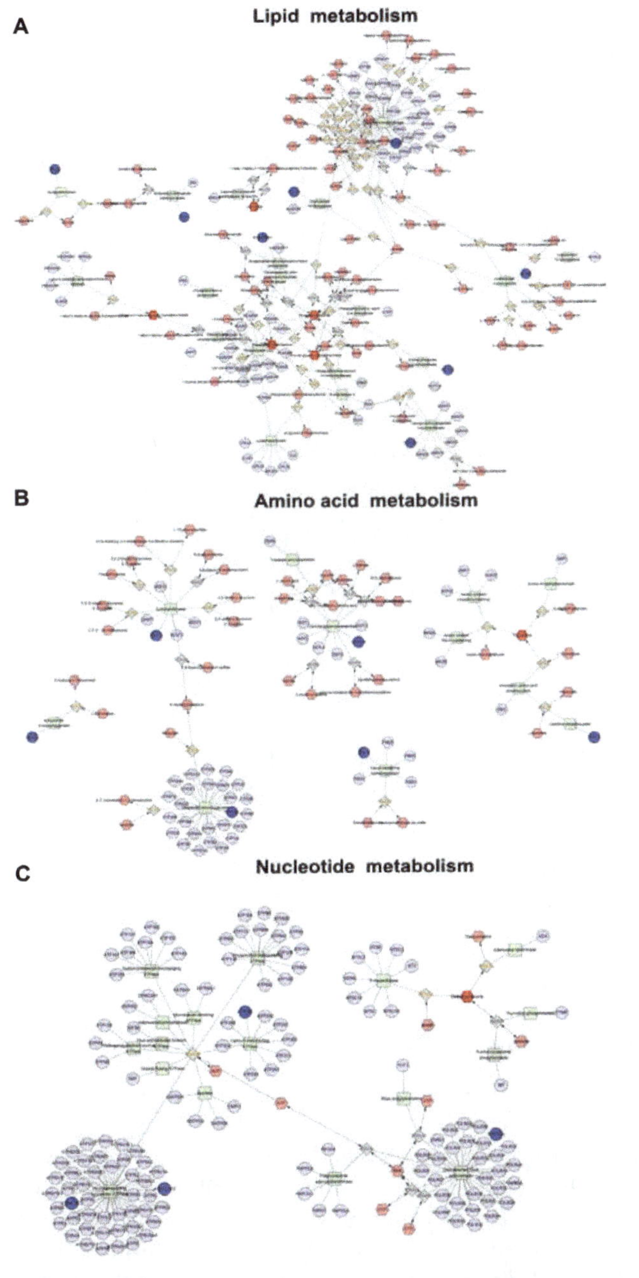

FIGURE 7 | Correlation networks construction, including lipid metabolism **(A)**, amino acid metabolism **(B)**, and nucleotide metabolism **(C)**, between the differential metabolites and differentially expressed genes. The dark red hexagonal represents detected metabolites, the shallow red hexagonal represents in-direct metabolites. The green square represents protein (enzyme). The blue circle represents genes that code for corresponding proteins.

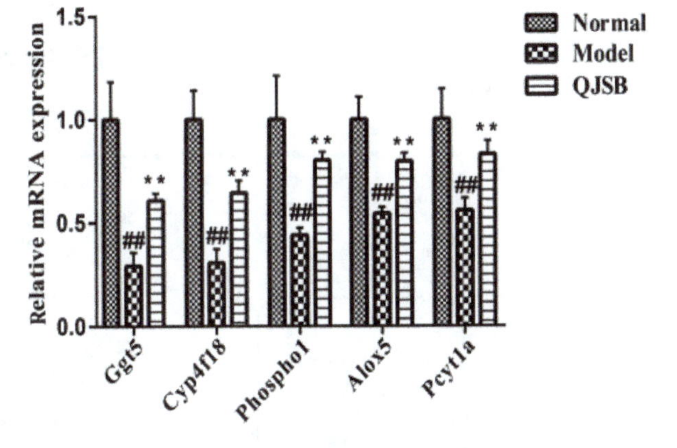

FIGURE 8 | The effects of QJSB on the expression of five lipid metabolism related genes (Ggt5, Cyp4f18, Phospho1, Alox5, and Pcyt1a) in bone marrow cells from leucopenia model mice. Data are presented as means ± SD. ## represents $P < 0.01$ vs. normal group and ** represents $P < 0.01$ vs. model group.

finally generate functionally mature cells such as lymphocytes, granulocytes, monocytes, and erythrocytes, et al. Among them, lymphocytes, including B and T cells, constitute a major proportion (more than 80%) of leukocytes (Dintzis and Treuting, 2011; O'Connell et al., 2015). B and T cells are the primary effector cells during the adaptive immune response (Medzhitov and Janeway, 1997; Iwasaki and Medzhitov, 2015). B cell receptor signaling pathway is involved in B lymphocyte proliferation, differentiation, survival and activation (Jacob et al., 2002; Schweighoffer et al., 2013; Reth and Nielsen, 2014). T cell activation is a vital event for immune system, and only the activated T cell can exert an efficient immune response. Cd3d and Tnfsf13b are key genes in these pathways. The protein encoded by Cd3d is part of the T-cell receptor/CD3 complex and is involved in T-cell activation and signal transduction. Cd3d-deficient patients show a complete block in T cell development. Deficiency of Cd3d also impairs T cell-dependent functions of B cells and causes severe immunodeficiency (de Saint Basile et al., 2004; Gil et al., 2011; Munoz-Ruiz et al., 2016). The protein encoded by Tnfsf13b plays roles in the survival and maturation of both of B and T cells (Pfister et al., 2011; Liu et al., 2016). Besides lymphocytes, both eosinophils and basophils are also involved in the immune response (Jacobsen et al., 2011; Voehringer, 2011). The imbalance of eosinophils and basophils might also affect the hematopoiesis (Tebbi et al., 1980; Enokihara et al., 1996; Schneider et al., 2010). In this study, the expression levels of Cd3d and Tnfsf13b were both up-regulated in QJSB group and recovered the abnormity of eosinophils and basophils induced by cyclophosphamide. These data indicate that QJSB might participate in the regulation of the immune effector process.

Although most HSCs normally exist in a quiescent or dormant state (Wilson et al., 2008), some of them divide and support the production of all mature blood cell types through multiple intermediate progenitor stages, during the steady state, and in response to urgencies to maintain blood cell number homeostasis (Busch et al., 2015; Sawai et al., 2016; Grinenko et al., 2018). Itgam is mainly involved in adhesion and migration of leukocytes. It is necessary for HSCs expansion *in vitro* and engraftment *in vivo* (Prashad et al., 2015). Patients with Itgam variants have reduced switched memory B-cell counts (Maggadottir et al., 2015). Ets1 is a key transcription factor required for CD8 T cell differentiation (Zamisch et al., 2009). It is a critical regulator of group 2 innate

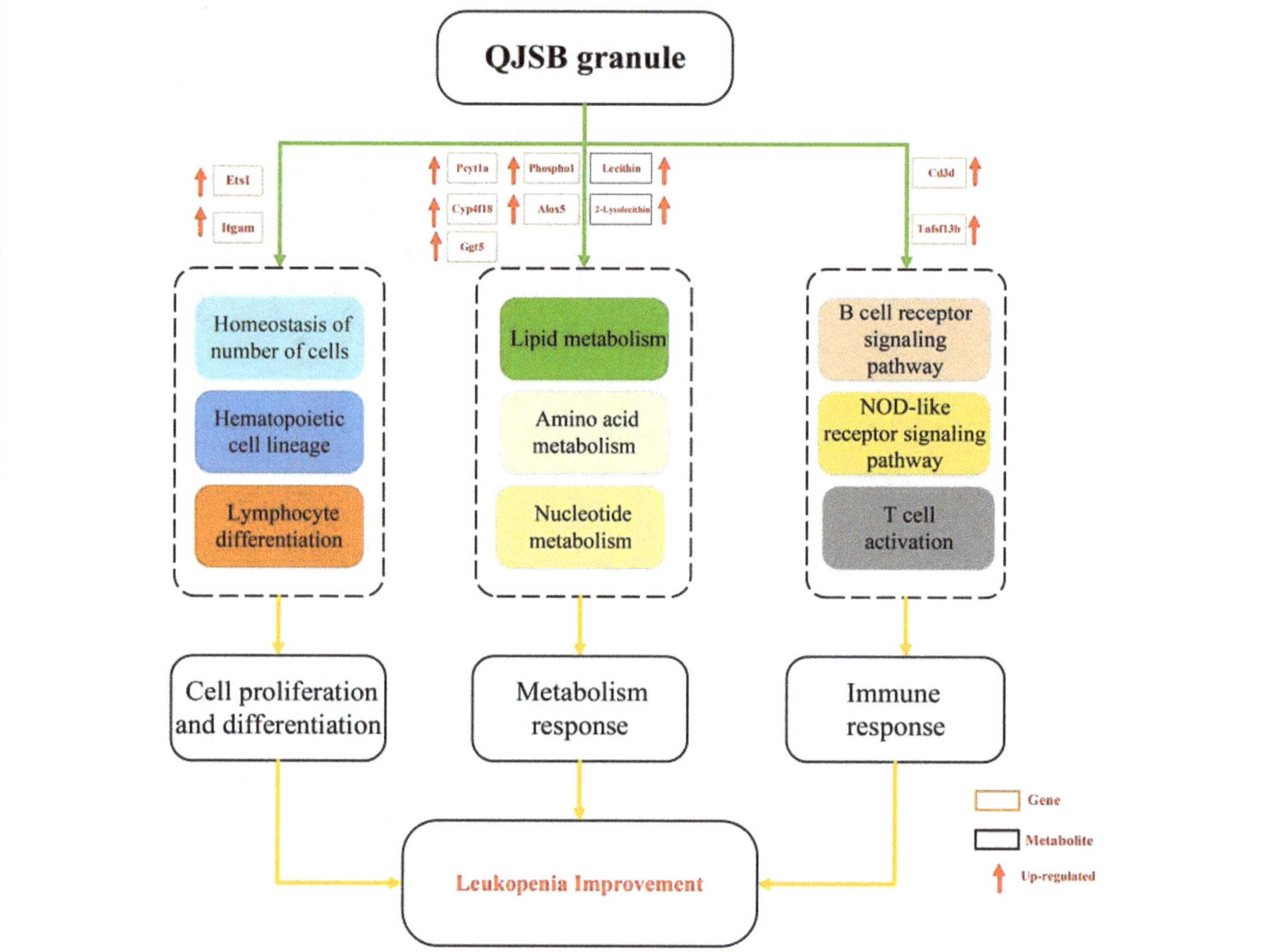

FIGURE 9 | Multi-pathways treatment mechanism of QJSB on leucopenia in mice. The orange rectangle represents the key gene and the black rectangle represents the key metabolite. Red arrow represents up-regulated.

lymphoid cells expansion and cytokines production (Zook et al., 2016). In this study, the different expression genes of Itgam and Ets1 are simultaneously enriched in QJSB group (vs. leucopenia group). These data indicate that HSCs expansion, lymphocyte differentiation and cytokines production may also be involved in the protective mechanism of QJSB.

Hematopoiesis-related cytokines are important factors for the regulation of hematopoietic function (Alexander, 1998). For example, IL-6 was first identified and characterized as a lymphocyte-stimulating factor according to its ability to promote the activation and population expansion of T cells, the differentiation and survival of B cells, and the regulation of the acute-phase response (Hunter and Jones, 2015). G-CSF, also known as colony-stimulating factor 3 (Csf3), is the major hematopoietic growth factor involved in the control of neutrophil development. G-CSF supports the proliferation, survival, and differentiation of neutrophilic progenitor cells *in vitro* and provides non-redundant signals for the maintenance of steady-state neutrophil levels *in vivo* (van de Geijn et al., 2003). G-CSF also participates in the development of other myeloid lineages, the mobilization of HSCs and myeloid cell migration (Liongue et al., 2009). To determine how G-CSF was regulated by QJSB, we constructed a subnetwork by extracting the links between G-CSF and differentially expressed genes under the treatment of QJSB from our background PPI network, i.e., the STRING network (**Supplementary Figure S2**). This network shows that G-CSF interacts with a group of differentially expressed genes, including Itgam, Il7r, Il18, Ccr2, Dpp4, Jun, and Ltf. Among these genes, Itgam and G-CSF receptor (CSF3R) are two markers of granulocyte differentiation and it was found that G-CSF could decrease Itgam expression (Lantow et al., 2013; Lin et al., 2015). IL-18 (interleukin-18) is involved in the hematopoietic progenitor cell growth and stimulates the secretion of IL-6 and the expression of G-CSF mRNA in splenic adherent cells (Ogura et al., 2001). Additionally, IL-18 treatment increases the serum G-CSF level in C57BL/6 mice (Kinoshita et al., 2011). It was reported that when immortalized bone marrow progenitors are induced by G-CSF to differentiate into mature neutrophils, the

CCR2 gene is strongly activated and CCR2 play a critical role in monocyte recruitment (Iida et al., 2005). G-CSF also increases CCR2 protein expression of THP-1 monocytes (Chen et al., 2008). As our data shows, Itgam was up-regulated while Il18 and Ccr2 were down-regulated by QJSB, a finding that was consistent with the decrease in the serum G-CSF level. Excessive activation and release of cytokines impair the hematopoietic function, and exhaust the production of hematopoietic factor (Hara et al., 2004). QJSB reversed the excessive exhaustion of certain cytokines induced by cyclophosphamide, which might be beneficial for the recovery of leucopenia.

Qi-Jing-Sheng-Bai granule also modulates the metabolism response, including lipid metabolism, amino acid metabolism and nucleotide metabolism. In lipid metabolism, the levels of metabolites such as phosphatidylcholine (lecithin) and 2-lysolecithin are elevated, and the expression of some genes encoding important metabolic enzymes like Pcyt1a, Phospho1, Cyp4f18, Alox5, and Ggt5 are also augmented by QJSB treatment. Additionally, RT-qPCR was performed to verify that QJSB upregulated their mRNA levels. Phosphatidylcholine participates in a series of biological activities such as biological membranes synthesis, cell proliferation and platelet activation (Ridgway, 2013; Li et al., 2014; O'Donnell et al., 2014). Metabolic enzymes encoded by Pcyt1a regulate the biological synthesis of phosphatidylcholine (Haider et al., 2018). The high expression of Pcyt1a causes elevated levels of phosphatidylcholine, which may result in accelerated biological membranes synthesis and cell proliferation of WBCs and platelets. Additionally, Cyp4f18, Alox5, and Ggt5 are involved in the processes of generation, transformation and degradation of leukotriene (Christmas et al., 2006; Rådmark et al., 2015). Thus, QJSB may promote lipid production by regulating lipid metabolism, and regulate immune and inflammatory responses by affecting the generation, transformation and degradation of leukotriene.

Amino acids and nucleotides are essential components of proteins and nucleic acids, respectively. They are indispensable for cell proliferation, survival and development. Leucogen and vitamin B4 are very commonly used for the treatment of leucopenia. Leucogen is an analog of cysteine while vitamin B4 is a precursor of adenine (Lecoq, 1957; Whelan, 2005; Zheng et al., 2006; Langhammer et al., 2011). Therefore, regulating amino acid metabolism and nucleotide metabolism have been confirmed to cure leucopenia. Our data indicate that QJSB participate in the biological synthesis and metabolism of energy, nutrition and genetic materials, which are essential for cell proliferation, development and maturation.

CONCLUSION

In summary, our data reveal the therapeutic mechanism of QJSB by integrative application of transcriptomics-based network pharmacology and metabolomics technologies. QJSB exerts protective effect against leucopenia in mice through participating in multi-pathways, mainly including accelerating cell proliferation and differentiation, regulating metabolism response pathways and modulating immunologic function.

ETHICS STATEMENT

All animal studies were performed according to the institutional ethical guidelines of animal care and were approved by the Committee on the Ethics of Animal Experiments of the Second Military Medical University, China.

AUTHOR CONTRIBUTIONS

ST, PH, and YG collected and analyzed the data, and drafted and revised the manuscript. JY, RW, and JZ collected and revised the manuscript. WZ and A-JL designed the study, collected the data, and revised the manuscript. All authors read and approved the final manuscript.

FUNDING

The work was supported by Professor of Chang Jiang Scholars Program, NSFC (81520108030 and 21472238), Shanghai Engineering Research Center for the Preparation of Bioactive Natural Products (16DZ2280200), the Scientific Foundation of Shanghai China (13401900103 and 13401900101), and the National Key Research and Development Program of China (2017YFC1700200).

SUPPLEMENTARY MATERIAL

FIGURE S1 | Distinct discrimination by comparison between Normal vs. Model **(A,C)**, Model vs. QJSB **(B,D)** either in ESI+ and ESI−. OPLS-DA was used to distinguish the cluster and its permutations plot was used to assess the current OPLS-DA model.

FIGURE S2 | The protein-protein network of Csf3 (G-CSF) with differentially expressed genes between QJSB and model group. Csf3 (G-CSF) was surrounded by differentially expressed genes based on the STRING database.

TABLE S1 | The primers of the key genes encoding important metabolic enzymes.

TABLE S2 | The top 300 differentially expressed genes were identified in Model vs. Normal, QJSB vs. Model and Leucogen vs. Model groups.

TABLE S3 | Summary of the LC-MS data sets used in OPLS-DA modeling. R2X (cum) represents the cumulative X-variation modeled after components, R2Y means the fraction of Y-variation modeled in the component, and Q2 expresses overall cross-validated R2Y for the component and is used to an estimate the model prediction. Cumulative values of R2X, R2Y, and Q2 close to 1 indicate an excellent model.

TABLE S4 | Differential metabolites of plasma in Model vs. Normal and QJSB vs. Model were identified by OPLS-DA on SIMCA software. RT is retention time on gas chromatograph. MZ is the ratio of protons and charge number. Fold change is the ratio of relative abundance of differential metabolites. The data were calculated by t test.

TABLE S5 | The active substances of absorbed prototype compounds in QJSB and theirs evidence.

REFERENCES

Aarts, M. J., Grutters, J. P., Peters, F. P., Mandigers, C. M., Dercksen, M. W., Stouthard, J. M., et al. (2013). Cost effectiveness of primary pegfilgrastim prophylaxis in patients with breast cancer at risk of febrile neutropenia. *J. Clin. Oncol.* 31, 4283–4289. doi: 10.1200/JCO.2012.48.3644

Alexander, W. S. (1998). Cytokines in hematopoiesis. *Int. Rev. Immunol.* 16, 651–682. doi: 10.3109/08830189809043013

Ballantyne, J. (2001). Amino acid metabolism. *Fish Physiol.* 20, 77–107. doi: 10.1016/S1546-5098(01)20004-1

Bender, D. A. (2012). *Amino Acid Metabolism*. Hoboken, NJ: John Wiley & Sons. doi: 10.1002/9781118357514

Busch, K., Klapproth, K., Barile, M., Flossdorf, M., Holland-Letz, T., Schlenner, S. M., et al. (2015). Fundamental properties of unperturbed haematopoiesis from stem cells in vivo. *Nature* 518, 542–546. doi: 10.1038/nature14242

Chen, Y.-K., Jiang, X.-M., and Gong, J.-P. (2008). Recombinant human granulocyte colony-stimulating factor enhanced the resolution of venous thrombi. *J. Vasc. Surg.* 47, 1058–1065. doi: 10.1016/j.jvs.2007.12.042

Christmas, P., Tolentino, K., Primo, V., Berry, K. Z., Murphy, R. C., Chen, M., et al. (2006). Cytochrome P-450 4F18 is the leukotriene B4 omega-1/omega-2 hydroxylase in mouse polymorphonuclear leukocytes: identification as the functional orthologue of human polymorphonuclear leukocyte CYP4F3A in the down-regulation of responses to LTB4. *J. Biol. Chem.* 281, 7189–7196. doi: 10.1074/jbc.M513101200

Cui, R., Chu, L., Liu, Z. Q., Xiao, Y. Y., Zhu, X. L., Chen, Y. J., et al. (2015). Hematologic toxicity assessment in solid tumor patients treated with cetuximab: a pooled analysis of 18 randomized controlled trials. *Int. J. Cancer* 136, 936–944. doi: 10.1002/ijc.29045

de Saint Basile, G., Geissmann, F., Flori, E., Uring-Lambert, B., Soudais, C., Cavazzana-Calvo, M., et al. (2004). Severe combined immunodeficiency caused by deficiency in either the delta or the epsilon subunit of CD3. *J. Clin. Invest.* 114, 1512–1517. doi: 10.1172/JCI22588

Dintzis, S., and Treuting, P. (2011). *Comparative Anatomy and Histology: A Mouse and Human Atlas*. Cambridge: Academic Press.

Dygai, A., Goldberg, V., Artamonov, A., Bekarev, A., Vereschagin, E., Madonov, P., et al. (2012). Effects and mechanisms of hemopoiesis-stimulating activity of immobilized oligonucleotides under conditions of cytostatic myelosuppression. *Bull. Exp. Biol. Med.* 152, 451–455. doi: 10.1007/s10517-012-1551-9

Enokihara, H., Koike, T., Nakamura, Y., Yamashiro, K., Tsuruoka, N., Saito, K., et al. (1996). Eosinophils negatively regulate eosinophilopoiesis by decreasing IL-5 levels. *Int. Arch. Allergy Immunol.* 111(Suppl. 1), 2–4. doi: 10.1159/000237403

Fang, H.-Y., Zeng, H.-W., Lin, L.-M., Chen, X., Shen, X.-N., Fu, P., et al. (2017). A network-based method for mechanistic investigation of shexiang baoxin pill's treatment of cardiovascular diseases. *Sci. Rep.* 7:43632. doi: 10.1038/srep43632

Gil, J., Busto, E. M., Garcillán, B., Chean, C., García-Rodríguez, M. C., Díaz-Alderete, A., et al. (2011). A leaky mutation in CD3D differentially affects αβ and γδ T cells and leads to a Tαβ−Tγδ+ B+ NK+ human SCID. *J. Clin. Invest.* 121, 3872–3876. doi: 10.1172/JCI44254

Grinenko, T., Eugster, A., Thielecke, L., Ramasz, B., Kruger, A., Dietz, S., et al. (2018). Hematopoietic stem cells can differentiate into restricted myeloid progenitors before cell division in mice. *Nat. Commun.* 9:1898. doi: 10.1038/s41467-018-04188-7

Gutteridge, W., and Coombs, G. (eds) (1977). "Nucleic Acid Metabolism," in *Biochemistry of Parasitic Protozoa*, (Berlin: Springer), 69–88. doi: 10.1007/978-1-349-15809-6_6

Haider, A., Wei, Y. C., Lim, K., Barbosa, A. D., Liu, C. H., Weber, U., et al. (2018). PCYT1A regulates phosphatidylcholine homeostasis from the inner nuclear membrane in response to membrane stored curvature elastic stress. *Dev. Cell* 45, 481.e8–495.e8. doi: 10.1016/j.devcel.2018.04.012

Hara, T., Ando, K., Tsurumi, H., and Moriwaki, H. (2004). Excessive production of tumor necrosis factor-alpha by bone marrow T lymphocytes is essential in causing bone marrow failure in patients with aplastic anemia. *Eur. J. Haematol.* 73:10. doi: 10.1111/j.1600-0609.2004.00259.x

Hunter, C. A., and Jones, S. A. (2015). IL-6 as a keystone cytokine in health and disease. *Nat. Immunol.* 16, 448–457. doi: 10.1038/ni.3153

Iida, S., Kohro, T., Kodama, T., Nagata, S., and Fukunaga, R. (2005). Identification of CCR2, flotillin, and gp49B genes as new G-CSF targets during neutrophilic differentiation. *J. Leuko. Biol.* 78, 481–490. doi: 10.1189/jlb.0904515

Iwasaki, A., and Medzhitov, R. (2015). Control of adaptive immunity by the innate immune system. *Nat. Immunol.* 16:343. doi: 10.1038/ni.3123

Jacob, A., Cooney, D., Pradhan, M., and Coggeshall, K. M. (2002). Convergence of signaling pathways on the activation of ERK in B cells. *J. Biol. Chem.* 277, 23420–23426. doi: 10.1074/jbc.M202485200

Jacobsen, E., Zellner, K., Colbert, D., Lee, N., and Lee, J. (2011). Eosinophils regulate dendritic cells and Th2 pulmonary immune responses following allergen provocation. *J. Immunol.* 187, 6059–6068. doi: 10.4049/jimmunol.1102299

Jiang, W.-Y. (2005). Therapeutic wisdom in traditional Chinese medicine: a perspective from modern science. *Trends Pharmacol. Sci.* 26, 558–563. doi: 10.1016/j.tips.2005.09.006

Kanehisa, M., and Goto, S. (2000). KEGG: kyoto encyclopedia of genes and genomes. *Nucleic Acids Res.* 28, 27–30. doi: 10.1093/nar/28.1.27

Kinoshita, M., Miyazaki, H., Ono, S., Inatsu, A., Nakashima, H., Tsujimoto, H., et al. (2011).). Enhancement of neutrophil function by IL-18 therapy protects burn-injured mice from MRSA infection. *Infect. Immun.* 79, 2670–2680. doi: 10.1128/IAI.01298-10

Langhammer, S., Fiebig, U., Kurth, R., and Denner, J. (2011). Increased neutralizing antibody response after simultaneous immunization with leucogen and the feline leukemia virus transmembrane protein. *Intervirology* 54, 78–86. doi: 10.1159/000318892

Lantow, M., Sivakumar, R., Zeumer, L., Wasserfall, C., Zheng, Y.-Y., Atkinson, M. A., et al. (2013). The granulocyte colony stimulating factor pathway regulates autoantibody production in a murine induced model of systemic lupus erythematosus. *Arthr. Res. Ther.* 15:R49. doi: 10.1186/ar4208

Lecoq, R. (1957). Anti-agranulocytic vitamin B4. *Int. Z Vitaminforsch Beih* 27, 291–300.

Li, H., Yue, R., Wei, B., Gao, G., Du, J., and Pei, G. (2014). Lysophosphatidic acid acts as a nutrient-derived developmental cue to regulate early hematopoiesis. *EMBO J.* 33, 1383–1396. doi: 10.15252/embj.201387594

Lin, Y., Li, D., Liang, Q., Liu, S., Zuo, X., Li, L., et al. (2015). miR-638 regulates differentiation and proliferation in leukemic cells by targeting cyclin-dependent kinase 2. *J. Biol. Chem.* 290, 1818–1828. doi: 10.1074/jbc.M114.599191

Liongue, C., Wright, C., Russell, A. P., and Ward, A. C. (2009). Granulocyte colony-stimulating factor receptor: stimulating granulopoiesis and much more. *Int. J. Biochem. Cell Biol.* 41, 2372–2375. doi: 10.1016/j.biocel.2009.08.011

Liu, H., Zhang, J., Li, J., Song, J., and Zhang, S. (2016). Molecular structure, distribution, and immunology function of TNFSF13B (BAFF) in Nile tilapia (*Oreochromis niloticus*). *Fish. Shellfish Immunol.* 51, 240–250. doi: 10.1016/j.fsi.2016.02.026

Liu, M., Tan, H., Zhang, X., Liu, Z., Cheng, Y., Wang, D., et al. (2014). Hematopoietic effects and mechanisms of Fufang e′ jiao jiang on radiotherapy and chemotherapy-induced myelosuppressed mice. *J. Ethnopharmacol.* 152, 575–584. doi: 10.1016/j.jep.2014.02.012

Love, M., Anders, S., and Huber, W. (2013). *Differential Analysis of RNA-Seq Data at the Gene Level Using the DESeq2 Package*. Heidelberg: European Molecular Biology Laboratory (EMBL).

Ma, Z.-C., Hong, Q., Wang, Y.-G., Tan, H.-L., Xiao, C.-R., Liang, Q.-D., et al. (2011). Effects of ferulic acid on hematopoietic cell recovery in whole-body gamma irradiated mice. *Int. J. Radiat. Biol.* 87, 499–505. doi: 10.3109/09553002.2011.548438

Maggadottir, S. M., Li, J., Glessner, J. T., Li, Y. R., Wei, Z., Chang, X., et al. (2015). Rare variants at 16p11.2 are associated with common variable immunodeficiency. *J. Allergy Clin. Immunol.* 135, 1569–1577. doi: 10.1016/j.jaci.2014.12.1939

Magge, R. S., and DeAngelis, L. M. (2015). The double-edged sword: neurotoxicity of chemotherapy. *Blood Rev.* 29, 93–100. doi: 10.1016/j.blre.2014.09.012

Medzhitov, R., and Janeway, C. A. Jr. (1997). Innate immunity: impact on the adaptive immune response. *Curr. Opin. Immunol.* 9, 4–9. doi: 10.1016/S0952-7915(97)80152-5

Meierhofer, D., Weidner, C., and Sauer, S. (2014). Integrative analysis of transcriptomics, proteomics, and metabolomics data of white adipose and liver tissue of high-fat diet and rosiglitazone-treated insulin-resistant mice identified pathway alterations and molecular hubs. *J. Proteo. Res.* 13, 5592–5602. doi: 10.1021/pr5005828

Munoz-Ruiz, M., Ribot, J. C., Grosso, A. R., Goncalves-Sousa, N., Pamplona, A., Pennington, D. J., et al. (2016). TCR signal strength controls thymic differentiation of discrete proinflammatory gammadelta T cell subsets. *Nat. Immunol.* 17, 721–727. doi: 10.1038/ni.3424

Ning, K., Zhao, X., Poetsch, A., Chen, W.-H., and Yang, J. (2017). Computational molecular networks and network pharmacology. *BioMed. Res. Int.* 2017:7573904. doi: 10.1155/2017/7573904

O'Connell, K. E., Mikkola, A. M., Stepanek, A. M., Vernet, A., Hall, C. D., Sun, C. C., et al. (2015). Practical murine hematopathology: a comparative review and implications for research. *Comp. Med.* 65, 96–113.

O'Donnell, V. B., Murphy, R. C., and Watson, S. P. (2014). Platelet lipidomics: modern day perspective on lipid discovery and characterization in platelets. *Circ. Res.* 114, 1185–1203. doi: 10.1161/CIRCRESAHA.114.301597

Ogura, T., Ueda, H., Hosohara, K., Tsuji, R., Nagata, Y., Kashiwamura, S.-I., et al. (2001). Interleukin-18 stimulates hematopoietic cytokine and growth factor formation and augments circulating granulocytes in mice. *Blood* 98, 2101–2107. doi: 10.1182/blood.V98.7.2101

Pfister, D. G., Ang, K.-K., Brizel, D. M., Burtness, B. A., Cmelak, A. J., Colevas, A. D., et al. (2011). Head and neck cancers. *J. Natl. Compr. Cancer Netw.* 9, 596–650. doi: 10.6004/jnccn.2011.0053

Prashad, S. L., Calvanese, V., Yao, C. Y., Kaiser, J., Wang, Y., Sasidharan, R., et al. (2015). GPI-80 defines self-renewal ability in hematopoietic stem cells during human development. *Cell Stem Cell* 16, 80–87. doi: 10.1016/j.stem.2014.10.020

Rådmark, O., Werz, O., Steinhilber, D., and Samuelsson, B. (2015). 5-Lipoxygenase, a key enzyme for leukotriene biosynthesis in health and disease. *Biochim. Biophys. Acta* 1851, 331–339. doi: 10.1016/j.bbalip.2014.08.012

Ratti, M., and Tomasello, G. (2015). Lipegfilgrastim for the prophylaxis and treatment of chemotherapy-induced neutropenia. *Expert Rev. Clin. Pharmacol.* 8, 15–24. doi: 10.1586/17512433.2015.984688

Reth, M., and Nielsen, P. (2014). Signaling circuits in early B-cell development. *Adv. Immunol.* 122, 129–175. doi: 10.1016/B978-0-12-800267-4.00004-3

Ridgway, N. D. (2013). The role of phosphatidylcholine and choline metabolites to cell proliferation and survival. *Crit. Rev. Biochem. Mol. Biol.* 48, 20–38. doi: 10.3109/10409238.2012.735643

Sawai, C. M., Babovic, S., Upadhaya, S., Knapp, D., Lavin, Y., Lau, C. M., et al. (2016). Hematopoietic stem cells are the major source of multilineage hematopoiesis in adult animals. *Immunity* 45, 597–609. doi: 10.1016/j.immuni.2016.08.007

Schneider, E., Thieblemont, N., De Moraes, M. L., and Dy, M. (2010). Basophils: new players in the cytokine network. *Eur. Cytok. Netw.* 21, 142–153. doi: 10.1684/ecn.2010.0197

Schweighoffer, E., Vanes, L., Nys, J., Cantrell, D., McCleary, S., Smithers, N., et al. (2013). The BAFF receptor transduces survival signals by co-opting the B cell receptor signaling pathway. *Immunity* 38, 475–488. doi: 10.1016/j.immuni.2012.11.015

Su, G., Burant, C. F., Beecher, C. W., Athey, B. D., and Meng, F. (2011). Integrated metabolome and transcriptome analysis of the NCI60 dataset. *BMC Bioinformatics* 12:S36. doi: 10.1186/1471-2105-12-S1-S36

Sun, C., Yang, J., Pan, L., Guo, N., Li, B., Yao, J., et al. (2018). Improvement of icaritin on hematopoietic function in cyclophosphamide-induced myelosuppression mice. *Immunopharmacol. Immunotoxicol.* 40, 25–34. doi: 10.1080/08923973.2017.1392564

Tebbi, C. K., Mahmoud, A. A., Polmar, S., and Gross, S. (1980). The role of eosinophils in granulopoiesis. I. Eosinophilia in neutropenic patients. *J. Pediatr.* 96(3 Pt 2):575.

van de Geijn, G. J., Aarts, L. H., Erkeland, S. J., Prasher, J. M., and Touw, I. P. (2003). Granulocyte colony-stimulating factor and its receptor in normal hematopoietic cell development and myeloid disease. *Rev. Physiol. Biochem. Pharmacol.* 149, 53–71. doi: 10.1007/s10254-003-0014-0

Voehringer, D. (2011). Basophils in allergic immune responses. *Curr. Opin. Immunol.* 23, 789–793. doi: 10.1016/j.coi.2011.09.005

Wang, X. (2006). Progress and future developing of the serum pharmacochemistry of traditional Chinese medicine. *Zhongguo Zhong Yao Za Zhi* 31, 789835–792835.

Whelan, W. (2005). Vitamin B4. *IUBMB Life* 57:125. doi: 10.1080/15216540500078939

Wilson, A., Laurenti, E., Oser, G., van der Wath, R. C., Blanco-Bose, W., Jaworski, M., et al. (2008). Hematopoietic stem cells reversibly switch from dormancy to self-renewal during homeostasis and repair. *Cell* 135, 1118–1129. doi: 10.1016/j.cell.2008.10.048

Wu, R., Lin, S., Wang, J., Tian, S., Ke, X., Qu, Y., et al. (2018). Rapid characterization of chemical constituents and metabolites of Qi-Jing-Sheng-Bai granule by using UHPLC-Q-TOF-MS. *J. Sep. Sci.* 41, 1960–1972. doi: 10.1002/jssc.201701310

Xu, W., Zhou, L., Ma, X., Chen, Y., Qin, B., Zhai, X., et al. (2011). Therapeutic effects of combination of paeoniflorin and albiflorin from paeonia radix on radiation and chemotherapy-induced myelosuppression in mice and rabbits. *Asian Pac. J. Cancer Prev.* 12, 2031–2037.

Zamisch, M., Tian, L., Grenningloh, R., Xiong, Y., Wildt, K. F., Ehlers, M., et al. (2009). The transcription factor Ets1 is important for CD4 repression and Runx3 up-regulation during CD8 T cell differentiation in the thymus. *J. Exp. Med.* 206, 2685–2699. doi: 10.1084/jem.20092024

Zhang, Y., Mao, X., Su, J., Geng, Y., Guo, R., Tang, S., et al. (2017). A network pharmacology-based strategy deciphers the underlying molecular mechanisms of Qixuehe Capsule in the treatment of menstrual disorders. *Chin. Med.* 12:23. doi: 10.1186/s13020-017-0145-x

Zhao, J., Jiang, P., and Zhang, W. (2009). Molecular networks for the study of TCM pharmacology. *Brief. Bioinform.* 11, 417–430. doi: 10.1093/bib/bbp063

Zheng, K. Y., Choi, R. C., Cheung, A. W., Guo, A. J., Bi, C. W., Zhu, K. Y., et al. (2011). Flavonoids from radix Astragali induce the expression of erythropoietin in cultured cells: a signaling mediated via the accumulation of hypoxia-inducible factor-1α. *J. Agric. Food Chem.* 59, 1697–1704. doi: 10.1021/jf104018u

Zheng, X. W., Qian, W., Hang, T. J., Ma, H. B., and Zhang, Z. X. (2006). Structures of leucogen and its related substances in solution state. *Yao Xue Xue Bao* 41, 675–679.

Zhi, K., Li, M., Bai, J., Wu, Y., Zhou, S., Zhang, X., et al. (2016). Quercitrin treatment protects endothelial progenitor cells from oxidative damage via inducing autophagy through extracellular signal-regulated kinase. *Angiogenesis* 19, 311–324. doi: 10.1007/s10456-016-9504-y

Zhou, N.-N., Zhao, Y.-Y., Zhai, L.-Z., Ruan, C.-M., Yang, Y.-P., Huang, Y., et al. (2018). The efficacy and toxicity of lobaplatin-contained chemotherapy in extensive-stage small-cell lung cancer. *J. Cancer* 9, 2232–2236. doi: 10.7150/jca.24557

Zook, E. C., Ramirez, K., Guo, X., van der Voort, G., Sigvardsson, M., Svensson, E. C., et al. (2016). The ETS1 transcription factor is required for the development and cytokine-induced expansion of ILC2. *J. Exp. Med.* 213, 687–696. doi: 10.1084/jem.20150851

8

Systems Pharmacology Study of the Anti-Liver Injury Mechanism of Citri Reticulatae Pericarpium

Jianxiong Wu[†], *Xietao Ye*[†], *Songhong Yang*[†], *Huan Yu* *, *Lingyun Zhong* * *and Qianfeng Gong* *

School of Pharmacy, Jiangxi University of Traditional Chinese Medicine, Nanchang, China

***Correspondence:**
Huan Yu
yuhuanhebei@163.com
Lingyun Zhong
ly1638163@163.com
Qianfeng Gong
gongqf2002@163.com

[†]*These authors have contributed equally to this work*

Liver diseases are mostly triggered by oxidative stress and inflammation, leading to extracellular matrix overproduction and prone to develop into liver fibrosis, cirrhosis and hepatocellular carcinoma. Liver injury (LI) refers to various pathogenic factors leading to the destruction of stem cells that then affect the liver's normal function, causing a series of symptoms and abnormal liver function indicators. Citri Reticulatae Pericarpium (CRP) is one of the most commonly used traditional Chinese medicines; it contains flavonoids including hesperidin, nobiletin, and tangeretin. CRP has antibacterial, antioxidant, and antitumor effects that reduce cholesterol, prevent atherosclerosis and decrease LI. Here we analyzed the components of CRP and their targets of action in LI treatment and assessed the relationships between them using a systems pharmacology approach. Twenty-five active ingredients against LI were selected based on ultra-performance liquid chromatography-quadrupole/time-of-flight mass spectrometry results and databases. The drug targets and disease-related targets were predicted. The 117 common targets were used to construct a protein-protein interaction network. We identified 1719 gene ontology items in LI treatment, including 1,525 biological processes, 55 cellular components, and 139 molecular functions. These correlated with 49 Kyoto Encyclopedia of Genes and Genomes pathways. These findings suggest that CRP may counteract LI by affecting apoptotic, inflammatory, and energy metabolism modules. *In vitro* experiments suggested that the mechanism may involve hesperidin and naringenin acting on CASP3, BAX, and BCL2 to affect the apoptosis pathway, attenuating liver fibrosis. Naringenin significantly inhibited AKT1 phosphorylation, which in turn mediated activation of the phosphoinositide 3-kinase-Akt signaling pathways against LI. This study provides a reference for systematically exploring the mechanism of CRP's anti-LI action and is also expands of the application of systems pharmacology in the study of traditional Chinese medicine.

Keywords: systems pharmacology, experiment verification, liver injury, mechanism of action, citri reticulatae pericarpium

INTRODUCTION

The pathogenetic events leading to liver injury (LI) include oxidative damage, apoptosis, disordered lipid metabolism, and mitochondrial dysfunction. LI refers to one or more results of organ damage, inflammation, bleeding, infection, or other symptoms. Alcohol use is a major predisposing factor for LI (Yang et al., 2020). The annual proportion of alcohol-induced LI has been increasing (Tsutsumi

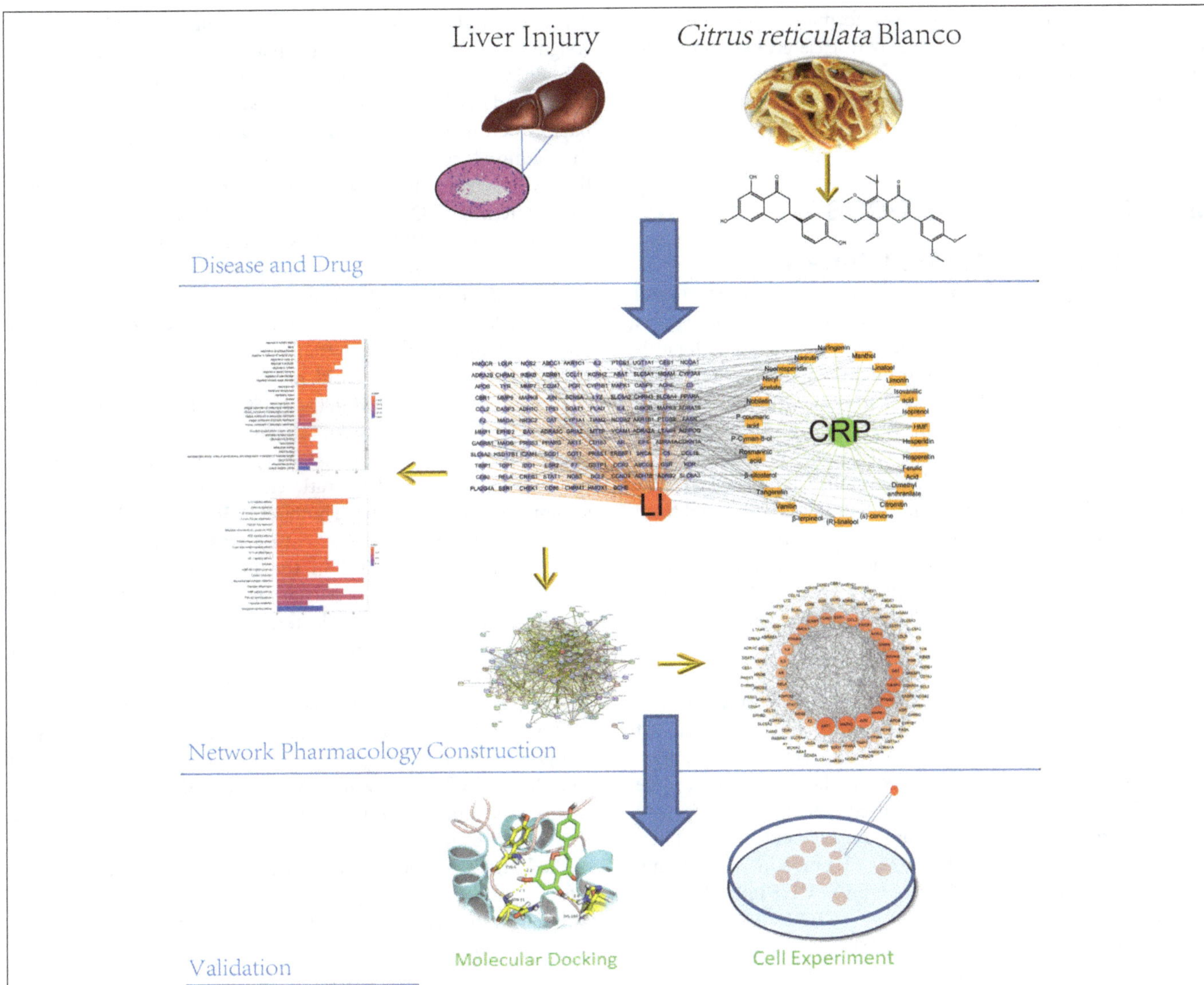

FIGURE 1 | A comprehensive strategy diagram for the study of the mechanism of CRP action on LI.

et al., 1994; Vatsalya et al., 2016). Excessive alcohol consumption often causes fatty acid imbalances that trigger liver inflammation.

Traditional Chinese medicine (TCM) is used to treat various diseases. Numerous studies have demonstrated that flavonoids and alkaloids components in TCM prevent or treat LI (Liu, 2016; Zhang et al., 2018). Citri Reticulatae Pericarpium (CRP, orange peel) is a dried and mature pericarp Citrus × aurantium L (Citrus × reticulata Blanco; Rutaceae) (Prc, 2015). CRP extract has excellent biological activity, and the citrus-rich extract is rich in polymethoxy flavonoids that regulate metabolism. CRP extract has excellent biological activity, and citrus-rich extracts rich in polymethoxy flavonoids reduce malnutrition (Zeng et al., 2020). CRP is used in TCM to treat nausea, vomiting, and anemia (Yu et al., 2018). Volatile oils and flavonoids in CRP are considered major components; these include narirutin, nobiletin, and hesperidin (Cui et al., 2019). These components act alone or in combination to combat inflammatory responses and lipid peroxidation, in turn attenuating oxidative stress-induced hepatocyte damage (Lin et al., 2019).

According to the TCM theory, LI is caused by damp heat; viruses invade the liver and lodge in the blood, resulting in liver loss and catharsis regulation. The spleen loses its health and transport capabilities, causing disordered *qi* and blood. CRP is bitter and pungent in taste, warm in nature; it regulates *qi* and dampness, eliminating phlegm and cough, stopping vomiting, eliminating food from the stomach, invigorating the spleen, soothing the liver, and promoting bile discharge (Prc, 2015). A typical TCM formula for treating liver disease is "Chaihu Shugan Powder," one of CRP's main components (Nie et al., 2020). TCM treatment reflects three points: overall, dynamic, and syndrome differentiation. Medications regulate bodily functions and balance them by eliminating pathogenic factors and strengthening vital energy.

Systems pharmacology is based on the theory of systems biology, integrating multi-disciplinary technologies such as multi-directional pharmacology, bioinformatics, and computer science to construct multi-level "disease-gene-target-drug" networks. This study analyzed and elucidated the links between CRP and LI using a modern systems pharmacology approach and *in vitro* experiments (**Figure 1**).

MATERIALS AND METHODS

Instruments and Herb Materials

While collecting and analyzing compounds, we used several instruments, including an ultra-pure liquid chromatograph (UPLC; Nexera X2 LC-30A, Shimadzu Corp. Kyoto, Japan)-hybrid triple-quadruple time-of-flight mass spectrometer (Triple TOF™5600+, AB Sciex, Toronto, Ontario, Canada) with an electrospray ionization source (ESI) and KQ-500 E ultrasonic cleaner (power 500 W, frequency 40 kHz Kunshan Ultrasonic Instrument Co., Ltd. Kunshan, China). The UPLC Titank C18 column (2.1 × 100 mm × 1.8 μm) was purchased from FLM Scientific Instruments Co., Ltd. (Guangzhou, China). Methanol, acetonitrile, and formic acid were purchased from ACS (Washington D.C. United States). Experimental water was ultrapure, obtained using a Milli-QB system (Bedford, MA, United States).

We obtained CRP medicinal materials (batch no. A162002–2) from the Jiangxi Xingan CRP planting base. They were formally identified by Professor Gong Qianfeng of Jiangxi University of TCM as dried and mature pericarps of Rutaceae plant oranges. The remaining samples were stored in the laboratory of the Jiangxi University of TCM. We used 22 standards (purity ≥98%) as references and in subsequent validation studies. Hesperidin (batch no. CHB18023), hesperetin (batch no. CHB180524), nobiletin (batch no. CHB180529), 3′-demethylnobiletin (batch no. CHB180131), 5-*o*-demethylnobiletin (batch no. CHB180321), narirutin (batch no. CHB:1809917), naringenin (batch no. CHB180914), sinensetin (batch no. CHB180126), isosinensetin (batch no. CHB180127), tangeretin (batch no. CHB190125), 5-hydroxy-4′,6,7,8-tetramethoxyflavon (batch no. CHB181119), 3,3′,4′,5,6,7,8-heptamethoxyflavone (batch no. CHB180120), 5,6,7,4′-tetramethoxyflavone (batch no. CHB190106), 5,7,4′-trimethoxyflavone (batch no. CHB181127), diosimin (batch no. CHB180125), diosmetin (batch no. CHB180312), poncirin (batch no. CHB180625), limonin (batch no. CHB180124), nomilin (batch no. CHB180315), naringenin chalcone (batch no. CHB180913), auraptene (batch no. CHB180529), and naringenin-7-O-β-D-glucoside (batch no. CHB181105) were all purchased from Chengdu Chroma-Biotechnology Co., Ltd. (Sichuan, China).

Screening of Active Compounds

Compounds Collected From UPLC-Q-TOF-MS/MS Analysis

Identification technology of compounds and metabolites in CRP has developed rapidly, and mass spectrometry identification is a common technical method (Zheng et al., 2013; Zeng et al., 2017; Li et al., 2019a). We added an appropriate amount of methanol to prepare standard solutions of 50–100 μg/ml and accurately weighed CRP powder (1.0 g), placed it in a conical flask containing 80 ml methanol, mixed it well, treated it with an ultrasound machine for 30 min, passed the solution through filter paper, then increased the volume to 100 ml, and finally filtered the solution through a 0.22 μm microporous membrane to obtain the CRP extraction solution. Ultra-Performance Liquid Chromatography-Quadrupole-Time-of-Flight Tandem Mass Spectrometry (UPLC-Q-TOF-MS/MS) conditions were as follows: chromatographic separation was performed at a flow rate of 0.25 ml/min at 40°C, and elution was performed with a linear gradient program according to various periods. The mobile phase system included solvent A (100% acetonitrile, v/v) and solvent B (0.01% formic acid in water, v/v). The process was solvent A (5–12%) for 5 min, (12–21%) for 10 min, (21–35%) for 10 min, (35–45%) for 11 min, (45–48%) for 4 min, (48–60%) for 1 min, (60–85%) for 9 min, (85–95%) for 1 min, (95%) for 2 min, (95–5%) for 1 min, and isocratic elution at 5% for 2.9 min. The ion source gases 1 and 2 were both set to 50 psi, curtain gas was set to 40 psi, ion spray voltage floating was set to 5500 V in the positive mode and 4500 V in the negative mode, ion source temperature was 500°C, collision energy was 40 V, collision energy spread was 15 V, declustering potential was 100 V, and nitrogen was used as a nebulizer and auxiliary gas. Samples were analyzed in both positive and negative ionization modes with a scanning mass-to-charge (m/z) range from 50 to 1,000. Data were collected in information-dependent acquisition mode and were analyzed using the Analyst TF 1.6 data acquisition workstation and PeakView®1.2 software. We compared the fragment ion information obtained for various compounds with that of the 22 standards and identified several CRP compounds. Also, we studied and analyzed the literature documenting fragment ion information of CRP components in detail carefully, matched it with our information of multiple compounds, and identified additional compounds.

Compounds Collected From Databases

To collect drug ingredients more thoroughly, we used The Encyclopedia of Traditional Chinese Medicine (http://www.tcmip.cn/ETCM), the Traditional Chinese Medicine Systems Pharmacology database and Analysis Platform (TCMSP, http://lsp.nwu.edu.cn/tcmsp.php), and the TCM database Taiwan (http://tcm.cmu.edu.tw). All three online databases were searched for compounds, using the Chinese name "ChenPi" and the Latin name *Citrus reticulata* Blanco.

Compound Identification Analysis

We integrated the collected compounds and established a CRP chemical composition. First, the concept of oral bioavailability (OB) was introduced. OB refers to the percentage of unmodified drug entering the circulatory system after oral administration, representing drug utilization efficiency. Higher OB correlates with a higher possibility of clinical usefulness (Lv W. et al., 2020). Drug-likeness (DL) refers to the potential of a compound to become a drug (Huang et al., 2017). Molecules with OB ≥ 30% or DL ≥ 0.18 are considered to have better pharmacological effects (Zhang M. et al., 2020). We referred to this principle to select active ingredients for the subsequent step of the analysis. Considering the special biological activities of some compounds, we included them in the final candidate component database.

Identification of the Related Targets and Gene Symbols of CRP Compounds

We used information in the TCMSP (http://lsp.nwu.edu.cn/tcmsp.php) and Swiss Target prediction (STP, https://www.swisstargetprediction.ch/) to extract protein targets for each CRP component (Mu et al., 2020). After removing redundant information, the targets that could interact with each CRP component were retained.

Acquisition of Liver Injury Gene Targets

The gene targets for LI was obtained from the GeneCards database (https://www.genecards.org/, version 4.9.0) and the Online Mendelian Inheritance in Man database (OMIM, http://www.omim.org/, updated on February 28, 2019) (Mu et al., 2020; Xu et al., 2020). We performed keyword searches using "liver injury" and carefully screened the results. Finally, we obtained genes associated with LI-related diseases.

Drug-Compounds-Genes-Disease Network Construction

To obtain overlapping targets, we first cross-contrasted CRP-related targets with LI-related targets. We then built a complex information network (D-C-G-D) based on the interactions among drugs (CRP), compounds, gene symbols, and disease (LI) using Cytoscape software (version 3.8.0) and drew a schematic diagram.

Protein-Protein Interaction Network Construction

PPI data were obtained from the STRING database (https://string-db.org/, Version 11.0, updated on January 19, 2019). The interaction relationships provided by STRING are based on the confidence score and can be used to filter and assess functional genomics data (Tao et al., 2020). The organism species was set to *Homo sapiens* (Human), and the merged gene symbols were analyzed. We also used the BioGPS database (https://biogps.org) to identify proteins' higher expression in some major organs (Gu et al., 2020). The heat map was generated using Heml software (version 1.0).

Gene Ontology and Kyoto Encyclopedia of Genes and Genomes Pathway Enrichment

Gene Ontology (GO) and Kyoto Encyclopedia of Genes and Genomes (KEGG) enrichment analyses were performed using R software (version 4.0.2). We used the R package "BiocGenerics," a classic and practical tool specially designed for biologists to conduct an in-depth analysis of these targets (Yu et al., 2012). All enriched entries were determined using the Bioconductor database (http://bioconductor.org/).

Computational Validation of Ingredients-Targets Interactions

Molecular docking is a drug design method that considers receptors' characteristics and the mode of interaction between receptors and drug molecules (Yang et al., 2019). We docked a variety of active components and key targets (BAX, BCL2, and caspase-3 [CASP3]) for a total of six component-target interactions. We obtained data from the RCSB Protein Data Bank (PDB, www.rcsb.org); the X-ray crystal structures of the key targets BAX, BCL2, and CASP3 were obtained and confirmed concerning the relevant literature; their PDB IDs were 1F16, 1G5M, and 5IBC, respectively. After processing targets and compounds using PyMOL software (version 1.3), docking work was performed using AUTODOCK VINA software (Version 1.1.2, Scripps Research, San Diego, CA, United States). The required input files for the AutoDock program were prepared using AutoDock tools.

Experimental Validation

Cell Culture

The LX-2 cell line was purchased from Beina Chuanglian Biotechnology Research Institute (HeNan, China). Cells were cultured in high-glucose Dulbecco's minimum essential medium (Solarbio, Beijing, China) containing 10% fetal bovine serum (Tianhang Biotechnology, Zhejiang, China) in a 37°C, 5% CO_2 incubator. Dimethyl sulfoxide was used to dissolve treatment compounds.

CCK-8 Assay for Cell Viability

Logarithmic growth phase cells were plated in 96-well plates (5×10^3 cells per well) and cultured overnight in a 37°C, 5% CO_2 incubator. The following day, various hesperidin and naringenin (0, 25, 50, 75, 100, and 125 μM) were added to fresh medium. After 12 h, the model and administration groups were incubated with 5 ng/ml transforming growth factor (TGF)-β1 for 24 h, and then 10 μL CCK-8 assay solution (Solarbio) was added to each well. A microplate reader (Nanjing Detie Experimental Equipment Co., Ltd. Nanjing, China) was used to measure the optical density (OD) value around 450 nm. Cell survival was calculated as: $\frac{Ab}{AC} \times 100\%$ (Ab and Ac stand for absorbance and absorbance of the control, respectively).

Real-Time Quantitative Polymerase Chain Reaction (qRT-PCR)

Total RNA was extracted using TRIzol® Reagent (Thermo Scientific, Waltham, MA, USA) and was reverse-transcribed with oligo-DT using HiScript™ Reverse transcriptase (Thermo Scientific) according to manufacturer instructions. The primers used were synthesized by Tsingke (Beijing, China). The sequences (forward and reverse, respectively), were as follows:

5′-CATGGGCTGGACATTGGACT-3′ and 5′-AAAGTAGGAGAGGAGGCCGT-3′ for BAX; 5′-TGAGTGCTCGCAGCTCATAC-3′ and 5′-TTCCCTGAGGTTTGCTGCAT-3′ for CASP3; 5′-CTTTGAGTTCGGTGGGGTCA-3′ and 5′-GAA

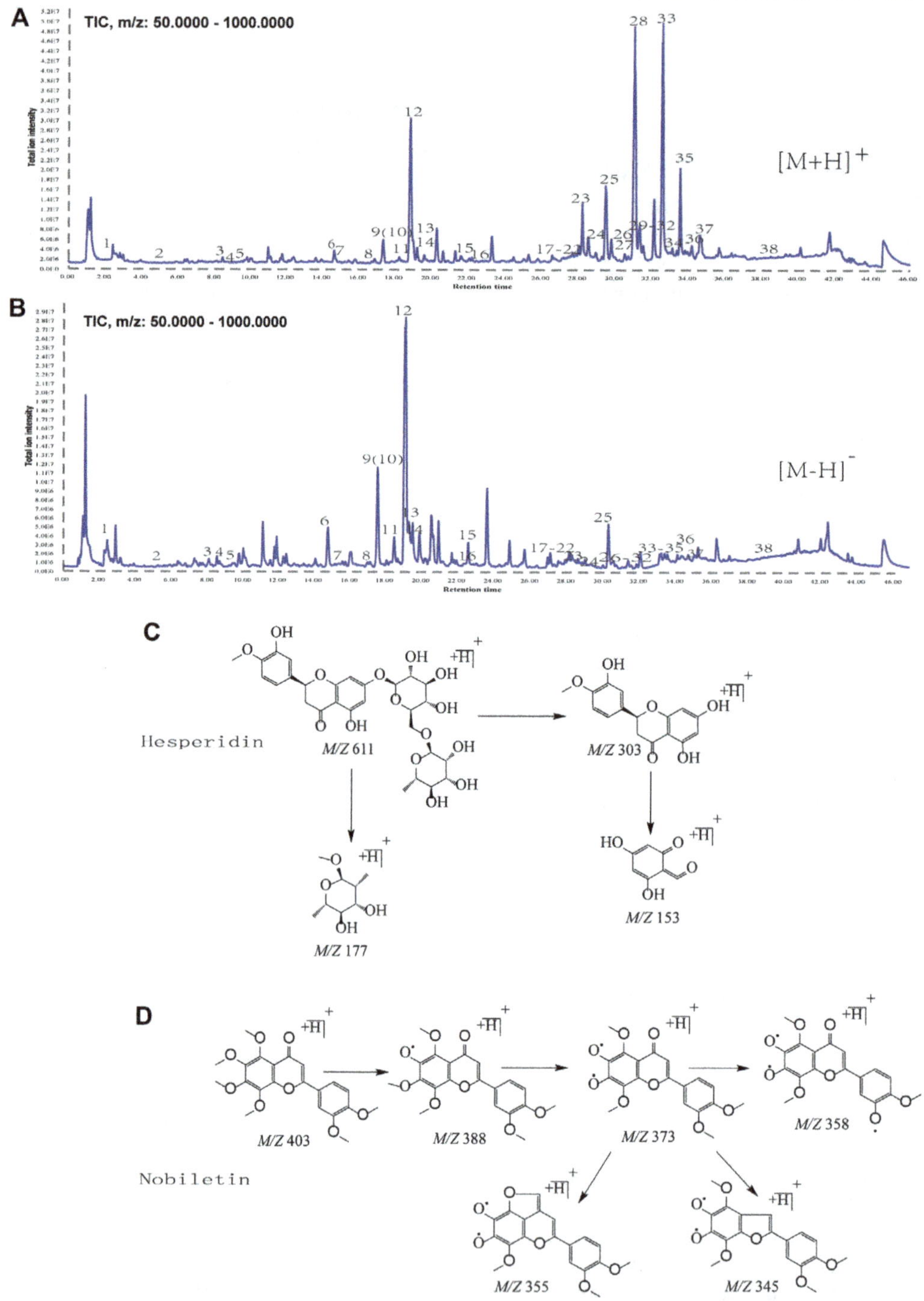

FIGURE 2 | (A, B) Total ion chromatograms of CRP obtained by UPLC/Q-TOF-MS/MS in positive and negative ion mode. **(C, D)** Fragmentation Law of hesperidin and nobiletin by Mass Spectrometry.

ATCAAACAGAGGCCGCA-3′ for BCL2; and 5′-GAAAGCCTG CCGGTGACTAA-3′ and 5′-TTCCCGTTCTCAGCCTTGAC-3′ for the internal control glyceraldehyde 3-phosphate dehydrogenase (GAPDH). The GenBank accession numbers of BAX, CASP3, BCL2, and GAPDH used were NM_001291428.2, NM_001354777.2, NM_000633.3, and NM_001256799.3, respectively. Reverse transcription reaction conditions were: 30°C 10 min, 42°C 60 min, 99°C 5 min, and 4°C 5 min. The synthesized cDNA was stored at −20°C for later use. Gene-expression data were normalized to that of the endogenous control GAPDH. The $2^{-\Delta\Delta}$ Ct method was used as the basis for relative gene expression.

TABLE 1 | CRP compounds identified by UPLC/Q-TOF-MS/MS.

No	Molecule name	Molecular formula	ESI-MS	Error (ppm)	tR/ min	ESI-MS/MS	References
1	Synephrine	$C_9H_{13}NO_2$ [M + H]$^+$	168.1018	−0.8	2.24	135.0679, 134.0601, 107.0498, 91.0554, 77.0405	Zheng et al. (2019)
2	Vanillic acid	$C_8H_8O_4$ [M-H]$^-$	167.03606	6.5	5.47	167.0302, 152.0135, 122.9371, 108.0229, 78.9459	Zheng et al. (2019)
3	Scopoletin	$C_{10}H_8O_4$ [M + H]$^+$	193.04982	1.5	8.35	193.0513, 178.0263, 150.0322, 133.0298, 122.0370	Zheng et al. (2020a)
4	Caffeic acid	$C_9H_8O_4$ [M-H]$^-$	179.03578	4.5	9.5	135.0469, 134.0400, 91.0000, 89.0556, 89.0438	Zheng et al. (2019)
5	Lucenin-2	$C_{27}H_{30}O_{16}$ [M + H]$^+$	611.1632	4.2	9.62	473.1115, 425.0908, 395.0796, 353.0682, 341.0691	Zheng et al. (2019)
6	Ferulic acid	$C_{10}H_{10}O_4$ [M-H]$^-$	193.05114	2.6	14.77	178.0267, 134.0387, 133.0308, 132.0217	Zheng et al. (2019)
7	Apigenin-8-C-glucoside	$C_{21}H_{20}O_{10}$ [M + H]$^+$	433.11435	3.3	15.18	433.1143, 415.1045, 397.0952, 313.0727, 283.0619	Zheng et al. (2019)
8	Diosmetin-6-C-glucoside	$C_{22}H_{22}O_{11}$ [M + H]$^+$	463.12507	3.4	16.75	445.1168, 427.1058, 367.0847, 343.0845, 313.0734	Zheng et al. (2019)
9	Narirutin	$C_{27}H_{32}O_{14}$ [M + H]$^+$	581.18783	2.3	17.35	273.3773, 273.0777, 195.0302, 153.0193, 85.0307	*
10	Naringenin-7-O-β-D-glucoside	$C_{21}H_{22}O_{10}$ [M + H]$^+$	435.12943	2	17.36	273.0777, 153.0195, 147.0452	*
11	Homoeriodictyol	$C_{16}H_{14}O_6$ [M + H]$^+$	303.08759	4.2	18.82	177.0560, 153.0195, 149.0611, 145.0299, 117.0351	Zheng et al. (2019)
12	Hesperidin	$C_{28}H_{34}O_{15}$ [M + H]$^+$	611.19883	2.9	18.83	303.0867, 177.0542, 153.0183	*
13	Diosimin	$C_{28}H_{32}O_{15}$ [M + H]$^+$	609.18374	3.8	19.2	302.2107, 301.9498, 301.7986, 301.5234, 301.0729	*
14	Scoparone	$C_{11}H_{10}O_4$ [M + H]$^+$	207.06564	2.2	19.59	207.0671, 191.0353, 163.0404, 151.0769, 107.0507	Zheng et al. (2020b)
15	Poncirin	$C_{28}H_{34}O_{14}$ [M + H]$^+$	595.20393	3	23.29	287.0929, 263.0568, 195.0303, 153.0191, 85.0305	*
16	Isosakuranetin	$C_{16}H_{14}O_5$ [M + H]$^+$	287.09258	4.1	23.3	153.0198, 161.0609, 133.0659, 287.0930	Zheng et al. (2019)
17	Naringenin	$C_{15}H_{12}O_5$ [M + H]$^+$	273.07576	0	26.47	153.0181, 147.0445, 119.0491, 91.0556	*
18	Naringenin chalcone	$C_{15}H_{12}O_5$ [M + H]$^+$	273.07632	2.1	26.52	153.0198, 147.0453, 119.0504, 91.0564	*
19	Diosmetin	$C_{16}H_{12}O_6$ [M + H]$^+$	301.07162	3.2	26.84	301.0740, 286.0501, 195.0457, 168.0066, 160.0530	*
20	Hesperetin	$C_{16}H_{14}O_6$ [M + H]$^+$	303.08759	4.2	27.38	177.0556, 153.0195, 145.0294, 117.0347, 303.0884	*
21	Jaceosidin	$C_{17}H_{14}O_7$ [M + H]$^+$	331.08241	3.6	27.8	331.0845, 316.0599, 301.0361, 273.0411, 168.0062	Zheng et al. (2020b)
22	Isosinensetin	$C_{20}H_{20}O_7$ [M + H]$^+$	373.12968	4	28.19	357.0974, 343.5625, 343.0819, 315.0865	*
23	3′-demethylnobiletin	$C_{20}H_{20}O_8$ [M + H]$^+$	389.12468	4.1	28.5	359.0765, 344.0532, 313.0713	*
24	6-Demethoxytangeretin	$C_{19}H_{18}O_6$ [M + H]$^+$	343.11925	4.8	29.44	313.0787, 285.0755, 181.0129, 153.0180, 313.5300	Zheng et al. (2020a)
25	Sinensetin	$C_{20}H_{20}O_7$ [M + H]$^+$	373.12979	4.3	29.5	357.0969, 343.0812, 339.0864, 329.1023, 312.0992	*
26	Limonin	$C_{26}H_{30}O_8$ [M + H]$^+$	471.20333	4.2	29.77	425.1981, 213.0922, 161.0605, 95.0146	*
27	5,7,4′-trimethoxyflavone	$C_{18}H_{16}O_5$ [M + H]$^+$	313.10816	3.6	30.51	298.0857, 297.0778, 270.0904, 269.0828	*
28	Nobiletin	$C_{21}H_{22}O_8$ [M + H]$^+$	403.13999	3.1	31.03	388.1125,373.0911, 358.0683, 355.0810, 345.0950	*
29	5,6,7,4′-tetramethoxyflavone	$C_{19}H_{18}O_6$ [M + H]$^+$	343.11934	5	31.32	327.0867, 313.0709, 299.0916, 282.0885	*
30	Nomilin	$C_{28}H_{34}O_9$ [M + H]$^+$	515.22891	2.6	31.51	515.2302, 469.2238, 205.0508, 187.0767, 161.0612	*
31	Chrysosplenetin B	$C_{19}H_{18}O_8$ [M + H]$^+$	375.10916	4.6	31.52	375.1096, 360.0862, 345.0623, 327.0518, 197.0095	Zheng et al. (2020b)
32	3,3′,4′,5,6,7,8-heptamethoxyflavone	$C_{22}H_{24}O_9$ [M + H]$^+$	433.15146	5	32.1	417.1202, 403.1035, 385.0935	*

(Continued on following page)

TABLE 1 | *(Continued)* CRP compounds identified by UPLC/Q-TOF-MS/MS.

No	Molecule name	Molecular formula	ESI-MS	Error (ppm)	tR/ min	ESI-MS/MS	References
33	Tangeretin	$C_{20}H_{20}O_7$ [M + H]$^+$	373.12991	4.6	32.55	344.2913, 343.0820, 328.0587, 325.0717, 297.0761	*
34	Obacunone	$C_{26}H_{30}O_7$ [M + H]$^+$	455.20774	-0.7	32.71	455.2080, 409.2024, 175.0760, 161.0601, 133.0643	Zheng et al. (2020a)
35	5-O-Demethylnobiletin	$C_{20}H_{20}O_8$ [M + H]$^+$	389.12458	3.8	33.52	373.0917, 359.0751, 341.0643, 197.0072	*
36	Atractylenolide II	$C_{15}H_{20}O_2$ [M + H]$^+$	233.1542	2.6	34.15	187.1494, 145.1024, 131.0865, 91.0556, 105.0709	Zheng et al. (2020b)
37	5-Hydroxy-4′,6,7,8-tetramethoxyflavone	$C_{19}H_{18}O_7$ [M + H]$^+$	359.11422	4.7	34.69	329.0675, 311.0570, 197.0093	*
38	Auraptene	$C_{19}H_{22}O_3$ [M + H]$^+$	299.16455	1.3	38.66	283.0539, 267.0223, 250.9903, 163.0404, 119.0488	*

Identified by comparison with standards.

Western Blot

LX-2 cells were collected, lyzed in radioimmunoprecipitation assay buffer, and then centrifuged at 13,000 rpm for 10 min at 4°C. Bicinchoninic acid protein analysis kits (Solarbio) were used to calculate the samples' protein concentrations based on standard curves. Protein samples (30 μg/sample) were added to the loading buffer, heated at 97°C for 6 min, and centrifuged at room temperature. After loading the samples, they were separated on 4% sodium dodecyl sulfate-polyacrylamide gels with voltage 150 V. The proteins were transferred to polyvinylidene membranes (Millipore, MA, United States) using a electroporation device. Next, the membranes were blocked with 5% skimmed milk powder in phosphate-buffered saline for 30 min. After incubation with a single antibody, a ChemiScope Mini 3,300 chemiluminescence imaging system (Shanghai, China) was used to image the blots. The primary antibodies were from Dingguo Changsheng Biotechnology Co., Ltd. (Beijing, China). Band intensity was analyzed using Quantity One software (version 4.6.6).

Statistical Analyses

The significance of results was determined based on one-way analysis of variance using Prism 8.0.1 software (Graph Pad Inc. San Diego, CA, United States). All experiments were performed in triplicate, and data are presented as mean ± SD. Differences were considered significant at $p < 0.05$.

RESULTS

Screening of Active Compounds Collected From UPLC-Q-TOF-MS/MS Analysis

We showed a typical total ion chromatogram of alcohol-soluble components extracted from CRP (**Figures 2A,B**) and the mass spectrometric cleavage law of hesperidin and nobiletin (**Figures 2C,D**). By sampling the primary mass spectrum, we determined each component's relative molecular weight and then obtained fragmentation information based on the secondary mass spectrum. Based on the retention time and mass spectrometric information of the standard material and the compounds reported in the literature, we identified a total of 38 compounds. Twenty-two of these (8, 9, 11, 12, 14, 16, 17, 18, 19, 21, 22, 24, 25, 26, 27, 28, 29, 31, 32, 34, 36, and 37) were identified through careful comparison of information between the samples and standard pure substances. The details are shown in **Supplementary Table S1**. Through the comparison of the multi-level fragment ion information recorded in the relevant literature and the analysis of the fragmentation law, the other 16 components were identified. **Table 1** presents the details of the 38 compounds.

Compounds Collected From Databases

We searched online databases commonly used for TCM ingredients, The Encyclopedia of Traditional Chinese Medicine (http://www.tcmip.cn/ETCM), Traditional Chinese Medicine Systems Pharmacology database and Analysis Platform (http://lsp.nwu.edu.cn/tcmsp.php), and the TCM database Taiwan (http://tcm.cmu.edu.tw) to produce a more comprehensive compound list (Yu et al., 2020; Zhu and Hou, 2020). We collected a total of 65 compounds from these databases as candidates for CRP studies (**Supplementary Table S2**).

Compound Identification Analysis

We collated the results of previous work, combined the components obtained using UPLC/Q-TOF-MS/MS analysis and all CRP components identified in online databases. After removing repeated items, we established a complete CRP internal compound composition library. To screen out the active ingredients of CRP, the classical absorption, distribution, metabolism, and excretion (ADME) parameters of OB and DL were used to screen them. We found five ingredients that met these conditions; however, this result was far below our expectations. CRP contains a large number of flavonoids, including hesperidin and naringin (Dong et al., 2010). Flavonoid glycosides are more easily absorbed after hydrolysis into flavonoid aglycones (Hostetler et al., 2012), and hesperidin is one of the typical constituents (Nectoux et al., 2019). The OB of hesperidin was 13.33%, which was <30%; however, it is an active compound that is significantly effective against LI (Adefegha et al., 2017; Elhelaly et al., 2019). Narirutin has an OB of 8.15% and a DL of 0.75. However, it alleviates LI by regulating protein

TABLE 2 | |Final selected compounds per the details of the active compounds in CRP.

NO.	Molecule name	Cas no.	Structure	References
1	β-sitosterol	83–46–5	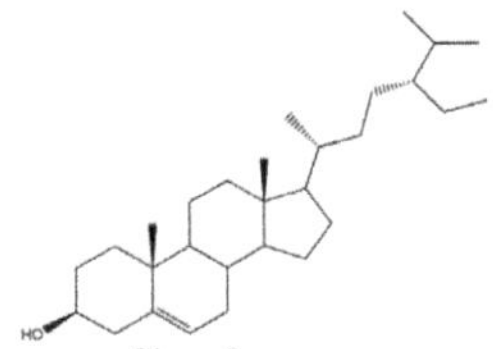	Luo et al. (2019)
2	Naringenin	480–41–1	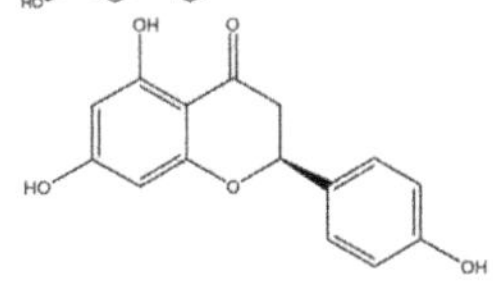	*
3	Hesperetin	520–33–2	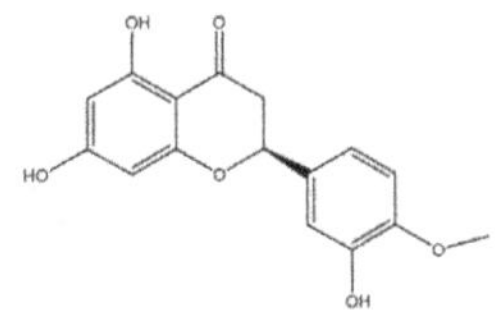	*
4	Citromitin	3570–71–6	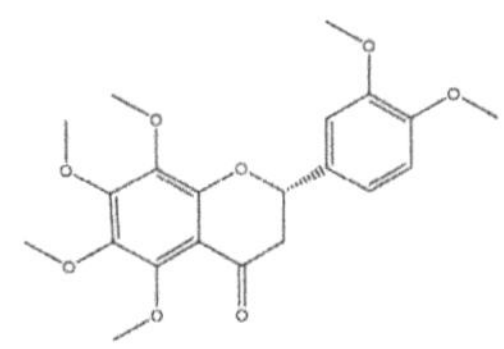	Luo et al., (2019)
5	Nobiletin	478–01–3	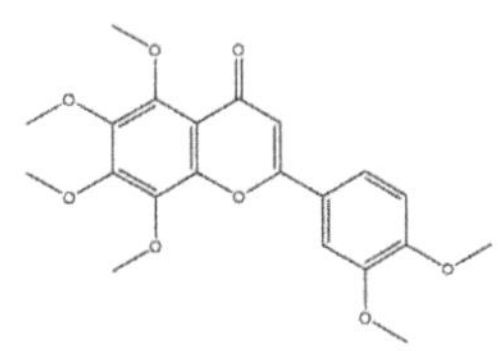	*
6	(R)-linalool	126–91–0	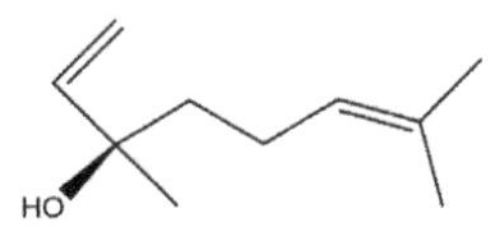	Johnson et al. (2019)
7	Isovanillic acid	645–08–9	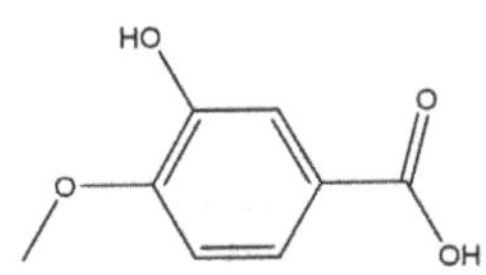	Zheng et al. (2019)
8	P-cymen-8-ol	1,197–01–9	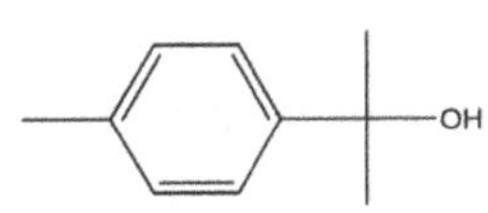	Yi et al. (2015)
9	Dimethyl anthranilate	85–91–6	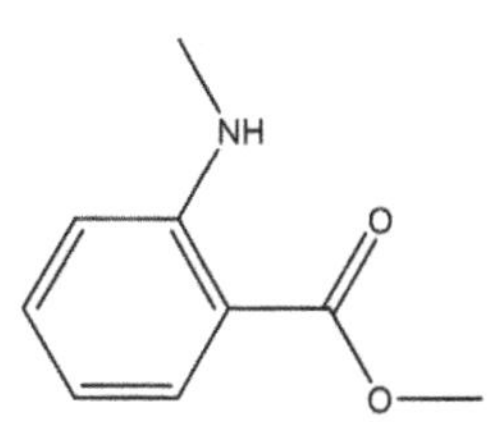	Li et al. (2019b)

(Continued on following page)

TABLE 2 | *(Continued)* |Final selected compounds per the details of the active compounds in CRP.

NO.	Molecule name	Cas no.	Structure	References
10	Isoprenol	763–32–6	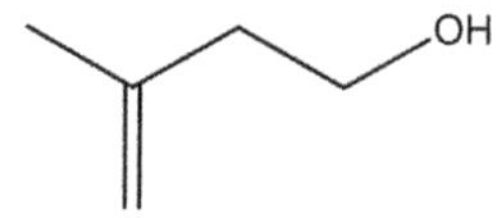	Run-Xia et al. (2013)
11	Neryl acetate	141–12–8	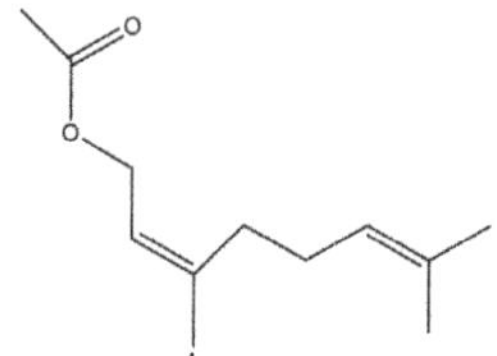	Yi et al. (2015)
12	Vanillin	121–33–5	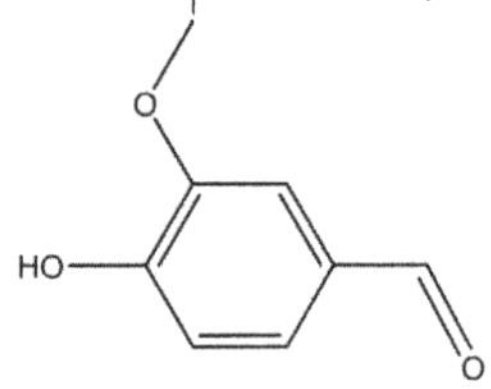	Zheng et al. (2020a)
13	β-terpineol	138–87–4	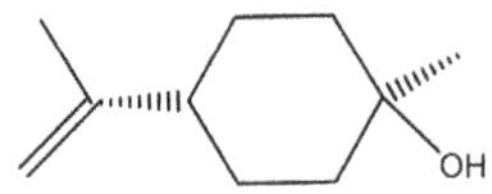	Qiao et al. (2008)
14	HMF	67–47–0	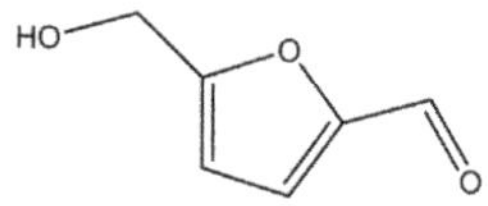	Xiao et al. (2009)
15	P-coumaric acid	501–98–4	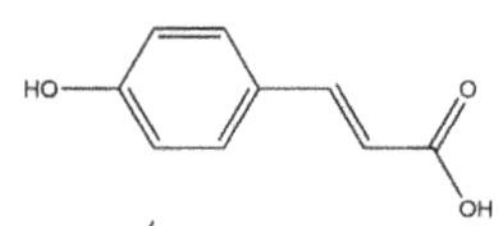	Feumba Dibanda et al. (2020)
16	Ferulic acid	1,135–24–6	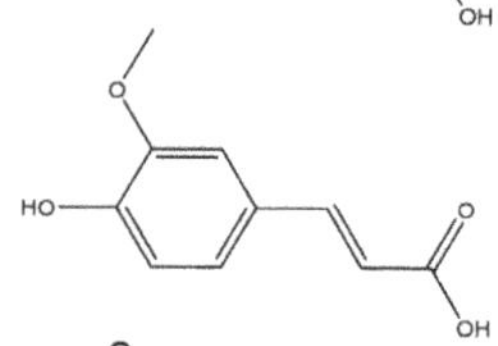	*
17	(S)-carvone	2244–16–8	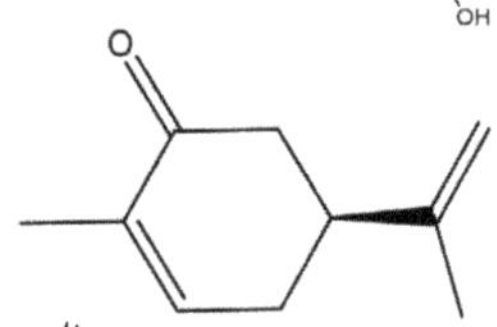	Wang et al. (2008)
18	Linalool	78–70–6	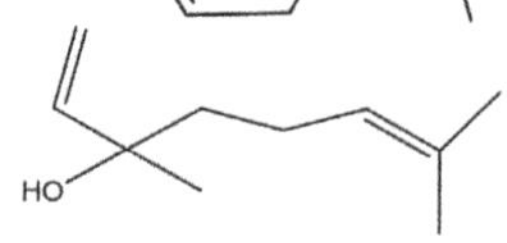	Lv et al. (2020b)
19	Menthol	2216–51–5	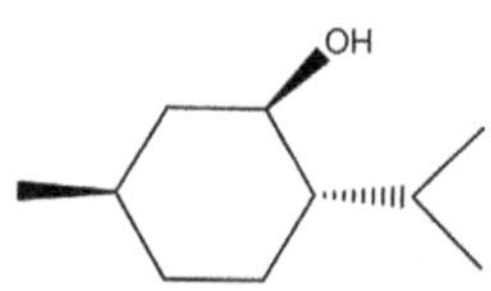	Kim et al. (2018)
20	Hesperidin	520–26–3	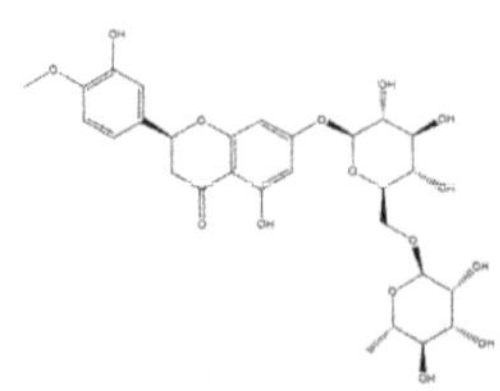	*

(Continued on following page)

TABLE 2 | *(Continued)* |Final selected compounds per the details of the active compounds in CRP.

NO.	Molecule name	Cas no.	Structure	References
21	Tangeretin	481–53–8	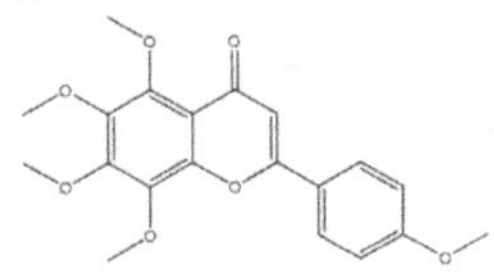	*
22	Rosmarinic acid	20,283–92–5	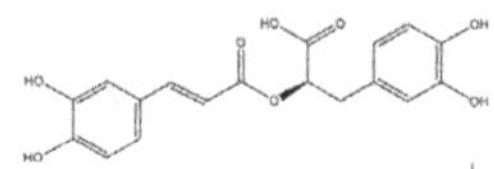	Feumba Dibanda et al. (2020)
23	Neohesperidin	13,241–33–3	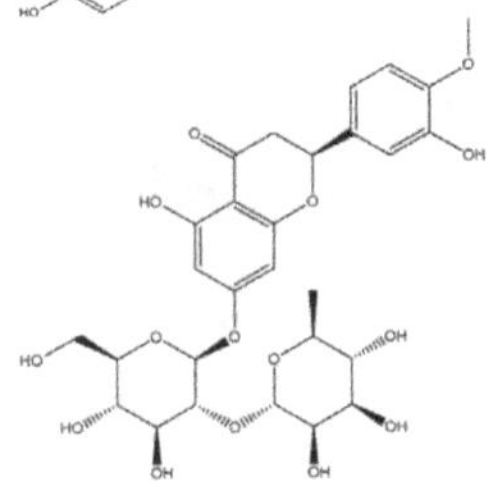	Zheng et al. (2020b)
24	Limonin	1,180–71–8	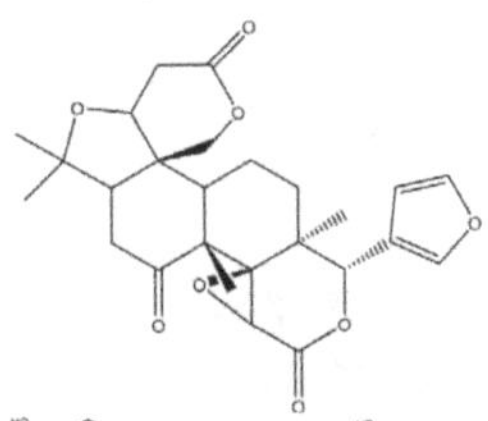	*
25	Narirutin	14,259–46–2	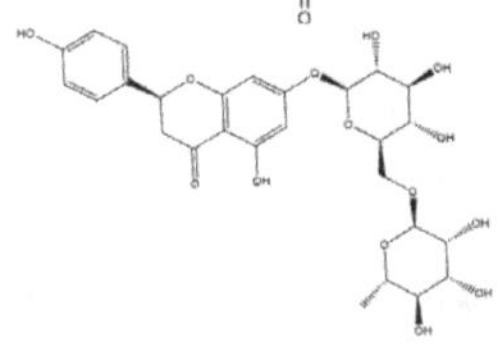	*

Identified using UPLC/Q-TOF-MS/MS.

phosphorylation in the mitogen-activated protein kinase (MAPK) pathway, which may be related to lipid metabolism (Jianping et al., 2019; Gao et al., 2020). Tangeretin has an OB of 21.38% and a DL of 0.43, but it can ameliorate oxygen-glucose deprivation-induced LI through the JNK signaling pathway (Wu et al., 2019). Rosmarinic acid has an OB of 1.38% and a DL of 0.35; it can activate the AMP-activated protein kinase (AMPK) pathway and inhibit inflammation through nuclear factor erythroid 2-related factor and nuclear factor-κB signaling and ameliorates obesity and LI (Gyhye et al., 2019). Another mechanism by which compounds counteract LI is antioxidation, and the candidate *p*-Cymen-8-ol has both antioxidant effects and antibacterial activity (Pires et al., 2006; Santana et al., 2009). Although some components have relatively low kinetic values, they have excellent biological activity; therefore, we still consider them active CRP components. For these reasons, we propose that as long as the candidate components in CRP have good biological activity and intersect with LI's target, they can be considered active CRP compounds for this indication. We selected 25 components as the final active compounds in the candidate compound library (**Table 2**).

Identification of Related Targets and Gene Symbols of Compounds in CRP

After we collected the relevant proteins from the TCMSP and STP databases, they were converted in the UniProt database, and redundant terms were removed to obtain 25 components in CRP and the 126 known associated target symbols (**Supplementary Table S3**).

Acquisition of Known Therapeutic Gene Targets for Liver Injury

A subset of the LI-related targets was obtained from the GeneCards database. We obtained 7372 known LI target symbols. Also, 92 known therapeutic target data for LI were obtained from OMIM. After eliminating redundancies, a total of 7442 known therapeutic targets for LI were collected (**Supplementary Table S4**).

Drug-Compounds-Genes-Disease Network Construction

We contrasted the obtained drug targets with disease-related genes to obtain their common cross genes. We constructed Venn

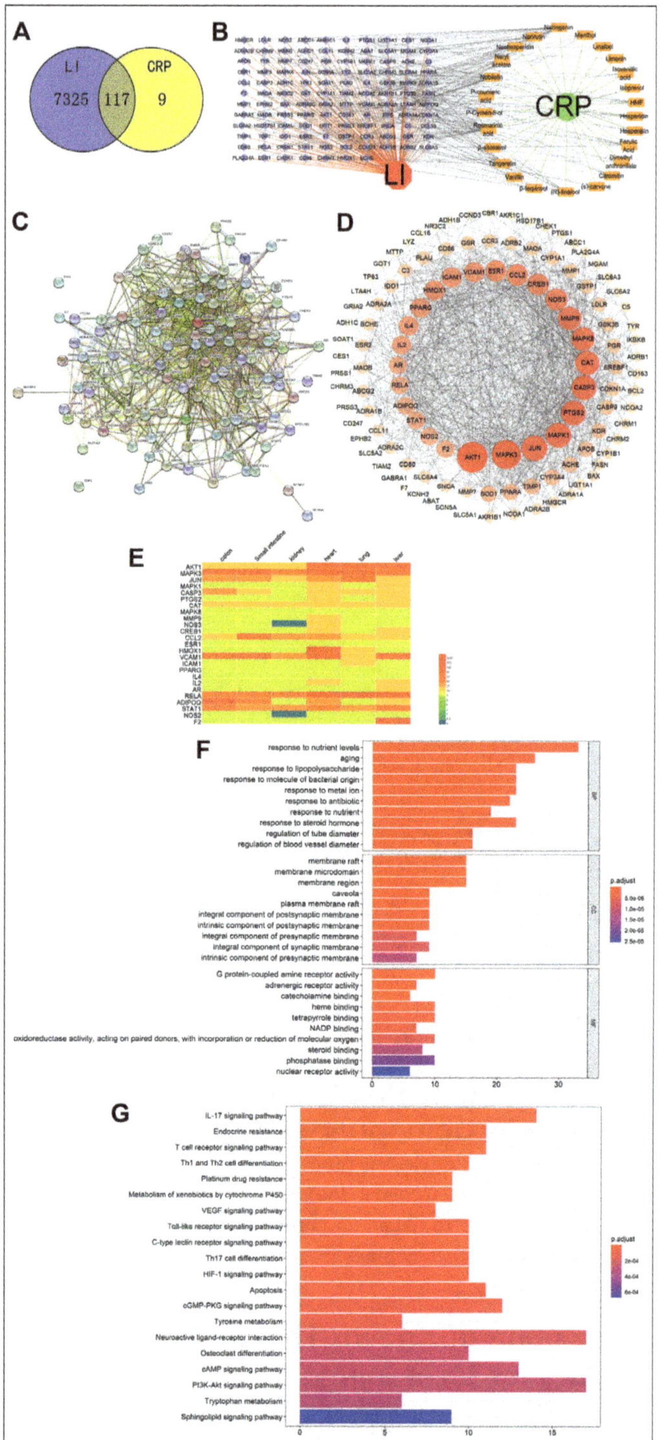

FIGURE 3 | (A) Venn diagram of related targets of CRP and LI. **(B)** D-C-G-D network. Green and red nodes indicate CRP and LI, respectively. Twenty-five orange nodes represent active ingredients in CRP; 117 blue nodes represent overlapping gene symbols between diseases and drugs, with edges indicating that nodes can interact; red edges indicate the action of LI with genes, green edges indicate the interaction of CRP with active ingredients, and gray edges indicate the interaction of active ingredients with genes. **(C)** The PPI network was obtained from the STRING database platform. **(D)** The PPI network is arranged according to degree value. **(E)** The *(Continued)*

diagrams (**Figure 3A**) with 117 overlaps of 7442 disease gene symbols and 126 drug-gene symbols. To intuitively demonstrate how CRP counteracts LI, we constructed a D-C-G-D network using Cytoscape software (**Figure 3B**). D-C-G-D details are in **Supplementary Table S5**.

Protein-Protein Interaction Network Construction

An action relationship map between genes was obtained after 117 overlapping genes were entered into the STRING online database (**Figure 3C**). These genes may be critical targets for LI treatment using CRP. The gene names are listed in **Supplementary Table S6**. After removing two free genes, we calculated the topological indices DC, BC, and CC for 115 genes. Degree (DC) indicates how much a gene is linked to other genes, suggesting that the gene may be necessary for the process of CRP counteracting LI. Detailed information about genes and topological indices is provided in **Supplementary Table S7**. We calculated the mean value of the 115 overlapping gene degrees to be 29.42. All genes with degree values >29.42 were selected, resulting in 25 core targets for interaction networks with other genes. After processing these associated targets using Cytoscape software, the inner loop of **Figure 3D** shows 25 genes with higher DC values. The deeper red color and large nodes indicate stronger correlations, and these may be critical genes for the CRP treatment of LI. To investigate LI and other major organs' connection, we considered these core targets' expression in various organs. According to the presented results of the heat map (**Figure 3E**), the 25 core targets' expression was generally similar in the main organs. For example, AKT1 and MAPK3 were highly expressed in the liver, heart, lung, kidney, small intestine, and colon, while expression levels of PPARG and IL4 were low in these organs. This finding suggests that, in addition to the liver, LI is also closely related to other organs, consistent with the fact that TCM considers the human body as a whole. The specific expression of these core targets in various organs is shown in **Supplementary Table S8**.

Gene Ontology and Kyoto Encyclopedia of Genes and Genomes Pathway Enrichment

To better summarize their specific functions, we performed GO enrichment analysis of 117 consensus genes and classified and elaborated them according to three modules: biological process (BP), cellular component (CC), and molecular function (MF), including 1525 GO terms for BP terms, 55 GO terms for CC terms, and 139 GO terms for MF terms, for a total of 1719

FIGURE 3 | expression of the core target in vital organs. Red and blue indicate higher and lower expression, respectively. **(F)** Bar graph of GO function enrichment of overlapping targets. **(G)** Bar graph of KEGG enrichment of overlapping targets. The *Y*-axis represents GO terms or KEGG pathways. The *X*-axis indicates the number of genes enriched in this pathway. The redder the color, the smaller the p. adjust value; it also indicates the reliability and importance. The bluer the color, the greater the p. adjust value.

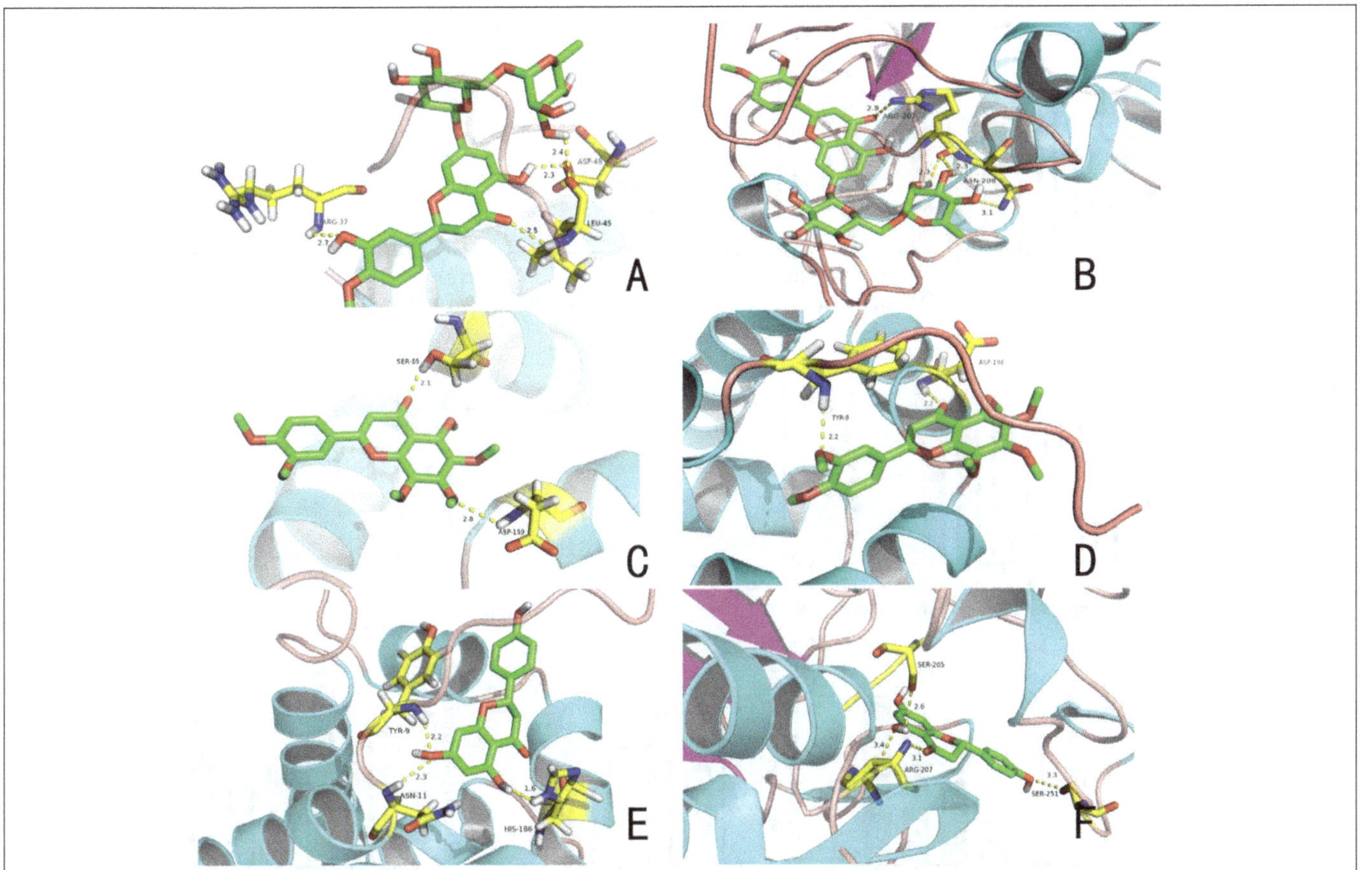

FIGURE 4 | Selected compounds' interactions with the targets. **(A)** Hesperidin with BAX, **(B)** hesperidin with CASP3, **(C)** nobiletin with BAX, **(D)** nobiletin with BCL2, **(E)** naringenin with BCL2, **(F)** naringenin with CASP3. The molecule is represented in a ball-stick model with atoms C, O, and N in green, red, and blue, respectively. Dashed lines indicate hydrogen bonds, and the numbers above represent distances in angstroms (Å).

enriched GO terms. Based on the p. adjust value ($p < 0.01$), we selected the first ten terms from small to large for the enrichment results of BP, CC, and MF (**Figure 3F**). The BP analysis results revealed essential ways in which genes participate in bodily processes. These processes involve responses to nutrient levels (GO: 0031667), aging (GO: 0007568), responses to lipopolysaccharide (GO: 0032496), responses to a molecule of bacterial origin (GO: 0002237), and responses to metal ion (GO: 0010038). CC analysis then identified the sites where these intersection genes function intracellularly and extracellularly, primarily involving membrane raft (GO: 0045121), membrane microdomain (GO: 0098857), membrane region (GO: 0098589), caveola (GO: 0005901), and plasma membrane raft (GO: 0044853). Similarly, from MF analysis, we understand the forms of protein and target binding, primarily involving G protein-coupled amine receptor activity (GO: 0008227), adrenergic receptor activity (GO: 0004935), catecholamine binding (GO: 1901338), heme-binding (GO: 0020037), and tetrapyrrole binding (GO: 0046906). Overall, GO enrichment analysis results suggest that most of the effects of CRP on the liver occur in cell proliferation, regulation of enzyme activity, and energy metabolism. The detailed results are in **Supplementary Table S9**.

To further identify CRP's potential pathways against LI, we also performed KEGG pathway enrichment analysis on 177 consensus genes, and the screen identified 49 pathways. For multiple pathways obtained by enrichment according to p. adjust ($p < 0.01$), we selected the top 20 paths for presentation (**Figure 3G**). The details of all KEGG pathway enrichment analyses are provided in **Supplementary Table S10.** Among these pathways, the interleukin (IL)-17 signaling pathway (hsa04657), endocrine resistance (hsa01522), the T cell receptor signaling pathway (hsa04660), Th1 and Th2 cell differentiation (hsa04658), platinum drug resistance (hsa01524), and others are critical pathways by which CRP acts on LI. Some of these are inflammatory pathways, some are apoptotic differentiation pathways, and others are receptor resistance pathways. Activation of inflammatory pathways such as IL-17 signaling (hsa04657) and tumor necrosis factor signaling (hsa04668) can significantly affect hepatocyte function (Yin and Feng, 2017; Doğanyiğit et al., 2020). Normal hepatocytes accelerate apoptosis after liver damage (Zhang T. et al., 2020). When CRP is administered to humans, the apoptosis pathway (hsa04210) may be affected by proteins such as BAX, BCL2, and CASP3 to maintain normal function. Liver function is also

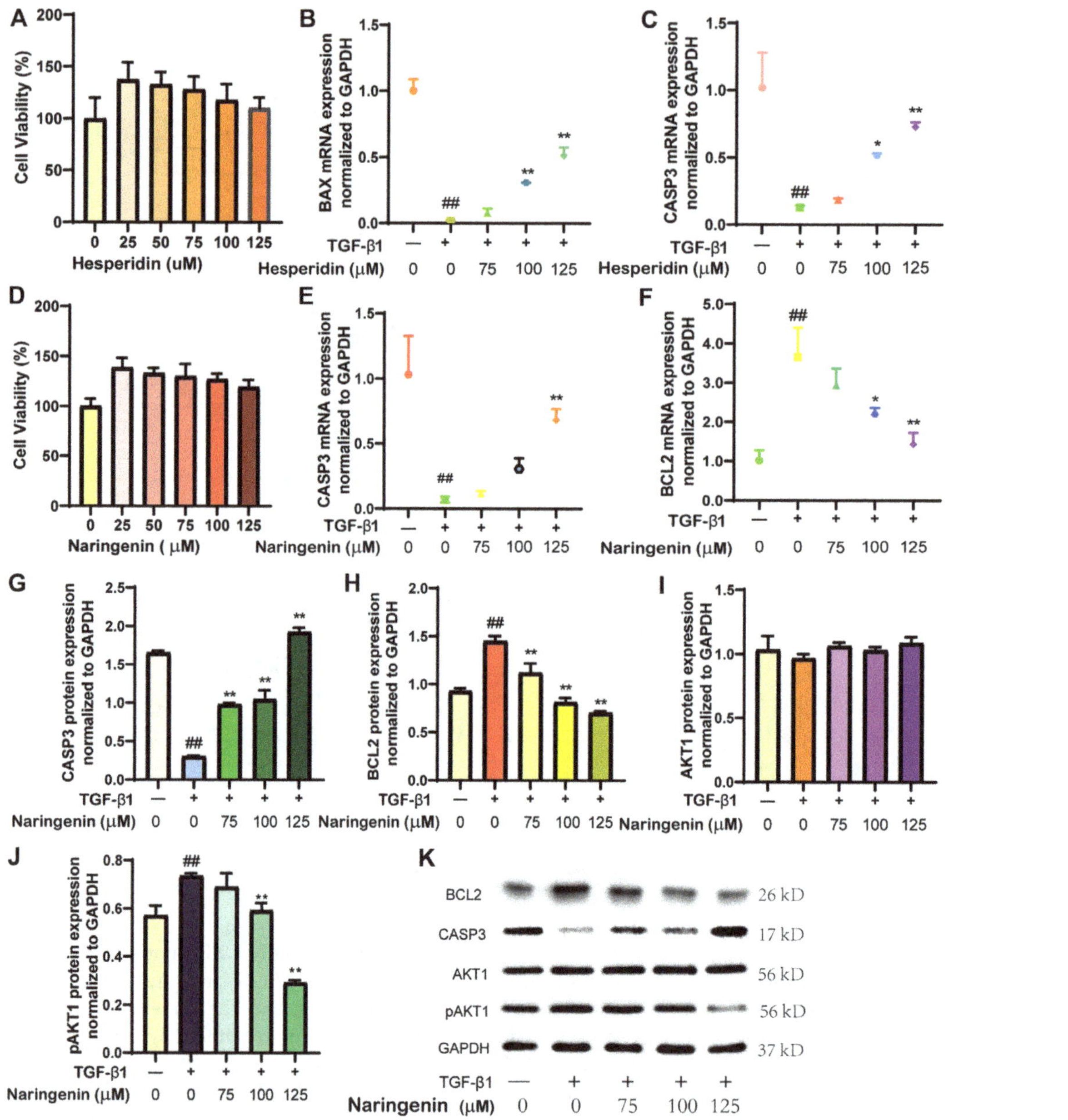

FIGURE 5 | Effect of hesperidin or naringenin on LX-2 cells. The effects of hesperidin **(A)** or naringenin **(D)** on LX-2 cell viability using the CCK-8 assay. mRNA expression of BAX **(B)**, CASP3 **(C, E)**, and BCL2 **(F)** were determined by qRT-PCR. Protein levels of CASP3 **(G)**, BCL2 **(H)**, AKT1 **(I)**, pAKT1 **(J)** were determined by western blot, with results of each group **(K)**. $^{\#}p< 0.05$, $^{\#\#}p< 0.01$ versus blank control group; $^{*}p< 0.05$, $^{**}p< 0.01$ vs. TGF-β1-treated group.

affected by the endocrine system, as endocrine resistance causes toxin-associated steatohepatitis (Clair, et al,2018).

Computational Validation of Ingredients-Targets Interactions

According to the GO and KEGG results, we found that CRP anti-LI is a biological process with multiple targets and pathways. Hesperidin is highly abundant in CRP and is a major active component (Xia et al., 2006). Nobiletin has suitable ADME parameters, suggesting that it may exhibit good drug performance during LI treatment. Based on PPI analysis, we know that some genes linked to naringenin have high metrics. We believe that components such as hesperidin, nobiletin, and naringenin simultaneously affect LI through common targets. Therefore, these compounds were subjected to molecular docking with apoptosis regulators BAX, CASP3, and BCL2 to test our hypothesis. The lower binding energy between molecules represents more potent force binding energy between them, and <0 kcal/mol favors the binding reaction (Shi et al., 2020).

According to the docking results, the binding energies of hesperidin to BAX and CASP3 were −8.2 and −8.6 kcal/mol, respectively; the binding energies of nobiletin to BAX and BCL2 were −5.9 and −7.7 kcal/mol, respectively; and the binding energies of naringenin to BCL2 and CASP3 were −7.7 and −7.2 kcal/mol, respectively. These results suggest that these compounds and their corresponding proteins have good binding. **Figure 4** shows the combinations. Multiple linkages were formed between hesperidin and three amino acid residues in BAX, ARG-37, LEU-45, and ASP-48, including a C-O double bond and strong binding of the amino group (**Figure 4A**). Hesperidin interacts with two amino acid residues ASN-208 and ARG-207, in CASP3 (**Figure 4B**). These results suggest that a compound simultaneously forms multiple bonds with different amino acids in a protein, allowing the drug to affect the protein. The molecular docking results for nobiletin with BAX and BCL2 are shown in **Figures 4C,D**, respectively. The C-O double bond on nobiletin binds to the -OH group on SER-55 and the other O atom is connected to the H atom on ASP-519 (**Figure 4C**). The two O atoms on nobiletin and the amino acid residue TYR-9 on BCL2 and the H atom on ASP-196 form two hydrogen bonds (**Figure 4D**). **Figures 4E,F** show the docking results of naringenin with BCL2 and CASP3, respectively. The naringenin molecule binds to three residues (ASN-11, TYR-9, and HIS-186) on BCL2 to form multiple hydrogen bonds (**Figure 4E**). Naringenin also forms strong hydrophobic binding with residues ARG-207, SER-205, and SER-251 in CASP3 (**Figure 4F**). Our analysis showed that hesperidin, nobiletin, and naringenin effectively acts on protein targets closely related to apoptotic effects.

Experimental Validation

Cell Viability

CCK-8 assays were performed to determine the effects of different doses of hesperidin and naringenin on LX-2 cell viability (**Figures 5A,D**). When hesperidin or naringenin was added at concentrations >75 μmol/L, cell proliferation was not significant, and viability remained high (100–130%). Based on this, three concentrations (75, 100, and 125 μmol/L) were selected for subsequent experiments.

Target Validation

TGF-β1-induced activation of LX-2 cells predisposes to liver fibrosis, resulting from chronic LI developing into cirrhosis that ultimately leads to liver failure (Bestion et al., 2020; Xiang et al., 2020). We chose hesperidin and naringenin to evaluate our prediction results further to validate changes in several relevant proteins in LX-2 cells with or without TGF-β1 (5 ng/ml) treatment. We performed qRT-PCR to determine the effect of hesperidin on BAX and CASP3 mRNA levels and that of naringenin on CASP3 and BCL2 mRNA levels. Western blot was used to measure naringenin's effect on CASP3, BCL2, ATK1, and pAKT1 protein levels. We found that mRNA levels of BAX and CASP3 were significantly lower after TGF-β1 treatment ($p < 0.01$, **Figure 5B,C,E**), BCL2 mRNA was significantly elevated ($p < 0.01$, **Figure 5F**), and mRNA levels of CASP3 and BCL2 were consistent with their protein expression results (**Figures 5G,H**). Compared with the group that only received TGF-β1 stimulation, The levels of multiple index proteins were adjusted to different extents after treatment with different concentrations of hesperidin or naringenin, which made the results obtained after compound treatment more similar to the normal group. Western blotting revealed that ATK1 was only weakly affected by TGF-β1 and naringenin; protein expression changes in each group were relatively stable (**Figure 5I**). Protein levels of pAKT1 increased rapidly after TGF-β1 treatment but decreased significantly after naringenin treatment (**Figure 5J**). This suggests that naringenin may have a more pronounced inhibitory effect on AKT1 phosphorylation. These data collectively suggest that CRP reduces LI by mediating cell apoptosis and protein phosphorylation and regulating BAX expression, CASP3, BCL2, and ATK1, all of which are consistent with our molecular docking results. The results support our predicted results based on systems pharmacology.

DISCUSSION

The liver is both a metabolic organ and an important mediator of immune function. LI may cause cancer, and the use of anti-cancer drugs may lead to more severe liver damage (Björnsson et al., 2020). TCM originates from nature and has few side effects, but its application and development have some limitations due to the complexity of the compositions and mechanisms of action. CRP is a pure, natural TCM that can also be used as a food, and a variety of compounds in CRP have been shown to have anti-proliferative effects on hepatoma cells (Chu et al., 2017).

In this study, we identified the active components and related targets of CRP. We linked them to LI-related targets to construct a D-C-G-D network that depicts links among 117 consensus genes and diseases. The PPI analysis showed complex interactions between 117 overlapping genes, and topological value analysis further indicated 25 core targets. We also examined these targets' expression relationships in the liver, heart, lung, kidney, small intestine, and colon. The results showed that their expression levels were similar in these organs that belong to the TCM category of "five viscera and six entrails." The theory of TCM posits that the viscera is an organic whole, the center of human life activities, and the organs work together to maintain the living body.

The GO analysis results revealed biological connections between drugs and diseases, and the BP enrichment clarified the response to the stimulation of external substances, such as response to acid chemical (GO:0001101). Hepatocytes are more sensitive to exogenous substance stimulation, and liver lesions develop when individuals regularly work in environments containing chemicals (Zhao et al., 2020). The CC analysis revealed the cellular environment in which the intersection protein or its product occurred, including membrane raft (GO: 0045121). Alcohol alters plasma membranes *in vitro*; preventing membrane raft oxidation is one approach to inhibit LI caused by excessive alcohol consumption (Chen et al., 2018). MF results suggest how intersection proteins or their products bind or function *in vivo* after the compound performs its action.

Among them, catecholamine binding (GO: 1901338) is related to the expression of genes, and catecholamine receptors' regulation prevents acute stress-induced LI (Zhu et al., 2014). We also found that a large number of GO terms were related to mitochondria, including regulation of mitochondrial membrane potential (hsa04210), apoptotic mitochondrial changes (GO: 0008637), and mitochondrial outer membrane permeabilization (GO: 0097345). This finding suggests that one of the critical mechanisms by which CRP ameliorates LI is to alter cellular energy metabolism (Xu et al., 2017; Dilberger et al., 2019).

The KEGG pathway enrichment results revealed that inflammatory and apoptotic pathways might be the primary CRP action pathways. CRP mediates the IL-17 signaling pathway by regulating targets such as PTGS2, MAPK3, and CASP3. PTGS2, also known as cyclooxygenase 2, extensively participates in hepatic inflammation induced by xenobiotics (Zhang et al., 2019). Through the D-C-G-D network, we know that hesperidin, nobiletin, and tangeretin are all involved in regulating PTGS2. The inhibition of PTGS2 mRNA expression is one of the manifestations of LI's acute inflammation resolution (Li et al., 2020). It also suggests that a protein can be affected by several compounds simultaneously. LX-2 cells are prone to proliferate faster, and this can lead to liver fibrosis (Bestion et al., 2020). Our *in vitro* results suggest that CRP can induce apoptosis in LX-2 cells by regulating targets such as BAX, BCL2, and CASP3, consistent with our finding that the apoptosis pathway (hsa04210) is affected by CRP. The liver has a unique regenerative capacity (Nejak-Bowen and Monga, 2011). Some cancer pathways are associated with uncontrolled cell growth, and their dysregulation can lead to liver cancer. The phosphoinositide 3-kinase (PI3K)-Akt signaling pathway (hsa04151) can be activated by a variety of cell stimulants and toxins and is potentially correlated with liver cancer (Shi et al., 2020). Our prediction results suggest that AKT1 has a high degree in this pathway, and the phosphorylated form is a biomarker for cancer and tumor biology (Balasuriya et al., 2020). Our *in vitro* validation experiments demonstrated that naringenin significantly inhibited AKT1 phosphorylation, which in turn mediated PI3K-Akt signaling pathways to counteract LI. This interesting finding will be the focus of our future study. Nobiletin in CRP inhibits hepatoma metastasis resulting from PI3K-Akt signaling and may become a new compound for liver cancer treatment (Shi et al., 2013). The western blot results indicated that naringenin significantly reduced pAKT1 levels, suggesting that it prevents LI exacerbation. Increased cytochrome P450 expression improves hepatocyte function (Lewis et al., 2020); xenobiotics' metabolism by cytochrome P450 (HSA00980) pathway was analyzed. We found that it resulted from naringenin, tangeretin, narirutin, and other compounds by affecting GSTP1, CYP1A1, and CBR1 targets.

We propose the following mechanism by which CRP counteracts LI. Hesperidin and naringenin in CRP affect the apoptosis pathway by acting on CASP3, BAX, and BCL2, reducing the likelihood of liver fibrosis. Naringenin significantly inhibits AKT1 phosphorylation, in turn mediating PI3K-Akt signaling to counteract LI. Systems pharmacology is a useful strategy to predict therapeutic mechanisms and identify new research directions. We acknowledge that the predictions and actual situations may be biased; however, they complement the *in vitro* findings, consistent with the molecular docking results that test the system pharmacology-based screening strategy's reliability from a different perspective.

CONCLUSION

Previous drug development models mainly followed the concept of "one drug, one gene, and one disease." In this study, modern technologies such as UPLC-Q-TOF-MS/MS and molecular docking were used to clarify the specific modes of the synergistic effects of multiple CRP components against LI, and provided convincing evidence. System pharmacology of TCM is an emerging multi-field interdisciplinary, but its development still has certain limitations. In addition to being an important reference for CRP in the treatment of liver diseases, our research also has many shortcomings. The specific interactions between all the drug components, proteins and multiple signal pathways involved in it need to be further studied. This approach of Systems pharmacology is a powerful new way to elucidate the mystery of TCM.

AUTHOR CONTRIBUTIONS

JW and QG conceived and designed the study. SY conceived and designed the *in vitro* experimental validation. JW, XY, and SY contributed equally to this work and shared first authorship. All authors have read and approved the final manuscript.

FUNDING

This study was supported by the National Traditional Chinese Medicine Standardization Project (ZYBZH-Y-JX-27).

ACKNOWLEDGMENTS

The authors are thankful to Jiangxi University of Traditional Chinese Medicine for assistance in conducting this study.

REFERENCES

Adefegha, S. A., Rosa Leal, D. B., Olabiyi, A. A., Oboh, G., and Castilhos, L. G. (2017). Hesperidin attenuates inflammation and oxidative damage in pleural exudates and liver of rat model of pleurisy. *Redox Rep.* 22 (6), 563–571. doi:10.1080/13510002.2017.1344013

Balasuriya, N., Davey, N. E., Johnson, J. L., Liu, H., Biggar, K. K., Cantley, L. C., et al. (2020). Phosphorylation-dependent substrate selectivity of protein kinase B (AKT1). *J. Biol. Chem.* 295 (24), 8120–8134. doi:10.1074/jbc.ra119.012425

Bestion, E., Jilkova, Z., Mège, J., Novello, M., Kurma, K., Ahmad Pour, S. T., et al. (2020). GNS561 acts as a potent anti-fibrotic and pro-fibrolytic agent in liver fibrosis through TGF-β1 inhibition[J]. *Ther. Adv. chronic Dis.* 11, 2040622320942042. doi:10.1177/2040622320942042

Björnsson, H. K., Sverrisdottir, A., and Bjornsson, E. (2020). 1088 drug-induced liver injury due to chemotherapeutic agents and other cancer medications. *A. Population Based Study[j]. Gastroenterol.* 158 (6).

Chen, Y., He, X., Yuan, X., Hong, J., Bhat, O., Li, G., et al. (2018). NLRP3 inflammasome formation and activation in nonalcoholic steatohepatitis: therapeutic target for antimetabolic syndrome remedy FTZ. *Oxid Med. Cel Longev* 2018, 2901871. doi:10.1155/2018/2901871

Chu, C-C., Chen, S-Y., Chyau, C-C., and Duh, P-D. (2017). Antiproliferative effect of sweet orange peel and its bioactive compounds against human hepatoma cells, *in vitro* and *in vivo*[J]. *J. Funct. Foods* 33. doi:10.1016/j.jff.2017.03.051

Clair, H. B., Pinkston, C. M., Rai, S. N., Pavuk, M., Dutton, N. D., et al. (2018). Liver disease in a residential cohort with elevated polychlorinated biphenyl exposures[J]. *Toxicol. Sci. : official J. Soc. Toxicol.* 164 (1), 39–49. doi:10.1093/toxsci/kfy076

Cui, Y., Zhao, J., Zhou, J., Tan, G., Zhao, Q., Zhang, Y., et al. (2019). Development of a sensitive monoclonal antibody-based indirect competitive enzyme-linked immunosorbent assay for analysing nobiletin in citrus and herb samples. *Food Chem.* 293, 144–150. doi:10.1016/j.foodchem.2019.04.101

Dilberger, B., Baumanns, S., Schmitt, F., Schmiedl, T., Hardt, M., Wenzel, U., et al. (2019). Mitochondrial oxidative stress impairs energy metabolism and reduces stress resistance and longevity of[J]. Oxidative medicine and cellular longevity of *C. elegans. Oxid Med. Cel Longev* 2019, 6840540. doi:10.1155/2019/6840540

Dong, P., Qiu, P., Zhu, Y., Li, S., Ho, C.-T., McClements, D. J., et al. (2010). Simultaneous determination of four 5-hydroxy polymethoxyflavones by reversed-phase high performance liquid chromatography with electrochemical detection. *J. Chromatogr. A* 1217 (5), 642–647. doi:10.1016/j.chroma.2009.11.097

Doğanyiğit, Z., Okan, A., Kaymak, E., Pandır, D., and Silici, S. (2020).Investigation of protective effects of apilarnil against lipopolysaccharide induced liver injury in rats via TLR 4/HMGB-1/NF-κB pathway. *Biomedicine & Pharmacotherapy*, 125, 109967. doi:10.1016/j.biopha.2020.109967

Elhelaly, A. E., Albasher, G., Alfarraj, S., Almeer, R., Bahbah, E. I., Fouda, M. M. A., et al. (2019). Protective effects of hesperidin and diosmin against acrylamide-induced liver, kidney, and brain oxidative damage in rats. *Environ. Sci. Pollut. Res.* 26 (34), 35151–35162. doi:10.1007/s11356-019-06660-3

Feumba Dibanda, R., Panyoo Akdowa, E., Rani P., A., Metsatedem Tongwa, Q., and Mbofung F., C. M. (2020). Effect of microwave blanching on antioxidant activity, phenolic compounds and browning behaviour of some fruit peelings. *Food Chem.* 302, 125308. doi:10.1016/j.foodchem.2019.125308

Gao, Y., Tian, Y., Zhang, X., Zhang, X., Duan, Z., Ren, F., et al. (2020). Magnesium isoglycyrrhizinate ameliorates concanavalin A-induced liver injury via the p38 and JNK MAPK pathway. *Immunopharmacology and immunotoxicology* 42 (5), 445–455. doi:10.1080/08923973.2020.1808984

Gu, S., Xue, Y., Gao, Y., Shen, S., Zhang, Y., Chen, K., et al. (2020). Mechanisms of indigo naturalis on treating ulcerative colitis explored by GEO gene chips combined with network pharmacology and molecular docking[J]. *Scientific Rep.* 10 (1), 15204. doi:10.1038/s41598-020-71030-w

Gyhye, Y., Myungsuk, K., Ahmad, R., Yang-Ju, S., Hong, C. R., Kim, S. M., et al. (2019). Lemon balm extract and its major chemical compound, rosmarinic acid, alleviate damages of liver in an animal model of nonalcoholic steatohepatitis (NASH) (P06-093-19)[J]. *Curr. Dev. Nutr.* 3 (Suppl. 1).

Hostetler, G., Riedl, K., Cardenas, H., Diosa-Toro, M., Arango, D., Schwartz, S., et al. (2012). Flavone deglycosylation increases their anti-inflammatory activity and absorption. *Mol. Nutr. Food Res.* 56 (4), 558–569. doi:10.1002/mnfr.201100596

Huang, J., Cheung, F., Tan, H.-Y., Hong, M., Wang, N., Yang, J., et al. (2017). Identification of the active compounds and significant pathways of yinchenhao decoction based on network pharmacology. *Mol. Med. Rep.* 16 (4), 4583–4592. doi:10.3892/mmr.2017.7149

Jianping, J., Li, Y., Zheng, S., Lixia, W., Letian, S., and Thomas, E. (2019). Hepatoprotective and anti-inflammatory effects of total flavonoids of Qu Zhi Ke (peel of Citrus changshan-huyou) on non-alcoholic fatty liver disease in rats via modulation of NF-κB and MAPKs[J]. *Phytomedicine : Int. J. phytotherapy phytopharmacology* 64.

Johnson, A., Hjelmeland, A., Heymann, H., and Ebeler, S. (2019). GC-Recomposition-Olfactometry (GC-R) and multivariate study of three terpenoid compounds in the aroma profile of Angostura bitters[J]. *Scientific Rep.* 9 (1), 7633. doi:10.1038/s41598-019-44064-y

Kim, J. H., Cha, J. Y., Shin, T. S., and Chun, S. S. (2018). Volatile flavor components of blended tea with fermented tea and herbs. *pnf* 23 (3), 245–253. doi:10.3746/pnf.2018.23.3.245

Lewis, B., Paula, S., Paine, S. W., Mellor, H. R., Abernethy, L., Littlewood, P., et al. (2020). Hydrostatic pressure regulates CYP1A2 expression in human hepatocytes via a mechanosensitive aryl hydrocarbon receptor-dependent pathway[J]. *Am. J. Physiol. Cel Physiol.* 318 (5).

Li, S.-Z., Guan, X.-M., Gao, Z., Lan, H.-C., Yin, Q., Chu, C., et al. (2019a). A simple method to discriminate Guangchenpi and Chenpi by high-performance thin-layer chromatography and high-performance liquid chromatography based on analysis of dimethyl anthranilate. *J. Chromatogr. B* 1126-1127, 121736. doi:10.1016/j.jchromb.2019.121736

Li, S.-Z., Zeng, S.-L., Wu, Y., Zheng, G.-D., Chu, C., Yin, Q., et al. (2019b). Cultivar differentiation of Citri Reticulatae Pericarpium by a combination of hierarchical three-step filtering metabolomics analysis, DNA barcoding and electronic nose. *Analytica Chim. Acta* 1056, 62–69. doi:10.1016/j.aca.2019.01.004

Li, Y., Chen, Y., Huang, X., Huang, D., Gan, H., Yao, N., et al. (2020). Tanshinol A ameliorates triton-1339W-induced hyperlipidemia and liver injury in C57bl/6J mice by regulating mRNA expression of lipemic-oxidative injury genes. *Lipids* 55 (2), 127–140. doi:10.1002/lipd.12217

Lin, Z.-H., Chan, Y.-F., Pan, M.-H., Tung, Y.-C., and Su, Z.-Y. (2019). Aged citrus peel (chenpi) prevents acetaminophen-induced hepatotoxicity by epigenetically regulating Nrf2 pathway. *Am. J. Chin. Med.* 47 (8), 1833–1851. doi:10.1142/s0192415x19500939

Liu, P. (2016). Inhibition of pathological angiogenesis of Chinese medicine against liver fibrosis. *Chin. J. Integr. Med.* 22 (8), 569–572. doi:10.1007/s11655-016-2468-3

Luo, Y., Zeng, W., Huang, K.-E., Li, D.-X., Chen, W., Yu, X.-Q., et al. (2019). Discrimination of Citrus reticulata Blanco and Citrus reticulata 'Chachi' as well as the Citrus reticulata 'Chachi' within different storage years using ultra high performance liquid chromatography quadrupole/time-of-flight mass spectrometry based metabolomics approach. *J. Pharm. Biomed. Anal.* 171, 218–231. doi:10.1016/j.jpba.2019.03.056

Lv, W., Lin, T., Ren, Z., Jiang, Y., Zhang, J., Bi, F., et al. (2020a). Rapid discrimination of Citrus reticulata 'Chachi' by headspace-gas chromatography-ion mobility spectrometry fingerprints combined with principal component analysis. *Food Res. Int.* 131, 108985. doi:10.1016/j.foodres.2020.108985

Lv, X., Xu, Z., Xu, G., Li, H., Wang, C., Chen, J., et al. (2020b). Investigation of the active components and mechanisms of Schisandra chinensis in the treatment of asthma based on a network pharmacology approach and experimental validation. *Food Funct.* 11 (4), 3032–3042. doi:10.1039/d0fo00087f

Mu, C., Sheng, Y., Wang, Q., Amin, A., Li, X., and Xie, Y. (2020). Potential compound from herbal food of rhizoma polygonati for treatment of COVID-19 analyzed by network pharmacology and molecular docking technology[J]. *J. Funct. Foods* 77, 104149. doi:10.1016/j.jff.2020.104149

Nectoux, A. M., Abe, C., Huang, S.-W., Ohno, N., Tabata, J., Miyata, Y., et al. (2019). Absorption and metabolic behavior of hesperidin (rutinosylated hesperetin) after single oral administration to sprague-dawley rats. *J. Agric. Food Chem.* 67 (35), 9812–9819. doi:10.1021/acs.jafc.9b03594

Nejak-Bowen, K. N., and Monga, S. P. S. (2011). Beta-catenin signaling, liver regeneration and hepatocellular cancer: sorting the good from the bad. *Semin. Cancer Biol.* 21 (1), 44–58. doi:10.1016/j.semcancer.2010.12.010

Nie, H., Deng, Y., Zheng, C., Pan, M., Xie, J., Zhang, Y., et al. (2020). A network pharmacology-based approach to explore the effects of Chaihu Shugan powder on a non-alcoholic fatty liver rat model through nuclear receptors. *J. Cel Mol Med* 24 (9), 5168–5184. doi:10.1111/jcmm.15166

Pires, A. M. L., Albuquerque, M. R. J. R., Nunes, E. P., Melo, V. M. M., Silveira, E. R., and Pessoa, O. D. L., (2006). Chemical composition and antibacterial activity of the essential oils of blainvillea rhomboidea (asteraceae)[J]. *Nat. Product. Commun.* 1 (5). doi:10.1177/1934578x0600100510

Prc, P. C. O. (2015). *Pharmacopoeia of the people's Republic of China[M]. 1.* Beijing: China Medical Science Press.

Qiao, Y., Xie, B., Zhang, Y., Zhang, Y., Fan, G., Yao, X., et al. (2008). Characterization of aroma active compounds in fruit juice and peel oil of jinchen sweet orange fruit (citrus sinensis (L.) osbeck) by GC-MS and GC-O. *Molecules* 13 (6), 1333–1344. doi:10.3390/molecules13061333

Run-Xia, G., Yu, Z., Xing-He, T., Feng, W., Wen, C., and Xiao-an, H. (2013). Change in essential oil composition of ponkan peels under different storage conditions[J]. Beijing: Food ence.

Santana, A. I., Vila, R., Espinosa, A., Olmedo, D., Gupta, M. P., and Cañiguera, S. (2009). Composition and biological activity of essential oils from Protium confusum[J]. *Nat. Prod. Commun.* 4 (10), 1401–1406. doi:10.1177/1934578x0900401017

Shi, M.-D., Liao, Y.-C., Shih, Y.-W., and Tsai, L.-Y. (2013). Nobiletin attenuates metastasis via both ERK and PI3K/Akt pathways in HGF-treated liver cancer HepG2 cells. *Phytomedicine* 20, 743–752. doi:10.1016/j.phymed.2013.02.004

Shi, P., Xie, Y., Xie, R., Lin, Z., Yao, H., and Wu, S. (2020). Acanthopanax senticosusAn integrated pharmacokinetic study of an extract preparation by combination of virtual screening, systems pharmacology, and multi-component pharmacokinetics in rats[J]. *Front. Pharmacol.* 11, 1295. doi:10.3389/fphar.2020.01295

Shi, Q., Xue, C., Yuan, X., and Yu, Z. (2020). Gene signatures and prognostic values of m1A-related regulatory genes in hepatocellular carcinoma[J]. *Scientific Rep.* 10 (1), 15083. doi:10.1038/s41598-020-72178-1

Tao, Q., Du, J., Li, X., Zeng, J., Tan, B., Xu, J., et al. (2020). Network pharmacology and molecular docking analysis on molecular targets and mechanisms of Huashi Baidu formula in the treatment of COVID-19. *Drug Dev. Ind. Pharm.* 46 (8), 1345–1353. doi:10.1080/03639045.2020.1788070

Tsutsumi, M., Wang, J.-S., and Takada, A. (1994). Microheterogeneity of serum glycoproteins in alcoholics: is desialo-transferrin the marker of chronic alcohol drinking or alcoholic liver injury?. *Alcohol. Clin. Exp. Res.* 18 (2), 392–397. doi:10.1111/j.1530-0277.1994.tb00031.x

Vatsalya, V., Song, M., Schwandt, M. L., Cave, M. C., Barve, S. S., George, D. T., et al. (2016). Effects of sex, drinking history, and omega-3 and omega-6 fatty acids dysregulation on the onset of liver injury in very heavy drinking alcohol-dependent patients. *Alcohol. Clin. Exp. Res.* 40 (10), 2085–2093. doi:10.1111/acer.13197

Wang, Y., Yi, L., Liang, Y., Li, H., Yuan, D., Gao, H., et al. (2008). Comparative analysis of essential oil components in Pericarpium Citri Reticulatae Viride and Pericarpium Citri Reticulatae by GC-MS combined with chemometric resolution method. *J. Pharm. Biomed. Anal.* 46 (1), 66–74. doi:10.1016/j.jpba.2007.08.030

Wu, C., Zhao, J., Chen, Y., Li, T., Zhu, R., Zhu, B., et al. (2019). Tangeretin protects human brain microvascular endothelial cells against oxygen-glucose deprivation-induced injury. *J. Cel Biochem* 120 (4), 4883–4891. doi:10.1002/jcb.27762

Xia, J., Kotani, A., Hakamata, H., and Kusu, F. (2006). Determination of hesperidin in Pericarpium Citri Reticulatae by semi-micro HPLC with electrochemical detection. *J. Pharm. Biomed. Anal.* 41 (4), 1401–1405. doi:10.1016/j.jpba.2006.02.030

Xiang, D., Zou, J., Zhu, X., Chen, X., Luo, J., Kong, L., et al. (2020). Physalin D attenuates hepatic stellate cell activation and liver fibrosis by blocking TGF-β/Smad and YAP signaling. *Phytomedicine* 78, 153294. doi:10.1016/j.phymed.2020.153294

Xiao, H., Yang, C. S., Li, S., Jin, H., Ho, C.-T., and Patel, T. (2009). Monodemethylated polymethoxyflavones from sweet orange (Citrus sinensis) peel Inhibit growth of human lung cancer cells by apoptosis. *Mol. Nutr. Food Res.* 53 (3), 398–406. doi:10.1002/mnfr.200800057

Xu, F., Liu, Y., Zhao, H., Yu, K., Song, M., Zhu, Y., et al. (2017). Aluminum chloride caused liver dysfunction and mitochondrial energy metabolism disorder in rat. *J. Inorg. Biochem.* 174, 55–62. doi:10.1016/j.jinorgbio.2017.04.016

Xu, H.-H., Li, S.-M., Xu, R., Fang, L., Xu, H., and Tong, P.-J. (2020). Predication of the underlying mechanism of Bushenhuoxue formula acting on knee osteoarthritis via network pharmacology-based analyses combined with experimental validation. *J. ethnopharmacology* 263, 113217. doi:10.1016/j.jep.2020.113217

Yang, Q., Han, B., Xue, J., Lv, Y., Li, S., Liu, Y., et al. (2020). Hexavalent chromium induces mitochondrial dynamics disorder in rat liver by inhibiting AMPK/PGC-1α signaling pathway. *Environ. Pollut.* 265, 114855. doi:10.1016/j.envpol.2020.114855

Yang, S., Zhang, J., Yan, Y., Yang, M., Li, C., Li, J., et al. (2019). Network pharmacology-based strategy to investigate the pharmacologic mechanisms of atractylodes macrocephala koidz. For the treatment of chronic gastritis. *Front. Pharmacol.* 10, 1629. doi:10.3389/fphar.2019.01629

Yi, L., Dong, N., Liu, S., Yi, Z., and Zhang, Y. (2015). Chemical features of Pericarpium Citri Reticulatae and Pericarpium Citri Reticulatae viride revealed by GC-MS metabolomics analysis. *Food Chem.* 186, 192–199. doi:10.1016/j.foodchem.2014.07.067

Yin, S., and Feng, D. (2017). IL-22 in liver inflammation, injury and repair[J]. *Liver Research.* 1 (3), 181-185. doi:10.1016/j.livres.2017.09.003

Yu, G., Wang, L.-G., Han, Y., and He, Q.-Y. (2012). clusterProfiler: an R Package for comparing biological themes among gene clusters. *OMICS: A J. Integr. Biol.* 16 (5), 284–287. doi:10.1089/omi.2011.0118

Yu, J.-W., Yuan, H.-W., Bao, L.-D., and Si, L.-G. (2020). Interaction between piperine and genes associated with sciatica and its mechanism based on molecular docking technology and network pharmacology. *Mol. Divers.* 25 (1), 233-248. doi:10.1007/s11030-020-10055-9

Yu, X., Sun, S., Guo, Y., Liu, Y., Yang, D., Li, G., et al. (2018). Citri Reticulatae Pericarpium (Chenpi): botany, ethnopharmacology, phytochemistry, and pharmacology of a frequently used traditional Chinese medicine. *J. ethnopharmacology* 220, 265–282. doi:10.1016/j.jep.2018.03.031

Zeng, S., Li, S., Xiao, P., Cai, Y., Chu, C., Chen, B., et al. (2020). Citrus polymethoxyflavones attenuate metabolic syndrome by regulating gut microbiome and amino acid metabolism[J]. *Sci. Adv.* 6 (1), eaax6208. doi:10.1126/sciadv.aax6208

Zeng, S.-L., Duan, L., Chen, B.-Z., Li, P., and Liu, E.-H. (2017). Chemicalome and metabolome profiling of polymethoxylated flavonoids in Citri Reticulatae Pericarpium based on an integrated strategy combining background subtraction and modified mass defect filter in a Microsoft Excel Platform. *J. Chromatogr. A* 1508, 106–120. doi:10.1016/j.chroma.2017.06.015

Zhang, H. Y., Wang, H. L., Zhong, G. Y., and Zhu, J. X. (2018). Molecular mechanism and research progress on pharmacology of traditional Chinese medicine in liver injury. *Pharm. Biol.* 56 (1), 594–611. doi:10.1080/13880209.2018.1517185

Zhang, L-Y., Zhan, D-L., Chen, Y-Y., Wang, W-H., He, C-Y., Lin, Y., et al. (2019). Aflatoxin B1 enhances pyroptosis of hepatocytes and activation of Kupffer cells to promote liver inflammatory injury via dephosphorylation of cyclooxygenase-2: an *in vitro*, *ex vivo* and *in vivo* study[J]. *Arch. Toxicol.* 93 (11). doi:10.1007/s00204-019-02572-w

Zhang, M., Yuan, Y., Zhou, W., Qin, Y., Xu, K., Men, J., et al. (2020a). Network pharmacology analysis of Chaihu Lizhong Tang treating non-alcoholic fatty liver disease. *Comput. Biol. Chem.* 86, 107248. doi:10.1016/j.compbiolchem.2020.107248

Zhang, T., Li, H., Wang, K., Xu, B., Chen, Z-N., and Bian, H. (2020b). Deficiency of CD147 attenuated non-alcoholic steatohepatitis progression in an NLRP3-dependent manner[J]. *Front. Cel. Dev. Biol.* 8, 784. doi:10.3389/fcell.2020.00784

Zhao, X., Chen, T., Wang, D., Du, Y., Wang, Y., Zhu, W., et al. (2020). Polybrominated diphenyl ethers and decabromodiphenyl ethane in paired hair/serum and nail/serum from corresponding chemical manufacturing workers and their correlations to thyroid hormones, liver and kidney injury markers. *Sci. Total Environ.* 729, 139049. doi:10.1016/j.scitotenv.2020.139049

Zheng, G., Chao, Y., Luo, M., Xie, B., Zhang, D., Hu, P., et al. (2020a). Construction and chemical profile on "activity fingerprint" of Citri Reticulatae Pericarpium from different cultivars based on HPLC-UV, LC/MS-IT-TOF, and principal component analysis*Evid. Based Complement. Alternat Med.*, 2020, 4736152. doi:10.1155/2020/4736152

Zheng, G., Liu, M., Chao, Y., Yang, Y., Zhang, D., Tao, Y., et al. (2020b). Identification of lipophilic components in Citri Reticulatae Pericarpium cultivars by supercritical CO fluid extraction with ultra-high-performance liquid chromatography-Q Exactive Orbitrap tandem mass spectrometry[J]. *J. Separat. Sci.* 43 (17), 3421–3440. doi:10.1002/jssc.202000490

Zheng, G.-D., Zhou, P., Yang, H., Li, Y.-s., Li, P., and Liu, E.-H. (2013). Rapid resolution liquid chromatography-electrospray ionisation tandem mass spectrometry method for identification of chemical constituents in Citri Reticulatae Pericarpium. *Food Chem.* 136 (2), 604–611. doi:10.1016/j.foodchem.2012.08.040

Zheng, Y. y., Zeng, X., Peng, W., Wu, Z., and Su, W. w. (2019). Characterisation and classification of Citri Reticulatae Pericarpium varieties based on UHPLC-Q-TOF-MS/MS combined with multivariate statistical analyses. *Phytochem. Anal.* 30 (3), 278–291. doi:10.1002/pca.2812

Zhu, N., and Hou, J. (2020). Exploring the mechanism of action Xianlingubao Prescription in the treatment of osteoporosis by network pharmacology. *Comput. Biol. Chem.* 85, 107240. doi:10.1016/j.compbiolchem.2020.107240

Zhu, Q., Gu, L., Wang, Y., Jia, L., Zhao, Z., Peng, S., et al. (2014). The role of alpha-1 and alpha-2 adrenoceptors in restraint stress-induced liver injury in mice[J]. *PloS one* 9 (3), e92125. doi:10.1371/journal.pone.0092125

9

Erxian Decoction Attenuates TNF-α Induced Osteoblast Apoptosis by Modulating the Akt/Nrf2/HO-1 Signaling Pathway

*Nani Wang[1,2], Hailiang Xin[3], Pingcui Xu[1,2], Zhongming Yu[1] and Dan Shou[1]**

[1] Department of Medicine, Tongde Hospital of Zhejiang Province, Hangzhou, China, [2] School of Pharmacy, Zhejiang Chinese Medical University, China, [3] School of Pharmacy, Second Military Medical University, China

***Correspondence:**
Dan Shou
shoudanok@163.com

Erxian decoction (EXD), a traditional Chinese medicine formula, has been used for treatment of osteoporosis for many years. The purpose of this study was to investigate the pharmacological effect of EXD in preventing osteoblast apoptosis and the underlying mechanism of prevention. Putative targets of EXD were predicted by network pharmacology, and functional and pathway enrichment analyses were also performed. Evaluations of bone mineral density, serum estradiol level, trabecular area fraction, serum calcium levels, and tumor necrosis factor (TNF)-α levels in ovariectomized rats, as well as cell proliferation assays, apoptosis assays, and western blotting in MC3T3-E1 osteoblasts were performed for further experimental validation. Ninety-three active ingredients in the EXD formula and 259 potential targets were identified. Functional and pathway enrichment analyses indicated that EXD significantly influenced the PI3K-Akt signaling pathway. *In vivo* experiments indicated that EXD treatment attenuated bone loss and decreased TNF-α levels in rats with osteoporosis. *In vitro* experiments showed that EXD treatment increased cell viability markedly and decreased levels of caspase-3 and the rate of apoptosis. It also promoted phosphorylation of Akt, nuclear translocation of transcription factor NF-erythroid 2-related factor (Nrf2), and hemeoxygenase-1 (HO-1) expression in TNF-α-induced MC3T3-E1 cells. Our results suggest that EXD exerted profound anti-osteoporosis effects, at least partially by reducing production of TNF-α and attenuating osteoblast apoptosis *via* Akt/Nrf2/HO-1 signaling pathway.

Keywords: network pharmacology, Erxian decoction, osteoporosis, Akt, tumor necrosis factor

INTRODUCTION

Osteoporosis is a skeletal disease characterized by imbalanced bone homeostasis, which leads to an increase in bone fragility and fracture risk (Liu et al., 2017). Development of osteoporosis is mainly due to the production of a large number of immune and hematopoietic factors in the bone microenvironment (Yu and Wang, 2016). These complex and interacting factors influence the formation and absorption of bone (Wei and Frenette, 2018). One of the most important factors in osteoporosis is tumor necrosis factor-alpha (TNF-α), which is the strongest bone resorption enhancer and also inhibits bone formation (Zhou et al., 2017a; Zhou et al., 2017b).

Erxian decoction (EXD) is a traditional Chinese medicine (TCM) formulation comprising six herbs: *Epimedium sagittatum* (Siebold & Zucc.) Maxim. (ES), *Curculigo orchioides* Gaertn. (CO), *Angelica sinensis* (Oliv.) Diels. (AS), *Phellodendron chinense* Schneid. (PC), *Anemarrhena asphodeloides* Bge. (AR), and *Morinda officinalis* How (MO). EXD has been used to treat osteoporosis for several decades (Wang et al., 2016). We previously reported that some components of EXD, such as icariin, curculigoside, and berberine, displayed inhibitory effects on osteoclastic bone resorption and positive effects on osteoblast proliferation (Wang et al., 2017a; Wang et al., 2017b). However, potential effects of EXD on TNF-α production and TNF-α-induced bone loss have not been investigated.

Recently, network pharmacology analyses have been used to investigate TCM formulas to predict the molecular targets and pathways of different diseases (Zhao and He, 2018). As a systems biology-based methodology, network pharmacology provides an effective approach for evaluating the multi-pharmacological effects of traditional medicines at the molecular level and for evaluating the interactions of chemical molecules and target proteins (Liu et al., 2016). In our previous study, network pharmacology was used to predict the mechanism for the effects of CO in the prevention and treatment of osteoporosis (Wang et al., 2017a; Wang et al., 2017b). In the current study, network pharmacology was combined with experimental validation to study the effects of EXD on TNF-α-induced bone loss and clarify the underlying mechanism.

MATERIALS AND METHODS

Instruments and Reagents

Double distilled water of at least 18.2 MΩ was purified by an ultrapure water system (Millipore Corporation, Boston, Massachusetts, USA). α-Modified minimum essential medium (α-MEM), phosphate buffered saline (PBS), trypsin, and fetal bovine serum (FBS) were purchased from Gibco (Gaithersburg, Maryland USA). TNF-α (purity >98%) was obtained from Sigma (St Louis, MO, USA).

Orcinol glucosid (>98%), palmatine (>99%), jatrorrhizine (>94%), berberine (>98%), protodioscin (>98%), baohuoside I (>99%), timosaponin BII (>99%), icariin (>98%), obacunone (>8%), curculigoside (>98%), anhydroicaritin (>98%), mangiferin (>98%), epimedin C (>98%), epimedin B (>98%), epimedin A (>98%), magnolflorine (>98%), and phellodendrine (>98%) standards were purchased from Aoke Biological Technology Co., LTD (Beijing, China). Ferulic acid (>98%) and naringin (>98%) were purchased from the National Institutes for Food and Drug Control (Beijing, China). Anemarsaponin B (>98%) was purchased from Yuanye Biological Technology Co. Ltd. (Shanghai, China).

The aerial parts of *E. sagittatum* (Siebold & Zucc.) Maxim. (Lot No: 170420, Drug name: Epimedii Folium) were obtained from Huadong Medicine Co. Ltd. (Zhejiang, China). The rhizomes of *C. orchioides* Gaertn. (Lot No: 1702074, Drug name: Curculiginis Rhizoma), the roots of *M. officinalis* How (Lot No: 1711067, Drug name: Morindae Officinalis Radix), the bark of *P. chinense* Schneid. (Lot No: 1710100, Drug name: Chinensis Cortex), and the rhizomes of *A. asphodeloides* Bge. (Lot No: 1710006, Drug name: Anemarrhenae Rhizoma) were obtained from Quzhou Nankong Chinese Medicine Co. Ltd. (Zhejiang, China). The roots of *A. sinensis* (Oliv.) Diels (Lot No: 1802011, Drug name: Angelicae Sinensis Radix) were obtained from Zhejiang Conba Pharmaceutical Co. Ltd. (Zhejiang, China).

Chemical Components of Herbs in Erxian Decoction

Chemical components of each herb in EXD were determined from the Traditional Chinese Medicine Systems Pharmacology (TCMSP) (Ru et al., 2014), TCM database @taiwan (Sanderson, 2011), Herbal Ingredients Targets (HIT), Traditional Chinese Medicine Integrated Database (TCMID) (Xue et al., 2013), and previous literature (Bian et al., 2013; Yu et al., 2013). The molecular properties of the herbs, including molecular weight (MW), Moriguchi octanol-water partition coefficient (AlogP), oral bioavailability (OB), drug-likeness (DL), number of donor atoms for H-bonds (nHDon), and number of acceptor atoms for H-bonds (nHAcc) were compared in **Table S1**.

Predication of Active Components and Targets

OB was used to monitor drug convergence during the ADME process, representing the percentage of an orally administered dose of unchanged drug that reached the systemic circulation (Simpson et al., 2009). DL was used for estimating how "drug-like" prospective compounds were a parameter that is applied in drug design to optimize pharmacokinetic and pharmaceutical properties (Gozalbes et al., 2010). EXD components were considered active if OB ≥30% and DL ≥0.18 (Wang et al., 2015). Validated targets of potential active components were determined from Therapeutic Target Database (Chen et al., 2002), TCMSP, Drug bank (Law et al., 2014), and STITCH (Kuhn et al., 2008).

Network Pharmacology Analyses

Gen Ontology (GO) function enrichment analysis and KEGG (Kyoto Encyclopedia of Genes and Genomes) pathway enrichment analysis were carried out using The Database for Annotation, Visualization and Integrated Discovery (DAVID) database (Huang et al., 2007). The interaction network of the potential active components and identified targets of EXD, as well as of enriched KEGG pathways, were visualized with Cytoscape v3.4.0 software (**Figure 1**).

Herbal Preparation

EXD extract was prepared by hot water extraction as previously described (Wang et al., 2017a; Wang et al., 2017b) with some modifications. Specifically, herbs were pulverized and 20 g of the powder of each herb (120 g total) was placed in

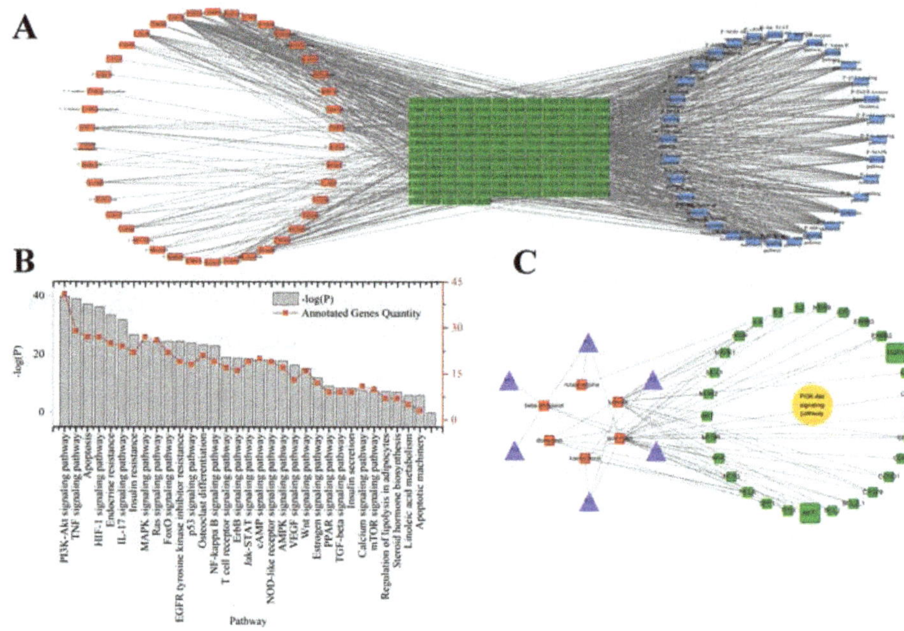

FIGURE 1 | (A) Potential active ingredient-target-pathways network of EXD acting on osteoporosis. The network was based on the interaction among ingredients in EXD, active components, and osteoporosis-related targets. Red nodes represented the ingredients; green nodes represented the targets; blue nodes represented the osteoporosis-related pathways. **(B)** KEGG pathways for potential targets of Erxian decoction. **(C)** The interaction among herbs, components, and targets in PI3K-Akt signaling pathway.

5-L triangular flasks. Samples were extracted twice with 2-L water (1 h each extraction) at 100°C. Extracted solutions were concentrated to 1 g (crude extract)/ml.

Animals and Treatment

Twelve-month-old female Wistar rats (weighting 350–400 g) were supplied by the Animal Center of the Zhejiang Academy of Traditional Chinese Medicine (Hangzhou, China). The rats were maintained in air-conditioned quarters at 24 ± 2°C and a relative humidity of 60 ± 5%. All protocols for animal experiments were approved in accordance with the Guide for the Care and Use of Laboratory Animals and were approved by the Bioethics Committee of Zhejiang Academy of Traditional Chinese Medicine.

Animals were body-weight matched and randomly assigned into several groups: 1) sham-operated group (Control group); 2) ovariectomy (OVX) group (Model group); and 3) three OVX operated groups with oral administration of EXD extract (EXD groups). The doses of EXD administered were 2, 4, and 6 g/kg/day in the low, middle, and high level to EXD groups, respectively. EXD administration was initiated 4 days after OVX operation and provided for 12 weeks.

Liquid Chromatographic Analysis

High-performance liquid chromatography (HPLC) was performed on a Thermo Fisher ultra-high-performance liquid chromatography 3000 system (Thermo Fisher Technologies, Waltham, MA, USA), comprising a dual pump, auto-sampler, ultraviolet (UV) detector and Chromeleon software equipped with a 4.6 × 250 mm ZORBAX Eclipse XDB C18 column (Agilent, Santa Clara, CA, USA). The column temperature was set at 30°C. The mobile phases of HPLC were composed of acetonitrile (A) and water (B). The analytical column was SHISEIDO Capcell Pak C18 (Tokyo, Japan). The gradient condition was as follows: 0–15 min, 95–80% B; 15–30 min, 80–60% B; 30–60 min, 60–40% B. The column flow rate was 1.00 ml/min. The wavelength of UV detection was set at 285 nm. The injection volume was 10 μl. The EXD extract was air-dried and the residue was dissolved to a final concentration of 5 mg/ml in a 1:9 mixture of acetonitrile and water. The diluted solution was passed through a 0.22-μM pore filter prior to HPLC analysis.

Histomorphology Assay

Left femurs were fixed in 10% formalin, embedded in paraffin, cut into 5-μm-thick sections, and finally stained with hematoxylin–eosin (HE) for histopathological analysis. At least 10 independent fields were assessed per sample in each treatment group. Trabecular area was measured according to the previous literature (Kloefkorn and Allen, 2016). Bone mineral density (BMD) was determined by Lunar dual-energy X-ray absorptiometry (GE, Boston, MA, USA) using the small animal scan mode.

Serum Biochemical Analysis

Blood was drawn from rats and centrifuged at 4°C, 5,000 × g for 10 min to collect the upper serum, and stored at −80°C.

The concentrations of serum calcium (Ca), estradiol (E_2), TNF-α, and caspase-3 were detected with commercial detection kits (Boster Biological Technology Co. Ltd, California, USA) in accordance with the manufacturers' protocols.

Immunohistochemistry Analysis

Osteocalcin expression in the right femur was examined by immunohistochemistry. Briefly, tissue sections were treated with 3% H_2O_2 to remove endogenous peroxidase, incubated with anti-osteocalcin antibody (ab13420, Abcam, Cambridge, UK) at 4°C overnight prior to addition of added secondary antibody (PV-6002, ZSGB-Bio, Beijing, China), incubated at 37° C for 30 min, then colored with DAB (diaminobenzidine) reaction staining. Finally, sections were evaluated by microscopy in a blinded manner.

MT3T3-E1 (5×10^6) cells were seeded in six-well plates and then treated with EXD extract or TNF-α as indicated. Cells were fixed with 4% paraformaldehyde in PBS (0.1 M, pH 7.4) for 15 min, permeabilized with 50 μg/ml digitonin in PBS for 5 min, blocked with 0.1% (v/v) gelatin in PBS for 30 min, and then incubated with primary antibodies for 1 h. After washing, cells were incubated with Alexa Fluor 488-conjugated goat anti-guinea pig and Alexa Fluor 647-conjugated goat anti-rabbit IgG secondary antibodies (Invitrogen, Waltham, MA, USA) for 30 min. Cells were imaged using a laser-scanning microscope (LSM510 META, Carl Zeiss, Oberkochen, Germany) with a Plan Apochromat 63 × NA 1.4 oil differential interference contrast objective lens.

Cell Culture and Treatment

MC3T3-E1 cells were cultured in α-MEM containing 10% FBS. All cells were washed with PBS before incubation with EXD or TNF-α. After reaching 85% confluence, the cells were treated with medium containing TNF-α and EXD according to the experimental design.

Cell Proliferation Assay

Cell viability was evaluated with commercially available 3-(4,5-dimethylthiazol-2-yl)-2,5-diphenyltetrazolium bromide (MTT) detection kits (Bio-Rad, Foster, California, USA) in accordance with the manufacturer's protocol. Briefly, treated cells were incubated 10% MTT solution at 37°C for 4 h, supernatants were removed, and the formazan crystals were dissolved in 150 μl DMSO (dimethyl sulfoxide). Absorbance was recoded at a wavelength of 490 nm.

Assay of Annexin V-EGFP/PI Apoptosis

Apoptosis was determined using the Annexin V-EGFP/PI Apoptosis Detection Kit (Jiancheng, Nanjing, China). MT3T3-E1 cells (5×10^6) were seeded in six-well plates and then treated with LY294002, EXD extract, or TNF-α according to the experimental design. Detection was performed using flow cytometric analysis (ACCURI C6, BD Bioscience, Franklin Lakes, NJ, USA).

Western Blot Analysis

MT3T3-E1 cells (5×10^6) were seeded in six-well plates and then treated with EXD extract or TNF-α according to the experimental design. Cells were extracted with lysis buffer for 30 min at 4°C and the supernatant containing total protein was harvested. Aliquots containing 50 μg of protein were separated by sodium dodecylsulfate polyacrylamide gel electrophoresis and transferred to a polyvinylidine difluoride membrane (Millipore, MA, USA). Membranes were soaked in blocking buffer (5% skimmed milk) for 2 h. The proteins were detected with primary antibodies overnight at 4°C, and then probed with HRP (horseradish peroxidase)-conjugated secondary antibody for 1 h at room temperature. Detection was performed with an enhanced chemiluminescence system (ECL, Beyotime, Haimen, China). The relative content of each protein of interest was calculated as the ratio of its optical density to that of β-actin in the same sample.

Statistical Analysis

All experiments were performed in triplicate and results are presented as mean ± SD. One-way ANOVA was used to assess statistical significance of differences between group means. A value of $p < 0.05$ was considered statistically significant.

RESULTS

Physicochemical Properties of Active Components in EXD

A total of 93 compounds present in EXD met the criteria for inclusion (OB ≥ 30% and DL index ≥ 0.18). MW, AlogP, HDon,

TABLE 1 | Properties of potential active ingredients from Erxian decoction.

Herb[a]	MW	AlogP	Hdon	Hacc	OB (%)	DL
ES	355.95 ± 111.69	3.36 ± 2.13*	2.77 ± 2.15*	5.27 ± 3.67**	48.36 ± 15.83	0.42 ± 0.23
CO	438.09 ± 184.08	4.77 ± 2.94	3.10 ± 2.88	4.80 ± 4.81**	46.01 ± 15.47	0.41 ± 0.29
MO	329.16 ± 88.24	3.51 ± 3.57	1.79 ± 1.45*	4.66 ± 3.07**	57.51 ± 28.23	0.36 ± 0.25
AS	407.69 ± 141.08	3.76 ± 2.05	2.53 ± 2.09*	4.95 ± 3.59*	51.66 ± 24.96	0.52 ± 0.28
PC	371.18 ± 97.28	4.16 ± 2.09	1.07 ± 1.47##	4.29 ± 2.03**	42.24 ± 10.80	0.60 ± 0.25##
AR	303.35 ± 94.34	5.71 ± 1.77#	0.40 ± 0.49#	0.40 ± 0.49##	52.37 ± 11.13	0.38 ± 0.31

[a]*Epimedium sagittatum (Siebold & Zucc.) Maxim. (ES), Curculigo orchioides Gaertn. (CO), Angelica sinensis (Oliv.) Diels. (AS), Phellodendron chinense Schneid. (PC), Anemarrhena asphodeloides Bge. (AR), Morinda officinalis How (MO).*

#$P < 0.05$, ##$P < 0.01$ compared to ES; *$P < 0.05$, **$P < 0.01$ compared to AR.

nHAcc, OB, and DL of all 93 compounds were determined to identify similarities and differences in the physicochemical properties of the components in each herb (**Table 1**). Herbal sources of these EXD components were determined from TCMSP, TCM database @taiwan, HIT, TCMID, and previous reports, as shown in **Table S1**. The structures of these potentially active components are presented in **Table S2**. The nHacc and DL of the components derived from ES were significantly different to those derived from PC, and the nHacc of compounds derived from AR were different from those from all other herbs.

Network Pharmacology Analysis of EXD

A total of 259 targets corresponding to active components in EXD were collected. Cytoscape was used to establish the chemical component-targets-pathway regulatory network of EXD, which showed correlation of 42 compounds, 150 targets, and 32 pathways, as shown in **Figure 1**. The network among PI3K-Akt pathway, the targets, and ingredients were presented in **Figure 1C**. According to the degree ranking in the network, the top 10 nodes were AKT1 (degree 108), TP53 (degree 102), IL6 (degree 99), VEGFA (degree 95),

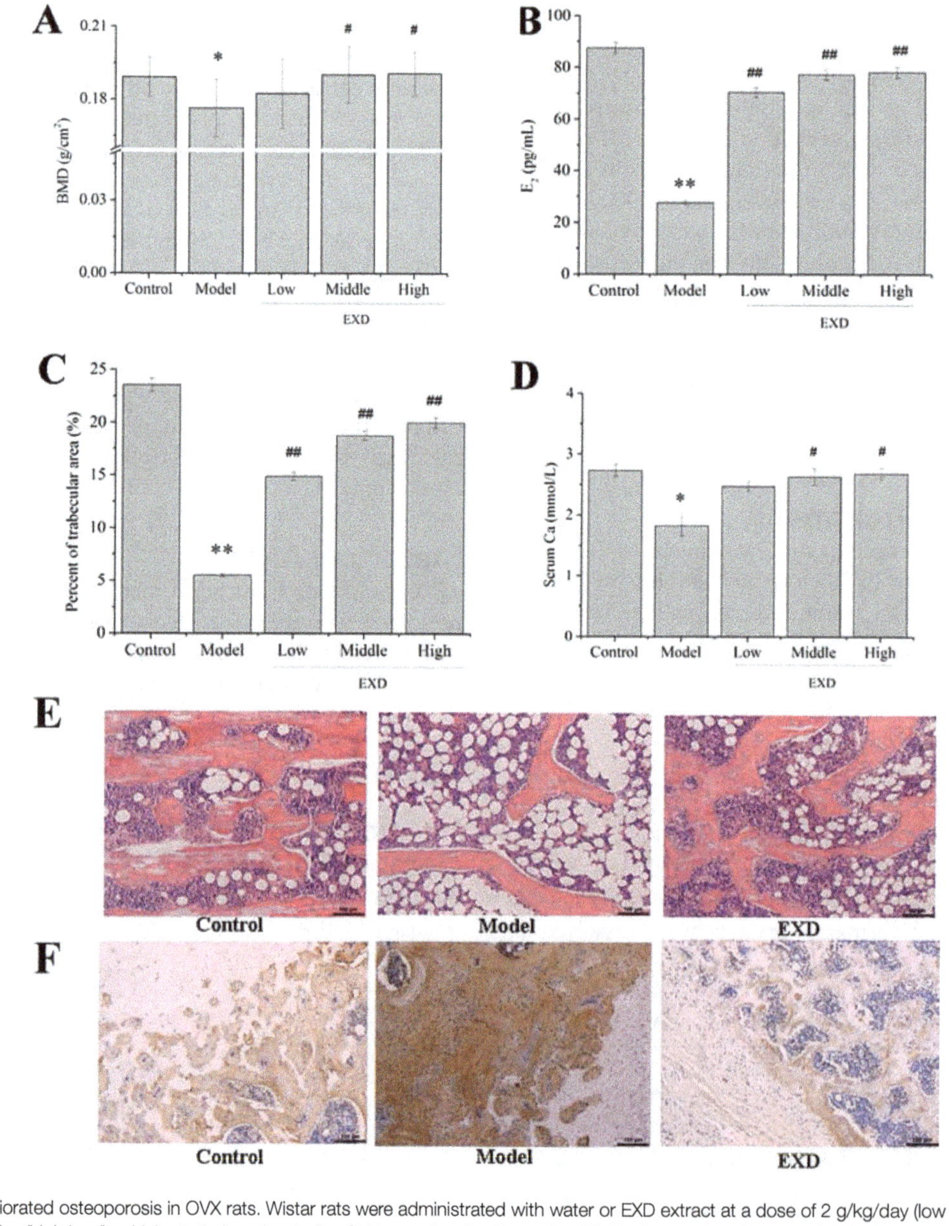

FIGURE 2 | EXD ameliorated osteoporosis in OVX rats. Wistar rats were administrated with water or EXD extract at a dose of 2 g/kg/day (low level), 4 g/kg/day (middle level), 6 g/kg/day (high level), which started on day 4 after OVX operation for 12 weeks. **(A)** The bone mineral density. **(B)** Serum estradiol level. **(C)** Percent of trabecular area. **(D)** Serum Ca level. **(E)** Representative images of femur stained with hematoxylin–eosin (magnification, ×200). Oral administration dose of EXD was 4 g/kg/day. **(F)** Representative images of femur stained with osteocalcin antibody (magnification, ×200). Oral administration dose of EXD was 4 g/kg/day. #P <0.05, ##P < 0.01 compared to the control group. *P < 0.05, **P < 0.01 compared to the model group.

CASP3 (degree 89), JUN (degree 88), PTGS2 (degree 86), MAPK8 (degree 85), MAPK1 (degree 83), and EGFR (degree 80). AKT1 appeared with the highest frequency and was correlated with 132 nodes, including 5 components, 19 KEGG pathways, and 108 targets. Among the 42 ingredients, luteolin from ES had the highest degree (degree 31). PI3K-Akt had the highest degree (40) in the signaling pathway. Six EXD components would have a close relationship with Akt signaling pathway. The network analysis suggested that the Akt pathway may play an important role in the anti-osteoporosis mechanism of EXD.

EXD Attenuated Osteoporosis in Ovariectomy Rats

Twenty dominant components in the EXD extract were quantified by HPLC-UV (**Figure S1**). These components ranged in concentration from 0.23 to 34.38 mg/L (**Table S3**), with icariin from ES, orcinol glucoside from CO, and epimedin B from ES being the most abundant compounds. As compared with the model group, BMD was significantly higher in the EXD group (**Figure 2A**). EXD treatment also increased the fraction of trabecular area of OVX rats, E_2 level, serum Ca, and bone formation (**Figures 2B–E**). As shown in **Figure 2F**, osteocalcin was negatively correlated with BMD, trabecular area, and E_2 level. It is possible that a high transformation type of osteoporosis was induced by OVX resulting in bone absorption being higher than bone formation (Zhou et al., 2017a; Zhou et al., 2017b). After EXD treatment, osteocalcin expression markedly reduced.

The level of TNF-α in the serum of the model group was 170% higher than in the control group (**Figure 3**). Compared with the model group, the EXD groups had an average 44% decrease in the TNF-α level.

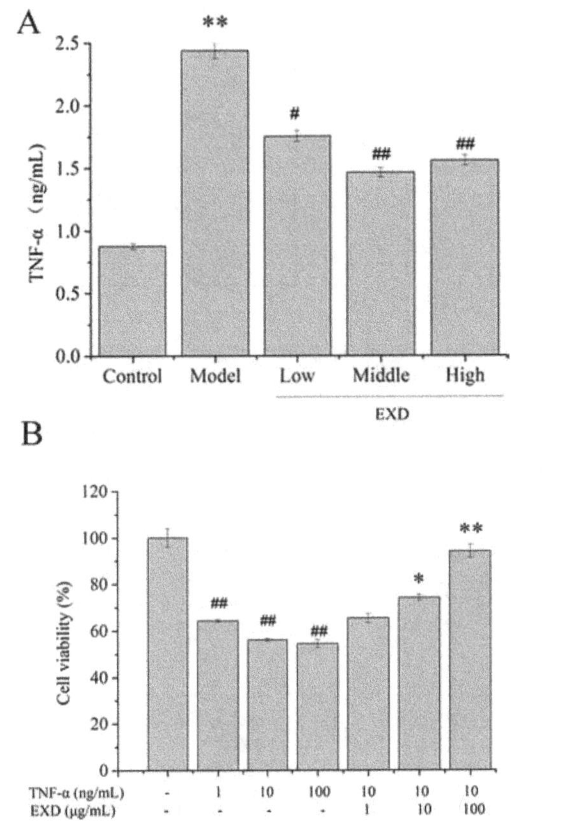

FIGURE 3 | (A) TNF-α level in ovariectomy rats. Wistar rats were administrated with water or EXD extract at a dose of 2 g/kg/day (low level), 4 g/kg/day (middle level), 6 g/kg/day (high level), which started on day 4 after OVX operation for 12 weeks. $^{\#}P$ <0.05, $^{\#\#}P$ < 0.01 compared to the control group. $^{*}P$ < 0.05, $^{**}P$ < 0.01 compared to the model group. **(B)** Effects of EXD on MC3T3-E1cell viability. Cells were induced by TNF-α. $^{\#}P$ <0.05, $^{\#\#}P$ < 0.01 compared to the control group. $^{*}P$ < 0.05, $^{**}P$ < 0.01 compared to the TNF-α group (10 ng/ml).

EXD Protects Osteoblasts Against TNF-α Induced Injury Through AKT/Nrf2/HO-1 Pathway

To investigate the potential effects of EXD on TNF-α-induced cytotoxicity in osteoblasts, MC3T3-E1 osteoblastic cells were treated with TNF-α or EXD in a range of concentrations (0.1–10 μM). Cell viability decreased after exposure to TNF-α and EXD treatment significantly protected MC3T3-E1 cell against TNF-α-induced injury in a dose-dependent manner (**Figure 3**).

EXD treatment reduced apoptosis after TNF-α exposure (**Figure 4**) and increased phosphorylation of AKT. It also significantly activated the expression of nuclear Nrf2 and HO-1, which were the essential downstream targets of Akt (**Figure 5**). PI3K inhibitor (LY294002) reduced both p-Akt and nuclear Nrf2 expression. A HO-1 inhibitor (ZnPP-IX) reduced the expression of HO-1 in the EXD-treated osteoblasts. Taken together, the above results indicated that EXD reduced TNF-α production and cell apoptosis, probably *via* activation of the Akt/Nrf2/HO-1 signaling pathway in TNF-α induced osteoblast.

DISCUSSION

EXD, a traditional Chinese medicinal formula, has been used widely for treating osteoporosis (Tong et al., 2012). However, the effect of EXD on osteoblast injury induced by TNF-α induced underlying mechanism has not been fully identified. In the current study, EXD treatment attenuated TNF-α production in OVX rat and protected osteoblasts against TNF-α-induced apoptosis. Our results suggest that EXD might attenuate osteoporosis at least partially by regulating the Akt/Nrf2/HO-1 signaling pathway (**Figure 6**).

In vivo investigation showed significantly decreased TNF-α serum levels after EXD treatment. Similarly, we showed that TNF-α reduced osteoblast activity and ALP activity *in vitro*, resulting in increased apoptosis and activation of caspase-3. The cleavage of caspase-3 is the final step of the process that initiates the apoptotic signaling (Wei and Frenette, 2018). However, EXD attenuated the increase of caspase-3 and TNF-α compared to the cell model. Thus, EXD treatment not only attenuated TNF-α production in the serum, but also protected osteoblasts against TNF-α-induced apoptosis.

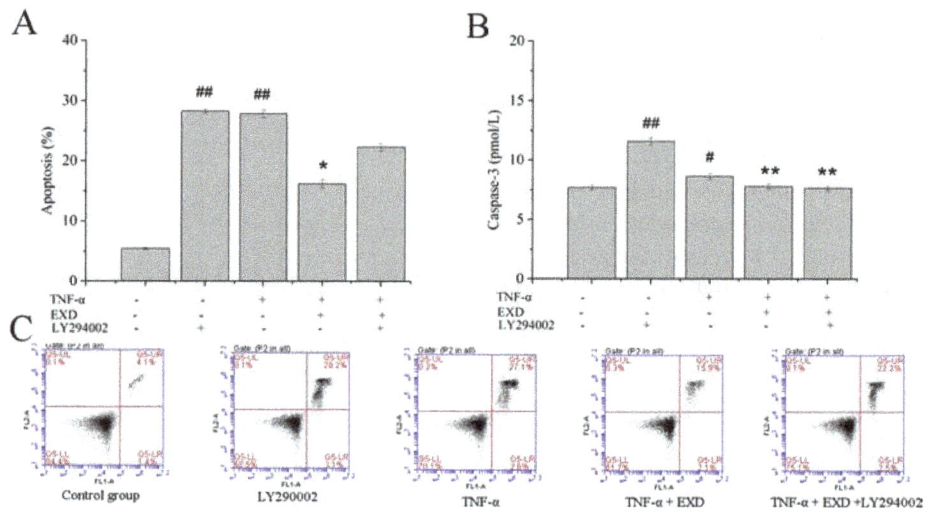

FIGURE 4 | Effect of EXD and selective inhibitor LY294002 on TNF-α-induced apoptosis in MC3T3-E1 cells. Cells were incubated with or without 20 μM LY294002, 100 μg/ml EXD, and 10 ng/ml TNF-α for 24 h. **(A)** Cell apoptosis rate. **(B)** Caspase-3 level. **(C)** Annexin V/PI staining results. $^{\#}P < 0.05$, $^{\#\#}P < 0.01$ compared to the control group. $^{*}P < 0.05$, $^{**}P < 0.01$ compared to the TNF-α group.

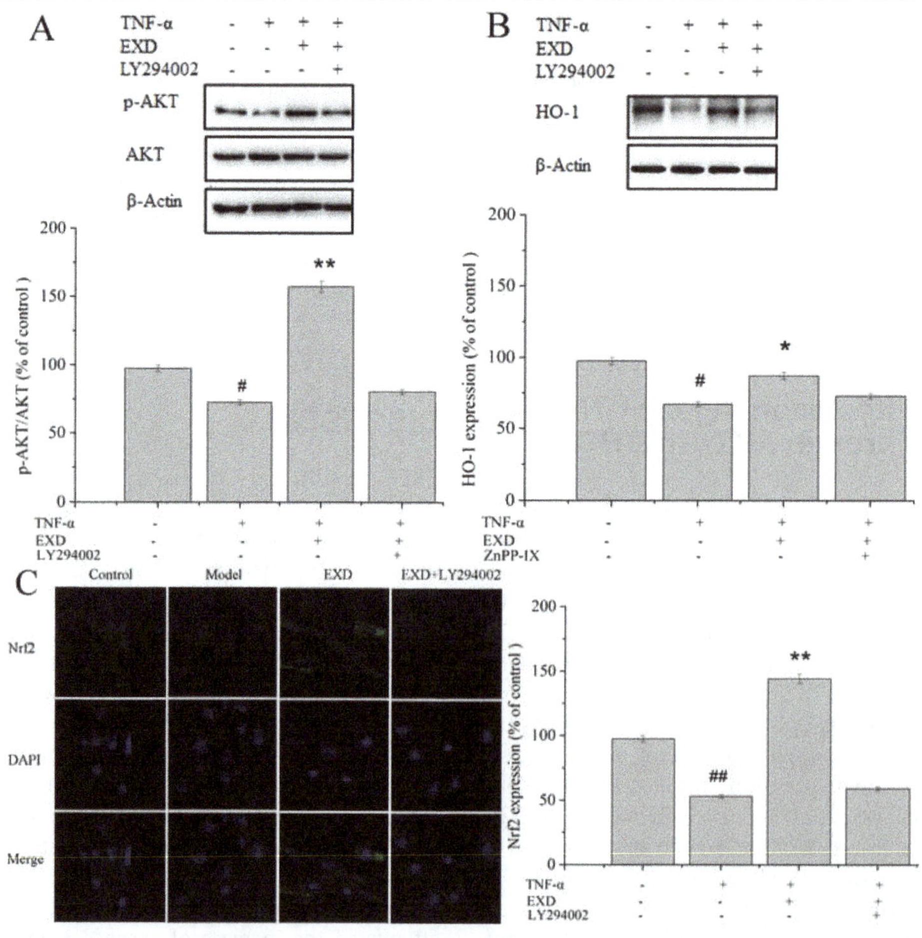

FIGURE 5 | Effect of EXD and selective inhibitor LY294002 on **(A)** AKT, **(B)** HO-1, and **(C)** Nrf2 expression (magnification, ×650). Cells were incubated with or without 20 μM LY294002, 5 μM ZnPP-IX, 100 μg/ml EXD, and 10 ng/ml TNF-α for 24 h. $^{\#}P < 0.05$, $^{\#\#}P < 0.01$ compared to the control group. $^{*}P < 0.05$, $^{**}P < 0.01$ compared to the TNF-α group.

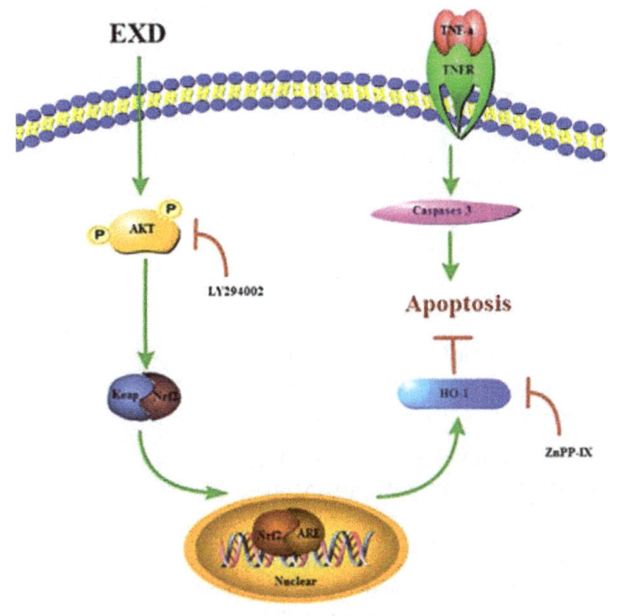

FIGURE 6 | A proposed signaling pathway involved in EXD against TNF-α-induced cell damage.

Molecular networks were constructed to demonstrate interactions between EXD ingredients, targets, and enriched pathways. Pathway and functional enrichment analyses indicate that EXD was primarily associated with the PI3K-Akt signaling pathway, which in turn was associated with 29 targets (**Figure 1**). Investigation of the correlation between PI3K-Akt activation and EXD-regulated osteoblast protection in the presence of TNF-α found results consistent with results from the network pharmacology study, i.e., EXD administration activated the PI3K-Akt pathway. A PI3K inhibitor (LY294002) reduced EXD-mediated protection of cell death and apoptosis (**Figure 4**), in accordance with the previous reports that activation of PI3K-Akt pathway attenuates osteoblast injury in osteoporosis (Vanella et al., 2010).

An increasing number of studies have indicated that TNF-α exposure significantly effects HO-1 expression, which is an essential anti-inflammatory molecule that regulates pro-inflammatory mediators (Chiu et al., 2016). Since the master upstream regulator of HO-1, Nrf2, is affected by the PI3K-Akt signaling pathway, we examined whether the Akt/Nrf2/HO-1 signaling pathway was involved in EXD mediated regulation of osteoblast apoptosis. EXD was found to increase the level of AKT phosphorylation and also promoted nuclear translocation of Nrf2, further increasing HO-1 expression. LY294002 inhibited nuclear translocation of Nrf2, and a HO-1 inhibitor (ZnPP-IX) reversed the EXD-mediated increase of HO-1 expression in TNF-α-induced osteoblasts. These observations suggest that EXD protected osteoblasts against TNF-α-induced apoptosis at least partially by activating the Akt/Nrf2/HO-1 signaling pathway.

Furthermore, the molecular network analysis predicted that six EXD components would have a close relationship with Akt signaling pathway, including kaempferol, luteolin, quercetin, beta-sitosterol, diosgenin, and rutaecarpine. The above six EXD compounds were derived from the traditional medicinal parts of six herbs in EXD. Three flavonoids (luteolin, kaempferol, and quercetin) could be isolated from the aerial parts of *E. sagittatum* (Siebold & Zucc.) Maxim. (Chen et al., 1996; Wang et al., 2010a; Wang et al., 2010b). Diosgenin was a spirostanol steroidal saponin, which could be obtained from the rhizomes of *A. asphodeloides* Bge. (Xia et al., 2017). These ingredients showed anti-osteoporosis effects *via* promotion of osteogenic differentiation and stimulation of mineralization in osteoblasts (Pang et al., 2006; Nash et al., 2015). Luteolin and kaempferol also had anti-apoptotic properties (Pang et al., 2006; Im et al., 2018). Beta-sitosterol existed in four herbs, including bark of *P. chinense* Schneid (Wang et al., 2009; Xue et al., 2015), roots of *M. officinalis* How. (Hong et al., 2009; Zhang et al., 2018), rhizomes of *A. asphodeloides* Bge. (Bian et al., 1996), and rhizomes of *C. orchioides* Gaertn. (Cao et al., 2009). Beta-sitosterol could promote the proliferation and mineralized nodule formation of osteoblasts (Chauhan et al., 2018). Rutaecarpine could be found in the fruit and bark of *P. chinense* Schneid. (Yan et al., 2017). Future investigations will evaluate the relationship between the above ingredients and the Akt/Nrf2/HO-1 signaling pathway.

CONCLUSIONS

In the current study, we showed that EXD protects osteoblasts against apoptosis following exposure to excess TNF-α and used network modeling to elucidate the underlying mechanism of this protection. EXD ameliorated osteoporosis and reduced TNF-α level in OVX rats in the dose range of 2–6 g/kg/day. Further studies will be carried out in order to explore the potential of EXD at a lower concentration range. Combining network pharmacology analysis with experimental verification *in vivo* and *in vitro*, we found that EXD may attenuate osteoporosis at least partially by reducing TNF-α production and regulating the Akt/Nrf2/HO-1 signaling pathway.

ETHICS STATEMENT

Twelve-month-old female Wistar rats (weighting 350-400 g) were supplied by the Animal Center of the Zhejiang Academy of Traditional Chinese Medicine (Hangzhou, China). The rats were maintained in air-conditional animal quarters at a temperature of 24 ± 2 °C and a relative humidity of 60 ± 5%. All protocols for animal experiments were approved in accordance with the regulations of experimental animal administration issued by the state commission of science and technology of the People's Republic of China.

AUTHOR CONTRIBUTIONS

NW designed and performed experimental procedures, including network pharmacology analysis and *in vitro* experiments. PX developed the osteoporosis rat models. HX helped with *in vivo* experiments and provided professional consultancy about pharmaceutical use. ZY assisted in preparing samples and provided medical materials. DS revised the manuscript critically for important intellectual content.

ACKNOWLEDGMENTS

The project was sponsored by the National Natural Science Foundation of China (No. 81603252, U1603283, 81873062), Zhejiang Provincial Natural Science Foundation of China (No. LQ17H280002), and the Open Fund Project of First-Class Discipline for Science of Chinese Pharmacy, Zhejiang Chinese Medical University (Ya2017008).

SUPPLEMENTARY MATERIAL

FIGURE S1 | (A) Typical chromatograms of the EXD extract and the standards. **(B)** The chemical structure of the peaks. Other information of the peaks was presented in **Table S3**.

REFERENCES

Bian, Q., Yang, H., Chan, C. O., Jin, D., Mok, D. K., and Chen, S. (2013). Fingerprint analysis and simultaneous determination of phenolic compounds in extracts of Curculiginis Rhizoma by HPLC-diode array detector. *Chem. Pharm. Bull.* 61 (8), 802–808. doi: 10.1248/cpb.c12-01058

Bian, J., Xu, S., Huang, S., and Wang, Z. (1996). A Study on the chemical constituents of Anemarrhena asphodeloides Bge. *Shenyang Yao Ke Da Xue Xue Bao* 13 (66), 34–40. doi: 10.1248/cpb.c12-01058

Cao, D., Han, T., Zheng, Y., Qin, L., and Zhang, Q. (2009). Phenolic glycosides and lignans components in Curculigo orchioides Gaertn. *Acad. J. Second Mil. Med. Univ.* 29 (2), 194–197. doi: 10.3724/SP.J.1008.2009.00194

Chen, C. C., Huang, Y. L., Sun, C. M., and Shen, C. C. (1996). New prenylflavones from the leaves of Epimedium sagittatum. *J. Nat. Prod.* 59 (4), 412–414. doi: 10.1021/np9601925

Chen, X., Ji, Z. L., and Chen, Y. Z. (2002). TTD: therapeutic target database. *Nucleic Acids Res.* 30 (1), 412–415. doi: 10.1093/nar/30.1.412

Chiu, P. R., Hu, Y. C., Hsieh, B. S., Huang, T. C., Cheng, H. L., Huang, L. W., et al. (2016). Osteoblasts activate the Nrf2 signaling pathway in response to arsenic trioxide treatment. *Int. J. Biochem. Cell Biol.* 79, 327–336. doi: 10.1016/j.biocel.2016.08.036

Chauhan, S., Sharma, A., Upadhyay, N. K., Singh, G., Lal, U. R., and Goyal, R. (2018). In-vitro osteoblast proliferation and in-vivo anti-osteoporotic activity of Bombax ceiba with quantification of lupeol, gallic acid and β-sitosterol by hptlc and hplc. *BMC Complement. Altern. Med.* 18 (1), 233–245. doi: 10.1186/s12906-018-2299-1

Gozalbes, R., Jacewicz, M., Annand, R., Tsaioun, K., and Pineda-Lucena, A. (2010). QSAR-based permeability model for drug-like compounds. *Bioorg. Med. Chem.* 18 (19), 7078–7084. doi: 10.1016/j.bmc.2010.08.003

Hong, Z., Hu, J., Yi, Y. T., and Yang, Z. M. (2009). Comparison on the volatile components in different years old Morinda officinalis. *J. Anhui Agric. Sci.* 37 (9), 4115–4117.

Huang, D. W., Sherman, B. T., Tan, Q., Kir, J., Liu, D., Bryant, D., et al. (2007). DAVID Bioinformatics Resources: expanded annotation database and novel algorithms to better extract biology from large gene lists. *Nucleic Acids Res.* 35, 169–175. doi: 10.1093/nar/gkm415

Im, E., Yeo, C., and Lee, E. O. (2018). Luteolin induces caspase-dependent apoptosis via inhibiting the AKT/osteopontin pathway in human hepatocellular carcinoma SK-Hep-1 cells. *Life Sci.* 209, 259–266. doi: 10.1016/j.lfs.2018.08.025

Kloefkorn, H. E., and Allen, K. D. (2016). Quantitative histological grading methods to assess subchondral bone and synovium changes subsequent to medial meniscus transection in the rat. *Connect. Tissue Res.* 58 (3-4), 373–385. doi: 10.1080/03008207.2016.1251425

Kuhn, M., von Mering, C., Campillos, M., Jensen, L. J., and Bork, P., (2008). STITCH: interaction networks of chemicals and proteins. *Nuclei Acids Research* 26, 684–688.

Law, V., Knox, C., Djoumbou, Y., Jewison, T., Guo, A. C., Liu, Y., et al. (2014). DrugBank 4.0: shedding new light on drug metabolism. *Nucleic Acids Res.* 42, 1091–1097. doi: 10.1093/nar/gkt1068

Liu, C., Ma, R., Wang, L., Zhu, R., Liu, H., Guo, Y., et al. (2017). Rehmanniae Radix in osteoporosis: a review of traditional Chinese medicinal uses, phytochemistry, pharmacokinetics and pharmacology. *J. Ethnopharmacol.* 198, 351–362. doi: 10.1016/j.jep.2017.01.021

Liu, T. G., Wan, Y. X., Zheng, Z. A., Bai, C., Yu, H., Deng, Q., et al. (2016). Study on mechanism of yinlai decoction's anti-inflammatory effects with the method of network pharmacology. *Acta Med. Mediterr.* 32 (4), 877–882. doi: 10.19193/0393-6384_2016_4_104

Nash, L. A., Sullivan, P. J., Peters, S. J., and Ward, W. E. (2015). Rooibos flavonoids, orientin and luteolin, stimulate mineralization in human osteoblasts through the Wnt pathway. *Mol. Nutr. Food Res.* 59 (3), 443–453. doi: 10.1002/mnfr.201400592

Pang, J. L., Ricupero, D. A., Huang, S., Fatma, N., Singh, D. P., Romero, J. R., et al. (2006). Differential activity of kaempferol and quercetin in attenuating tumor necrosis factor receptor family signaling in bone cells. *Biochem. Pharmacol.* 71, 818–826. doi: 10.1016/j.bcp.2005.12.023

Ru, J., Li, P., Wang, J., Zhou, W., Li, B., Huang, C., et al. (2014). TCMSP: a database of systems pharmacology for drug discovery from herbal medicines. *J. Cheminform.* 6 (1), 13. doi: 10.1186/1758-2946-6-13

Sanderson, K. (2011). Databases aim to bridge the East-West divide of drug discovery. *Nat. Med.* 17 (12), 1531. doi: 10.1038/nm1211-1531a

Simpson, D. S., Lovell, K. M., Lozama, A., Han, N., Day, V. W., Dersch, C. M., et al. (2009). Synthetic studies of neoclerodane diterpenes from Salvia divinorum: role of the furan in affinity for opioid receptors. *Org. Biomol. Chem.* 7 (18), 3748–3756. doi: 10.1039/b905148a

Tong, Y., Sze, S. W., Cheung, H. P., Lu, J., Zhang, K. Y., and Ip, C. W. (2012). Anti-osteoporotic effects of multiple herbal components in erxian decoction. A Chinese medicinal formula. *Planta Med.* 78 (11), 1117–1117. doi: 10.1055/s-0032-1320562

Vanella, L., Kim, D. H., Asprinio, D., Peterson, S. J., Barbagallo, I., Vanella, A., et al. (2010). HO-1 expression increases mesenchymal stem cell-derived osteoblasts but decreases adipocyte lineage. *Bone* 46 (1), 236–243. doi: 10.1016/j.bone.2009.10.012

Wang, M., Ji, T., Yang, J. B., and Su, Y. L. (2009). Studies on the chemical constituents of *Phellodendron chinense*. *Zhong Yao Cai* 32 (2), 208–210. doi: 10.13863/j.issn1001-4454.2009.02.026

Wang, N., Zhang, Q., Xin, H., Shou, D., and Qin, L. (2017a). Osteoblast cell membrane chromatography coupled with liquid chromatography time-of-flight mass spectrometry for screening specific active components from traditional Chinese medicines. *J. Sep. Sci.* 40, 4311–4319. doi: 10.1002/jssc.201700688

Wang, N., Zhao, G., Zhang, Y., Wang, X., Zhao, L., Xu, P., et al. (2017b). A network pharmacology approach to determine the active components and potential targets of Curculigo orchioides in the treatment of osteoporosis. *Med. Sci. Monit.* 23, 5113–5122. doi: 10.12659/MSM.904264

Wang, S., Tong, Y., Ng, T. B., Lao, L., Lam, J. K. W., and Zhang, K. Y. (2015). Network pharmacological identification of active compounds and potential actions of erxian decoction in alleviating menopause-related symptoms. *Chin. Med.* 10 (1), 19–31. doi: 10.1186/s13020-015-0051-z

Wang, S. W., Cheung, H. P., Tong, Y., Lu, J., Ng, T. B., Zhang, Y. B., et al. (2016). Steroidogenic effect of erxian decoction for relieving menopause via the p-Akt/PKB pathway *in vitro* and *in vivo*. *J. Ethnopharmacol.* 100, 196–197. doi: 10.1016/j.maturitas.2017.03.255

Wang, Y. K., Hong, Y. J., Wei, M., Wu, Y., Huang, Z. Q., Chen, R. Z., et al. (2010a). Curculigoside attenuates human umbilical vein endothelial cell injury induced by H2O2. *J. Ethnopharmacol.* 132 (1), 233–239. doi: 10.1016/j.jep.2010.08.008

Wang, Y., Wang, Y., Guo, Z., Jin, Y., Zhang, X., Wang, L., et al. (2010b). Identification of prenyl flavonoid glycosides and phenolic acids in Epimedium koreanum Nakai by Q-TOF-MS combined with selective enrichment on "click oligo (ethylene glycol)" column. *J. Pharm. Biomed. Anal.* 51 (3), 606–616. doi: 10.1016/j.jpba.2009.09.033

Wei, Q., and Frenette, P. S. (2018). Niches for hematopoietic stem cells and their progeny. *Immunity* 48 (4), 632–648. doi: 10.1016/j.immuni.2018.03.024

Xia, Y., Gong, F., Guo, X., Liang, J., and Kuang, H. (2017). Fragmentation patterns of five spirostanol steroidal saponins. *Acta Chin. Med. Pharmacol.* 45 (5), 10–13. doi: 10.19664/j.cnki.1002-2392.2017.05.003

Xue, J., Zhang, H., Sun, Y., Mi, Y. Y., Kuang, H., and Wang, Q. (2015). Composition and difference of fatty acid components in phellodendro Chinese and Phellodendron amurense. *Guizhou Agric. Sci.* 43 (8), 220–222.

Xue, R., Fang, Z., Zhang, M., Yi, Z., Wen, C., and Shi, T. (2013). Tcmid: traditional Chinese medicine integrative database for herb molecular mechanism analysis. *Nucleic Acids Res.* 41, 1089–1095. doi: 10.1093/nar/gks1100

Yan, C., Zhang, Y., Wang, X., and Luo, H. (2017). Chemical constituents and anti-tumor activity from the fruits of *Phellodendron chinense* Schneid. *Nat. Prod. Res. Dev.* 29, 1270–1276. doi: 10.16333/j.1001-6880.2017.8.002

Yu, B., and Wang, C. Y. (2016). Osteoporosis: the result of an 'aged' bone microenvironment. *Trends Mol. Med.* 22 (8), 641–644. doi: 10.1016/j.molmed.2016.06.002

Yu, X., Tong, Y., Huang, W., Sze, S. C., Zhong, L., Lau, C. B., et al. (2013). Erxian decoction, a traditional Chinese herbal formula, inhibits angiogenesis in human umbilical vein endothelial cells. *Biol. Pharm. Bull.* 36 (5), 754–763. doi: 10.1248/bpb.b12-00860

Zhang, J. H., Xin, H. L., Xu, Y. M., Shen, Y., He, Y. Q., Yeh, H., et al. (2018). Morinda officinalis How.—a comprehensive review of traditional uses, phytochemistry and pharmacology. *J. Ethnopharmacol.* 213, 230–255. doi: 10.1016/j.jep.2017.10.028

Zhao, R. L., and He, Y. M. (2018). Network pharmacology analysis of the anti-cancer pharmacological mechanisms of Ganoderma lucidum extract with experimental support using Hepa1-6-bearing C57 BL/6 mice. *J. Ethnopharmacol.* 210, 287–295. doi: 10.1016/j.jep.2017.08.041

Zhou, J., Liao, Y., Xie, H., Liao, Y., Zeng, Y., Li, N., et al. (2017a). Effects of combined treatment with ibandronate and pulsed electromagnetic field on ovariectomy-induced osteoporosis in rats. *Bioelectromagnetics* 38 (1), 31–40. doi: 10.1002/bem.22012

Zhou, X., Li, Z., and Zhou, J. (2017b). Tumor necrosis factor α in the onset and progression of leukemia. *Exp. Hematol.* 45, 17–26. doi: 10.1016/j.exphem.2016.10.005

10

Exploring the Critical Components and Therapeutic Mechanisms of Perilla frutescens L. in the Treatment of Chronic Kidney Disease via Network Pharmacology

Chen Yong[1], Zhengchun Zhang[2], Guoshun Huang[1], Yang Yang[1], Yiye Zhu[1], Leilei Qian[3], Fang Tian[4], Li Liu[4], Qijing Wu[1], Zhongchi Xu[1], Chong Chen[1], Jing Zhao[1], Kun Gao[1] and Enchao Zhou[1]**

[1]Division of Nephrology, Affiliated Hospital of Nanjing University of Chinese Medicine, Jiangsu Province Hospital of Chinese Medicine, Nanjing, China, [2]Division of Nephrology, JiangYan Hospital affiliated to Nanjing University of Chinese Medicine, Taizhou, China, [3]Division of Nephrology, The People's Hospital of Rugao, Rugao, China, [4]Research Center of Chinese Medicine, Jiangsu Province Hospital of Chinese Medicine, Nanjing, China

***Correspondence:**
Kun Gao
dr.gaokun@outlook.com
Enchao Zhou
zhouenchao@njucm.edu.cn

Chronic kidney disease (CKD) is a chronic progressive disease that seriously threatens human health. Some patients will continue to progress into the CKD stage 3–5 (also called chronic renal failure), which is mainly manifested by a decline in renal function and multi-system damage. *Perilla frutescens (L.) Britton. (Lamiaceae)* is one of the most widely used traditional Chinese medicine (TCM) herbs in CKD, especially in CKD stage 3–5. But its active components and mechanisms are still unclear. In this study, we used network pharmacology to analyze the active components of *P. frutescens* and the main therapeutic targets for intervention in CKD stage 3–5. Then, the key components were selected for enrichment analysis and identified by high performance liquid chromatograph (HPLC). Finally, we verified the critical components through molecular docking, and *in vitro* experiments. The results show that 19 main active components of *P. frutescens* were screened, and 108 targets were intersected with CKD stage 3–5. The PPI network was constructed and found that the core nodes AKT1, TP53, IL6, TNF, and MAPK1 may be key therapeutic targets. Enrichment analysis shows that related targets may be involved in regulating various biological functions, and play a therapeutic role in CKD stage 3–5 by regulating apoptosis, T cell receptor, and PI3K-AKT signaling pathways. Molecular docking indicates that the key active components were well docked with its corresponding targets. Five active components were identified and quantified by

Abbreviations: ADR, adriamycin; BP, biological process; CASP3, caspase 3; CC, cellular component; CCND1, cyclin D1; CKD, chronic kidney disease; CRF, chronic renal failure; DL, drug-like; EGFR, epidermal growth factor receptor; EPO, erythropoietin; ERK 1/2, extracellular signal-regulated kinase 1/2; HIF-1α, hypoxia inducible factor-1α; HPLC, high performance liquid chromatograph; IL6, interleukin 6; JNK, c-Jun N-terminal kinase; MAPK, mitogen-activated protein kinase; MF, molecular function; MMP9, matrix metalloproteinase 9; NAC, N-acetyl-L-cysteine; NCOA2, nuclear receptor coactivator 2; NF-κB, nuclear factor-κ-gene binding; NRK-52E, normal rat tubular proximal epithelial cell; OB, oral bioavailability; PARP1, poly (ADP-ribose) polymerase 1; PFAE, P. frutescens aqueous extracts; PI3K, phosphoinositide 3-kinase; PPI, protein-protein interaction; PTGS 2, prostaglandin-endoperoxide synthase 2; ROS, reactive oxygen species; TCM, traditional Chinese medicine; TCR, T cell receptor; TEC, tubular epithelial cell; TLR, Toll-like receptor; TNF, tumor necrosis factor; TP53, tumor protein 53; VEGF, vascular endothelial growth factor.

HPLC. According to the results, luteolin was selected as the critical component for further verification. *In vitro* experiments have shown that luteolin can effectively alleviate adriamycin (ADR)-induced renal tubular apoptosis and suppress AKT and p53 phosphorylation. The effects of luteolin to reduce apoptosis may be mediated by inhibiting oxidative stress and downregulating the mitogen-activated protein kinase (MAPK) and p53 pathways. In general, we screened and analyzed the possible active components, therapeutic targets and pathways of *P. frutescens* for treating CKD. Our findings revealed that luteolin can reduce renal tubular epithelial cell apoptosis and may be the critical component of *P. frutescens* in the treatment of CKD. It provides references and direction for further research.

Keywords: Perilla frutescens L., chronic kidney disease, network pharmacology, luteolin, critical component, therapeutic mechanism

INTRODUCTION

Chronic kidney disease (CKD) stage 3–5 is traditionally referred to as chronic renal failure (CRF). CKD is a chronically progressive clinical syndrome that mainly manifests as kidney damage and can involve multiple organs throughout the body. It is the common end stage of various kidney diseases. Various factors lead to decompensation of renal function, resulting in the retention of water, electrolyte and metabolites, acid-base balance disorder, and other systemic injuries. CKD is characterized by a long course, complicated conditions, difficult treatment, and poor prognosis. It seriously affects the quality of life and health, and brings a heavy economic and health burden to the family and society (Qiu et al., 2017). There is an urgent need to find new and effective therapeutic strategies to slow the progression of CKD.

Traditional Chinese medicine (TCM) provides an alternative treatment for CKD. Several studies have demonstrated the safety and efficacy of TCM in CKD (Song et al., 2019; Xi et al., 2020). The use of TCM in nephrology has attracted interest. Herbs are an important part of TCM intervention. Some herbs can effectively delay the progression of CKD and reduce the incidence of complications through synergistic effects with a variety of pharmacodynamic substances. A series of studies have addressed the value of TCM herbs in CKD therapy. The delayed progression of CKD that has been described mainly involves reduced oxidative stress, inhibition of the inflammatory response, reduced renal cell apoptosis, and alleviation of renal fibrosis (Lu et al., 2018; Wang et al., 2018; Fu and Hu, 2019; Zhao et al., 2019). In addition, there is a mutual crosstalk among these pharmacological effects, which reflects the multi-target effects of TCM herbs.

The leaf of *Perilla frutescens (L.) Britton. (Lamiaceae)* is used to treat patients with CKD (especially stage 3–5) in the clinic (Guangtang and Huiman, 2017). The treatment can significantly delay the progression of CKD. In TCM theory, it can disperse the poison in the blood and harmonize the digestive system. Our team previously confirmed that a TCM formulation composed mainly of *P. frutescens* can significantly improve renal function and increase the estimated glomerular filtration rate (Yang and Enchao, 2015). *In vitro* and *in vivo* experiments have confirmed that it can alleviate the oxidative damage of renal tubular epithelial cells, reduce renal mesangial cell dysfunction, and delay renal fibrosis (Yiye et al., 2019; Kim and Kim, 2019). However, the active components of *P. frutescens* and details of its effects for treating CKD are still unclear.

Network pharmacology refers to the use of computer simulations and high-throughput analytical methods to reveal complex pharmacological behaviors (Xinqiang et al., 2020). In TCM research, the process mainly includes identifying related genes of the disease treated by TCM herbs and constructing a network model to evaluate the influence of TCM herbs on disease networks. Especially concerning TCM intervention in chronic and complex diseases, such as CKD, it is helpful to clarify the mechanism and confirm the specific targets and herbs. Molecular docking is a technology that screens active components through computer simulations of ligand binding to a target (Xinqiang et al., 2020). This technology is widely used in drug design and screening, as well as in structure-based virtual screening and ligand research. Combining the technology with network pharmacology can verify the analysis results in terms of the molecular structure.

In this study, we applied network pharmacology to systematically explore the main active components, targets and pharmacological mechanisms of *P. frutescens* for treating CKD. The binding ability of the key active components to the corresponding targets was analyzed by molecular docking. The screened components were quantified by HPLC and verified by *in vitro* experiments. So as to further identify the critical components of *P. frutescens* and evaluate its effects on kidney injury.

MATERIALS AND METHODS

Collection and Screening of Main Active Components of *P. frutescens*

A search for all chemical components of *P. frutescens* was conducted in the traditional Chinese medicine systems pharmacology (TCMSP) database (http://lsp.nwu.edu.cn/index.php) using "zisu" as the key word. Filter criteria included database ADME (absorption, distribution, metabolism, excretion) parameters, select oral bioavailability (OB) ≥30%, and drug-likeness (DL) ≥0.18. In addition, the search focused on components that were effective in the relevant literature but did not meet the above screening criteria to supplement. Finally, the main active components of *P. frutescens* were identified.

Target Prediction of the Main Active Components

The predicted targets of the main active components were retrieved from the TCMSP database. They were entered into the Uniport database (http://www.uniprot.org/) with the species restricted to "Human." The official gene name of all target proteins was checked one-by-one. The genes constituted the predicted targets of the main active components.

Collection of Targets Related to CKD

A search for target genes related to CKD stages 3–5 was performed in the Gene cards database (https://www.genecards.org/) with the keyword "chronic renal failure" (because CKD stages 3–5 are traditionally termed CRF). Due to the excessive number of CRF-related targets, a score ≥10 was used as the threshold to screen the main targets related to CKD stage 3–5 for further research.

Acquiring Targets of Main Active Components for CKD Treatment

Venny 2.1.0 (http://bioinfogp.cnb.csic.es/tools/venny/index.html) software was used to obtain the intersection of the predicted targets of *P. frutescens* and the main targets of CKD stage 3–5. A Venn diagram was drawn. The intersection genes were possible relevant targets for the treatment of CKD with *P. frutescens*.

Construction and Analysis of the Network Model of Main Active Components-CKD Treatment Related Targets

The main active components and the corresponding CKD stage 3–5 related targets were imported into Cytoscape3.6.0 software. The main active components-targets network model was drawn. Then, the Network Analyzer plugin was used to analyze the network topology and to calculate the degree, betweenness centrality, and closeness centrality parameter values. The larger the value, the more important the node is in the network, enabling the clarification of the core components and targets of *P. frutescens* in the treatment of CKD.

Construction and Modular Analysis of Protein-Protein Interaction (PPI) Network Model

The core targets in the network model were imported into the String11.0 database (https://string-db.org/) with species limited to "homo sapiens." The highest confidence protein score value was >0.7. Unconnected single proteins were removed to obtain the PPI diagram of these core targets. The relevant action information of these targets was imported into Cytoscape 3.6.0 software to construct a network model and perform topological analysis, and adjust the node size, color, and edge thickness according to the value of the degree and combined score. The degree value was used as a reference to filter out the key nodes in the PPI network and draw a bar graph. At the same time, the MCODE plugin for protein modular analysis was used to set Degree Cutoff = 2, Node Score Cutoff = 0.2, K-Core = 5, Max.Depth = 100, and to screen out key protein modules in the PPI network.

Enrichment Analysis of Gene Ontology (GO) and Signaling Pathway

The relevant targets were imported into Cytoscape3.6.0 software. The ClueGO and CluePedia plugins were used to annotate the GO biological functions of these targets, including the enrichment of cellular components (CCs) and molecular functions (MFs). The analysis was set with a p-value ≤0.01 as the criterion to screen out the main biological functions of the core targets. The network model was established and a pie chart drawn.

Target information was imported into the DAVID6.8 online analysis platform (https://david.ncifcrf.gov/) for enrichment analysis of biological processes (BPs) and signaling pathways. The criterion and background were both "homo sapiens." The GO-BP and Kyoto Encyclopedia of Genes and Genomes (KEGG) databases were used to enrichment analyze the BPs and pathways related to the targets. The smaller the p-value, the higher the degree of enrichment. Therefore, the main BPs and pathways of *P. frutescens* for CKD stage 3–5 treatment were selected using the criterion of p <0.01. The enrichment results were visualized by software R language 4.0.3 and clusterProfiler package.

Molecular Docking Verification

The three-dimensional structure of the main active components of *P. frutescens* was downloaded from the PubChem database (https://pubchem.ncbi.nlm.nih.gov/) and OpenBabel software was used to convert it to the mol2 format. The complex crystal structure containing the original ligand of the key targets in the PPI network from the RSCB PDB database (http://www.rcsb.org/) was imported into the Pymol software to separate the receptor protein and the ligand molecule, followed by pretreatments such as dehydration. After importing the active components and corresponding potential therapeutic targets into Pyrx0.8 software for pretreatment and energy optimization, Autodock vina was used for molecular docking. The crystal box was selected to maximize the coverage of the entire receptor and active site. The binding affinities of receptors and ligands were analyzed and the docking results were compared with those of the original ligand.

Preparation of *P. frutescens* Aqueous Extracts

P. frutescens leaves (lot no. 200501, place of origin: Liu'an, China) was purchased from Anhui Dabie Mountain Traditional Chinese

Medicine Decoction Pieces Co. Ltd (Liu'an, China), and all herbs meet the standards of the Chinese Pharmacopoeia 2015. We weighed out 1200 × g of decoction pieces of *P. frutescens* leaves and extracted them twice with water. Firstly, the herb was immersed in 12,000 ml water and heated for 1 h at 100°C. 9000 ml of filtrate was obtained. After filtration, boiled herb was added 8000 ml water and heated for 1 h again. Then, we got 6800 ml of filtrate. The two filtrates were mixed and concentrated to obtain *P. frutescens* Aqueous Extracts (PFAE). Finally, PFAE solvent was prepared into freeze-dried powder by vacuum freeze-drying method. The PFAE freeze-dried powder was dissolved in water for use in the experiments. The quality and component validation were examined with fingerprint analysis *via* high performance liquid chromatograph (HPLC).

HPLC Analysis

A Waters e2695 HPLC (on-line degasser, quaternary pump, automatic sampler, and UV detector), with a Kh-500de ultrasonic cleaner (Kunshan Hechuang Ultrasonic Instrument), Sartorius CPA225D electronic balance (Nanjing Yimanelli Instrument and Equipment), and a C18 (250 mm, 4.6 mm, 5 m) chromatographic column were used in this analysis. Luteolin (lot no. B20888, HPLC≥98%), rosmarinic acid (lot no. B20862, HPLC≥98%), caffeic acid (lot no. B50428, HPLC≥98%), perilla aldehyde (lot no. B21699, HPLC≥98%) and (+)-catechin (lot no. B21722, HPLC≥98%) were purchased from Shanghai Yuanye Biotechnology (Shanghai, China).

200 mg of PFAE freeze-dried powder was weighed and resolved in 1 ml 80% methanol, then eddy mixed for 10 min. After centrifugation at 13,000 rpm for 10 min, the supernatant was taken for HPLC analysis. Five reference sample substances were accurately weighed and dissolved in methanol to prepare a standard solution. The concentration of each component was 0.5 mg/ml.

The chromatographic method was as follows: A Dubhe C18 chromatographic column (4.6 mm × 250 mm, 5 μm) was employed. The mobile phase was acetonitrile (A) - 0.1% acetic acid (B). Linear gradient elution: 0–17 min, 15%A, 17–20 min, 15%A, 20–25 min, 20%A, 25–30 min, 20%A, 30–38 min, 28%A, 38–40 min, 28%A, 20%A, 40–45 min, 35% A, 45–50 min, 35%A ~ 40%A, 50–60 min, 40%A ~ 15%A. The volumetric flow rate was 1 ml/min, the column temperature was 25 C, the detection wavelength was 330 nm, and the operation time was 60 min. After each run, the chromatographic column was balanced with the initial mobile phase for 20 min to ensure the stability of peak extraction.

10 μl of the reference solution and test solution were accurately absorbed and injected into the liquid chromatograph. The chromatographic peaks, retention time and peak area were recorded within 60 min.

Experimental Verification

We have screened and identified some components in *P. frutescens* through network pharmacology and HPLC. Therefore, we conducted *in vitro* experiments to further verify whether these components can effectively reduce kidney damage. Luteolin is a key component in network pharmacological model, and molecular docking model shows that it binds well to corresponding therapeutic targets. In addition, it has also been identified and quantified in the PFAE by HPLC. Therefore, luteolin was selected as the representative active component for subsequent *in vitro* experiments. According to the network pharmacological analysis, luteolin inhibits CKD progression mainly by regulating apoptosis. Previous studies have successfully established a tubular epithelial cell (TEC) injury model using adriamycin (ADR), which promotes TEC apoptosis. The model confirmed that the mechanism is closely related to oxidative stress and the mitogen-activated protein kinase (MAPK) pathway, which is an important form of renal pathology in CKD stage 3–5. Therefore, *in vitro*, ADR was used to disrupt renal TECs to construct a kidney injury model. Subsequent treatment with luteolin was performed to assess whether it can reduce apoptosis and regulate the expression of AKT, p53, and IL6. Oxidative stress, MAPK pathway and PI3K-AKT pathway are the most common and important ways related to apoptosis. Therefore, we further detected them to explore the mechanism by which luteolin reduces apoptosis.

Reagents

Luteolin (lot no. HY-N0162, 98.15%) was purchased from MedChemExpress (Shanghai, China). ADR hydrochloride (lot no. S120812, 99.13%) was purchased from Selleck Chemicals (Shanghai, China). Fetal bovine serum (FBS) was purchased from Thermo Fisher Scientific (Waltham, MA, United States), as were phosphate buffered saline (PBS), 0.25% trypsin-EDTA, antibiotic-antimycotic (Anti-Anti, 100×), and Dulbecco's modified Eagle medium/F-12 (DMEM/F-12). Cell Counting Kit-8 (CCK-8) was obtained from APExBIO (Houston, TX, United States). Dimethyl sulfoxide (DMSO) was purchased from Sigma-Aldrich (St. Louis, MO, United States). Antibodies to phosphorylated (p)-p38 MAPK (Thr180/Tyr182) (lot no. 4511), p-extracellular signal-regulated kinase (ERK)1/2 (Thr202/Tyr204) (lot no. 4370), p-stress-activated protein kinase/c-Jun N-terminal kinase (SAPK/JNK) (Thr183/Tyr185) (lot no. 4668), p-AKT (Ser473) (lot no. 4060), p53 (lot no. 2524), p-p53 (Ser15) (lot no. 9284), Caspase3 (lot no. 9662), and Cleaved Caspase-3 (lot no. 9664) were procured from Cell Signaling Technology (Shanghai, China). Antibodies to AKT (lot no. 10176-2-AP), p38 MAPK (lot no. 14064-1-AP), JNK (lot no. 24164-1-AP), Bcl-2 (lot no. 26593-1-AP), Bax (lot no. 50599-2-Ig), and β-actin (lot no. 66009-1-Ig), horseradish peroxidase (HRP)-conjugated Affinipure goat anti-mouse IgG (H+L) (lot no. SA00001-1), and HRP-conjugated Affinipure goat anti-rabbit IgG (H+L) (lot no. SA00001-2) were purchased from Proteintech (Wuhan, China). Antibodies to p-AKT (Thr308) (lot no. AF0016), p-phosphoinositide 3-kinase (PI3K) p85 (Tyr458) [Tyr467]/p55 (Tyr199) (lot no. AF0016), Interleukin 6 (IL6) (lot no. DF6087), ERK1/2 (lot no. AF0155) and poly (ADP-ribose) polymerase 1 (PARP1) (lot no. DF7198) were from Affinity Biosciences (Cincinnati, OH, United States). N-acetyl-L-cysteine (NAC) (lot no. S0077, >99%), reactive oxygen species (ROS) assay kit, BCA protein assay kit, One Step TdT-Mediated dUTP Nick End Labeling (TUNEL) Apoptosis Assay Kit, and 4,6-diamidino-2-phenylindole (DAPI) staining solution were purchased from Beyotime Biotechnology (Shanghai, China). The Annexin V fluorescein isothiocyanate/propidium iodide (FITC/PI) apoptosis kit was purchased from Multi Sciences (Hangzhou, China).

Cell Line and Culture

Normal rat tubular proximal epithelial cell lines (NRK-52E) were obtained from the University of Yamanashi (Yamanashi, Japan). The cells were maintained in DMEM/F-12 supplemented with 5% FBS, 100 U/ml penicillin G, and 100 mg/ml streptomycin, and incubated at 37°C in 5% CO_2. The cells at approximately 80–90% confluency were digested and passaged.

Cell Morphology and Viability

NRK-52E cells were digested and seeded in 96-well plates at 1×10^4 cells per well. After 24 h of incubation, the cells were cultured in a serum-free medium and stimulated with ADR (2 μg/ml) in the absence and presence of PFAE (5 mg/ml) or luteolin (10 μM/L). After 24 h of treatment, changes in cell morphology and number were observed by inverted phase-contrast microscopy using model CKX41 microscope (Olympus, Tokyo, Japan). Then, the medium was discarded, and 100 μl serum-free medium containing 10% CCK-8 was added to each well. After incubating for another 1 h, the absorbance was measured using a model ELx800 spectrometer (BioTek Instruments, Winooski, VT, United States) at a wavelength of 450 nm. Cell viability is expressed as a percentage of the control.

Detection of Production of ROS

ROS production was detected using an ROS detection kit. Briefly, cells were seeded in a 12-well plate and incubated for 24 h. ADR, luteolin, and NAC were used to stimulate the cells according to the experimental protocol. The fluorescent probe 2′,7′-dichlorofluorescin diacetate (DCFH-DA) was diluted with serum-free medium at a ratio of 1:1000 to obtain a final concentration of 10 μmol/L. The medium was removed and 500 μl of diluted DCFH-DA was added to each well. Cells were incubated at 37°C for 20 min and washed thrice with serum-free medium. Fluorescent images were visualized and captured with a standard green fluorescence cube using a model Ts2R inverted fluorescence microscope (Nikon, Tokyo, Japan). Fluorescence images were analyzed quantitatively using ImageJ software (1.52a; NIH, Bethesda, MD, United States).

Fluorescence Staining of Apoptotic Cells

TUNEL staining kit and DAPI staining solution were used to assess the presence of apoptotic cells. Briefly, the cells were incubated and treated in accordance with the experimental protocol, washed once with PBS, and fixed with 4% paraformaldehyde for 30 min. Then, they were permeabilized with 0.3% Triton X-100 in PBS for another 30 min and washed three times with PBS. Fifty microliters of TUNEL staining solution were added to each well and incubated in the dark for 1 h at 37°C. Then, cells were washed three times with PBS and 100 μl of DAPI staining solution was added to each well, followed by incubation in the dark for 10 min and washing with PBS. Finally, cell fluorescent images were captured using a fluorescence microscope (Nikon Ni-U, DS-Qi2) equipped with standard red and ultraviolet fluorescence cubes. Fluorescent images were analyzed quantitatively using ImageJ software (1.52a).

Flow Cytometry Analysis to Detect Apoptosis

An Annexin V-FITC/PI apoptosis assay kit was used to detect apoptosis. Briefly, the cells were washed with PBS and digested with trypsin for 3 min. Then, serum-containing medium was added to terminate the digestion. Each sample was centrifuged and the supernatant was discarded. Five hundred microliters of 1× binding buffer were added to resuspend the cells, followed by 5 μl Annexin V-FITC and 10 μl PI to each tube. After incubation for 10 min protected from light on ice, a FACSCelesta flow cytometer (BD, Santa Clara, CA, United States) was used to analyze the percentage of apoptotic cells.

Western Blot Analysis

After incubation and intervention, the cells were lysed in RIPA buffer supplemented with 2% protease and phosphatase inhibitor cocktail for 20 min on ice. After sonication, the samples were centrifuged at 4°C for 20 min, and each supernatant was collected for subsequent experiments. The total protein concentration was determined using a BCA protein assay kit. Equal amounts of protein (20 μg) were separated by 10 or 12% sodium-dodecyl sulfate-polyacrylamide gel electrophoresis (SDS-PAGE). The resolved proteins were electrophoretically transferred to polyvinylidene difluoride (PVDF) membranes (Millipore, Billerica, MA, United States). The membranes were blocked with 5% non-fat dried milk in PBS containing Tween (PBST) buffer for 1 h at room temperature, washed thrice with PBST, and incubated with primary antibodies overnight at 4°C. The membranes were washed again and incubated with HRP-conjugated anti-rabbit or anti-mouse IgG for 1 h at room temperature. The bands were flushed with chemiluminescent HRP substrate and imaged using a chemiluminescence system (ChemiDoc™ XRS+ with Image Lab Software; Bio-Rad, Hercules, CA, United States). Western blot images were analyzed quantitatively using ImageJ software (1.52a). β-actin was also assayed to confirm equal loading of proteins.

Statistical Analyses

Statistical analyses were performed using SPSS version 19.0 (IBM, Armonk, NY, United States). All values are expressed as mean ± standard deviation (SD). Comparisons of two populations were made using unpaired 2-tailed Student's t-test. For multiple groups, statistical significance was determined using one-way analysis of variance (ANOVA) followed by Dunnett's test. Statistical significance was set at $p<0.05$.

RESULTS

Main Active Components and Targets of *P. frutescens*

A total of 328 chemical components of *P. frutescens* were retrieved from the TCMSP database. Use of OB ≥30% and DL ≥0.18 as the

TABLE 1 | Main active components of *P. frutescens*.

Code	Compound name	CAS	OB%	DL
C1	Bishomo-gamma-linolenic acid	1783-84-2	44.11	0.2
C2	(s)-Carvone	2244-16-8	47.43	0.03
C3	11,14-Eicosadienoic acid, methyl ester	2463-02-7	39.67	0.23
C4	ZINC03860434	117-81-7	43.59	0.35
C5	Beta-sitosterol	83-46-5	36.91	0.75
C6	Beta-carotene	7235-40-7	37.18	0.58
C7	Clionasterol	83-47-6	36.91	0.75
C8	Cholesterin	57-88-5	37.87	0.68
C9	Cirtrusin C	18604-50-7	40.52	0.23
C10	(+)-Catechin	154-23-4	54.83	0.24
C11	Cyanin	523-42-2	47.42	0.76
C12	Gondoic acid	5561-99-9	30.7	0.2
C13	Caffeic acid	501-16-6	25.76	0.05
C14	Rosmarinic acid	20283-92-5	1.38	0.35
C15	Luteolin	491-70-3	36.16	0.25
C16	Caryophellene	87-44-5	23.79	0.09
C17	Linolenic acid ethyl ester	1191-41-9	46.1	0.2
C18	Perilla aldehyde	18031-40-8	39	0.03
C19	Perilla ketone	553-84-4	81.94	0.03

OB, oral bioavailability; DL, drug-likeness.

screening criteria yielded 14 active components. An analysis of the published literature revealed that although (s) – carvone (Alasanea and Liu, 2017), caffeic acid (Tyszka-Czochara et al., 2018), rosmarinic acid (Colica et al., 2018), caryophellene (Sharma et al., 2016), perilla aldehyde (Song et al., 2018), and perilla ketone (Roellecke et al., 2017) did not meet the aforementioned OB and DL screening criteria, *in vivo* and *in vitro* experiments were validated. Therefore, these components were included to result in 19 main active components (C20 Supraene did not retrieve the predicted target, and so was excluded in further research) (**Table 1** and **Supplementary Figure S1**). The predicted targets of the active components were searched for in the TCMSP database, and the predicted targets in the Uniport database were checked to obtain 225 targets of the main active components. Of these, 141 unique targets were finally obtained after deduplication.

Main Targets Related to CKD

The relevant targets of CKD stage 3–5/CRF were searched for in the Gene cards database with a score ≥10 as the screening criterion. The search resulted in 2263 main targets.

Key Targets of *P. frutescens* in Treatment of CKD

The predicted targets of *P. frutescens* were mapped to the main targets related to CKD stage 3–5 using Venny2.1.0 software. A Venn diagram was constructed (**Figure 1A**). A total of 108 intersection targets were obtained. These may be the key targets of *P. frutescens* for CKD treatment.

Main Active Components-Targets Network Model

The main active components and key targets of *P. frutescens* were imported into Cytoscape 3.6.0, to build a main active component-target network model. The model included 160 nodes and 225 edges. In this model, 19 active components are shown as diamond-shaped yellow nodes, 141 targets are blue square nodes, and the edges represent the interaction between the components and the targets (**Figure 1B**). The Network Analyzer plugin was used to perform network topology analysis and to calculate the degree, betweenness centrality and closeness centrality parameter values. The median of the degree was one. Therefore, we chose degree >2 (i.e., more than twice the median) as the criterion to filter out the core nodes in the network model, including 12 components and 18 targets (**Supplementary Table S1**).

Further analysis of the nodes in the table revealed that the highest degree among the main active components was C15 (luteolin), with 57 targets. In descending order, C5 (β-sitosterol) corresponded to 37 targets, C14 (rosmarinic acid) had 32 targets, C13 (caffeic acid) corresponded to 22 targets, and C6 (β-carotene) had 21 targets. The target is the key to the pharmacological effect of the component, so it is speculated that luteolin, β-sitosterol, and rosmarinic acid are the key components of *P. frutescens* in the treatment of CKD stage 3–5. Among the target nodes, the highest degree was prostaglandin-endoperoxide synthase 2 (PTGS2), which targeted 11 components. Subsequently, in descending order, PTGS1 and nuclear receptor coactivator 2 (NCOA2) all targeted eight components, heat shock protein 90 (HSP90) is connected to five active components. The biological functions related to these key targets were mainly related to inflammation, immunity, metabolism, and others, suggesting that *P. frutescens* may exert its pharmacological effects on CKD through the aforementioned approaches.

Additionally, the network model found that 18 active components targeted at least two targets, and 41 targets were connected to at least two components. There was a large amount of cross-coincidence between each component and target. These results reflect the multi-component, multi-target effects of *P. frutescens*.

PPI Network Model

The relevant targets of *P. frutescens* for treating CKD stage 3–5 were imported into String 11.0, under the condition of "homo sapiens." The highest confidence protein score value was set as >0.7, a PPI network was constructed, and unrelated individual proteins were removed. The network included 105 targets and 736 interactions. The PPI network information was imported into Cytoscape3.6.0 to build a network model, and the Network Analyzer plugin was used to analyze network characteristics. By adjusting the node color and size according to the degree, the greater the degree, the larger was the node. The thickness of the side was revised according to the Combine score: the larger the Combine score, the thicker the side (**Figure 2A**).

We selected degree ≥20 as the criterion. Twenty-seven key proteins in the PPI network were selected (**Figure 2B**), including AKT1, tumor protein 53 (TP53), IL6, tumor necrosis factor (TNF), MAPK1, JUN, vascular endothelial growth factor A (VEGFA), epidermal growth factor receptor

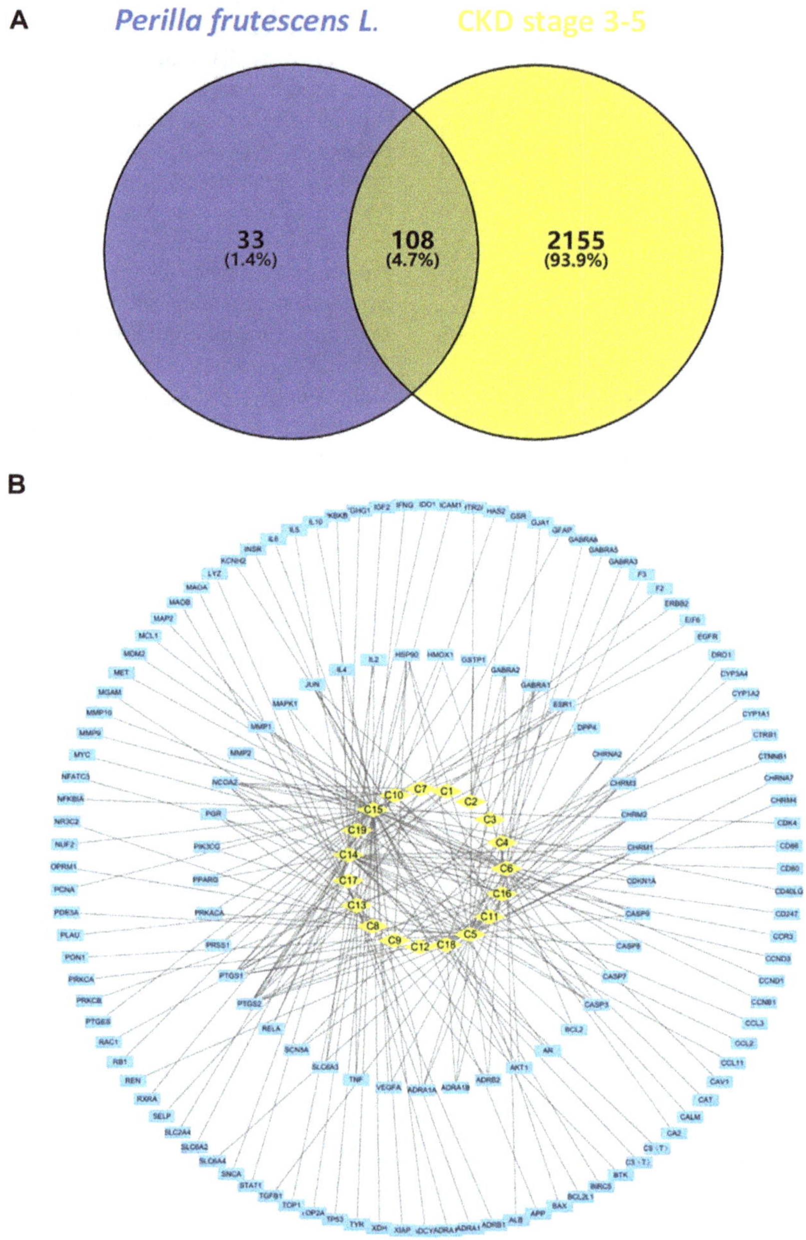

FIGURE 1 | Construction and analysis of the network model of Perilla frutescens *L.* in the treatment of chronic kidney disease (CKD). **(A)** Relevant targets of *P. frutescens* in the treatment of CKD stages 3–5. The predicted targets of main active components were mapped to the main targets of CKD stages 3–5, and 108 relevant targets were obtained. **(B)** Main active components-targets network model. The main active components, targets, and their interaction relationships were imported into Cytoscape3.6.0 software to construct the network model. The yellow diamond represents the active components, the blue square represents the targets, and the lines represents the interaction relationships.

(EGFR), caspase 3 (CASP3), cyclin D1 (CCND1), MYC, RELA, matrix metalloproteinase 9 (MMP9), IL2, PTGS2, and others, implicating these targets as the main targets of *P. frutescens* in the treatment of CKD stage 3–5.

The PPI network is modular, and the functional module is the basic unit of protein function. Modular analysis can simplify the complex protein network, which is conducive to further research on the biological and pharmacological functions of the protein. Therefore, the MCODE plugin in the Cytoscape software was used to perform modular analysis of the PPI network, with Degree Cutoff = 2, Node Score Cutoff = 0.2, K-Core = 5, and Max. Depth = 100. Two key protein modules were identified. Protein module A contained 20 targets and 101 interactions. Protein module B contained 25 targets and 99 interactions (**Figure 2C**).

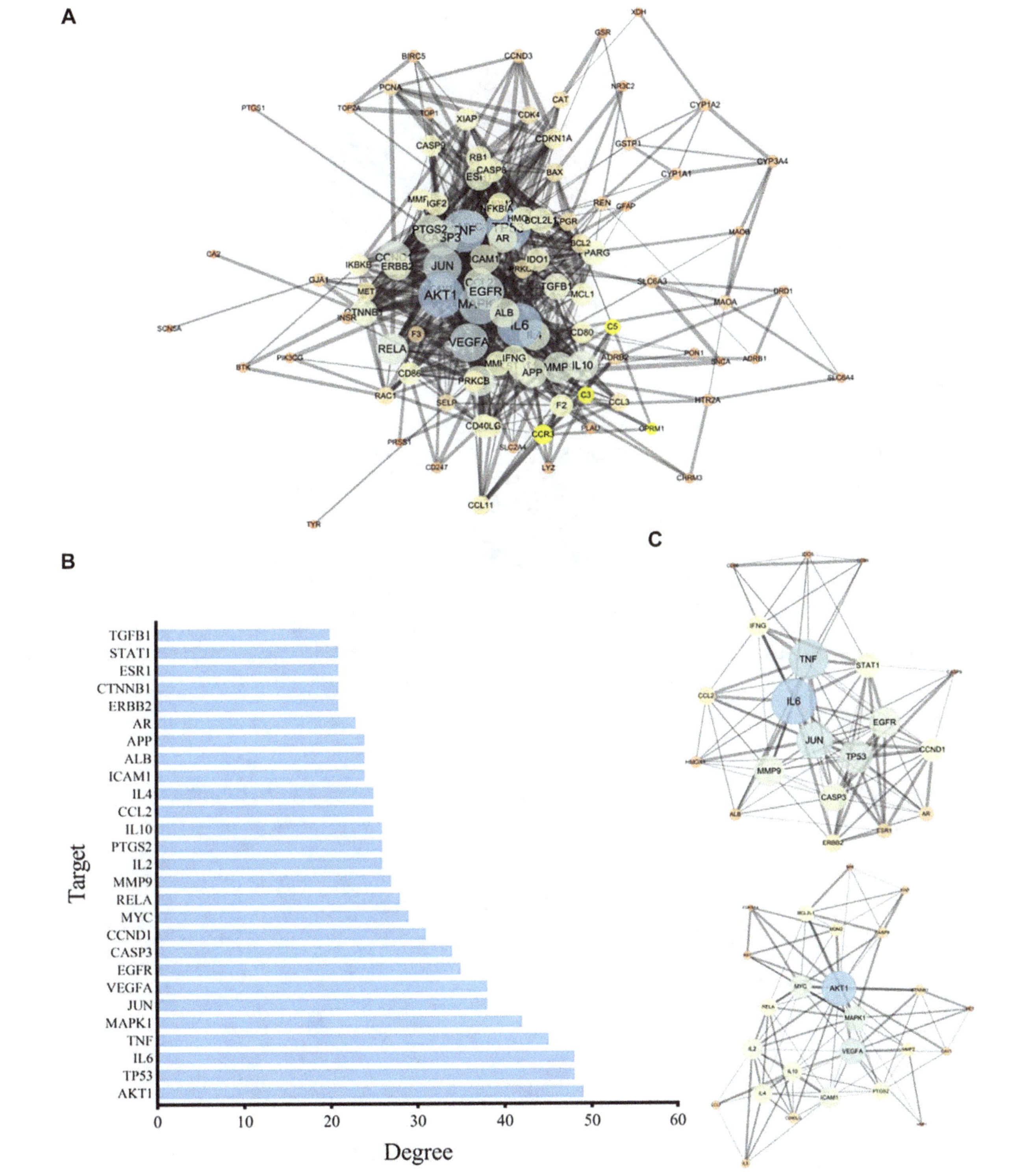

FIGURE 2 | Construction and analysis of the protein-protein interaction (PPI) network. **(A)** The PPI network model. The related targets of *P. frutescens* for the treatment of CKD stages 3–5 were imported into the String 11.0 database to construct the PPI network. The PPI network information was input into Cytoscape 3.6.0 software to construct the PPI network model and adjusted according to the network topology analysis. **(B)** Key nodes in PPI network model. The key nodes in the PPI network model were screened with Degree ≥20, 27 key proteins in the PPI network were selected. **(C)** Key modules in the PPI network model. Modular analysis of the PPI network was carried out by using MCODE plugin. Two key protein modules were screened. Module A contains 20 targets and 101 interactions and module B contains 25 targets and 99 interactions.

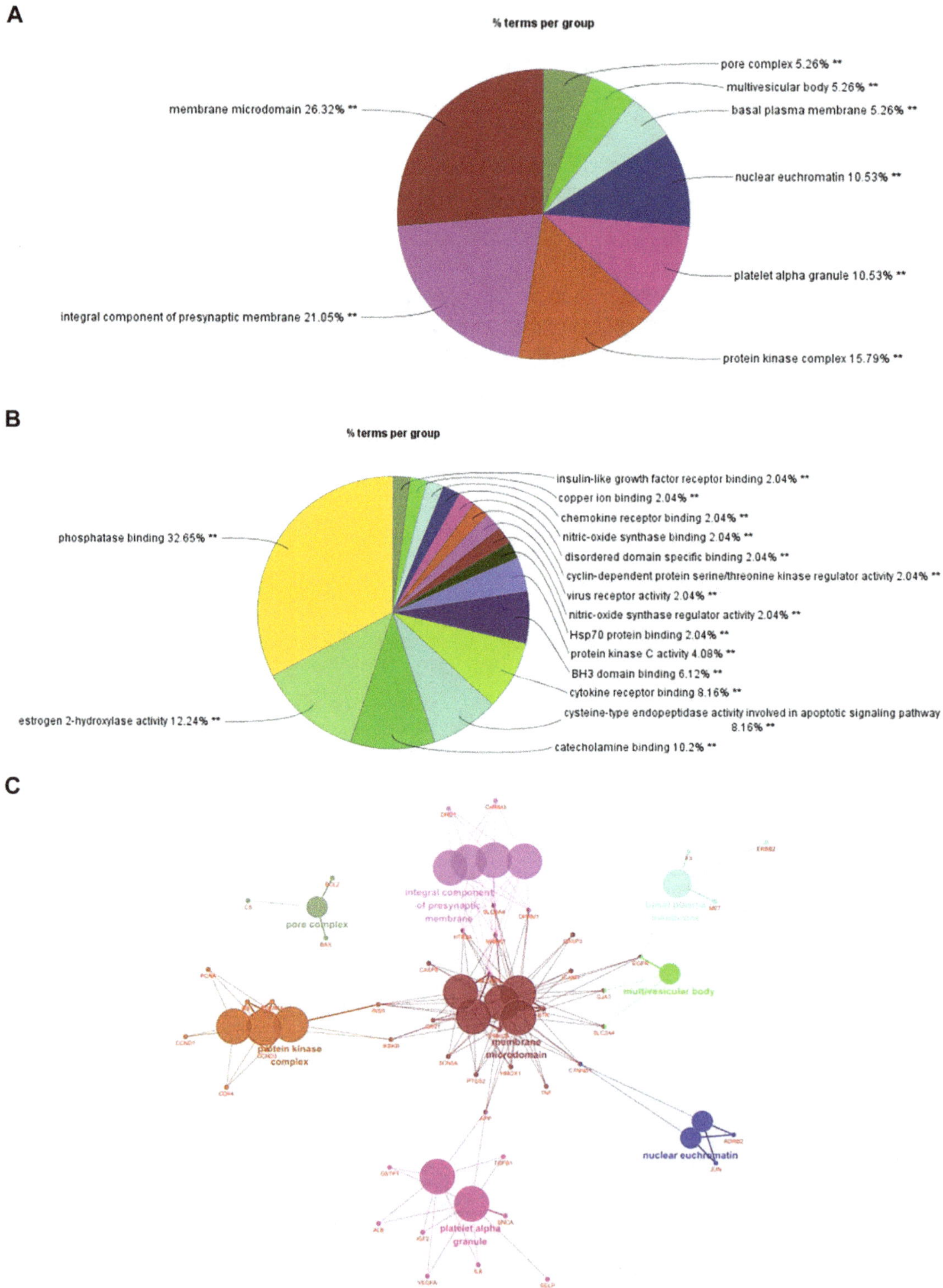

FIGURE 3 | Enrichment analysis of cellular component (CC) and molecular function (MF). **(A)** Enrichment analysis of CC. Targets ($n = -105$) in the PPI network were imported into Cytoscape 3.6.0 software. The enrichment analysis of CC was carried out with a p-value ≤ 0.01. A pie chart and network model of the mainly enriched related CCs were obtained. **(B)** Enrichment analysis of MF. According to the same methods and criteria of CC enrichment analysis, the enrichment analysis of MF was carried out to obtain the main related MFs. **(C)** The network model of CC enrichment analysis. The enrichment analysis of CC was selected as a representative to construct the network model by using Cytoscape 3.6.0 software.

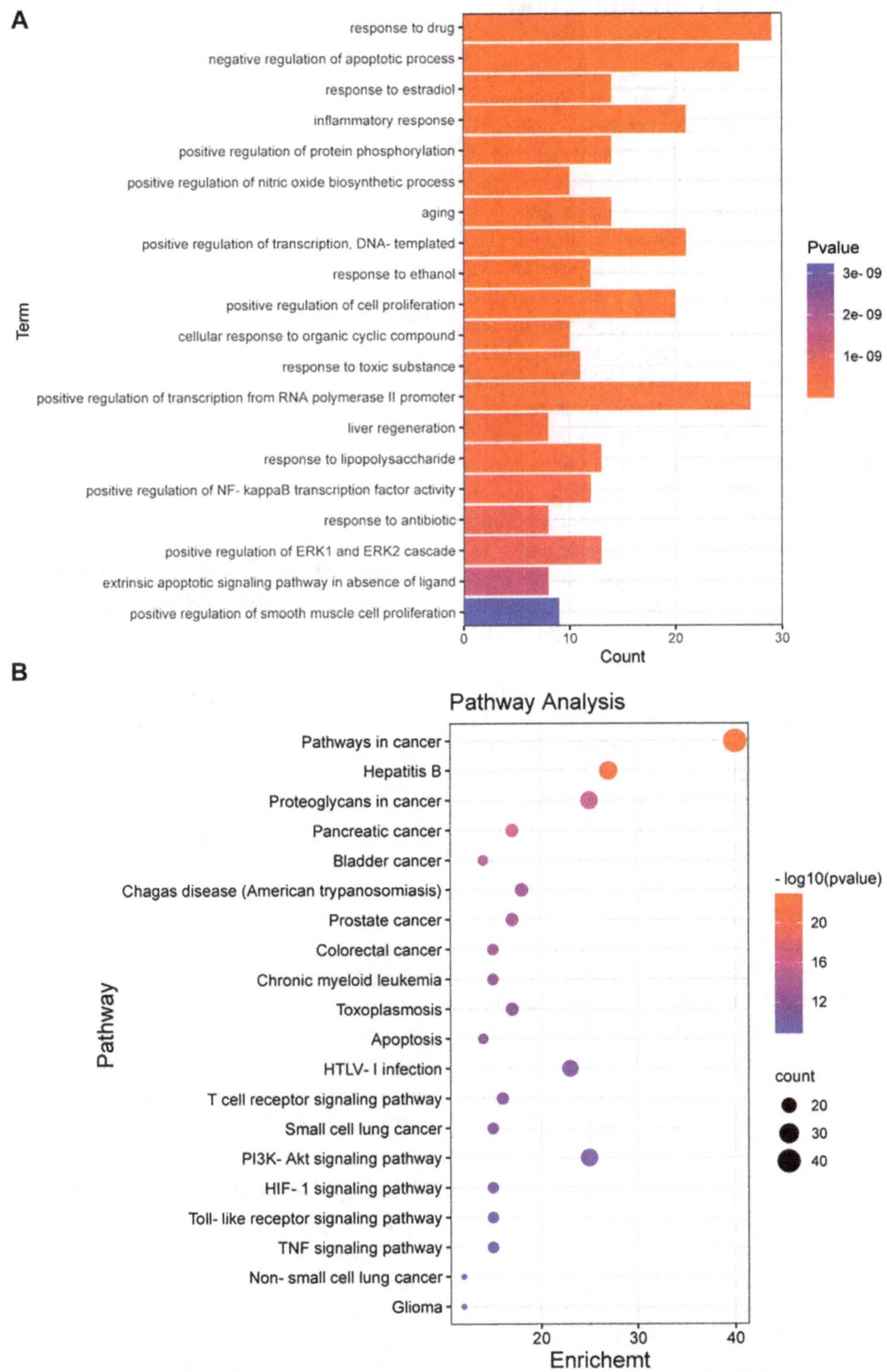

FIGURE 4 | Enrichment analysis of biological process (BP) and KEGG signaling pathway. **(A)** Enrichment analysis of BP. The 105 targets in PPI network were imported into David6.8 online analysis platform for enrichment analysis of BP. The top 20 BPs were selected to draw the bar graph. **(B)** Enrichment analysis of KEGG signaling pathway. The analysis was carried out according to the same methods and criteria of BP enrichment analysis. The top 20 signaling pathways were selected to draw the bubble diagram.

Enriched Gene Biological Functions and Signaling Pathways

We imported 105 targets in the PPI network into Cytoscape3.6.0 software and used ClueGO and CluePedia plugins for enrichment analysis of CC and MF. A $p \leq 0.01$ was the screening parameter. A pie chart was drawn (**Figures 3A,B**). CCs mainly included membrane microdomains, integral components of presynaptic membranes, protein kinase complexes, platelet alpha granules, nuclear euchromatin, basal plasma membrane, multivesicular body, and pore complex. MFs mainly involved phosphatase binding, estrogen 2-hydroxylase activity, catecholamine binding, cysteine-type endopeptidase activity involved in the apoptotic signaling pathway, cytokine receptor binding, BH3 domain binding, protein kinase C activity, HSP70 protein binding, nitric oxide synthase regulator activity, virus receptor activity, cyclin-dependent protein serine/threonine kinase regulator activity, disordered domain-specific binding, nitric oxide synthase binding, chemokine receptor binding, copper ion binding, and insulin-like growth factor receptor binding. Enrichment analysis of CCs was selected as a representative to construct a network model (**Figure 3C**). Multiple targets were connected to at least two CCs, which are the key nodes in the network. The findings provided further evidence of the multi-target, multi-effect characteristics of *P. frutescens*.

A total of 105 targets were imported into the DAVID6.8 online analysis platform for the enrichment analysis of BP and KEGG signaling pathways. With $p < 0.01$ as the screening criterion, 254 BPs and 101 pathways were obtained. The first 20 BPs and pathways were selected using the clusterProfiler package in R language to draw bar graphs and bubble diagrams (**Figures 4A,B** and **Supplementary Figures S2A,B**). In the bubble diagram, the node size represents the gene number: the larger the node, the more genes corresponding to the node. The color of the node represents the *p*-value. The smaller the *p*-value, the redder the color; otherwise, the values were depicted in shades of blue. The ordinate represents the BP or pathway name corresponding to the node, and the abscissa represents the fold enrichment. The greater the fold enrichment, the higher the degree of gene enrichment. BPs were observed to be mainly related to the response to drugs, negative regulation of apoptotic process, response to estradiol, inflammatory response, positive regulation of protein phosphorylation, positive regulation of nitric oxide biosynthesis process, aging, positive regulation of transcription, response to ethanol, positive regulation of cell proliferation, cellular response to organic cyclic compounds, response to toxic substances, positive regulation of transcription from RNA polymerase II promoter, positive regulation of nuclear factor-kappa B (NF-κB) transcription factor activity, and positive regulation of ERK1 and ERK2 cascade. Enriched pathways related to CKD stages 3–5 mainly included the apoptosis signaling pathway, T cell receptor (TCR) signaling pathway, PI3K-AKT signaling pathway, hypoxia inducible factor-1 (HIF-1) signaling pathway, Toll-like receptor (TLR) signaling pathway, and TNF signaling pathway. Thus, *P. frutescens* may play a therapeutic role in CKD stages 3–5 by regulating the above multiple pathways.

TABLE 2 | Molecular docking of active components and corresponding targets in *P. frutescens*.

Component	Target	Binding Affinity (kJ/mol)
Luteolin	PTGS2	−9.3
	AKT1	−8.5
	p53	−6.9
	TNF-α	−8.9
	MAPK1	−8.8
	IL6	−7.5
	JUN	−8.7
β-sitosterol	PTGS2	−11.8
	JUN	−11.6
Rosmarinic acid	PTGS2	−6.7
	MAPK1	−7.9
Caffeic acid	PTGS2	−7.2
	TNF-α	−6.8
β-carotene	PTGS2	−9.0
	AKT1	−8.9
	JUN	−9.5

Docking of Core Components and Corresponding Main Targets of *P. frutescens*

The key components in the component-target network were selected as the ligand, and the corresponding core node as the receptor. Imported Pyrx was used for preprocessing, and Autodock vina was used for molecular docking (**Table 2**). Binding affinity <0 meant that the receptor and ligand bound spontaneously: the lower the value, the greater the binding affinity. The binding energies of the targets, PTGS2, AKT1, p53, TNF-α, MAPK1, IL6, JUN, and their original ligands were −11.6, −8.7, −4.3, −9.7, −9.8, −4.5, −9.6 kJ/mol, respectively. The binding capacity of each key component and corresponding target was similar to that of the original ligand. We selected luteolin, the most critical component in the network model, and performed molecular docking and visual analysis through Schrödinger Maestro and Pymol2.1 (**Figures 5A,B**). These results verified that the main active components of *P. frutescens* may play a therapeutic role in CKD by acting on their corresponding key targets.

Quality Control and Component Validation of PFAE

As shown in **Figure 6**, five chemical components in PFAE were detected by HPLC, including luteolin ($C_{15}H_{10}O_6$; CAS: 491-70-3), rosmarinic acid ($C_{18}H_{16}O_8$; CAS: 20283-92-5), caffeic acid ($C_9H_8O_4$; CAS: 501-16-6), perilla aldehyde ($C_{10}H_{14}O$; CAS: 18031-40-8) and (+)-catechin ($C_{15}H_{14}O_6$; CAS: 154-23-4). Luteolin, rosmarinic acid and caffeic acid are the main active components of *P. frutescens*, and the content is large. Therefore, the concentrations of these three components in different preparations were measured for quality control.

In addition, these components identified by HPLC were coincident with those screened from the TCMSP database. And according to the results of network pharmacological

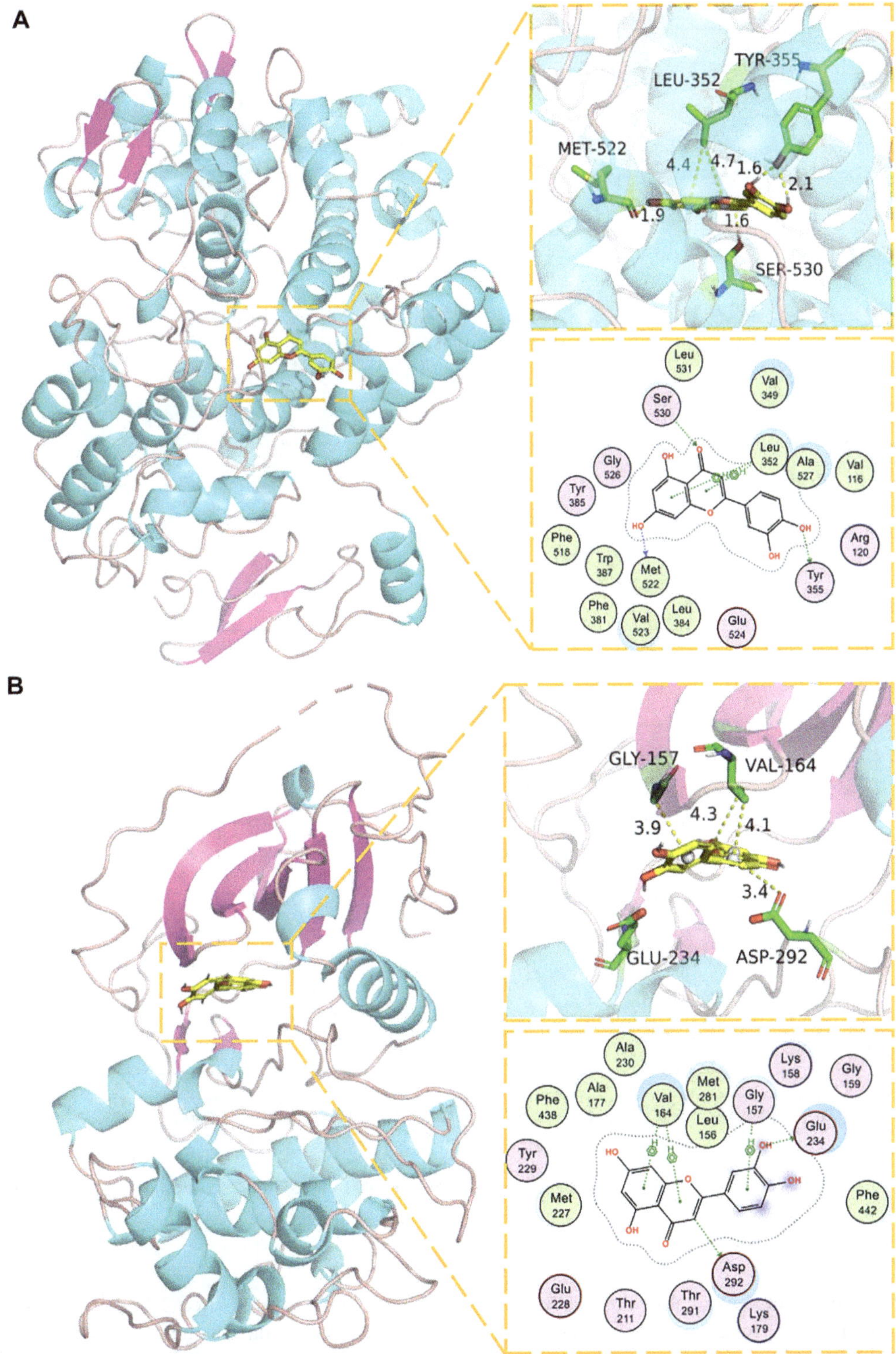

FIGURE 5 | Molecular docking model of luteolin and corresponding targets. **(A)** Molecular docking mode of luteolin and PTGS1. The backbone of protein was rendered in tube and colored in bright blue. Luteolin is rendering by yellow. Yellow dash represents hydrogen bond distance or π-stacking distance. **(B)** Molecular docking mode of luteolin and AKTI. The backbone of protein was rendered in tube and colored in bright blue. Luteolin is rendering by yellow. Yellow dash represents hydrogen bond distance or π-stacking distance.

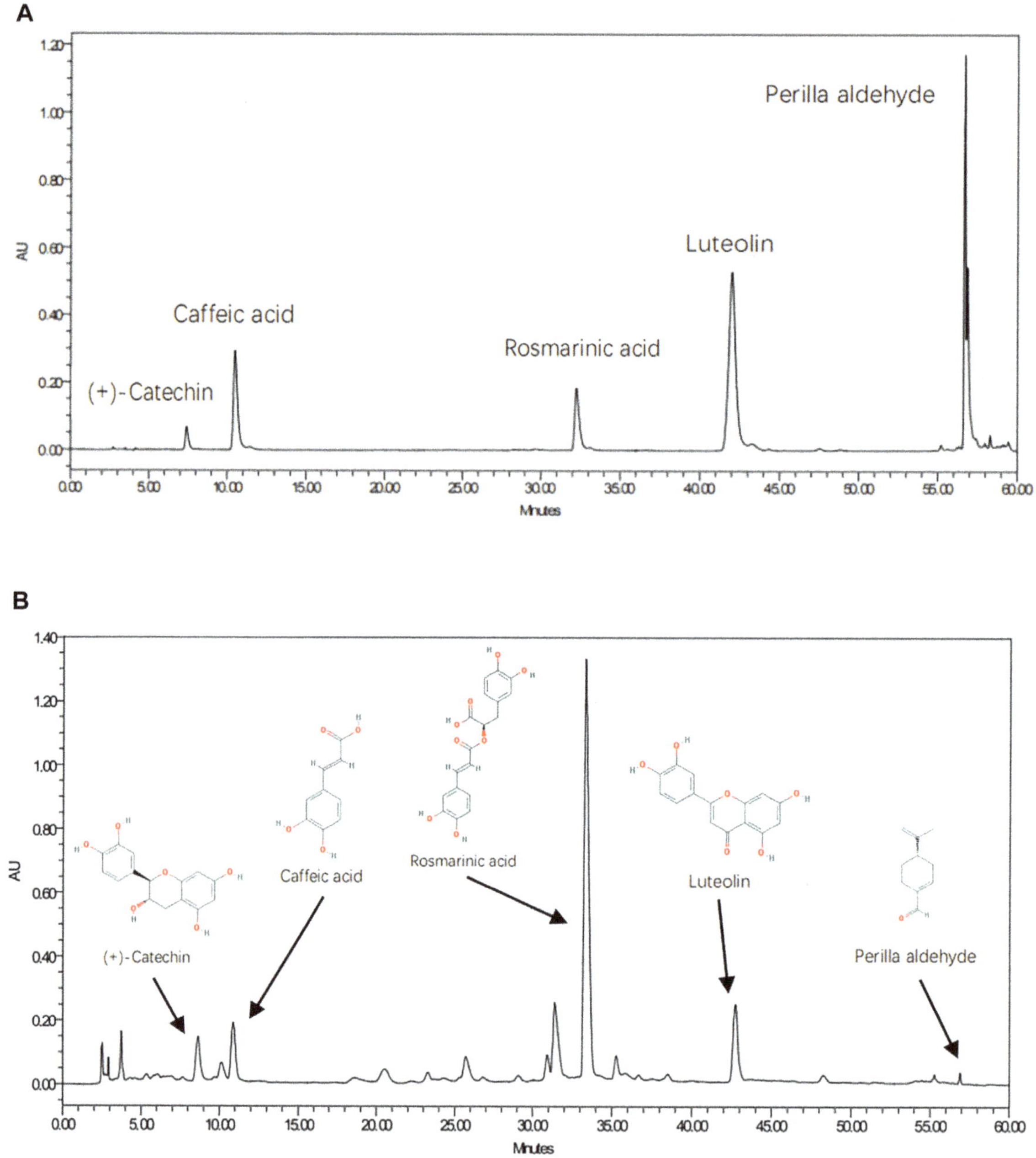

FIGURE 6 | Quality Control and Component Validation of P. frutescens Aqueous Extracts (PFAE) by HPLC. **(A)** Chromatograms of mixed standards. **(B)** PFAE samples.

analysis, these five components were also the main active components in the network model of *P. frutescens* for treating CKD.

Luteolin Reduces Adriamycin-Induced Renal Tubular Cell Injury

According to the HPLC results, we calculated that the concentration of luteolin in the PFAE was about 0.15 mg/ml, which provided the basis for further study of its therapeutic effects. Luteolin-pretreated NRK-52E cells were examined to assess the effect on cell morphology and viability. Compared with the control group, the number of cells in the ADR (2 μg/ml) group was reduced, the cells were shrunken and deformed, and some damaged cells floated in the culture (**Supplementary Figures S3A,B**). Compared with the ADR group, the number of cells was increased in the PFAE (5 mg/ml) and luteolin (10 μM/L) pretreatment groups, and the cell morphology was normal (**Figure 7A**). Cell viability was measured using the CCK-8 assay. Compared with the ADR group, the cell viability in the

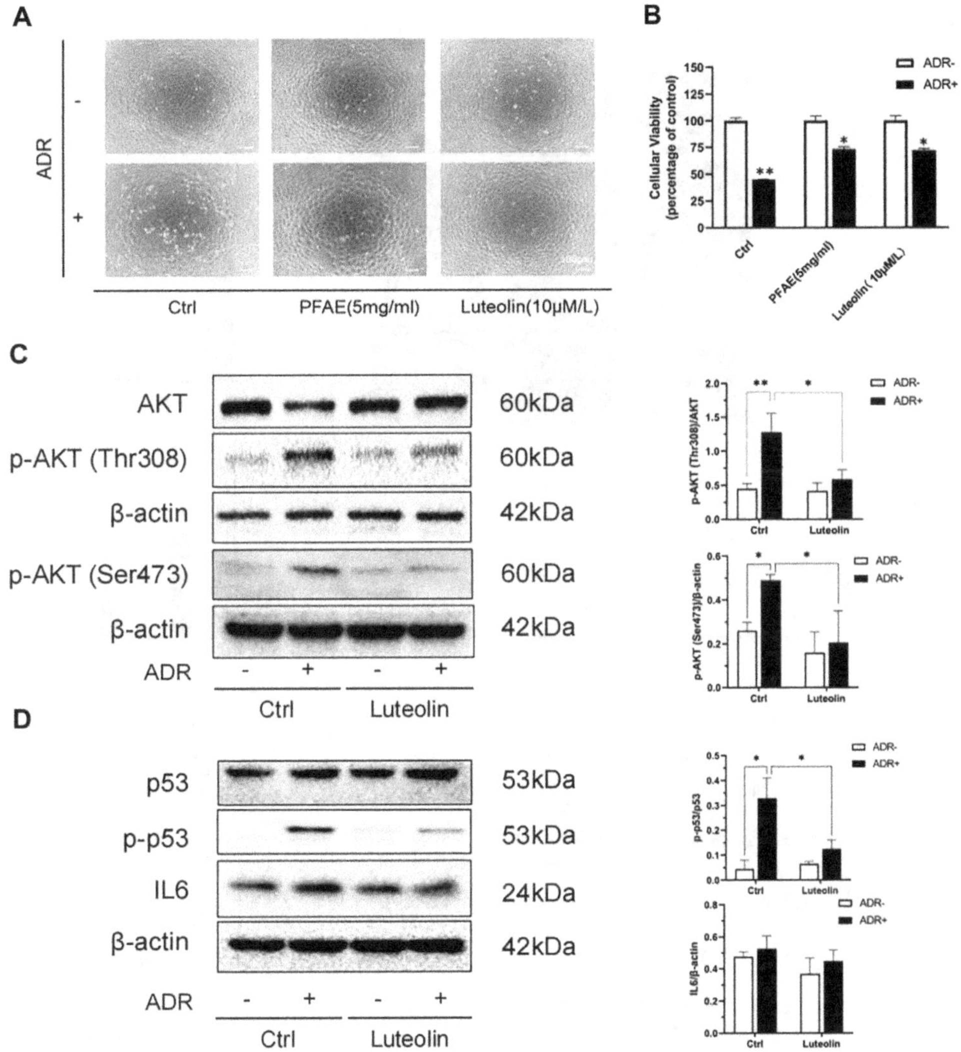

FIGURE 7 | Luteolin alleviates Adriamycin (ADR)-induced renal injury and modulates AKT phosphorylation. (A) Effects of luteolin on the morphological changes of ADR-induced NRK-52E cells. Pretreated NRK-52E cells with FPAE (5 mg/ml) or luteolin (10 μM/L) for 1 h and then stimulated with ADR (2 μg/ml) for 24 h. Morphological changes of cells were observed by inverted phase-contrast microscopy (magnification ×100). **(B)** Effects of luteolin on cellular viability of ADR injury model. NRK-52E cells were exposed to the indicated concentrations of ADR with or without luteolin Cell viability was measured by the CCK-8 assay. Data are expressed as the percentages of living cells against the control (mean ± SD, $n = 3$; *p <0.05 versus ADR in Ctrl. **p <0.01 versus Ctrl) **(C)** Effects of luteolin on the phosphorylation of AKT in ADR-injured cells. NRK-52E cells were pretreated with luteolin for 1 h and then challenged with ADR for another 24 h. Cellular lysates were subjected to western blot analysis of AKT, phosphorylated AKT and B actin Statistical analysis of phosphorylated AKT is shown on the right (mean ± SD, $n = 3$; *p <0.05, **p <0.01) **(D)** Effects of luteolin on the expression of p53 and IL6 in ADR-injured cells. NRK-52E cells were pretreated with luteolin for 1 h and then incubated with ADR for another 6 h. Cellular lysates were subjected to western blot analysis of p53, phosphorylated p53, IL6 and β-actin. Statistical analysis of phosphorylated p53 and IL6 are shown on the right (mean ± SD, $n = 3$; *p <0.05).

PFAE+ADR and luteolin+ADR groups was significantly increased. Therefore, PFAE and luteolin (the key component of *P. frutescens*) can attenuate ADR-induced cell injury (**Figure 7B**).

Luteolin Modulates the Phosphorylation of AKT and P53

AKT participates in a variety of physiological processes in the body, including cell proliferation, apoptosis, protein translation, and glucose metabolism. It plays an important role in various kidney diseases. AKT is the core protein in the PPI network, and molecular docking has revealed good binding ability between luteolin and AKT. We used ADR to construct an *in vitro* renal tubular injury model and found that it can significantly increase the phosphorylation of AKT. Upon the addition of luteolin was added, and this promotion was effectively inhibited (**Figure 7C**).

At the same time, TP53 and IL6 are also key targets of the PPI network model. P53 (the expressed protein of TP53) is a key protein that regulates the cell cycle. It is closely related to cell self-repair and cell apoptosis. IL6 is regarded as a pro-inflammatory cytokine, which plays a key role in the immune

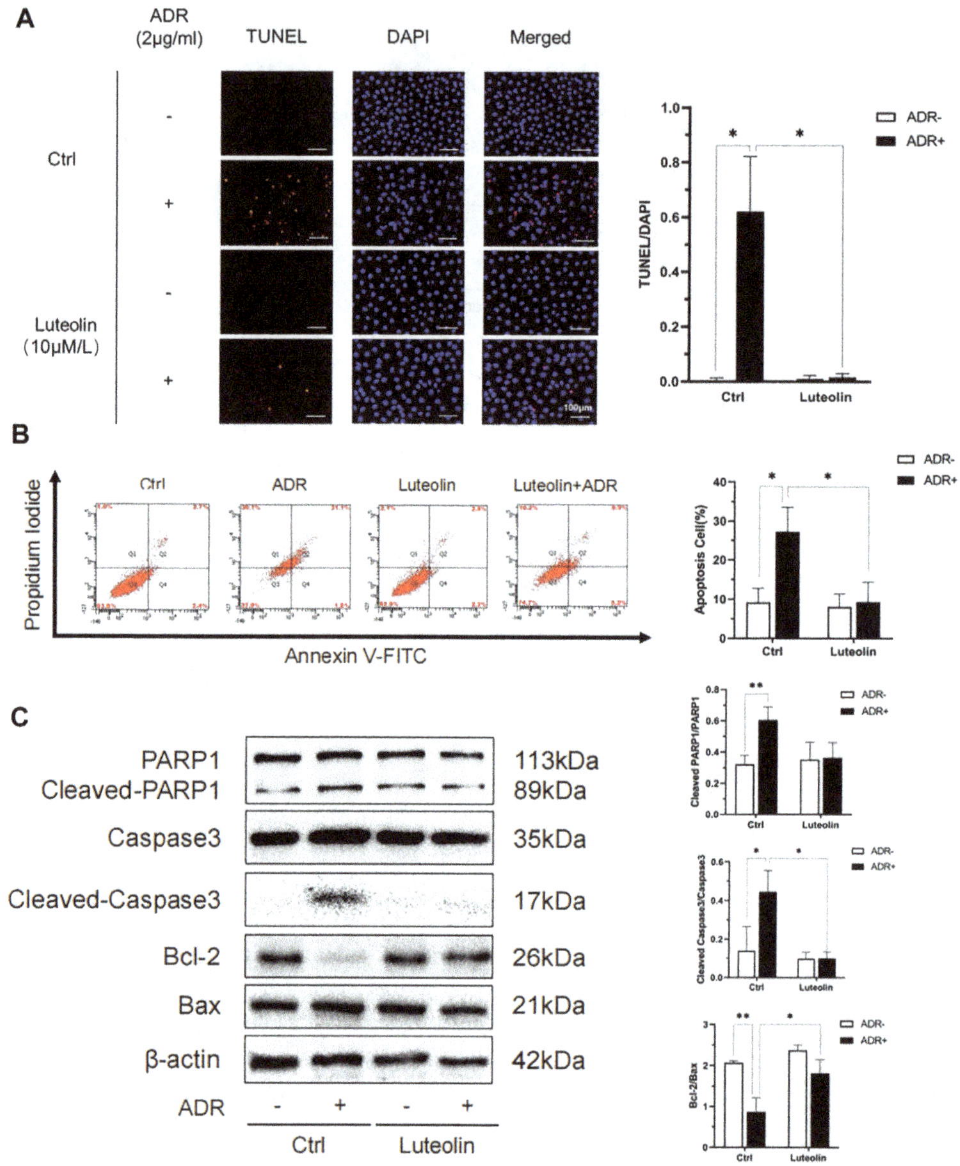

FIGURE 8 | Luteolin reduces ADR-induced apoptosis. **(A)** Effects of luteolin in ADR-induced apoptosis by TUNEL and DAPI staining assay. NRK-52E cells were incubated with ADR for 24 h in the presence and absence of luteolin. Apoptotic cells were detected by TUNEL and DAPI staining. Fluorescence staining was observed by fluorescence microscope (magnification ×200) and the analysis result on the right was expressed as the percentages of dead cells compared with the Ctrl (mean ± SD, $n = 3$; $^{*}p < 0.05$) **(B)** Effects of luteolin in apoptosis as measured by flow cytometry. NRK-52E cells were pretreated with luteolin for 1 h and stimulated with ADR for another 24 h. Apoptotic cells were detected by flow cytometry using Annexin V-FITC/PI. Flow cytometry data is shown on the right (mean ± SD, $n = 3$; $^{*}p < 0.05$). **(C)** Effects of luteolin on expression of apoptosis-related proteins. NRK-52E cells were pretreated with luteolin for 1 h and incubated with ADR for another 24 h. Cellular lysates were analyzed by western blot targeting Cleaved-PARPI, Cleaved Caspase3, Bcl-2 and Bax. Statistical analysis of western blot results are shown on the right (mean ± SD, $n = 3$; $p < 0.05$, $^{**}p < 0.01$).

response and inflammation. Both p53 and IL6 are involved in the development of CKD, and can aggravate renal injury by inducing apoptosis, promoting inflammation, accelerating cell senescence and other ways (Amdur et al., 2016; Juvet et al., 2020; Wang et al., 2020). Therefore, we also detected the phosphorylation level of p53 and the expression of IL6. The results showed that luteolin can significantly reduce ADR-induced p53 phosphorylation, but had no significant effect on IL6 (**Figure 7D**). These results indicate that AKT and p53 may be the targets of luteolin in reducing ADR-mediated kidney damage.

Luteolin Mitigates ADR-Elicited Apoptosis

TUNEL + DAPI staining and flow cytometry analysis were performed to verify the anti-apoptotic role of luteolin in NRK-52E cells treated with ADR. The apoptosis rate in the luteolin+ADR group was significantly lower than that in the ADR group (**Figures 8A,B**). We further tested the expression of apoptosis-related

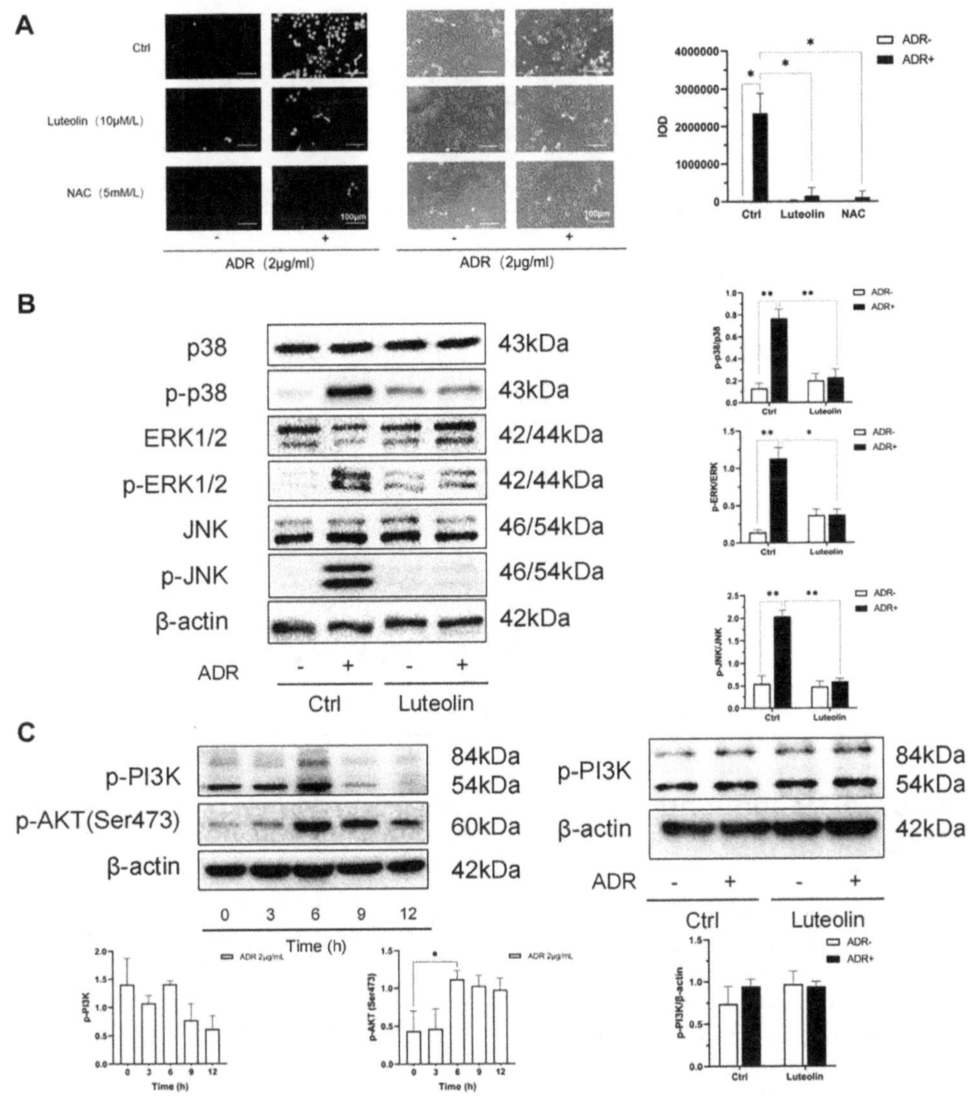

FIGURE 9 | Oxidative stress and MAPK pathway may be the mechanism of luteolin to ameliorate apoptosis. **(A)** Effects of luteolin on ROS production. NRK-52E cells were pretreated with luteolin and NAC (5 mM/L) for 1 h and then stimulated with ADR for another 4 h. ROS staining was observed by florescence microscope (magnification ×200). The fluorescence intensity represents the ROS production level. Statistical analysis data is shown at the bottom (mean ± SD, $n = 3$; $^{*}p < 0.05$). **(B)** The regulatory effects of luteolin on MAPK pathway related proteins. NRK-52E cells were pretreated with luteolin for 1 h and incubated with ADR for 24 h. Cellular lysates were subjected to western blot analysis for phosphorylated p38 ERK1/2 and JNK. Densitometric analysis of these phosphorylated proteins are shown on the right (mean ± SD, $n = 3$; $^{*}p < 0.05$, $^{**}p < 0.01$). **(C)** Effects of ADR on phosphorylated PI3K and AKT. NRK-52E cells were stimulated with ADR for different periods. Then, the expression of phosphorylated PI3K and AKT was detected by western blot Densitometric analysis of these proteins are shown at the bottom (mean ± SD, $n = 3$; $^{*}p < 0.05$). **(D)** The regulatory effects of luteolin on p-PI3K. NRK-52E cells were pretreated with luteolin for 1 h and stimulated with ADR for another 6 h Cellular lysates were subjected to western blot analysis for phosphorylated PI3K. Densitometric analysis is shown at the bottom (mean ± SD, $n = 3$).

proteins, including PARP1, Caspase3, Bcl-2, and Bax. Compared with the ADR group, these apoptotic proteins were significantly down-regulated in the luteolin+ADR group (**Figure 8C**). These data show that luteolin mitigated ADR-induced apoptosis.

Luteolin Relieves Oxidative Stress Induced by ADR

Oxidative stress is one of the important mechanisms in cell apoptosis and plays a key role in the pathological process of CKD. The overproduction of ROS is the initial factor of oxidative stress. We tested ROS production using an immunofluorescence probe. As shown in **Figure 9A**, after 4 h of incubation, ADR significantly increased the generation of ROS (green), whereas pretreatment with luteolin or NAC antioxidant suppressed the ADR-induced overproduction of ROS. Furthermore, compared with the NAC pretreated group, there was no significant difference in the inhibitory effect of luteolin on ROS induced by ADR. These outcomes suggest that luteolin effectively inhibits ADR-induced apoptosis *via* suppression of ROS overproduction.

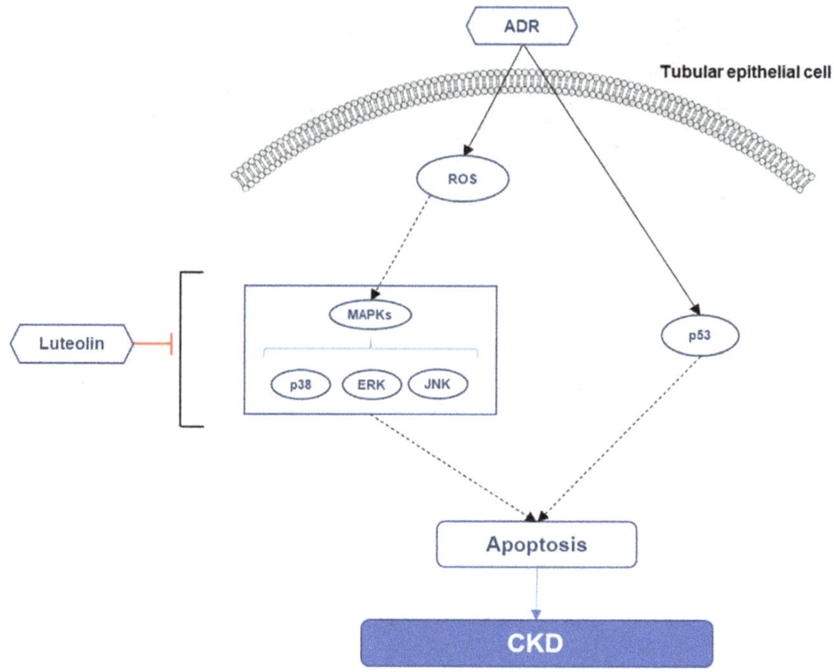

FIGURE 10 | Possible mechanism of luteolin alleviating the apoptosis of renal tubular epithelial cells.

Luteolin Attenuated ADR-Induced Apoptosis by Regulating MAPK and P53 Pathways

According to the results of network pharmacology analysis, luteolin inhibits apoptosis to protect the kidneys against multiple insults. The MAPKs are critical in apoptosis and usually activated by oxidative stress. Thus, we focused on the MAPK pathway to assess the role of luteolin. As shown in **Figure 9B**, ADR significantly promoted the activation of MAPK families (ERK1/2, p38, and JNK) in renal tubular cells, whereas pretreatment of cells with luteolin effectively reduced the phosphorylation of p38, ERK1/2, and JNK. These results suggest that the regulation of MAPK pathways may mediate the protective effect of luteolin on ADR-induced kidney damage, and can be regarded as a link between oxidative stress and apoptosis.

PI3K-Akt pathway plays an important role in cell apoptosis, and it is also one of the top pathways in the KEGG enrichment analysis. We have found that luteolin can reduce the phosphorylation of AKT. Therefore, we further detected the phosphorylation of PI3K. The results showed that the effect of luteolin on PI3K phosphorylation did not reach statistical significance (**Figures 9C,D**). According to the results, the role of PI3K-Akt pathway in luteolin's reduction of apoptosis has not been clarified, and the reason why the changes of PI3K and AKT are not completely parallel needs to be further studied.

The p53 pathway is also closely related to cell apoptosis. In **Figure 7D**, we have found that luteolin can inhibit the phosphorylation of P53. Therefore, down-regulation of the p53 pathway may also be an important mechanism by which luteolin alleviates apoptosis.

Finally, we summarized the possible mechanism of luteolin to reduce the apoptosis of renal tubular cells (**Figure 10**). Additionally, the key pathway maps of MAPK and P53 were also retrieved from KEGG database to provide reference for further in-depth exploration of the mechanism (**Supplementary Figures S4A,B**).

DISCUSSION

Network pharmacological analyses have demonstrated that the main active components of *P. frutescens* are luteolin, β-sitosterol, rosmarinic acid, caffeic acid, and β-carotene. These components can play a therapeutic role in kidney disease by regulating immunity, inflammation, and metabolism (Fuyuno et al., 2018; Huang et al., 2018; Wei et al., 2018). Through their intersection with renal injury-related genes, 108 targets were presently identified. Analysis of these related targets revealed that the core nodes in the PPI network included AKT1, TP53, IL6, TNF, MAPK1, JUN, VEGFA, EGFR, CASP3, CCND1, MYC, RELA, MMP9, IL2, and PTGS2. These are involved in the immune response, inflammation, cell proliferation, and apoptosis. They are closely related to the development and prognosis of CKD. The findings suggest that the above proteins may be the main targets of *P. frutescens* in the treatment of CKD. At the same time, the analysis of the main active component-target network and PPI network revealed the complex and close relationships between each component and target, which are connected to each other in a variety of ways.

GO enrichment analysis revealed that these targets are involved in the composition of various CCs, which regulate the activity of various kinases, nuclear receptors, transcription factors, and the binding capacity of cytokine receptors, chemokine receptors, catecholamines, phosphatases, and proteases. The CCs may have therapeutic roles in CKD stage 3–5 by affecting BPs, such as regulation of transcription and apoptosis, protein phosphorylation, inflammatory response, aging, and cell proliferation.

The enrichment analysis of the KEGG signaling pathway showed that *P. frutescens* slows the progression of CKD by regulating the apoptosis, TCR, PI3K-AKT, HIF-1, TLR, and TNF signaling pathways. Apoptosis disorders are closely associated with CKD. Apoptosis signaling pathways mainly include MAPK, NF-κB, PI3K-AKT, and others, which are closely related to CKD and jointly induce activation of downstream caspase families. These pathways induce abnormal apoptosis of renal TECs and vascular endothelial cells and mediate the continuous progression of the disease. As an important part of cellular immunity, T cells mediate the immune response of the body, promote the release of inflammatory factors and aggravate the inflammatory response. Moreover, the TCR signaling pathway can also regulate Treg differentiation, which plays a crucial role in maintaining homeostasis and physiological function (Li and Rudensky, 2016). The PI3K/AKT pathway is closely related to cell growth and proliferation. Regulation of this pathway can affect renal mesangial cell proliferation and extracellular matrix secretion (Son et al., 2020). Chronic hypoxia is an important pathological factor in CKD. Under hypoxia, the expression of HIF-1α increases, which activates the transcription of downstream factors, such as VEGF and erythropoietin, and improves the hypoxic status of the body (Mudaliar et al., 2013). The inflammatory response is key to the deterioration of CKD. TLR is a ligand-activated membrane-bound receptor that mainly causes an inflammatory response by activating NF-κB. TLR also initiates a downstream signaling cascade reaction, which leads to renal TEC injury and aggravates renal function (Miyata et al., 2013). TNF-α is the most important cytokine in the TNF family. It can initiate downstream biological reactions, such as inflammation and apoptosis, by binding to TNF receptor 1 on the cell surface, including participation in the induction of the caspase family mediated apoptosis and activation of NF-κB, p38, ERK, and other signaling pathways to promote downstream inflammatory responses (Akdis et al., 2016).

It should be noted that, the targets of these active components overlap and cross in multiple pathways and biological functions. For example, the apoptosis signaling pathway in enrichment analysis contained 14 key targets, and the HIF-1 signaling pathway also had 15 targets. Conversely, many targets are involved in multiple biological functions and signaling pathways too. AKT, a key node in the network model, is involved in 45 of all 254 enriched BPs. And it also contributes to 59 enriched signaling pathways, such as apoptosis pathway, HIF-1 pathway, and PI3K-Akt pathway. Recently, research has found that the frequently used herb pairs tend to have shorter distances compared to random herb pairs, and the center distance determined at the ingredient level improves the discrimination of top-frequent herb pairs from random herb pairs (Wang et al., 2021). It provides us with an effective methodological reference, whether in exploring the rules of classic TCM formulas, herb combination, or pharmacological analysis. In supplementary materials **Supplementary Table S1**, we also enumerated some network topology characteristics of the active components and targets, such as Betweenness Centrality and Closeness Centrality. But we have not yet conducted an in-depth and comprehensive discussion on it. This network pharmacology modeling provides a new perspective and method for our follow-up research, and help us to better explore the space of herbal combinations more effectively.

Molecular docking was used to verify the binding ability of the main active components and their corresponding therapeutic targets. The binding ability was good, which further reflected the therapeutic effect of the main active components of *P. frutescens*.

Luteolin, rosmarinic acid, caffeic acid, perilla aldehyde and (+)-catechin were detected by HPLC to construct PFAE fingerprint. These components were also coincident with the aforementioned components obtained from TCMSP database and network pharmacological analysis.

Finally, we selected luteolin, a key component of *P. frutescens*, to verify the mechanism of kidney protection *in vitro*. Accumulating evidence has suggested that luteolin exhibits anti-oxidation, anti-inflammatory, and anti-fibrotic effects (Alekhya et al., 2019). Previous studies have reported that luteolin can reduce renal ischemia-reperfusion injury, lipopolysaccharide or cisplatin induced acute kidney injury, and angiotensin-induced renal injury (Domitrović et al., 2013; Xin et al., 2016; Hong et al., 2017; Liu et al., 2021), but there are few studies on its pharmacological mechanism in CKD. In our study, we found that luteolin can significantly mitigate apoptosis induced by ADR and modulated the phosphorylation of AKT and p53. Meanwhile, the detection of oxidative stress and the key pathway closely related to apoptosis revealed that luteolin can inhibit oxidative stress and down-regulate MAPK pathway. These results suggest that the MAPK and p53 pathways could be the key mechanisms by which luteolin exerts its anti-apoptotic pharmacological effects.

In conclusion, in this study, we clarified the multi-component, multi-target, multi-pathway effects of *P. frutescens* by network pharmacological analysis. Luteolin, the critical component of *P. frutescens*, was identified by network pharmacology and HPLC. *In vitro* experiments, we verified that both luteolin and *P. frutescens* can effectively reduce renal tubular injury, and investigated the mechanism by which luteolin alleviates kidney injury. Luteolin can reduce ADR-induced apoptosis of TECs. Anti-oxidation, down-regulate MAPKs phosphorylation and inhibition of the p53 pathway could be the key mechanisms in it. Our findings revealed that luteolin may be the essential component of *P. frutescens* for treating CKD stage 3–5, which provides a basis and direction for further mechanism research. At the same time, the results also enriched and improved the pharmacological research of *P. frutescens*. It will also help us perform in-depth research on the herb and related formula in the future. However, in this study, we did not verify specific interrelationships between these pathways and apoptosis. We are planning experiments to clarify the specific mechanisms by adding positive control agents, gene transfection and *in vivo* experiments. In addition, we mainly focus on a single component called luteolin. The interaction between various components and targets constitutes the clinical therapeutic effect of TCM, and it is also the feature and advantage of TCM treatment. Recently, researchers have continuously constructed a variety of new network pharmacology models and platforms, thus providing effective strategies for us to better explore herb pairs and formulas (Zhou et al., 2016; Bu et al., 2020; Wang et al., 2021). Therefore, more in-depth studies on drug-drug interactions and combinations might be needed in the future, so as to more comprehensively elucidate the clinical efficacy mechanism of TCM.

AUTHOR CONTRIBUTIONS

EZ conceived and designed the experiments. CY, ZZ, GH, YY, YZ, and LQ performed the experiments. CY, GH, and KG analyzed the data. EZ, FT, LL, QW, ZX, CC, and JZ participated in intellectual discussions. CY, KG, and EZ wrote the manuscript. All authors approved the final version of the manuscript.

FUNDING

This work was supported by the National Natural Science Foundation of China (81873270 to EZ, 81873259 to KG, and 81904115 to JZ), the Science Project of Jiangsu Province Hospital of Traditional Chinese Medicine (Y2018RC17 to EZ), the Top Talents Training Program of Jiangsu Province (WSN-012 to EZ), Advantage Discipline Project of Nanjing University of Chinese Medicine (ZYX03KF076 to EZ), Graduate Research and Practice Innovation Project (SJCX21_0735 to CY), and the Medical International Cooperation Project of Nanjing Municipal Science and Technology Bureau (202002051 to EZ).

ACKNOWLEDGMENTS

The authors thank Prof. Hongzhi Qiao and Yinping Mao of the School of Pharmacy, Nanjing University of Chinese Medicine for the HPLC analysis of PFAE and professional consultation on pharmacology.

REFERENCES

Akdis, M., Aab, A., Altunbulakli, C., Azkur, K., Costa, R. A., Crameri, R., et al. (2016). Interleukins (From IL-1 to IL-38), Interferons, Transforming Growth Factor β, and TNF-α: Receptors, Functions, and Roles in Diseases. *J. Allergy Clin. Immunol.* 138 (4), 984–1010. doi:10.1016/j.jaci.2016.06.033

Alekhya Sita, G. J., Gowthami, M., Srikanth, G., Krishna, M. M., Rama Sireesha, K., Sajjarao, M., et al. (2019). Protective Role of Luteolin Against Bisphenol A-Induced Renal Toxicity Through Suppressing Oxidative Stress, Inflammation, and Upregulating Nrf2/ARE/HO-1 Pathway. *IUBMB Life* 71 (7), 1041–1047. doi:10.1002/iub.2066

Alsanea, S., and Liu, D. (2017). BITC and S-Carvone Restrain High-Fat Diet-Induced Obesity and Ameliorate Hepatic Steatosis and Insulin Resistance. *Pharm. Res.* 34 (11), 2241–2249. doi:10.1007/s11095-017-2230-3

Amdur, R. L., Feldman, H. I., Gupta, J., Yang, W., Kanetsky, P., Shlipak, M., et al. (2016). Inflammation and Progression of CKD: The CRIC Study. *Clin. J. Am. Soc. Nephrol.* 11 (9), 1546–1556. doi:10.2215/CJN.13121215

Bu, D., Xia, Y., Zhang, J., Cao, W., Huo, P., Wang, Z., et al. (2021). FangNet: Mining Herb Hidden Knowledge from TCM Clinical Effective Formulas Using Structure Network Algorithm. *Comput. Struct. Biotechnol. J.* 19, 62–71. doi:10.1016/j.csbj.2020.11.036

Colica, C., Di Renzo, L., Aiello, V., De Lorenzo, A., and Abenavoli, L. (2018). Rosmarinic Acid as Potential Anti-inflammatory Agent. *Rev. Recent Clin. Trials.* 13 (4), 240–242. doi:10.2174/157488711304180911095818

Domitrović, R., Cvijanović, O., Pugel, E. P., Zagorac, G. B., Mahmutefendić, H., and Škoda, M. (2013). Luteolin Ameliorates Cisplatin-Induced Nephrotoxicity in Mice through Inhibition of Platinum Accumulation, Inflammation and Apoptosis in the Kidney. *Toxicology* 310, 115–123. doi:10.1016/j.tox.2013.05.015

Fu, X. J., and Hu, S. Y. (2019). Shenduning Granule Attenuates Renal Injury from Oxidative Stress Through the Nuclear Factor Erythroid 2-Related Factor 2/Antioxidant Response Element Pathway. *Pharmacology* 103 (5-6), 236–245. doi:10.1159/000494981

Fuyuno, Y., Uchi, H., Yasumatsu, M., Morino-Koga, S., Tanaka, Y., Mitoma, C., et al. (20182018). Perillaldehyde Inhibits AHR Signaling and Activates NRF2 Antioxidant Pathway in Human Keratinocytes. *Oxid. Med. Cel Longev.* 2018, 9524657. doi:10.1155/2018/9524657

Guangtang, D., and Huimin, W. (2017). Experience in the Treatment of Chronic Renal Failure by Bupi Yishen Therapy. *Chin. J. Integr. Trad. West. Nephrol.* 18 (09), 818–819. doi:10.3969/j.issn.1009-587X.2017.09.023

Hong, X., Zhao, X., Wang, G., Zhang, Z., Pei, H., and Liu, Z. (20172017). Luteolin Treatment Protects Against Renal Ischemia-Reperfusion Injury in Rats. *Mediators Inflamm.* 2017, 9783893. doi:10.1155/2017/9783893

Huang, X., Xi, Y., Pan, Q., Mao, Z., Zhang, R., Ma, X., et al. (2018). Caffeic Acid Protects Against IL-1β-induced Inflammatory Responses and Cartilage Degradation in Articular Chondrocytes. *Biomed. Pharmacother.* 107, 433–439. doi:10.1016/j.biopha.2018.07.161

Juvet, C., Siddeek, B., Yzydorczyk, C., Vergely, C., Nardou, K., Armengaud, J. B., et al. (2020). Renal Programming by Transient Postnatal Overfeeding: The Role of Senescence Pathways. *Front. Physiol.* 11, 511. doi:10.3389/fphys.2020.00511

Kim, H. R., and Kim, S. Y. (2019). Perilla Frutescens Sprout Extract Protect Renal Mesangial Cell Dysfunction Against High Glucose by Modulating AMPK and NADPH Oxidase Signaling. *Nutrients* 11 (2), 356. doi:10.3390/nu11020356

Li, M. O., and Rudensky, A. Y. (2016). T Cell Receptor Signalling in the Control of Regulatory T Cell Differentiation and Function. *Nat. Rev. Immunol.* 16 (4), 220–233. doi:10.1038/nri.2016.26

Liu, Y. S., Yang, Q., Li, S., Luo, L., Liu, H. Y., Li, X. Y., et al. (2021). Luteolin Attenuates Angiotensin II-induced R-enal D-amage in A-polipoprotein E-deficient M-ice. *Mol. Med. Rep.* 23 (2), 157. doi:10.3892/mmr.2020.11796

Lu, J., Liu, X., Liao, Y., Wang, D., Chen, J., and Li, S. (2018). Jian-Pi-Yi-Shen Formula Regulates Inflammatory Cytokines Production in 5/6 Nephrectomized Rats via Suppression of NF-Kb Activation. *Evid. Based Complement. Alternat Med.* 2018, 7203547. doi:10.1155/2018/7203547

Miyata, T., Suzuki, N., and van Ypersele de Strihou, C. (2013). Diabetic Nephropathy: Are There New and Potentially Promising Therapies Targeting Oxygen Biology? *Kidney Int.* 84 (4), 693–702. doi:10.1038/ki.2013.74

Mudaliar, H., Pollock, C., Komala, M. G., Chadban, S., Wu, H., and Panchapakesan, U. (2013). The Role of Toll-like Receptor Proteins (TLR) 2 and 4 in Mediating Inflammation in Proximal Tubules. *Am. J. Physiol. Ren. Physiol.* 305 (2), F143–F154. doi:10.1152/ajprenal.00398.2012

Qiu, Z., Zheng, K., Zhang, H., Feng, J., Wang, L., and Zhou, H. (2017). Physical Exercise and Patients with Chronic Renal Failure: A Meta-Analysis. *Biomed. Res. Int.* 2017, 7191826. doi:10.1155/2017/7191826

Roellecke, K., Jäger, V. D., Gyurov, V. H., Kowalski, J. P., Mielke, S., Rettie, A. E., et al. (2017). Ligand Characterization of CYP4B1 Isoforms Modified for High-Level Expression in *Escherichia coli* and HepG2 Cells. *Protein Eng. Des. Sel* 30 (3), 205–216. doi:10.1093/protein/gzw075

Sharma, C., Al Kaabi, J. M., Nurulain, S. M., Goyal, S. N., Kamal, M. A., and Ojha, S. (2016). Polypharmacological Properties and Therapeutic Potential of β-Caryophyllene: A Dietary Phytocannabinoid of Pharmaceutical Promise. *Curr. Pharm. Des.* 22 (21), 3237–3264. doi:10.2174/1381612822666160311115226

Song, Y., Liu, W., Tang, K., Zang, J., Li, D., and Gao, H. (2020). Mangiferin Alleviates Renal Interstitial Fibrosis in Streptozotocin-Induced Diabetic Mice Through Regulating the PTEN/PI3K/Akt Signaling Pathway. *J. Diabetes Res.* 2020, 9481720. doi:10.1155/2020/9481720

Song, Y., Sun, R., Ji, Z., Li, X., Fu, Q., and Ma, S. (2018). Perilla Aldehyde Attenuates CUMS-Induced Depressive-like Behaviors via Regulating TXNIP/TRX/NLRP3 Pathway in Rats. *Life Sci.* 206, 117–124. doi:10.1016/j.lfs.2018.05.038

Song, Z., Qin, T., Pan, Y., Wu, L., Liu, T., and Hua, Q. (2019). Shenkang Injection Improves Coagulation in Patients with Chronic Kidney Disease: A Systematic Review and Meta-Analysis. *J. Tradit. Chin. Med.* 39 (4), 451–458. doi:10.19852/j.cnki.jtcm.2019.04.001

Tyszka-Czochara, M., Bukowska-Strakova, K., Kocemba-Pilarczyk, K. A., and Majka, M. (2018). Caffeic Acid Targets AMPK Signaling and Regulates Tricarboxylic Acid Cycle Anaplerosis while Metformin Downregulates HIF-1α-Induced Glycolytic Enzymes in Human Cervical Squamous Cell Carcinoma Lines. *Nutrients* 10 (7), 841. doi:10.3390/nu10070841

Wang, C., Hou, X. X., Rui, H. L., Li, L. J., Zhao, J., Yang, M., et al. (2018). Artificially Cultivated *Ophiocordyceps Sinensis* Alleviates Diabetic Nephropathy and its Podocyte Injury via Inhibiting P2X7R Expression and NLRP3 Inflammasome Activation. *J. Diabetes Res.* 2018, 1390418. doi:10.1155/2018/1390418

Wang, M., Yang, J., and Wang, C. (2020). Shen Shuai II Recipe Attenuates Apoptosis in 5/6 Renal Ablation/Infarction Rats by Inhibiting P53 and the Mitochondrial Pathway of Apoptosis. *Oxid Med. Cel Longev* 2020, 7083575. doi:10.1155/2020/7083575

Wang, N., Du, N., Peng, Y., Yang, K., Shu, Z., Chang, K., et al. (2020). Network Patterns of Herbal Combinations in Traditional Chinese Clinical Prescriptions. *Front. Pharmacol.* 11, 590824. doi:10.3389/fphar.2020.590824

Wang, Y., Yang, H., Chen, L., Jafari, M., and Tang, J. (2021). Network-based Modeling of Herb Combinations in Traditional Chinese Medicine. *Brief Bioinform* 22, bbab106. doi:10.1093/bib/bbab106

Wei, Y., Chen, J., Hu, Y., Lu, W., Zhang, X., Wang, R., et al. (20182018). Rosmarinic Acid Mitigates Lipopolysaccharide-Induced Neuroinflammatory Responses Through the Inhibition of TLR4 and CD14 Expression and NF-Kb and NLRP3 Inflammasome Activation. *Inflammation* 41 (2), 732–740. doi:10.1007/s10753-017-0728-9

Xi, Y., Lu, X., Zhu, L., Sun, X., Jiang, Y., He, W., et al. (2020). Clinical Trial for Conventional Medicine Integrated with Traditional Chinese Medicine (TCM) in the Treatment of Patients with Chronic Kidney Disease. *Medicine (Baltimore)* 99 (21), e20234. doi:10.1097/MD.0000000000020234

Xin, S. B., Yan, H., Ma, J., Sun, Q., and Shen, L. (2016). Protective Effects of Luteolin on Lipopolysaccharide-Induced Acute Renal Injury in Mice. *Med. Sci. Monit.* 22, 5173–5180. doi:10.12659/MSM.898177

Xinqiang, S., Yu, Z., Ningning, Y., Erqin, D., Lei, W., and Hongtao, D. (2020). Molecular Mechanism of Celastrol in the Treatment of Systemic Lupus Erythematosus Based on Network Pharmacology and Molecular Docking Technology. *Life Sci.* 240, 117063. doi:10.1016/j.lfs.2019.117063

Yang, S., and Enchao, Z. (2015). Clinical Study of "Yishen Jiedu Decoction" Combined with Long Range Intermittent Traditional Chinese Medicine Enema in Treatment of 30 Patients with Chronic Kidney Disease Stage 3-4. *Jiangsu J. Trad. Chin. Med.* 47 (11), 29–31. Available at: https://d.wanfangdata.com.cn/periodical/ChlQZXJpb2RpY2FsQ0hJTmV3UzIwMjExMDI2Eg1qc3p5MjAxNTExMDEyGgg3aDJmNXhzNg%3D%3D

Yiye, Z., Enchao, Z., Kun, G., Huang, G-s., Li, W., and Xia, P. (2019). Protective Effect and Mechanism of Aqueous Extract of Perillae Folium on Adriamycin-Induced Oxidative Injury in HK-2 Cell. *Chin. J. Exp. Traditional Med. Formulae* 25 (12), 50–57. doi:10.13422/j.cnki.syfjx.20191238

Zhao, J., Chan, Y. C., He, B., Duan, T. T., and Yu, Z. L. (2019). A Patent Herbal Drug Yi-Shen-Hua-Shi Granule Ameliorates C-BSA-Induced Chronic Glomerulonephritis and Inhabits TGFβ Signaling in Rats. *J. Ethnopharmacol* 236 (23), 258–262. doi:10.1016/j.jep.2019.02.044

Zhou, W., Wang, J., Wu, Z., Huang, C., Lu, A., and Wang, Y. (2016). Systems Pharmacology Exploration of Botanic Drug Pairs Reveals the Mechanism for Treating Different Diseases. *Sci. Rep.* 6, 36985. doi:10.1038/srep36985

11

A Novel Antiplatelet Aggregation Target of Justicidin B Obtained from *Rostellularia Procumbens* (L.) Nees

Yan-Fang Yang[1,2,3†], Song-Tao Wu[1†], Bo Liu[1,2,3], Zhou-Tao Xie[1], Wei-Chen Xiong[1], Peng-Fei Hao[1], Wen-Ping Xiao[1], Yuan Sun[1], Zhong-Zhu Ai[1,2,3], Peng-Tao You[1,2,3] and He-Zhen Wu[1,2,3*]*

[1] Faculty of Pharmacy, Hubei University of Chinese Medicine, Wuhan, China, [2] Key Laboratory of Traditional Chinese Medicine Resources and Chemistry of Hubei Province, Wuhan, China, [3] Collaborative Innovation Center of Traditional Chinese Medicine of New Products for Geriatrics Hubei Province, Wuhan, China

***Correspondence:**
Song-Tao Wu
songt1wu@163.com
He-Zhen Wu
hezh_wu@163.com

†These authors have contributed equally to this work.

The present study explored the possible bioactive ingredients and target protein of *Rostellularia procumbens* (L.) Nees. Firstly, we found that the ethyl acetate extraction obtained from *R. procumbens* could inhibit platelet aggregation. Then, gene chip was used to investigate differentially expressed genes and blood absorption compounds were investigated using high performance liquid chromatography-mass spectrometry characterization (LC-MS). Depending on the results of gene chip and LC-MS, the targets of blood absorption compounds were predicted according to the reverse pharmacophore matching model. The platelet aggregation-related genes were discovered in databases, and antiplatelet aggregation-related gene targets were selected through comparison. The functions of target genes and related pathways were analyzed and screened using the DAVID database, and the network was constructed using Cytoscape software. We found that integrin $\alpha_{IIb}\beta_3$ had a highest degree, and it was almost the intersection of all pathways. Then, blood absorption compounds were screened by optical turbidimetry. Western blot (WB) revealed that justicidin B separated from the ethyl acetate fraction may inhibit the expression of integrin $\alpha_{IIb}\beta_3$ protein. For the first time, we used Prometheus NT.48 and MST to detect the stability of this membrane protein to optimize the buffer and studied the interaction of justicidin B with its target protein. To our best knowledge, this is the first report to state that justicidin B targets the integrin $\alpha_{IIb}\beta_3$ protein. We believe that our findings can provide a novel target protein for the further understanding of the mechanism of *R. procumbens* on platelet aggregation.

Keywords: justicidin B, integrin $\alpha_{IIb}\beta_3$, platelet aggregation, gene chip, LC-MS, network pharmacology, Prometheus NT.48, microscale thermophoresis

INTRODUCTION

Integrin $\alpha_{IIb}\beta_3$ is a major platelet-surface receptor for the regulation of platelet aggregation and thrombosis. Fibrinogen is attached to the integrin $\alpha_{IIb}\beta_3$ protein of one platelet and is linked to the integrin $\alpha_{IIb}\beta_3$ protein of another platelet. At the same time, the platelets are grouped together to cause a platelet aggregation cascade. Therefore, integrin $\alpha_{IIb}\beta_3$ is a key protein for platelet aggregation (Coller and Shattil, 2008; Yun et al., 2016; Andrews and Gardiner, 2017; Bender et al., 2017; Chatterjee and Gawaz, 2017).

Rostellularia procumbens (L.) Nees (Acanthaceae) is widely distributed in the Taiwan Province and the southwest provinces and has been proven to have a huge potential for the development of Chinese medicine owing to its plant resources, chemical constituents, pharmacological action, and clinical application. It has complex chemical composition (Savithramma et al., 2007; Joshi and Joshi, 2000; Committee, 2011).

In addition, reports have shown that *R. procumbens* has significant pharmacological properties such as anti-viral and anti-tumoral (Chen et al., 1995; Corrêa and Alcântara, 2012). It has also been noted that aqueous extracts of *R. procumbens* decrease platelet aggregation (Chen et al., 1996). According to preliminary experiments, ethyl acetate extract is the active fraction. Animal experimentation conducted analyze this fraction. Then, gene chip was used to investigate differentially expressed genes. Blood absorption compounds were investigated using LC-MS. Targets of blood absorption compounds were predicted according to the reverse pharmacophore matching model. The platelet aggregation-related genes were found in databases, and antiplatelet aggregation-related gene targets were selected through comparison. The functions of target genes and related pathways were analyzed and screened using the DAVID database, and the network of antiplatelet aggregation effect of blood absorption compounds was constructed using Cytoscape software. However, the detailed molecular interaction between justicidin B and its target is still unknown. Firstly, blood absorption compounds were screened by optical turbidimetry. Prometheus NT.48 is used to detect protein stability and screen buffer (Maschberger et al.). Then, we compared the two models of microscale thermophoresis (MST) and used NT.115 to verify the interaction between the compound and the integrin $\alpha_{IIb}\beta_3$ protein (van den Bogaart et al., 2012; Batoulis et al., 2016; Sparks and Fratti, 2019; Vinothkannan Ravichandran et al., 2018).

In this study, according to preliminary experiments, blood absorption compounds of *R. procumbens* were screened by serum pharmacological. Gene chip and network pharmacology were used to find the target. Then, the interaction between justicidin B and the membrane protein integrin $\alpha_{IIb}\beta_3$ was verified by Western blot (WB) and MST. It would lay the groundwork for understanding the molecular mechanism involved in the inhibition of platelet aggregation by *R. procumbens.*

MATERIALS AND METHODS

Chemical and Materials

The ethyl acetate extract was obtained from the Key Laboratory for Traditional Chinese Medicine Resources and Chemistry of Hubei Province (Chen, 2012; Su, 2014; Wu et al., 2013) [ethyl acetate (EtOAc), Lichrosolv, purity ≥ 99.9%]. Acetonitrile (ACN) was of LC-MS grade and was purchased from Thermo-Fisher (Pittsburgh, PA, USA). Deionized water was made available in-lab using a Milli-Q purification instrument (Millipore, Bedford, MA, USA). 5-Hydroxytryptophan was obtained from National Institutes for Food and Drug Control (China). Thrombin was purchased from BioMed Lublin, Poland. Arachidonic acid (AA), bovine serum albumin (BSA), adenosine diphosphate (ADP), β-acetyl-γ-O-hexadecyl-L-α-phospharidylcholine hydrate (PAF), 12-O-tetradecanoylphorbol-13-acetate (PMA), and dimethyl sulfoxide (DMSO) were purchased from Sigma (St. Louis, MO, USA). RNeasy Mini Kit and RNase-free DNase I were purchased from QIAGEN. Pico Reagent Kit, GeneChip90 Hybridization, Wash, and Stain Kit were purchased from Affymetrix. Integrin $\alpha_{IIb}\beta_3$ monoclonal antibody was purchased from SAB (Maryland, USA), and β-actin and anti-mouse IgG were purchased from Cell Signaling (Boston, USA).

Experimental Animals

SD male rats (190–230 g) were randomly divided into two groups of 16 animals per group, treated orally as follows: control group received 0.5% CMC-Na, groups of ethyl acetate extract (97.20 g/ml) (fasting for 12 h before intragastric administration, administered by intragastric administration at 1 ml/200 mg twice a day for 3 days). After the last administration for 1.5 h, we took 5–8 ml of blood from the femoral artery. All experimental procedures were approved by Animal Care and Use Committee of Institute of Materia Medica, People's Republic of China.

Extraction and Detection of Total RNA in Two Groups of Platelets

The platelet of the control group and ethyl acetate group at 4°C and 12,000 rpm was centrifuged for 10 min using RNeasy Mini Kit separation of total RNA. The RNA concentration and A260/A280 ratio were determined using an SMA 3000 microspectrophotometer (Meriton, China). The results showed that the ratio was 2.00:2.05, indicating a high purity of the extracted RNA, which was deemed suitable for subsequent analysis. After this, a total of 1 μg RNA was used for 1% agarose gel electrophoresis. The ratio of 28S/18S was then determined using a JS-380A Bioanalyzer (Shanghai, China) to determine the quality of RNA. If the RNA integrity number (RIN) > 7.0 and 28S/18S > 0.7, samples were transcribed by a Pico Reagent Kit. Following this, samples were prepared using a GeneChip90 Hybridization, Wash, and Stain Kit (Affymetrix, Thermo Fisher Scientific, Inc.). Then, chips were scanned using a GeneChip Scanner 3000 (Affymetrix, Thermo Fisher Scientific, Inc.).

Detection of Blood Absorption Compounds

Justicidin B, chinensinaphthol methyl ether, and 6'-hydroxy justicidin B were weighed accurately, and 1 mg/ml control solution with methanol was prepared. The control solution was stored at 4°C for use. The supernatant that was treated by solid phase microextraction cartridge was collected and dried by nitrogen after centrifugation (12,000 r/min, 10 min). Before the liquid injection, 200 μl acetonitrile was used for redissolution and the supernatant was determined by HPLC-DAD-ESI-MS after filtration.

The chromatography analysis was performed on an Agilent XDB-C18 column (150 mm × 4.6 mm, 4 μm) at 25°C; the mobile phase was a mixture of aqueous solutions containing water (A) and acetonitrile (B). The gradient elution procedure was made as follows: 0–14 min, 26% B; 14–51 min, 26–38.5% B; 51–80 min, 38.5% B. The injection volume was 100 µl, and the flow rate was 1 ml/min. The wavelength of 190–690 nm was used for the detection. Mass spectrometry detection was set as follows: capillary temperature, 200°C; source voltage, 4.5 kV for the positive ion mode. The mass range was from 50 to 1,600. Blood absorption compounds were identified by accurate mass, MS/MS ion fragment pattern, and retention time of LC and then were validated by available standard.

Prediction and Analysis of Differentially Expressed Target Genes

Based on the results of the gene chip and LC-MS, we conducted a network pharmacology study. The PharmMapper Server (http://lilab.ecust.edu.cn/pharmmapper/index.php) is a freely accessed web server used to identify potential target candidates for given probe blood absorption compounds using a pharmacophore mapping approach. GeneCards (https://www.genecards.org/) and MalaCards (http://www.malacards.org/) were used for potential target screening from the results of gene chip. All potential target genes were collected and uploaded to the DAVID (https://david.ncifcrf.gov/summary.jsp) database. Following this, the functions and signaling pathways of target genes as well as pathway enrichment were investigated *via* Gene Ontology (GO; http://geneontology.org/) and Kyoto Encyclopedia of Genes and Genomes (KEGG) pathway analyses (http://www.genome.jp/kegg/ko.html).

Construction of the Network

The blood absorption compounds and target genes were imported into Cytoscape 3.6.1 software to build an active compound/target gene/pathway network and an active compound/platelet aggregation-related target gene network. The blood absorption compounds and target genes were input as the node. If there was a connection between two nodes, edge was used to show the connection.

The network was then analyzed with the network analyze function. High degree gene targets in the protein interaction network were analyzed. According to the results of KEGG enrichment, the pathways with higher counts were selected to analyze their key targets. Meanwhile, the genes suitable for the analysis of the targets were obtained through comparative analysis from the literature and database.

Screening of Active Compounds Inhibiting Platelet Aggregation

Platelet-rich plasma (PRP) was prepared by centrifugation of fresh blood at 200×*g* for 10 min at room temperature and aspirating the supernatant. Platelet-poor plasma was then sedimented by centrifugation of residual blood at 800×*g* for 10 min at room temperature. Blood platelet aggregation was monitored by platelet turbidity, with 0% aggregation calibrated as the absorbance of platelet-poor plasma and 100% aggregation as the absorbance of PRP. PRP was incubated with the drug at 37°C for 20 min and then stimulated with AA, ADP, thrombin, PAF, and PMA. The aggregation of PRP (preincubated with the tested plant fraction) in response to 10 µM inducer was recorded using an aggregometer (LBY-NJ4).

Western Blotting to Detect Integrin $\alpha_{IIb}\beta_3$

Just like 2.7, we got PRP what were split into four groups: blank control group, inducer group, justicidin B induction group, and the last group received aspirin. Different groups were cultured 1.5 h, and the incubator was set to 5% CO_2 at 37°C. Then, platelets were washed with PBS twice, harvested, and lysed in RIPA buffer containing protease inhibitors on ice for 60 min. The protein concentration was determined by the BCA method. Next, protein samples (18 µg) were equally loaded onto SDS-PAGE and electrotransferred to PVDF membranes. Subsequently, the membranes were blocked with 5% non-fat milk for 1 h and incubated overnight with primary antibodies. The membranes were washed with TBST buffer three times and then incubated with secondary antibodies for 1 h at 25°C. The membranes were then rinsed three times with blocking solution and visualized by the ECL detection system.

NT. LabelFree Analysis

Since integrin $\alpha_{IIb}\beta_3$ is a membrane protein, we used NT. LabelFree to prevent the label from affecting the results. Titration series with ligand concentrations varying between 0 and 1,000 mM were prepared in the Prometheus NT.48 optimized buffer (**Figure S1**). SD-test (the automatic pre-detection of MST to detect the stability of protein signal) was required before measurement.

Approximately, 3 µl was loaded into NT.LabelFree standard-treated capillaries (Nanotemper). MST experiments were performed at 40% MST (infra-red laser) power and 60% LED power at 25°C using the Monolith NT.LabelFree Instrument (Nanotemper). Ratios between normalized initial fluorescence and after temperature-jump and thermophoresis were calculated and averaged from five to nine independent runs. Means of fluorescence intensity obtained by the MST measurements were fitted, and the resultant Kd values were given together with an error estimation from the fit by the built-in formula of the analysis software.

NT.115 Analysis

The fluorescence of the ligand interfered with the result. This was further exacerbated when using label-free thermophoresis owing to the additional noise present in measuring fluorescence in ranges where inherent fluorescence of the protein itself is measured. After the SD-test experiment verified that the label had little effect on the protein, we used NT.115 for measurement.

All the compounds were analyzed with the concentration gradient of 50 µM with 20 µM of CviR that was labeled Monolith NTTM Protein Labeling Kit RED–NHS (Cat Nr: L001) before instrumental analysis. LED power was 20% and Prometheus NT.48 optimized buffer was used only for the analysis.

Analysis was performed on Monolith Nano Temper (NT)115 and its accessory, i.e., standard-treated 4-µl volume glass capillaries were employed to measure the molecular interaction (Nano Temper Technologies GmbH, Munich, Germany). Means of fluorescence intensity obtained by the MST measurements were fitted, and the resultant Kd values were given together with an error estimation from the fit by the built-in formula of NT1.5.41 analysis software.

RESULTS

Microarray Results

Compared with the control group, hundreds of genes were revealed to be differentially expressed in platelet in EtOAc extract group (**Table 1**). In EtOAc extract group, PLCB2, PRKCA, GNAQ, MAPK10, MAPK8, MAPK11, MAPK14, GNAI2, PIK3CG, and PIK3R1 were markedly down-regulated in the model group compared with the control group.

The Blood Absorptions Compounds of EtOAc Extract

All samples were analyzed by LC-MS according to chromatographic conditions. By comparing the relative retention time and UV absorption spectra of the chromatographic peaks of the test solution and the mixed control solution, the information of the mass spectrometry fragmentation, combined with the preliminary research results and literature of the laboratory, we can confirm that 6'-hydroxy justicidin B, justicidin B, and chinensinaphthol methyl ether are the prototype compounds of the ethyl acetate extract in the blood (**Figure 1**, **Table 2**).

Prediction and Analysis of the Target Genes

All potential target genes were synthesized and uploaded to the DAVID database for KEGG pathway annotation and GO enrichment. The threshold was set as $P \leq 0.05$, and the pathways or gene functions with higher count were analyzed. The top 10 pathways were graphed by GraphPad Prism 6 (**Figure 2**).

KEGG pathway annotation showed that 30 of the 31 potential target genes were enriched (96.8%) and involved 62 pathways, and 27 of these pathways were significantly correlated with the target genes ($P \leq 0.05$). The following pathways had the largest number of genes involved: Platelet activation (11, 35.5%), Rapl signaling pathway (12, 38.7%), Focal adhesion (9, 29.0%), Proteoglycans in cancer (8, 25.8%), PI3K-Akt signaling pathway (7, 22.6%), and Pathways in cancer (7, 22.6%). GO enrichment analysis showed that the number of genes involved in the CC (Cell Components), MF (Molecular Function), and BP (Biological Process) targets was 31 (100%). CC enrichment was mainly involved in following target genes: extracellular exosome (19, 61.3%), plasma membrane (16, 51.6%), and cytosol (14, 45.2%). MF enrichment was mainly involved in the following target genes: protein binding (25, 80.6%), ATP binding (9, 29.0%), and enzyme binding (8, 25.8%). BP enrichment was mainly involved in the following target genes: platelet aggregation (5, 16.1%), platelet activation (6, 19.4%), and blood coagulation (6, 19.4%).

TABLE 1 | The top different 50 genes of platelet expression between the ethyl acetate extract group and blank group.

Rank	Gene symbol	Gene annotation
1	PRKACG	Protein kinase, cAMP-dependent, catalytic, gamma
2	PRKCA	Protein kinase C, alpha
3	ADCY5	Adenylate cyclase 5
4	PLCB2	Phospholipase C, beta 2
5	PLCB4	Phospholipase C, beta 4
6	NFKB1	Nuclear factor of kappa light polypeptide gene enhancer in B-cells 1
7	TJP1	Tight junction protein 1
8	CTNNB1	Catenin (cadherin-associated protein), beta 1
9	ENPP3	Ectonucleotide pyrophosphatase/ phosphodiesterase 3
10	GLB1	Galactosidase, beta 1
11	GJA1	Gap junction protein, alpha 1
12	ADCY4	Adenylate cyclase 4
13	CYP2C9	Cytochrome P450, family 2, subfamily C, polypeptide 9
14	CDC42	Cell division cycle 42
15	MAPK10	Mitogen-activated protein kinase 10
16	MAPK8	Mitogen-activated protein kinase 8
17	CYP4A11	Cytochrome P450, family 4, subfamily A, polypeptide 11
18	PIK3CG	Phosphoinositide-3-kinase, catalytic, gamma polypeptide
19	NT5E	5'-Nucleotidase, ecto
20	PTGS1	Prostaglandin-endoperoxide synthase 1
21	STAT1	Signal transducer and activator of transcription 1
22	PIK3R1	Phosphoinositide-3-kinase, regulatory subunit 1
23	PLD2	Phospholipase D2
24	PIK3CD	Phosphoinositide-3-kinase, catalytic, delta polypeptide
25	MAOB	Monoamine oxidase B
26	GSK3B	Glycogen synthase kinase 3 beta
27	MAPK11	Mitogen-activated protein kinase 11
28	MAPK14	Mitogen-activated protein kinase 14
29	EGFR	Epidermal growth factor receptor
30	VEGFA	Vascular endothelial growth factor A
31	ATF4	Activating transcription factor 4
32	CRKL	v-crk sarcoma virus CT10 oncogene homolog
33	PPP2CB	Protein phosphatase 2, catalytic subunit, beta isozyme
34	PPP2R1A	Protein phosphatase 2, regulatory subunit A, alpha
35	GBA	Glucosidase, beta, acid
36	IMPAD1	Inositol monophosphatase domain containing 1
37	HK2	Hexokinase 2
38	HK3	Hexokinase 3
39	CYP3A4	Cytochrome P450, family 3, subfamily A, polypeptide 4
40	ITGB2	Integrin, beta 2 (complement component 3 receptor 3 and 4 subunit)
41	UGT2B7	UDP glucuronosyltransferase 2 family, polypeptide B7
42	SMAD3	SMAD family member 3
43	RAF1	cdna:known gene:ENSG00000132155
44	CYP2B6	Cytochrome P450, family 2, subfamily B, polypeptide 6
45	PLB1	Phospholipase B1
46	ACAA2	Acetyl-CoA acyltransferase 2
47	GNAI1	G protein, alpha inhibiting activity polypeptide 1
48	GNAI2	G protein, alpha inhibiting activity polypeptide 2
49	ACAA2	Acetyl-CoA acyltransferase 2
50	GNAQ	G protein, alpha q polypeptide

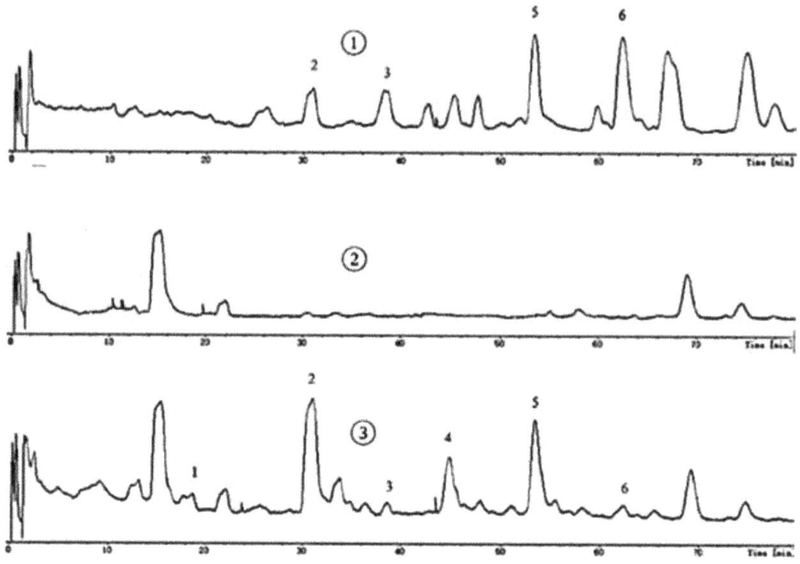

FIGURE 1 | Mass spectrometry.

TABLE 2 | HPLC-DAD-ESI-MS data and identification of the compounds *in vitro* and *in vivo*.

Peak	TR/ min	MW	Molecular formula	*In vitro* compounds (*m/z*)	Blood absorptions compounds (*m/z*)	Identification
1	18.8	352	$C_{20}H_{16}O_6$	—	353.1012, 335.0896, 325.0494, 307.0914	ProcumbenosideL conversion compound
2	31.0	380	$C_{21}H_{16}O_7$	381.0975,363.0875, 337.1063,279.0969, 137.0161	381.1050, 363.0880, 337.1122, 279.0973, 137.0189	6'-Hydroxy justicidin B
3	38.6	410	$C_{22}H_{18}O_8$	411.1084,393.0962, 274.0833, 137.0189	411.1064, 393.0958, 274.0819, 137.0177	6'-Hydroxy justicidin A
4	44.8	410	$C_{22}H_{18}O_8$	433.0881,411.1051, 393.0939,381.0966, 244.5356	433.0878, 411.1049, 393.1009, 381.0866, 244.5389	6'-Hydroxy justicidin C
5	53.4	364	$C_{21}H_{16}O_6$	365.1105,335.0881, 321.1084, 291.0983	365.1105, 335.0881, 321.1084, 291.0983	Justicidin B
6	62.4	394	$C_{22}H_{18}O_7$	395.1194,381.0905, 365.0982,351.1203, 244.0503	417.0942, 395.1110, 381.1024, 351.1185, 244.0505	Chinensinaphthol methyl ether

Construction of the Network

According to the results of gene chip, target genes in the top 10 pathways and compounds were selected to construct an active compound/target gene/pathway network and an active compound/platelet aggregation-related target gene network (**Figure 3**). The network diagram shows the synergistic effect of various compounds on multiple targets when *R. procumbens* plays a role in antiplatelet aggregation effects.

The network analyze tool was used to analyze the network, and genes with higher degree were associated with more genes. It can be considered that the corresponding protein of the genes plays an important role in central correlation when *R. procumbens* plays an antiplatelet aggregation role. The integrin $\alpha_{II}b\beta3$ (integrin $\alpha_{II}b\beta3$ is a protein that in humans is encoded by the ITGA2B and ITGB3 gene) had the highest degree; it was the intersection of all platelet-related pathways.

The results were compared with those of the KEGG pathway analysis and combined with the literature study. Integrin $\alpha_{IIb}\beta_3$ was selected as the target for the binding validation experiment.

Screening of Active Compounds

Platelet with four kinds of inducers was stimulated, and platelet aggregation was detected after being incubated by these isolated blood absorption compounds. The platelet aggregation inhibition rate (MIR) was calculated to indicate the inhibitory activity of the drug. Results showed that those justicidin B groups had higher maximum aggregation compared with others. The remaining compounds showed different degrees of antiplatelet aggregation (**Table 3**, **Figure 4**).

Integrin $\alpha_{IIb}\beta_3$ Expression in PRP

We investigated whether justicidin B had a regulatory effect on integrin $\alpha_{IIb}\beta_3$ expression. As shown in **Figure 4**, the integrin $\alpha_{IIb}\beta_3$ level was significantly increased on the inducer group

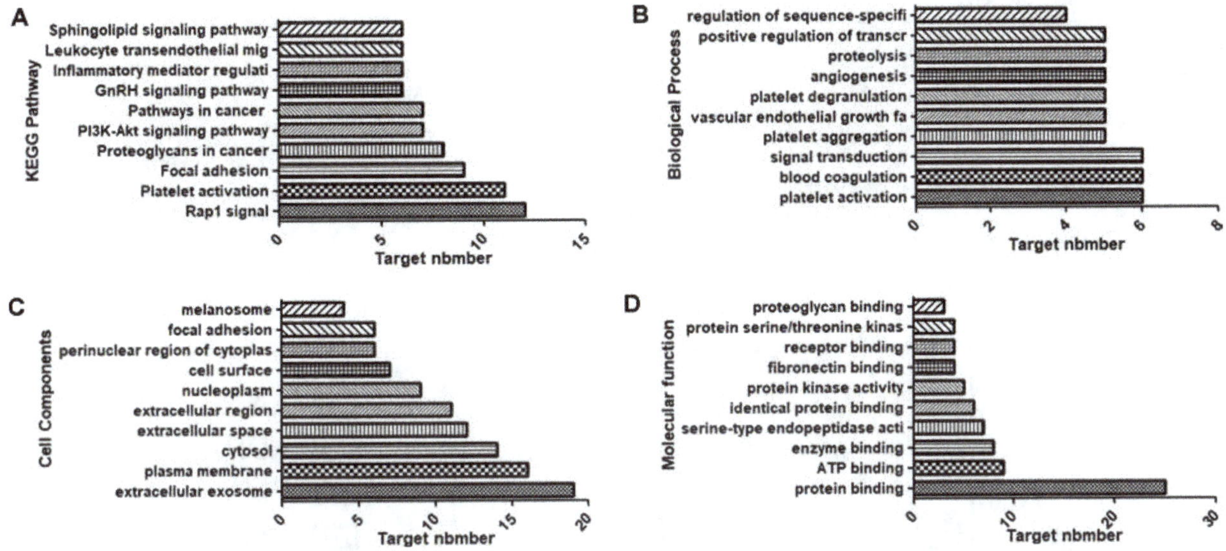

FIGURE 2 | Top 10 components of the KEGG pathway and GO enrichment analyses. **(A)** KEGG pathways. **(B)** Biological process. **(C)** Cell components. **(D)** Molecular function.

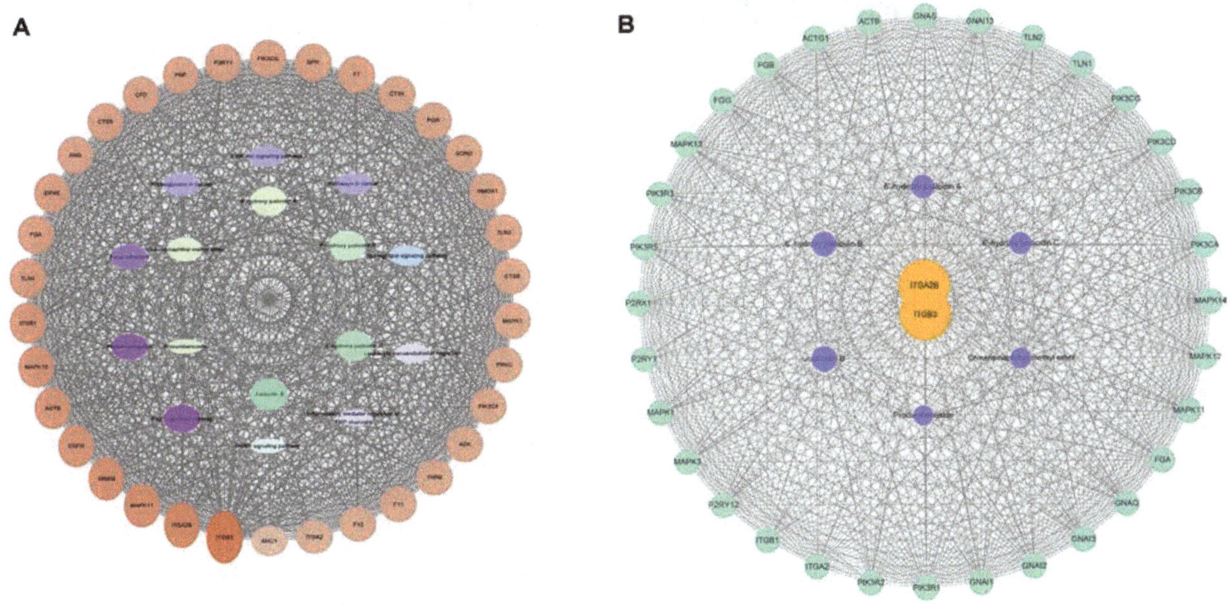

FIGURE 3 | Network diagram constructed by Cytoscape. **(A)** Network diagram of active components/target genes/enrichment pathways. **(B)** Network diagram of active components/platelet aggregation-related target genes.

($P < 0.01$, versus control group). More remarkably, justicidin B produced a dramatically inhibited effect on integrin $\alpha_{IIb}\beta_3$ level (versus inducer group, $P < 0.01$, **Figure 5**).

NT. LabelFree

MST experiments were performed to detect the molecular interaction between inhibitor and integrin $\alpha_{IIb}\beta_3$. Owing to the influence of ligand fluorescence, we obtained unsatisfactory results under the SD-test pass condition, accompanied by large errors (**Figure 6**).

NT.115

The SD-test verified that the label had less effect on the protein. We used NT.115 for the experiment. As differences in

TABLE 3 | MIR (%) of different compounds.

Compounds (x ± SD, n = 3)	MIR (%)				
	AA	ADP	PMA	PAF	Thrombin
Aspirin	93.43 ± 2.81	93.88 ± 1.75	71.26 ± 1.21	7.22 ± 2.51	34.59 ± 0.77
Chinensinaphthol methyl ether	67.94 ± 1.27	43.12 ± 2.74	42.22 ± 1.16	18.40 ± 0.12	1.04 ± 1.51
Justicidin B	97.04 ± 0.85	61.26 ± 1.05	19.18 ± 1.28	27.87 ± 1.39	30.76 ± 2.27
6'-Hydroxy justicidin B	36.53 ± 1.29	36.46 ± 1.01	70.69 ± 1.25	4.13 ± 0.95	0.50 ± 0.74

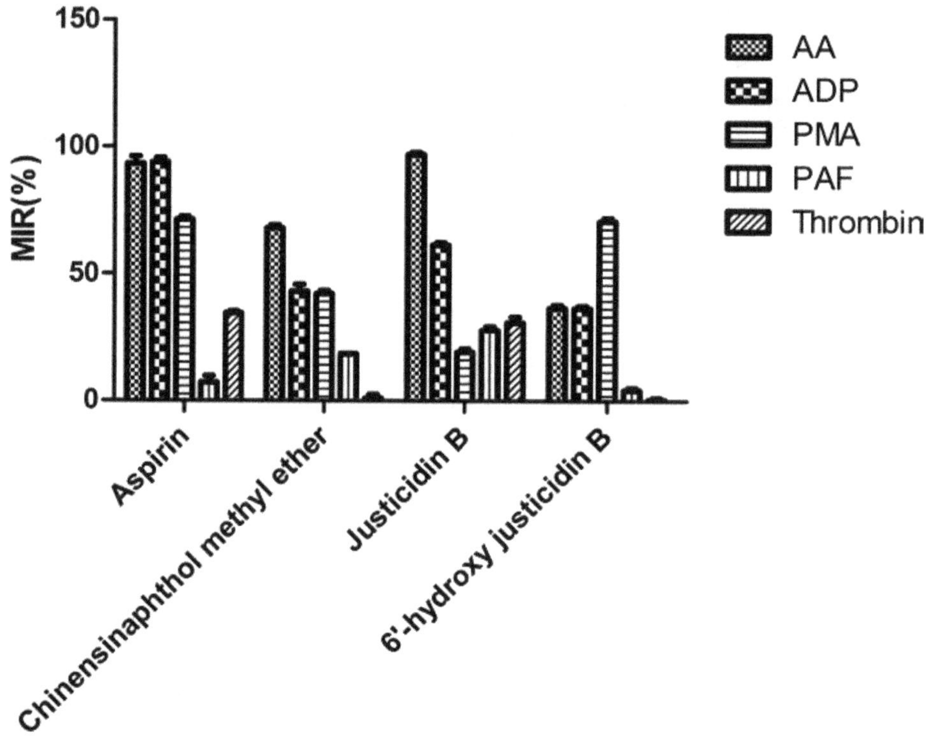

FIGURE 4 | MIR (%) of different compounds.

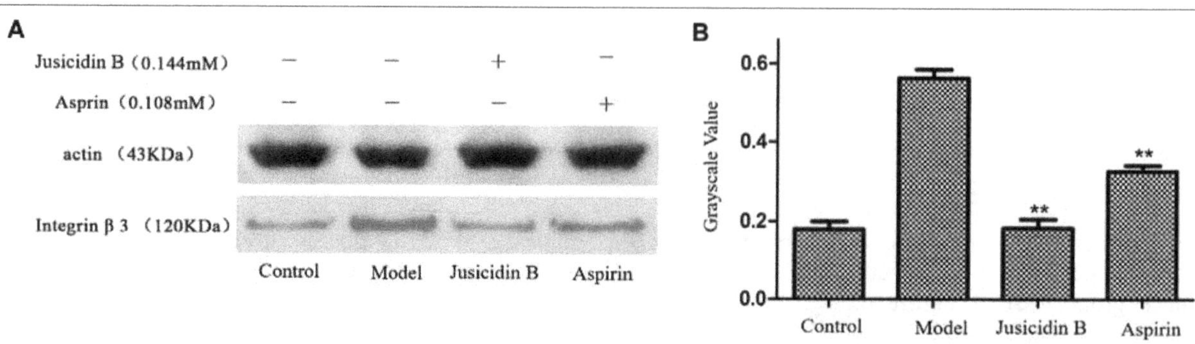

FIGURE 5 | The influence of justicidin B on integrin $\alpha_{IIb}\beta_3$ protein. **(A)** Western blot. **(B)** Grayscale value.

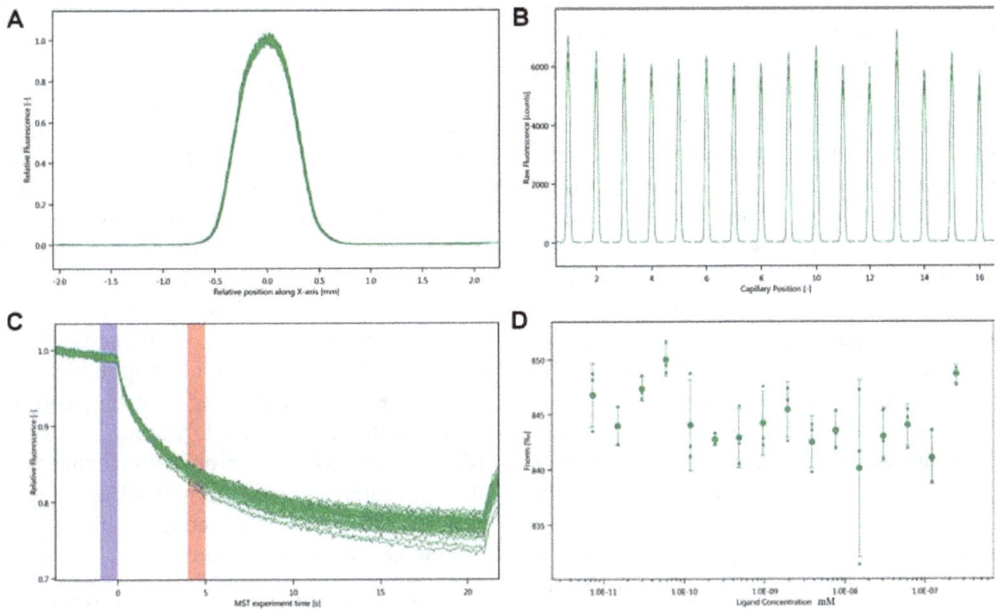

FIGURE 6 | Molecular interaction of integrin $\alpha_{IIb}\beta_3$ using NT. LabelFree analysis. **(A)** SD-TEST capillary shap. **(B)** SD-TEST capillary scan. **(C)** MST time traces of 16 different justicin B concentrations (ranging from 0.00748 to 245 µM). **(D)** Dependence of the MST signal on the justicin B concentration (measured 30 s after turning on heating; data from **C**).

normalized fluorescence of the bound and unbound state allow determination of the fraction bound, the dissociation constant was thus calculated. All values were multiplied by a factor of 1,000, which yielded the relative fluorescence change in per thousand. The Kd values of justicin B were 35.017 ± 5.9014 µm (**Figure 7**).

DISCUSSION

R. procumbens has been used in herbal medicines for promoting blood circulation and pain relief. Modern pharmacological studies have shown that *R. procumbens* has a good antiplatelet aggregation effect (Chen et al., 1996). According to preliminary

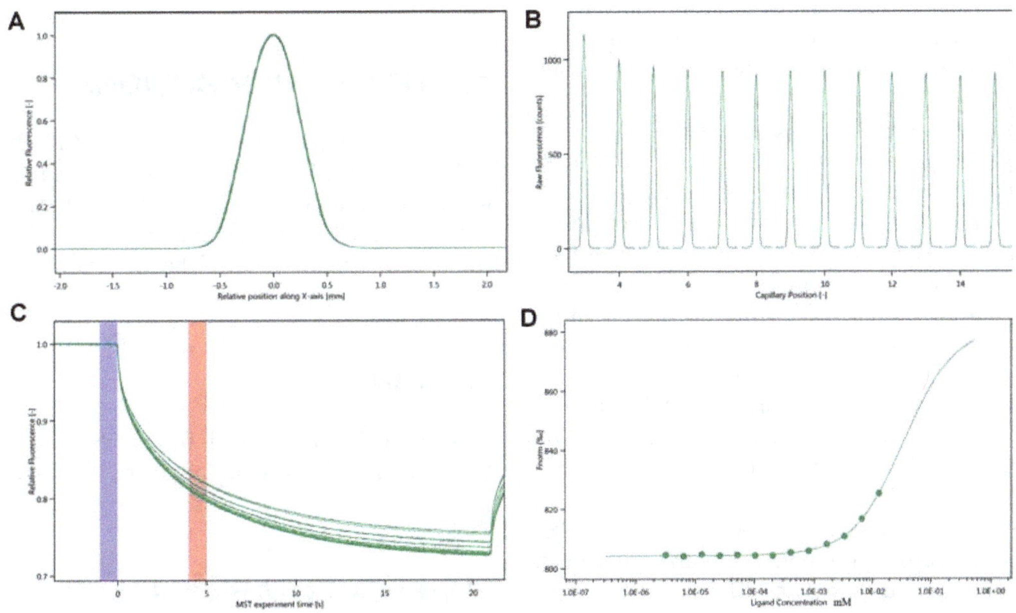

FIGURE 7 | Molecular interaction of integrin $\alpha_{IIb}\beta_3$ using NT. 115 analysis. **(A)** SD-TEST capillary shap. **(B)** SD-TEST capillary scan. **(C)** MST time traces of 16 different justicin B concentrations (ranging from 0.0032 to 13.1 mM). **(D)** Dependence of the MST signal on the justicin B concentration (measured 30 s after turning on heating; data from **C**).

experiments, ethyl acetate extract is the active fraction. However, the chemical composition of this plant material is quite complex. Therefore, it was difficult to determine the active ingredient and target protein by using traditional methods.

The animal experiment was utilized for further verification. Results of gene chip illustrated that ethyl acetate extract could inhibit Gq–PLC–PKC pathway and Gi–PI3K–MAPK pathway. The down-regulation of GNAI1 gene related to the regulation of AC kinase was also observed, indicating that the ethyl acetate site can reduce inhibitory effect of Gi and enhance the activity of AC kinase. This result indicated that the ethyl acetate site could regulate the GI–AC–CAMP signaling pathway. Above all, ethyl acetate might inhibit platelet aggregation by inhibiting Gq–PLC–PKC, Gi–PI3K–MAPK, and other signaling pathways.

In order to further explore the material basis of *R. procumbens*, the blood absorption compounds of *R. procumbens* were screened by serum pharmacological method. Based on the results of the gene chip and LC-MS, GO enrichment analysis found that the targets involved extracellular exosome, plasma membrane, extracellular space, cytosol, and other cell compartments. At the molecular level, the targets were involved in protein binding, enzyme binding, ATP binding, and other molecular activities, and they were related to platelet aggregation, platelet activation, and platelet degranulation. It indicated that the drug may inhibit platelet aggregation by binding to membrane proteins, affecting its energy utilization and activation. The pathway enrichment results also indicated that *R. procumbens* may play an antiplatelet aggregation role by inhibiting the key targets of the platelet activation signaling pathway, such as integrin $\alpha_{IIb}\beta_3$. It was the intersection of all platelet-related pathways. Proteoglycans in cancer, PI3K–Akt signaling pathway, and so on also suggest that justicidin B may affect the expression and activity of cancer-related proteins by binding integrin $\alpha_{IIb}\beta_3$.

Then, we use optical turbidimetry to measure the activity of three isolated blood absorption compounds. We found that justicidin B is the most active compound. Then, WB experiment verified this fact. It is well known that membrane proteins are less stable, and this has shown to have a massive impact on the MST (NT.LabelFree) experiment (Chasis and Mohandas, 1986). To identify optimal test and storage conditions for the membrane protein integrin $\alpha_{IIb}\beta_3$, the protein was subjected to a thermal unfolding formulation screen of the Prometheus NT.48 (supplementary material). NanoTemper's on-the-fly technology allows to measure 48 samples in parallel, providing more than 10 data points per minute. Formulation developments benefit from ultra-high resolution that are not compromised by aggregation but, at the same time, offer ease of use. Prometheus NT.48 results suggest that Hepes is the best detergent. The onset for ratio of Hepes-DDM is 46.1°C, which is higher than other buffers. This attempt was not reported before.

MST is a powerful technique to measure biomolecular interaction that are based on thermophoresis—the movement of molecules in a temperature gradient. This technique was reported to be highly sensitive such that it allows precise quantification of molecular interaction (Jerabek-Willemsen et al., 2014). Because of the influence of ligand fluorescence, we obtained unsatisfactory results, accompanied by relatively large errors. The results of the Prometheus NT.48 experiment showed that the protein stability was relatively good, and the labeled protein SD-test was qualified; hence, we experimented further with NT.115 and obtained better results. MST results suggest that the selected compound has potential molecular interaction with integrin $\alpha_{IIb}\beta_3$. The Kd value of justicin B was 35.017 ± 5.9014 μm. These data suggest that justicin B has a good interaction with integrin $\alpha_{IIb}\beta_3$. According to Seidel et al. (2013), the fitting curve may be either S-shaped or mirror S-shaped. The standard symbol of MST amplitude (change in normalized fluorescence) depends on the chemistry of the compound that is titrated, its binding site, and the conformational change induced upon binding. Justicin B shows a positive slope suggesting a strong conformational change induced upon complex formation. Probably its interaction plays a major role in conformational change. We speculate that it might interfere with the platelet aggregation mechanism by negatively influencing the conformational changes required for the integrin $\alpha_{IIb}\beta_3$ activation.

Taken together, our results demonstrate that the ethyl acetate extract plays an anti-platelet aggregation role through integrin $\alpha_{IIb}\beta_3$, and justicin B, which is the most active blood absorption compound, targets it. We believe that our findings would provide a better foundation for further understanding of the mechanism of *R. procumbens* intervention in platelet aggregation.

ETHICS STATEMENT

This study was carried out in accordance with the recommendations of Animal Care and Use Committee of Institute of Materia Medica, China.

AUTHOR CONTRIBUTIONS

H-ZW conceived the study. H-ZW and Y-FY designed the study. S-TW performed the experiments and the data analysis, and wrote the manuscript. Y-FY, W-CX, BL, P-FH, W-PX, YS, Z-ZA, P-TY, and Z-TX revised the manuscript. All the authors read and approved the final version of the manuscript.

FUNDING

This research was funded by the National Natural Science Foundation of China, grant number 31570343.

SUPPLEMENTARY MATERIAL

FIGURE S1 | Thermal unfolding curves. **(A)** Thermal unfolding curves in presence of Hepes and pbs. **(B)** Thermal unfolding curves in presence of Ttis. Insets show the detergent dependence of the first unfolding transition midpoint (Tm1).

REFERENCES

Andrews, R. K., and Gardiner, E. E. (2017). Basic mechanisms of platelet receptor shedding. *Platelets* 28, 319–324. doi: 10.1080/09537104.2016.1235690

Batoulis, H., Schmidt, T. H., Weber, P., Schloetel, J.-G., Kandt, C., and Lang, T. (2016). Concentration dependent ion-protein interaction patterns underlying protein oligomerization behaviours. *Sci. Rep.* 6, 24131. doi: 10.1038/srep24131

Bender, M., Stegner, D., and Nieswandt, B. (2017). Model systems for platelet receptor shedding. *Platelets* 28, 325–332. doi: 10.1080/09537104.2016.1195491

Chasis, J. A., and Mohandas, N. (1986). Erythrocyte membrane deformability and stability: two distinct membrane properties that are independently regulated by skeletal protein associations. *J. Cell. Biol.* 103, 343–350. doi: 10.1083/jcb.103.2.343

Chatterjee, M., and Gawaz, M. (2017). Clinical significance of receptor shedding-platelet GPVI as an emerging diagnostic and therapeutic tool. *Platelets.* 28, 362–371. doi: 10.1080/09537104.2016.1227062

Chen, Q.-J. (2012). *The preliminary study of anti-chronic nephritis from Rostellularia procumbens (L.)* Nees. [dissertation]. Hubei: Hubei University of Chinese Medicine.

Chen, C.-C., Lin, C.-F., Huang, Y.-L., Ko, F.-N., and Teng, C.-M. (1995). Bioactive constituents from the flower buds and peduncles of Lindera megaphylla. *J. Natural. Prod.* 58, 1423–1425. doi: 10.1021/np50123a013

Chen, C.-C., Hsin, W.-C., Ko, F.-N., Huang, Y.-L., Ou, J.-C., and Teng, C.-M. (1996). Antiplatelet arylnaphthalide lignans from Justicia procumbens. *J. Natural. Prod.* 59, 1149–1150. doi: 10.1021/np960443+

Coller, B. S., and Shattil, S. J. (2008). The GPIIb/IIIa (integrin αIIbβ3) odyssey: a technology-driven saga of a receptor with twists, turns, and even a bend. *Blood* 112, 3011–3025. doi: 10.1182/blood-2008-06-077891

Committee FoCE (2011). *Flora of China (Curcurbitaceae through Valerianaceae with Annonaceae and Berberidaceae)* vol. 19. Beijing & St Louis: Fl China Science Press & Missouri Botanical Garden Press, 1–884.

Corrêa, G. M., Alcântara, AFdC. (2012). Chemical constituents and biological activities of species of Justicia: a review. *Rev. Bras. Farmacogn.* 22, 220–238. doi: 10.1590/S0102-695X2011005000196

Jerabek-Willemsen, M., André, T., Wanner, R., Roth, H. M., Duhr, S., Baaske, P., et al. (2014). MicroScale thermophoresis: interaction analysis and beyond. *J. Mol. Struc.* 1077, 101–113. doi: 10.1016/j.molstruc.2014.03.009

Joshi, A. R., and Joshi, K. (2000). Indigenous knowledge and uses of medicinal plants by local communities of the Kali Gandaki Watershed Area, Nepal. *J. Ethnopharmacol.* 73, 175–183. doi: 10.1016/S0378-8741(00)00301-9

Maschberger, M., Resch, H. M., Duhr, S., and Breitsprecher, D. Exploring protein stability by nanoDSF.

Savithramma, N., Sulochana, C., and Rao, K. (2007). Ethnobotanical survey of plants used to treat asthma in Andhra Pradesh, India. *J. Ethnopharmacol.* 113, 54–61. doi: 10.1016/j.jep.2007.04.004

Seidel, S. A., Dijkman, P. M., Lea, W. A., van den Bogaart, G., Jerabek-Willemsen, M., Lazic, A., et al. (2013). Microscale thermophoresis quantifies biomolecular interactions under previously challenging conditions. *Methods.* 59, 301–315. doi: 10.1016/j.ymeth.2012.12.005

Sparks, R. P., and Fratti, R. (2019). "Use of microscale thermophoresis (MST) to measure binding affinities of components of the fusion machinery," in: *SNAREs*. Springer, 191–198. doi: 10.1007/978-1-4939-8760-3_11

Su, W.-Y. (2014). *Study on chemical constituents of Rostellularia procumbens (L.)* Nees. [dissertation]. Hubei: Hubei University of Chinese Medicine.

van den Bogaart, G., Meyenberg, K., Diederichsen, U., and Jahn, R. (2012). Phosphatidylinositol 4, 5-bisphosphate increases Ca2+ affinity of synaptotagmin-1 by 40-fold. *J. Biol. Chem.* 287, 16447–16453. doi: 10.1074/jbc.M112.343418

Vinothkannan Ravichandran, L. Z., Wang, H., Yu, G., Zhang, Y., and Li, A. (2018). Virtual screening and biomolecular interactions of CviR-based quorum sensing inhibitors against Chromobacterium violaceum. *Front. Cell. Inf. Microbiol* 8, 1–13. doi: 10.3389/fcimb.2018.00292

Wu, H.-Z., Zhang, Y.-Q., Zhang, B.-W., Yan, B., and Yang, Y.-F. (2013). Study on chemical constituents of Rostellularia procumbens (L.) Nees. *Hubei. J. Trad. Chin. Med.* 35, 68–69.

Yun, S.-H., Sim, E.-H., Goh, R.-Y., Park, J.-I., and Han, J.-Y. (2016). Platelet activation: the mechanisms and potential biomarkers. *BioMed. Res. Int.* 2016, 1–15. doi: 10.1155/2016/9060143

12

The Study on the Mechanism of Hugan Tablets in Treating Drug-Induced Liver Injury Induced by Atorvastatin

Shujing Lv[†], *Honghong Yu*[†], *Xinyue Liu and Xiaoyan Gao* *

School of Chinese Materia Medica, Beijing University of Chinese Medicine, Beijing, China

***Correspondence:**
Xiaoyan Gao
gaoxiaoyan@bucm.edu.cn

[†]These authors have contributed equally to this work and share first authorship

Atorvastatin is a widely used lipid-lowering drug in the clinic. Research shows that taking long-term atorvastatin has the risk of drug-induced liver injury (DILI) in most patients. Hugan tablets, a commonly used drug for liver disease, can effectively lower transaminase and protect the liver. However, the underlying mechanism of Hugan tablets alleviating atorvastatin-induced DILI remains unclear. To address this problem, comprehensive chemical profiling and network pharmacology methods were used in the study. First, the strategy of "compound–single herb–TCM prescription" was applied to characterize the ingredients of Hugan tablets. Then, active ingredients and potential targets of Hugan tablets in DILI treatment were screened using network pharmacology, molecular docking, and literature research. In the end, the mechanism of Hugan tablets in treating atorvastatin-induced DILI was elucidated. The results showed that Hugan tablets can effectively alleviate DILI induced by atorvastatin in model rats, and 71 compounds were characterized from Hugan tablets. Based on these compounds, 271 potential targets for the treatment of DILI were predicted, and 10 key targets were chosen by characterizing protein–protein interactions. Then, 30 potential active ingredients were screened through the molecular docking with these 10 key targets, and their biological activity was explained based on literature research. Finally, the major 19 active ingredients of Hugan tablets were discovered. In addition, further enrichment analysis of 271 targets indicated that the PI3K-Akt, TNF, HIF-1, Rap1, and FoxO signaling pathways may be the primary pathways regulated by Hugan tablets in treating DILI. This study proved that Hugan tablets could alleviate atorvastatin-induced DILI through multiple components, targets, and pathways.

Keywords: Hugan tablets, drug-induced liver injury, UPLC-Q-TOF-MS/MS, network pharmacology, molecular docking

INTRODUCTION

Hyperlipidemia widely affects the health of the elderly nowadays and is recognized as a social problem (Townsend et al., 2019). In the treatment of hyperlipidemia, atorvastatin is a commonly prescribed lipid-lowering drug (Black, 2002). However, studies showed that the long-term use of atorvastatin could cause serious side effects, represented by liver injury, in which case the level of liver

---

Abbreviations: ASH, Artemisiae Scopariae Herb; BR, Bupleuri Radix; DILI, drug-induced liver injury; IR, Isatidis Radix; MB, mung bean; PFS, Pulvis Fellis Suis; SCF, Schisandrae Chinensis Fructus.

transaminase of the patient would be increased (Clarke and Mills, 2006; Deedwania et al., 2007). Therefore, drug research on decreasing the side effects of statins is of great significance.

In recent years, traditional Chinese medicine (TCM) has made significant breakthroughs in the treatment of drug-induced liver injury (DILI), such as the application of Hugan tablets (Yao et al., 2018). The prescription of Hugan tablets is composed of six medicinal herbs, namely, Bupleuri Radix (BR, derived from *Bupleurum chinense* DC. or *Bupleurum scorzonerifolium* Willd.), Artemisiae Scopariae Herba (ASH, derived from *Artemisia capillaris* Thunb.), Schisandrae chinensis Fructus [SCF, derived from *Schisandra chinensis* (Turcz.) Baill.], Isatidis Radix (IR, derived from *Isatis tinctoria* L.), Pulvis Fellis Suis (PFS, derived from *Sus scrofa domestica* Brisson), and mung bean [MB, derived from *Vigna radiata* (L.) R. Wilczek]. Clinically, Hugan tablets can reduce the level of liver transaminase such as aspartate transaminase (AST), alanine transaminase (ALT), and total bilirubin (TBIL) and is used for chronic hepatitis and early liver cirrhosis (Liu et al., 2019). However, whether Hugan tablets have a therapeutic effect on atorvastatin-induced liver injury remains unclear, and its mechanism of action has not yet been elucidated.

Network pharmacology has been successfully applied to the construction of networks that characterize the relationship between drugs, targets, and diseases, and it has played an active role in the research of TCM prescriptions due to its integrity and systematicness (Hopkins, 2008). However, a major challenge restricting its application is the accurate characterization of active ingredients. At present, most of the network pharmacology studies are based on the components reported in the database yet do not experimentally investigate the content of ingredients, which is closely related to the medicinal effects. Therefore, in this study, the strategy of "compound–single herb–TCM prescription" based on ultrahigh-performance liquid chromatography coupled with a quadrupole time-of-flight tandem mass spectrometry (UPLC-Q-TOF-MS/MS) (Xing et al., 2017) was applied to characterize the ingredients of Hugan tablets, which provides a solid material foundation for the follow-up network pharmacology and molecular docking.

In this study, the effect of Hugan tablets on the treatment of DILI was validated in rat models and then the ingredients of Hugan tablets were characterized. Based on this material basis, the major active ingredients and targets of Hugan tablets were selected by network pharmacology, molecular docking, and literature research. At last, the potential mechanism of Hugan tablets was analyzed (**Figure 1**). This study demonstrated the huge potential of TCM for ameliorating the side effects of chemical drugs.

MATERIALS AND METHODS

Chemicals and Reagents

Atorvastatin calcium tablets (batch No. 170518) were obtained from Jialin Pharmaceutical (Beijing, China). AST, ALT, TBIL, and alkaline phosphatase (ALP) assay kits were obtained from Beckman Kurt Experimental System Co., Ltd. (Suzhou, China). Hugan tablets (batch No. 201710078), BR, ASH, SCF, IR, PFS, and MB were obtained from Sunflower Pharmaceutical Group Co., Ltd. (Harbin, China).

Mass spectrometry–grade acetonitrile, methanol, and formic acid were obtained from Fisher Scientific. The reference standards of quercetin, rutin, scopoletin, hyperoside, scoparone, chlorogenic acid, saikosaponin B2, schisantherin A, schisandrin A, schisandrin B, schisandrin C, schisandrol A, schisandrol B, and schisanhenol were obtained from Chengdu Purifa Technology Development Co., Ltd. (Chengdu, China). Chenodeoxycholic acid (CDCA) was obtained from Shanghai Yuanye Biotechnology Co., Ltd. (Shanghai, China). Vitexin was obtained from Shanghai Aladdin Biochemical Technology Co., Ltd. (Shanghai, China). Saikosaponin A, proline, and hyodeoxycholic acid (HDCA) were obtained from the National

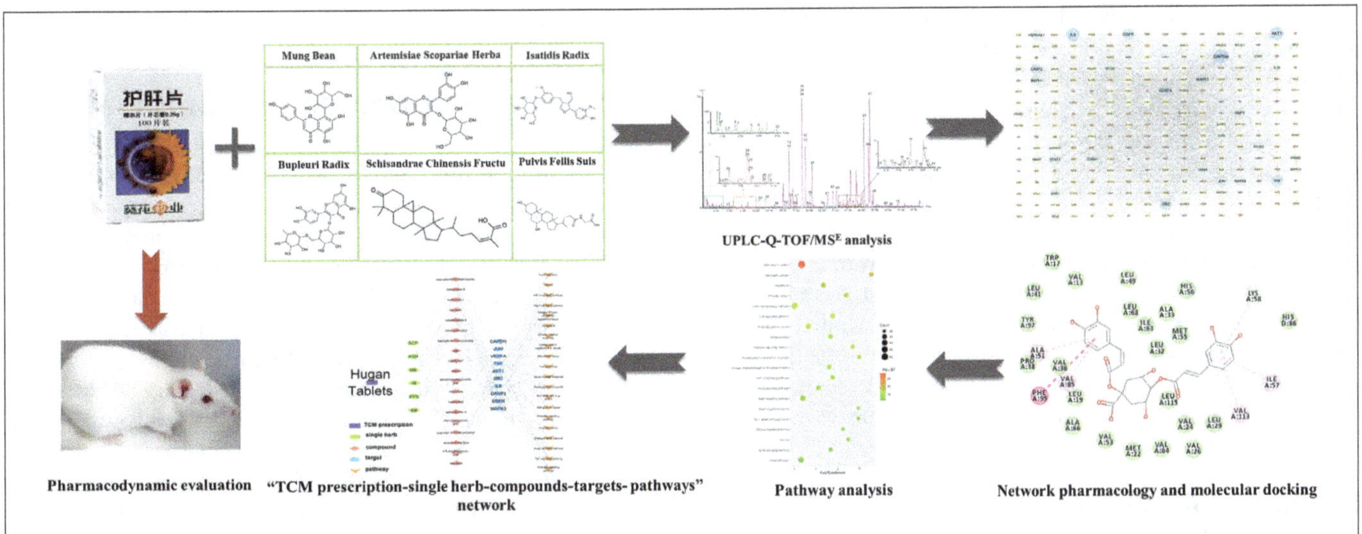

FIGURE 1 | Flowchart for the investigation of the mechanism of Hugan tablets in treating drug-induced liver injury induced by atorvastatin.

Institutes for Food and Drug Control (Beijing, China). Arginine was obtained from Shanghai Macklin Biochemical Co., Ltd. (Shanghai, China). The purity of all standards was over 98%, as determined by HPLC analysis.

Animals

Male Sprague Dawley (SD) rats weighing 190–210 g were raised in the Animal Experimental Center of Beijing University of Chinese Medicine. Animal experiments were approved by the Animal Care and Ethics Committee of Beijing University of Chinese Medicine (approval number: BUCM-4-2018091304-3,023). The environmental temperature was controlled at 21–25°C with a relative humidity of 55–65% (12 h/12 h day/night cycle), and the pads were changed four times a week. Rats were allowed to adapt to the environment for 7 days with free food and water before the experiment.

Pharmacological Experiment Design and Preparation of Bio-Samples

For the dosage of Hugan tablets, according to the clinical dosage, 0.504 g kg^{-1}·d^{-1} was set as the low dosage, and the double-dose 1.008 g kg^{-1}·d^{-1} was set as the high dosage. The dosage of atorvastatin calcium tablets suspension was 50 mg kg^{-1}.

At the beginning, 68 SD rats were randomly assigned into three groups: 34 in the atorvastatin group, 17 in the control group, and 17 in the prevention group. The atorvastatin group received the intragastric administration of atorvastatin calcium tablet suspension. The prevention group received the intragastric administration of atorvastatin calcium tablet suspension plus high-dose Hugan tablets at the same time. The control group was given water of the same volume. After 50 days, the rats in the initial atorvastatin group were identified as successful models and were subsequently divided into two groups randomly, with some rats remaining within the atorvastatin group and the others moved to the treatment group. The treatment group received the intragastric administration of high-dose Hugan tablets, instead of atorvastatin calcium tablet suspension. Finally, there were four groups of experimental animals. The continuous administration was conducted for 14 days. After the last administration, all rats were fasted for 12 h and given water freely. Then, once the rat was anesthetized with chloral hydrate, blood was drawn from the main abdominal vein and the liver was peeled off as soon as possible to evaluate the efficacy of the Hugan tablets.

The blood samples were centrifuged at 3,000 rpm for 15 min to separate serum for biochemical analysis. Serum ALT, AST, ALP, and TBIL levels were measured with a CX4 Pro automatic biochemical analyzer (Beckman Coulter Inc., United States). The left lateral lobe of the liver was fixed in 10% formalin, then embedded in paraffin, sectioned, and stained with hematoxylin–eosin (HE). An optical microscope was used to observe the histological sections.

Statistical Analysis

SPSS software 17.0 (SPSS Inc., Chicago, United States) was used for statistical analysis. All data are presented as mean ± SD. Differences between multiple groups were examined using the one-way ANOVA. The LSD-t test was adopted to compare the data between two groups. The significance levels were $^{*}p < 0.05$, $^{**}p < 0.01$.

Preparation of Sample and Reference Solution for LC-MS/MS

Hugan tablets composed of 4.2 g BR, 4.2 g ASH, 4.2 g IR, 2.2 g SCF, 0.3 g PFS, and 0.2 g MB. First, Hugan tablets, BR, ASH, SCF, IR, PFS, and MB were crushed. Then, 2.0 g of powder was accurately weighed and transferred to a 50-ml triangular flask with plug, in which 25 ml of 70% methanol was added. After 1 h ultrasound-assisted extraction, the extract solution was centrifuged at 12,000 r/min for 10 min and then filtered through a 0.22-μm filter membrane before qualitative analysis. Every single standard solution was prepared by dissolving accurately weighed standards in methanol and stored at 4°C in the dark.

UPLC-Q-TOF-MS/MS Analysis

The analysis was performed on a Waters ACQUITY UPLC I-Class system coupled with the Waters SYNAPT G2-Si Mass Spectrometer *via* an electrospray ionization (ESI) interface. Chromatographic separation was performed using an ACQUITY UPLC BEH C18 column (2.1 × 100 mm, 1.7 μm) held at 40°C, and the flow rate was 0.3 ml/min. The mobile phases consisted of 0.1% formic acid aqueous solution (A) and acetonitrile (B), using a linear gradient program as follows: 0–9 min, 2–20% B; 9–12 min, 20–30% B; 12–17 min, 30–40% B; 17–24 min, 40–42% B; 24–38 min, 42–98% B; and 38–40 min, 98% B.

The optimal mass spectrometer parameters were employed as follows: capillary voltage, 3 kV; cone voltage, 40 V; source temperature, 100°C; desolvation gas temperature, 300°C; and desolvation gas flow, 600 L/h. MS measurement was obtained in the MS^E mode, and the collision energy of low energy function and high energy function was set at 6 V and 20–40 V, respectively. The acquisition mass range was 50–1,200 Da in both negative and positive ion modes. Data were acquired and analyzed by Waters MassLynx V4.1 and Waters UNIFI 1.71 software.

Identification of Compounds in Hugan Tablets

The identification procedure was mainly divided into five steps (Wang et al., 2016; Wang et al., 2017). 1) The mass spectrometry data were collected using the aforementioned methods. 2) A database of chemical compounds of each medicinal herb in Hugan tablets (including the name, molecular formula, and structural formula of each compound) was built by the SciFinder database (https://www.cas.org/products/scifinder), the ChemSpider database (http://www.chemspider.com/), and relevant literature reports. 3) The peaks were screened preliminarily by the UNIFI™ platform based on the in-house database and the self-built database. The known compounds were validated further based on the accurate mass, fragment ions, neutral losses, retention behaviors, reference standards, and previous reports. 4) For the potential novel compounds, based on the accurate mass, fragment ions, characteristic fragments, and retention behaviors, possible structures were obtained by combining UniFi's Elucidate function with the literature, ChemSpider, Mass Bank (https://massbank.eu/MassBank/), and other databases, and then entered them into UniFi software for further verification. 5) The compounds in single herb were identified and then the ingredients in the TCM prescription were characterized by comparing the peaks in prescription with the corresponding peaks in each single herb.

Target Collection

The potential targets of the compounds in Hugan tablets were searched from SwissTargetPrediction (http://www.swisstargetprediction.ch/) (Gfeller et al., 2014) and TCMSP (Ru et al., 2014). The biological targets related to DILI were selected from the Online Mendelian Inheritance in Man (OMIM, http://www.omim.org/) and the GeneCards database (https://www.genecards.org/). The protein names of these targets were converted into their official gene names via UniProtKB (http://www.uniprot.org/). Then, the Venn diagram was drawn to obtain the intersected drug-related targets and the disease-related targets, which are potential targets for Hugan tablets to treat DILI.

Pathway Enrichment of Potential Targets

The Database for Annotation, Visualization, and Integrated Discovery (DAVID, http://david.abcc.ncifcrf.gov/home.jsp, version 6.8) was employed to analyze the KEGG pathways of the predicted targets. The R package ggplot2 was used to create the bubble plot.

Protein–Protein Interaction Network Construction

All potential targets were uploaded into the STRING database (http://string-db.org/) (Szklarczyk et al., 2017) to analyze their interactions. The PPI data were imported into Cytoscape v3.7.1 (http://cytoscape.org/) to construct a PPI network and perform topological analysis. The top 10 targets ranked by degree were selected to screen the potential active ingredients of Hugan tablets based on molecular docking.

Screening of Active Ingredients of Hugan Tablets

The crystal structures of the ten key proteins were downloaded from the RCSB (http://www.rcsb.org/) database. Discovery Studio 4.0 (DS) LibDock was used to molecularly dock the compounds of Hugan tablets with the ten target proteins. For the target protein with the original co-crystal ligand available, the cutoff value was the LibDock score of the protein and its corresponding original ligand (Rao et al., 2007). For the protein without original co-crystal ligand, the cutoff value was the LibDock score of the protein and its corresponding approved positive drug (Hu et al., 2012). Compounds with a higher LibDock score than the cutoff value were considered potential active ingredients of Hugan tablets. Then, literature investigation into the potential active ingredients was carried out to obtain information on the hepatoprotective effects of these ingredients and their contents in a single herb, so as to eliminate some false-positive results of virtual screening and finally screen the major active ingredients of Hugan tablets.

"TCM Prescription-Single Herb-Compounds-Targets-Pathways" Network Construction

The potential active ingredients, key target proteins, and corresponding top 20 pathways obtained by the previous screening were imported into Cytoscape 3.6.1 software, and the "Merge" plug-in in Cytoscape software was used to construct the "TCM prescription–single herb–compounds–targets–pathways" network of Hugan tablets in the treatment of DILI.

RESULTS

Evaluation of the Preventive and Therapeutic Effects of Hugan tablets

The serum levels of ALT, AST, ALP, and TBIL were the biochemical factors most commonly used to evaluate the liver function (Boone et al., 2005; Kwo et al., 2017; Lei et al., 2020). Compared with the control group, the serum levels of ALT, AST, ALP, and TBIL of the atorvastatin group were significantly increased ($p < 0.01$) (**Figure 2A**), which indicated that the model was successfully established. Before dosing of atorvastatin, the preventive administration of Hugan tablets could significantly reduce the levels of ALT, TBIL, AST, and ALP in rats with DILI. The amelioration effect was further observed as levels of ALT and TBIL, which showed no significant difference from the control group, while AST and ALP levels are still significantly higher than those of normal rats ($p < 0.05$; $p < 0.01$). After dosing of atorvastatin, the therapeutic administration of Hugan tablets significantly reduced the ALT, AST, and TBIL levels of the DILI model rats and made the TBIL level comparable to normal rats, while the levels of ALT and AST did not reach the normal level. Taken together, the results showed that Hugan tablets had significant ameliorating effects on DILI. However, in the results of HE staining, no significant alteration in the liver tissues was observed among the control group, atorvastatin group, prevention group, and treatment group, indicating that the degree of injury is light, and it has not yet been reflected in the pathology (**Figure 2B**).

Identification of Compounds in Hugan Tablets

To investigate the underlying mechanisms of Hugan tablets in the DILI induced by atorvastatin, the ingredients of Hugan tablets were clarified. A problem for the analysis of TCM prescriptions was that if the compounds were identified directly, the peak with a high response might depress the small peak, thus increase the difficulty of identification. Therefore, the strategy of "compounds-single herb-TCM prescription," which was successfully developed in our previous research, was used to characterize the ingredients of Hugan tablets (Wang et al., 2017). First, the reference substances of various analogies in

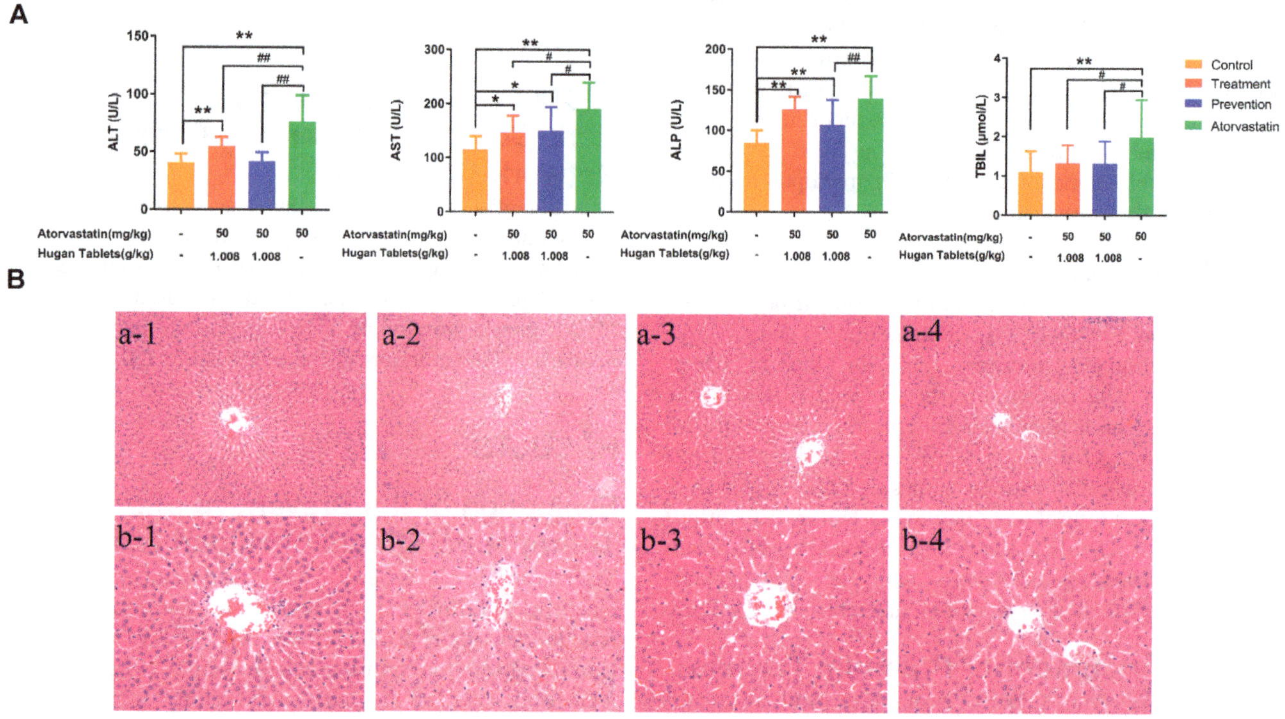

FIGURE 2 | Efficacy of Hugan tablets in ameliorating DILI. **(A)** Effects of Hugan tablets on alleviating elevated serum ALT, AST, ALP, and TBIL, resulting from atorvastatin-induced liver injury ($n_{Control} = 13$; $n_{Treatment} = 10$; $n_{Prevention} = 15$; $n_{Atorvastatin} = 12$). Data are presented as mean ± SD. $^{*}p < 0.05$, $^{**}p < 0.01$ vs. control group, $^{\#}p < 0.05$, $^{\#\#}p < 0.01$ vs. atorvastatin group. **(B)** Histomorphology of liver tissues of rats in different groups (HE, a × 200, b × 400). 1: control group; 2: atorvastatin group; 3: prevention group; 4: treatment group.

each herb were analyzed by high-resolution mass spectrometry (HRMS), and the diagnostic ions and fragmentation rules were summarized. By using data post-processing methods such as extracting diagnostic ions, comparing fragment pathways, and filtering neutral loss, the components in each single herb were identified. Then, the ingredients in the TCM prescription were characterized by comparing the peaks in the prescription with those identified in each single herb. The base peak chromatograms (BPCs) of Hugan tablets in both positive and negative ion modes are presented in **Figure 3**. In addition, the BPC of Hugan tablets and its medicinal herb is shown in **Supplementary Figure S1**.

Take the identification of a compound in ASH as an example, in the BPC of ASH (**Figure 4B**), the F2 peak ($1.56e^6$) with a higher response was observed, while at the same retention time, the F1 peak response in the BPC of Hugan tablets (**Figure 4A**) was lower ($2.37e^4$). Therefore, first, F2 can be identified to infer F1 due to the same retention time. F2 provided the precursor ion of $[M + H]^+$ at *m/z* 465.1029, as well as fragment ions at *m/z* 303.0487 $[M + H\text{-}C_6H_{10}O_5]^+$, *m/z* 153.0182 $[M + H\text{-}C_{14}H_{16}O_8]^+$, and *m/z* 137.0241 $[M + H\text{-}C_{14}H_{16}O_9]^+$, which were characteristic fragment ions of flavonols (**Figure 4C**). Thus, F2 was confirmed as hyperoside by comparing with the MS^n data and retention time of the reference standard. The possible cleavage pathway of hyperoside is shown in **Figure 4D**. This method can not only effectively identify compounds with low content but also increase the reliability of compound identification in the TCM prescription.

We have comprehensively characterized 71 compounds of Hugan tablets, including 11 flavonoids and their glycosides, 8 triterpene saponins, 3 coumarins, 29 lignans, 8 organic acids, 5 bile acids, 3 nucleic acids, and 4 other compounds. The retention time and the MS^n data of the characterized compounds are summarized in **Supplementary Table S1**.

Potential Targets of Hugan Tablets in Treating Drug-Induced Liver Injury

Among the 71 compounds, 832 drug targets were searched from the SwissTargetPrediction and TCMSP databases. A total of 1,117 disease targets of DILI were obtained from the OMIM and Genecards databases. Then, the Venn diagram was drawn to obtain 271 overlapped targets (**Figure 5A**), which are potential targets for Hugan tablets in treating DILI. For specific target information, see **Supplementary Table S2**.

Protein–Protein Interaction Network Analysis

The 271 potential targets were introduced into STRING to obtain the information on predicted interaction, and Cytoscape software was used to construct and analyze the PPI network (**Figure 5B**). Network topology analysis was performed to get the degree value of these targets. The targets with a higher degree may represent the key targets for the treatment of DILI by Hugan tablets. Thus, the top ten targets

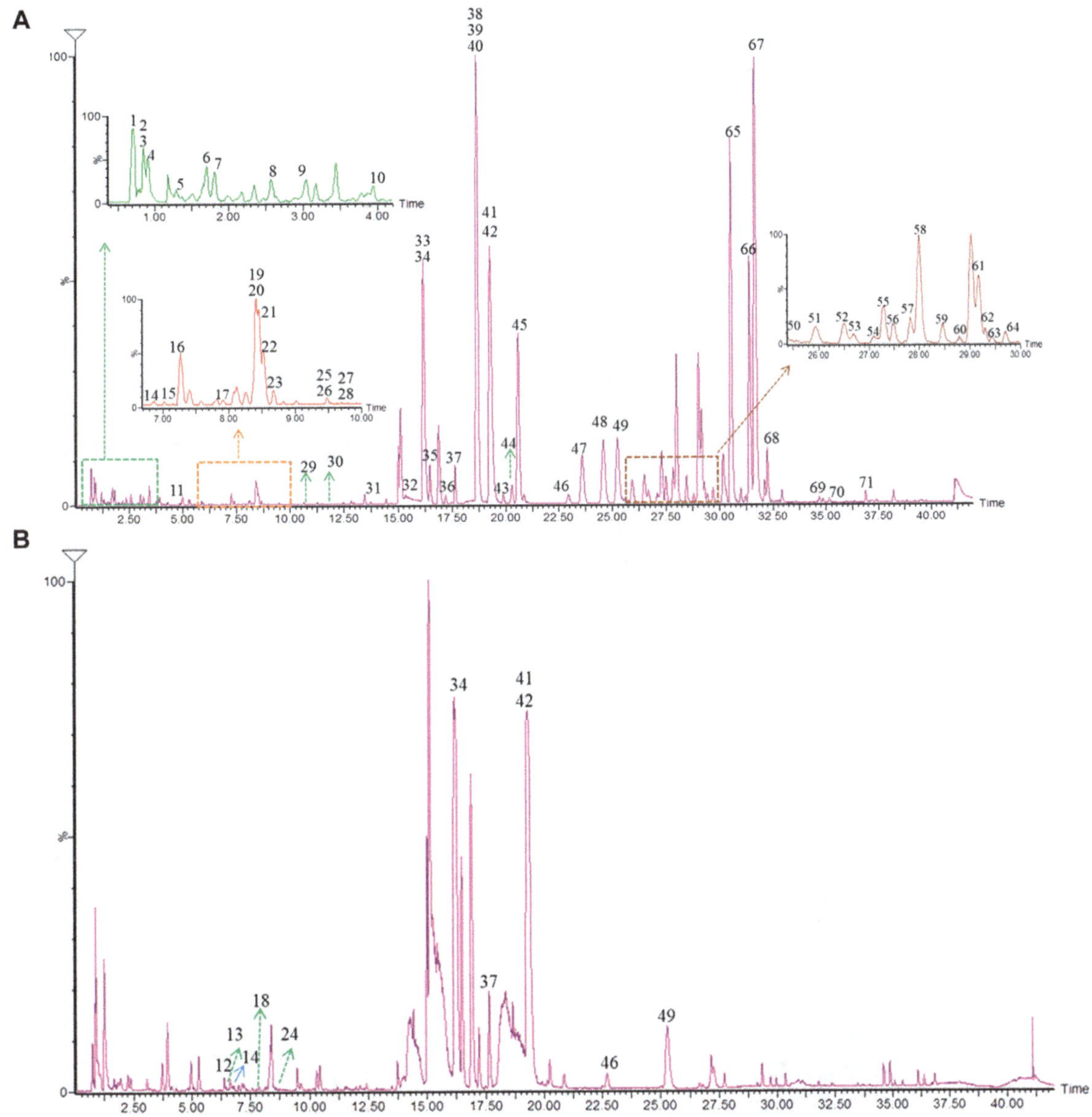

FIGURE 3 | BPC of Hugan tablets in both positive **(A)** and negative **(B)** ion modes.

ranked by degree value were collected, namely, GAPDH, IL6, AKT1, VEGFA, TNF, EGFR, SRC, MAPK3, CASP3, and JUN (**Table 1**).

Active Ingredients of Hugan Tablets

The molecular docking score can reflect the affinity of the compound and the target, which can be used to virtually screen the compounds more likely to interact with potential targets. Based on molecular docking, 30 compounds with a higher LibDock score than the cutoff value were considered as potential active ingredients of Hugan tablets (**Supplementary Table S3**). Detailed information of the docking scores and cutoff values are presented in **Supplementary Table S4**.

Next, we conducted literature research on the biological activities of 30 potential active ingredients and their content in a single herb, and excluded the ingredients with little content or whose biological activity related to liver protection has not been verified. Finally, 19 active ingredients of Hugan tablets were screened out (**Table 2**), including 10 flavonoids, 5 phenylpropanoids, 1 triterpenoid saponin, 2 and 1 tetracyclic triterpenoid. It was found that the active ingredients in Hugan tablets mainly exhibit antioxidant, anti-inflammatory, and liver fibrosis–inhibiting effects, to play a role in protecting the liver. It is worth noting that most of the 10 flavonoids belong to flavonols, suggesting that the introduction of the 3-hydroxyl group in the flavonoid core structure may be important for their liver-protecting activity.

Pathway Analysis

Based on the DAVID database, a pathway enrichment analysis of targets was performed to identify the potential pathways intervened by Hugan tablets administration. A total of 139

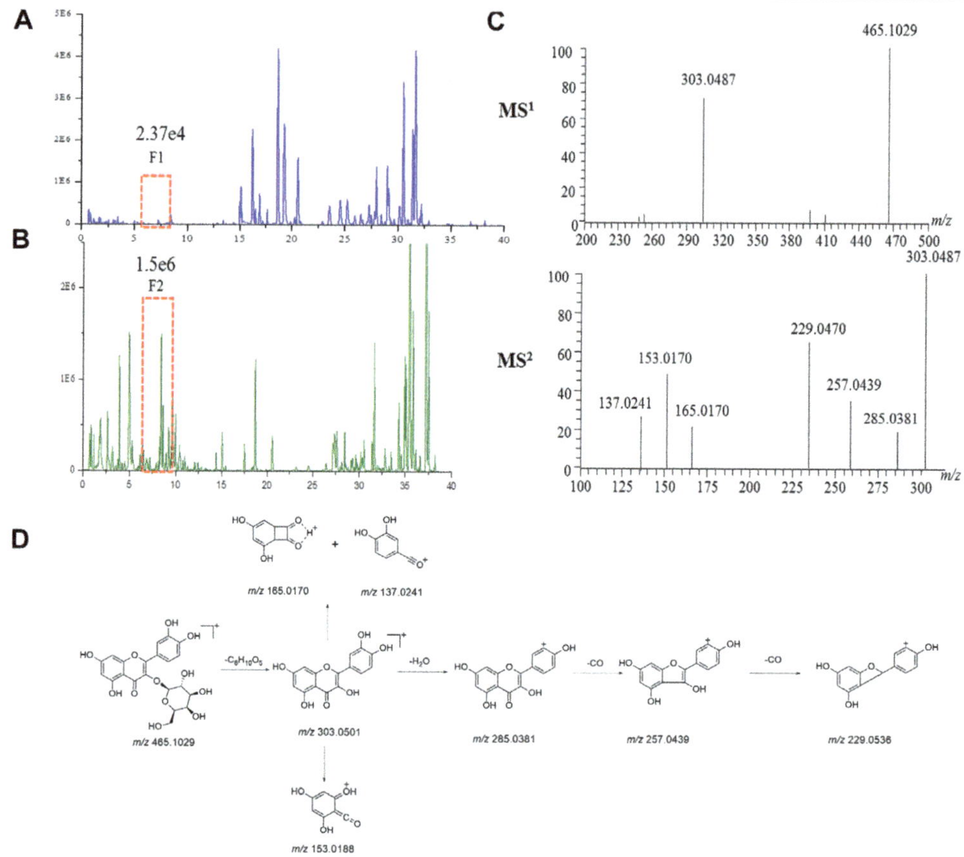

FIGURE 4 | Identification of compounds in Hugan tablets. Chromatograms of common components in Hugan tablets **(A)** and BR **(B)** in positive ion mode **(C)** The MS^1 spectrum and MS^2 spectrum of F2. **(D)** The fragmentation pathway of hyperoside.

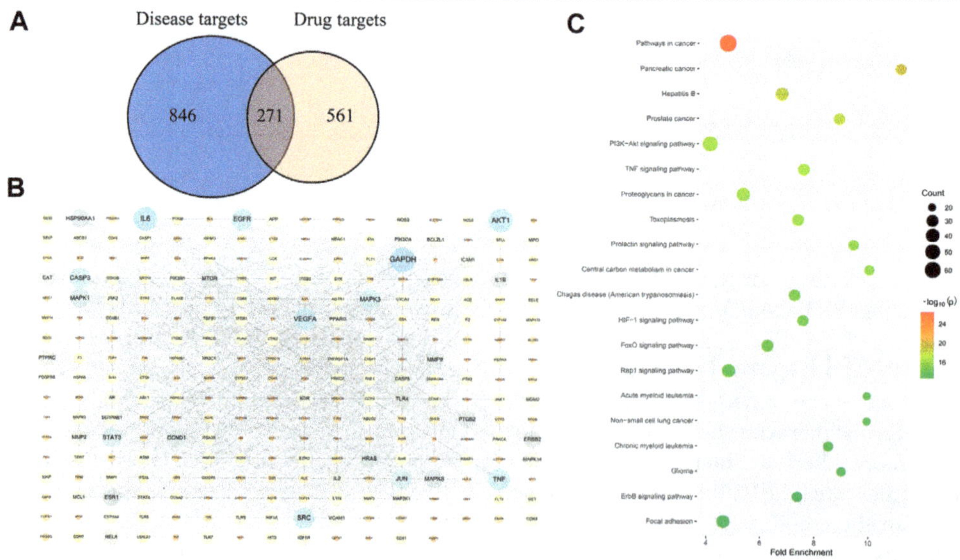

FIGURE 5 | Network pharmacology–based analysis of the treatment of DILI with Hugan tablets. **(A)** Common targets of Hugan tablets and DILI. **(B)** PPI network of potential targets. **(C)** KEGG pathway enrichment results.

TABLE 1 | Ten key targets of Hugan tablets in treating DILI.

NO.	Gene symbol	Uniprot Id	Description	Degree	Pdb
1	GAPDH	P04406	Glyceraldehyde-3-phosphate dehydrogenase	183	1U8F
2	IL6	P05231	Interleukin-6	172	1ALU
3	AKT1	P31749	RAC-alpha serine/threonine-protein kinase	172	6HHF
4	VEGFA	P15692	Vascular endothelial growth factor A	155	4QAF
5	TNF	P01375	Tumor necrosis factor	149	7KP9
6	EGFR	P00533	Epidermal growth factor receptor	146	3POZ
7	SRC	P12931	Proto-oncogene tyrosine-protein kinase src	144	2H8H
8	MAPK3	P27361	Mitogen-activated protein kinase 3	140	4QTB
9	CASP3	P42574	Caspase-3	139	1GFW
10	JUN	P05412	Transcription factor AP-1	130	5FV8

potential pathways were obtained, with a cutoff *p*-value of 0.05, and the top 20 pathways (with the lowest *p*-values) are shown in **Figure 5C**. The number of targets contained in each pathway suggests that Hugan tablets mainly exert its protective effect on DILI by regulating the PI3K-Akt, TNF, HIF-1, Rap1, and FoxO signaling pathways.

"TCM Prescription–Single Herb–Compounds–Targets–Pathways" Network Construction

According to the 19 potential active ingredients, 10 key targets, and corresponding top 20 pathways screened earlier, the "TCM prescription–single herb–compounds–targets–pathways" network of Hugan tablets in the treatment of DILI was constructed (**Figure 6**). In this network, the target(s) and the pathway(s) that the compound(s) in Hugan tablets act on could be summarized comprehensively. For example, compounds such as clemastanin B, rutin, 4,5-dicaffeoylquinic acid, and chlorogenic acid may act on the PI3K-Akt signaling pathway by binding IL6, AKT1, VEGFA, or MAPK3.

Besides, it could be found that drug–target interactions exist not only in the mode of "single target binding to multiple compounds" but also in the mode of "single compound binding to multiple targets". For example, MAPK3 can bind to clemastanin B, kaempferol-3-*O*-rutinoside, quercetin-3-*O*-robinobioside, rutin, and 4,5-dicaffeoylquinic acid, while rutin acts on AKT1, EGFR, SRC, MAPK3, and CASP3, which were involved in multiple pathways. This indicated that Hugan tablets influenced DILI by comprehensive regulation of multiple compounds, targets, and pathways.

DISCUSSION

The research on the mechanism of TCM has always been challenging because it contains multiple components, targets, and pathways. Network pharmacology explores the relationship between drugs and diseases from a global perspective by constructing networks and is an ideal tool for studying the pharmacology of TCM for the treatment of diseases.

In order to provide a solid pharmacodynamic prerequisite and material basis for network pharmacology, we verified the efficacy of Hugan tablets in a model of atorvastatin-induced liver injury and then identified 71 compounds from Hugan tablets. Based on network pharmacology, molecular docking, and literature research, 19 active ingredients, 10 key targets, and some important pathways of Hugan tablets anti-DILI were obtained, and a "TCM prescription–single herb–compounds–targets–pathways" network was constructed.

Liver injury is usually accompanied by inflammatory responses. Inflammatory factors such as transforming growth factor-beta (TGF-β) and tumor necrosis factor (TNF) are key inflammatory regulators in the progress of the liver disease, which can cause or aggravate liver cell damage (Jaeschke, 2006; Kubes and Jenne, 2018). Therefore, inhibition of inflammation is of great significance for the prevention and treatment of liver injury. In the acute tissue injury stage, the dysregulated TNF-α signaling can activate an inflammatory cascade to trigger excessive release of cytokines/chemokines and cell death (Lai et al., 2019). Therefore, Hugan tablets may regulate TNF signaling pathway through IL-6, AKT1, TNF, MAPK, CASP3, and JUN, thereby inhibiting inflammation and protecting the liver cells from apoptosis. It has been reported that the knockout of repressor and activator protein (Rap1) reduced the hepatic damage and hepatic inflammatory response (Li et al., 2016). So, it is speculated that Hugan tablets may inhibit the Rap1 signaling pathway by acting on AKT1, VEGFA, EGFR, SRC, and MAPK3, thereby preventing inflammation and protecting the liver.

Oxidative stress is closely related to almost all human liver diseases. The FoxO signaling pathway is involved in cell apoptosis induced by oxidative stress, and studies have shown that FoxO3 has a pro-apoptotic effect on liver cell under oxidative stress (Tao et al., 2013). Therefore, Hugan tablets may regulate the FoxO3 signaling pathway by acting on the targets of IL6, AKT1, EGFR, and MAPK3 to alleviate the apoptosis of the liver cells under oxidative stress.

In addition, liver injury and inflammation cause the activation of the liver tissue immune system for tissue repair. When the repair is excessive and out of control, hepatic stellate cells (HSCs) are activated (Puche et al., 2013; Higashi et al., 2017), and the extracellular matrix (ECM) secreted by them is excessively deposited in the liver, resulting in abnormal liver structure and liver function. This process can also be called liver fibrosis (Jiang et al., 2017). Studies have shown that the activation of the PI3K-Akt signaling pathway can promote the proliferation of HSC, thereby accelerating the occurrence and development of liver fibrosis (Zhang et al., 2019; Du et al., 2020). Therefore, Hugan tablets may inhibit the activation of the PI3K-Akt signaling pathway

TABLE 2 | Screening results of active ingredients of Hugan tablets.

Type of compounds	Compounds	CAS	Molecular formula	Structural formula	Herb source	Biological activity	References
Flavonoids	Hyperoside	482–36–0	$C_{21}H_{20}O_{12}$	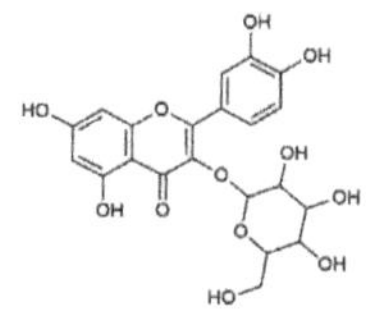	BR, ASH	It suppresses hepatic oxidative stress by activating endogenous antioxidant mechanisms and protects against liver fibrosis	Niu et al. (2017), Guo et al. (2019)
	Kaempferol-3-*O*-rutinoside	17,650–84–9	$C_{27}H_{30}O_{15}$	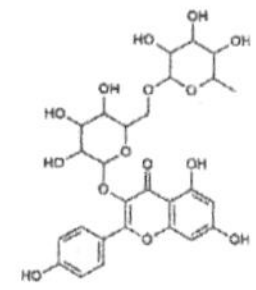	ASH	It probably mediates a strong hepatoprotective effect *via* the reduction of oxidative stress and apoptotic cell death	Wang et al. (2015)
	Quercetin-3-*O*-robinobioside	52,525–35–6	$C_{27}H_{30}O_{16}$	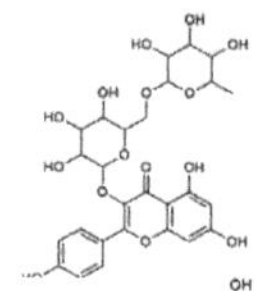	ASH	It has high antioxidant activity	Zhu et al. (2020)
	Rutin	153–18–4	$C_{27}H_{30}O_{16}$	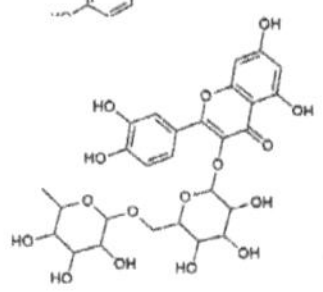	BR, MB, ASH	It ameliorates hepatic injury *via* the IL-6/STAT3 pathway, and interfering with oxidative stress, inflammation, and apoptosis	Hafez et al. (2015), Caglayan et al. (2019)
	Narcissin	604–80–8	$C_{28}H_{32}O_{16}$	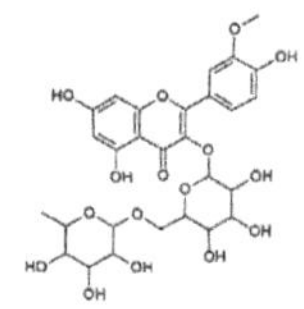	BR, ASH	It reveals significant antioxidant and hepatoprotective effects	Gevrenova et al. (2015)
	Kaempferol-3-*O*-rhamnoside	482–39–3	$C_{21}H_{20}O_{10}$	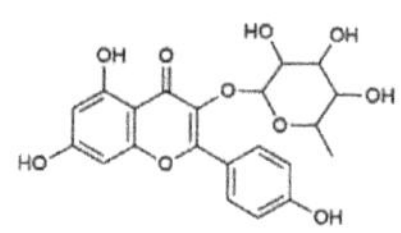	ASH	It has a hepatoprotective effect on the lipopolysaccharide/d-galactosamine–induced acute liver failure	Hu et al. (2018)
	Isoquercitrin	21,637–25–2	$C_{21}H_{20}O_{12}$	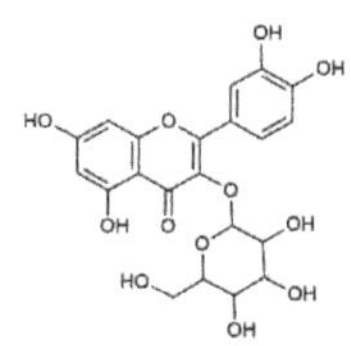	BR, ASH, MB	It protects the liver though inhibition of oxidative stress, nitrosative stress, and inflammation	Xie et al. (2016)
	Vitexin	3,681–93–4	$C_{21}H_{20}O_{10}$	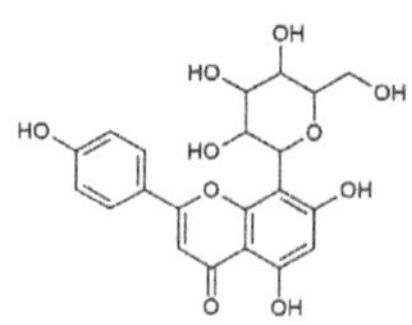	MB	It ameliorates the liver disease by inhibiting inflammation	Li et al. (2020)
	Capillarisin	56,365–38–9	$C_{16}H_{12}O_7$	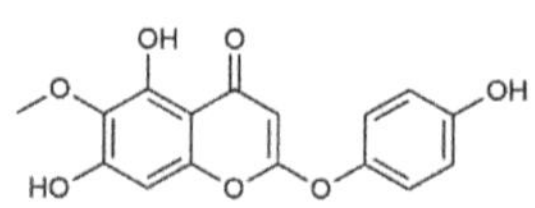	ASH	It suppresses oxidative stress and prevents liver apoptosis primary hepatocytes *via* the reduction of HO-1 expression and inactivation of its downstream target NF-κB	Lee et al. (2009)
	Quercetin	117–39–5	$C_{15}H_{10}O_7$	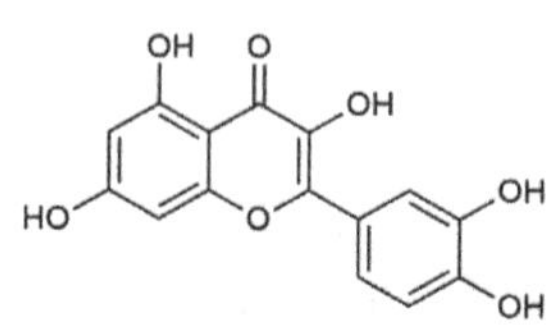	BR	It significantly minimizes oxidative stress as well as inflammatory response in hepatic cells	Lee et al. (2019)

(Continued on following page)

TABLE 2 | *(Continued)* Screening results of active ingredients of Hugan tablets.

Type of compounds	Compounds	CAS	Molecular formula	Structural formula	Herb source	Biological activity	References
Phenylpropanoids	Indigoticoside A	143,663–00–7	$C_{26}H_{34}O_{11}$	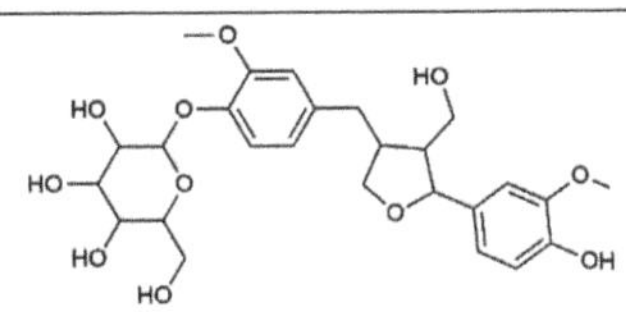	RI	It has a strong antioxidant activity	Xiao et al. (2014)
	Clemastanin B	112,747–98–5	$C_{32}H_{44}O_{16}$	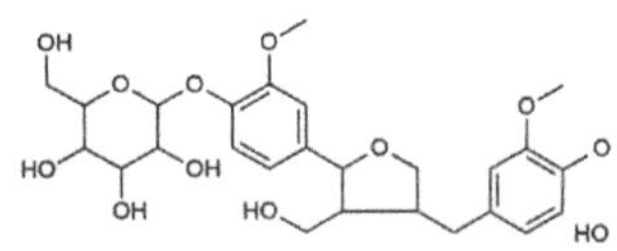	IR	It has a strong antioxidant activity	Xiao et al. (2014)
	Scoparone	120–08–1	$C_{11}H_{10}O_4$	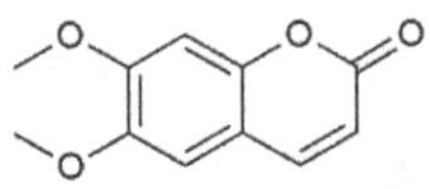	BR, ASH	It attenuates hepatic stellate cell activation through inhibiting TGF-β/Smad signaling pathway	Liu and Zhao, (2017)
	4,5-Dicaffeoylquinic acid	57,378–72–0	$C_{25}H_{24}O_{12}$	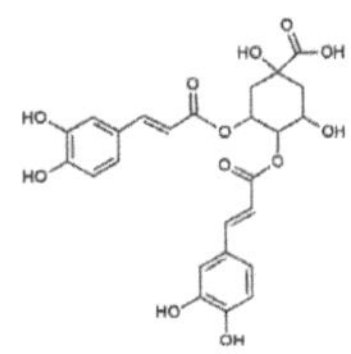	ASH	It is the anti-inflammatory and anti-HBV components in ASH.	Tan et al. (2008); Zhao et al. (2014)
	Chlorogenic acid	327–97–9	$C_{16}H_{18}O_9$	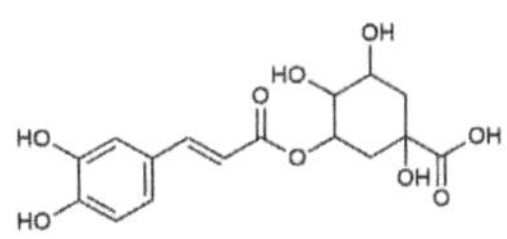	BR, ASH	It inhibits liver injury and might be related with antioxidant and anti-inflammatory	Shi et al. (2016)
Triterpenoid saponins	Saikosaponin A	20,736–09–8	$C_{42}H_{68}O_{13}$	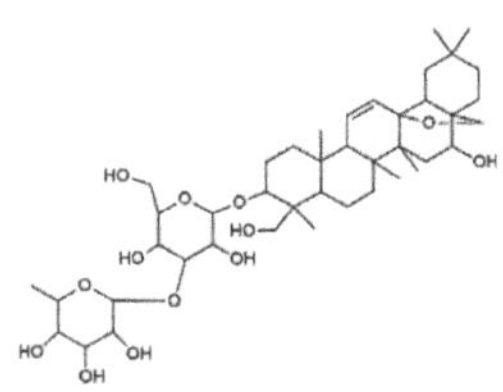	BR	It downregulates BMP-4 expression and inhibits hepatic stellate cell activation to inhibit liver fibrosis; it inhibits the expression of hepatic pro-inflammatory cytokines and the NF-κB signal pathway and increases the expression of anti-inflammatory cytokine IL-10, thereby inhibiting liver injury	Wang et al. (2013), Wu et al. (2008)
Bile acids	Glycochenodeoxycholic acid	640–79–9	$C_{26}H_{43}NO_5$	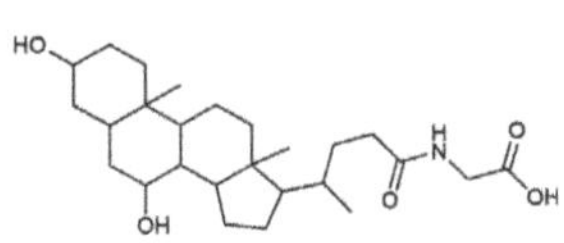	PFS	It shows a strong association with fibrosis	Kwan et al. (2020)
	Chenodeoxycholic acid	474–25–9	$C_{24}H_{40}O_4$	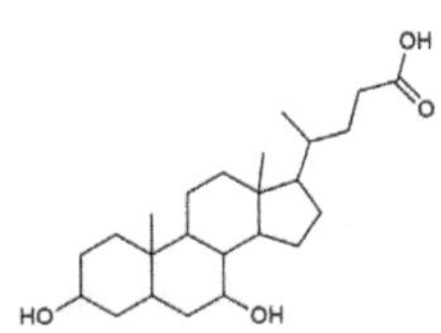	PFS	It ameliorates liver fibrosis by inhibiting TIMP-1 expression resulting from activation of farnesoid X receptor	Kang et al. (2012)
Tetracyclic triterpenoids	Schisandronic acid	55,511–14–3	$C_{30}H_{46}O_3$	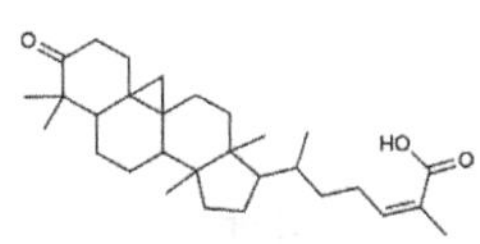	SCF	It has an antioxidant activity	Tasneem et al. (2021)

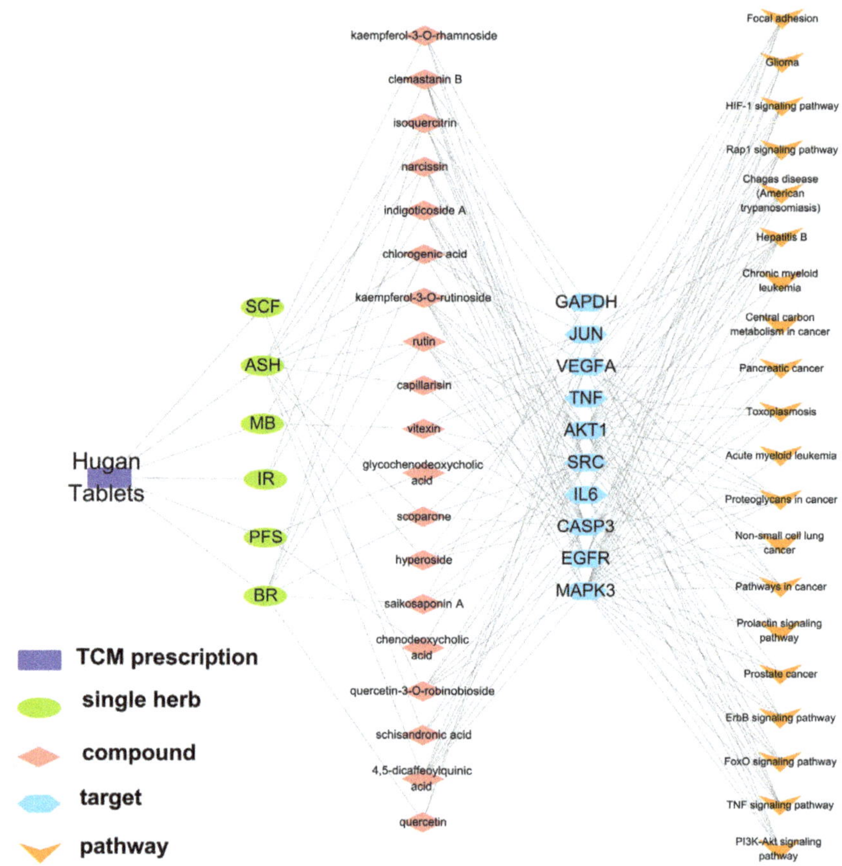

FIGURE 6 | Network diagram of "TCM prescription–single herb–compounds–targets–pathways."

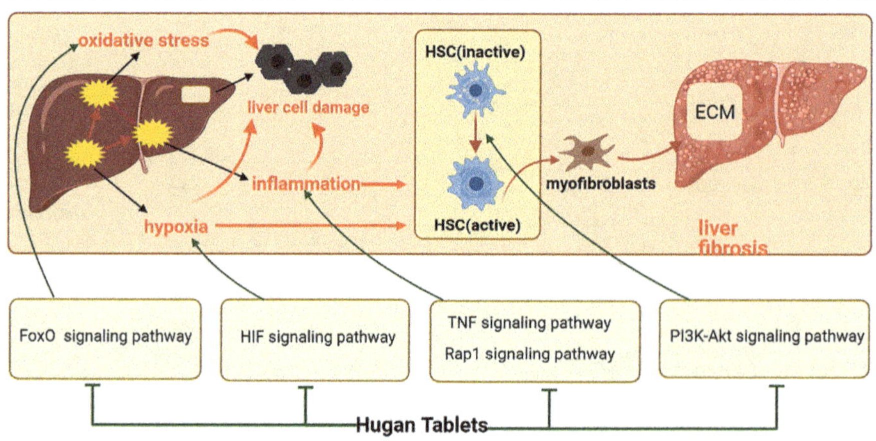

FIGURE 7 | Potential mechanism of Hugan tablets in treating DILI.

through IL-6, AKT1, VEGFA, EGFR, and MAPK3, thereby inhibiting the activation of HSCs and delaying the occurrence of liver fibrosis. In the early stage of the disease, liver injury can also cause local tissue hypoxia, which can aggravate the cell damage and inflammation and promote liver fibrosis. These effects are mediated by hypoxia-inducible factor (HIF) (Rosmorduc and Housset, 2010), so Hugan tablets may regulate the HIF signaling pathway by regulating the expression of GAPDH, IL-6, AKT1, VEGFA, and MAPK3, so as to alleviate the adverse effects of hypoxia to protect the liver. In summary, Hugan tablets may alleviate DILI by resisting oxidative stress and inhibiting inflammation and hepatic fibrosis (**Figure 7**). However, this study still has limitations, for example, the key targets and pathways of Hugan tablets need to be verified by *in vivo* and *in vitro* experiments.

CONCLUSION

In this study, it was found that Hugan tablets can effectively alleviate atorvastatin-induced DILI. Seventy-one compounds in Hugan tablets were characterized, which provided an important basis for elucidating the substance basis of Hugan tablets. Network pharmacological analysis results indicated that Hugan tablets could inhibit inflammatory and alleviate hepatic fibrosis through the comprehensive regulation of multiple compounds, targets, and pathways, thereby achieving an anti-DILI effect.

AUTHOR CONTRIBUTIONS

XG designed and conceptualized this study. SL and XL drafted the article. SL and HY conducted the experiments and data analysis.

FUNDING

This work was supported by the project "From the analysis of traditional Chinese medicine to the discovery of the effective components of traditional Chinese medicine for the prevention and treatment of metabolic diseases" (2020-JYB-ZDGG-033).

ACKNOWLEDGMENTS

The authors are thankful to the Special Project of Ministry of Education (China) for the assistance in conducting this study.

REFERENCES

Black, D. M. (2002). A General Assessment of the Safety of HMG CoA Reductase Inhibitors (Statins). *Curr. Atheroscler. Rep.* 4 (1), 34–41. doi:10.1007/s11883-002-0060-0

Boone, L., Meyer, D., Cusick, P., Ennulat, D., Bolliger, A. P., Everds, N., et al. (2005). Selection and Interpretation of Clinical Pathology Indicators of Hepatic Injury in Preclinical Studies. *Vet. Clin. Pathol.* 34 (3), 182–188. doi:10.1111/j.1939-165x.2005.tb00041.x

Caglayan, C., Kandemir, F. M., Darendelioğlu, E., Yıldırım, S., Kucukler, S., and Dortbudak, M. B. (2019). Rutin Ameliorates Mercuric Chloride-Induced Hepatotoxicity in Rats via Interfering with Oxidative Stress, Inflammation and Apoptosis. *J. Trace Elem. Med. Biol.* 56, 60–68. doi:10.1016/j.jtemb.2019.07.011

Clarke, A. T., and Mills, P. R. (2006). Atorvastatin Associated Liver Disease. *Dig. Liver Dis.* 38 (10), 772–777. doi:10.1016/j.dld.2006.04.013

Deedwania, P., Stone, P. H., Bairey Merz, C. N., Cosin-Aguilar, J., Koylan, N., Luo, D., et al. (2007). Effects of Intensive versus Moderate Lipid-Lowering Therapy on Myocardial Ischemia in Older Patients with Coronary Heart Disease. *Circulation* 115 (6), 700–707. doi:10.1161/CIRCULATIONAHA.106.654756

Du, Z., Lin, Z., Wang, Z., Liu, D., Tian, D., and Xia, L. (2020). SPOCK1 Overexpression Induced by Platelet-Derived Growth Factor-BB Promotes Hepatic Stellate Cell Activation and Liver Fibrosis through the Integrin α5β1/PI3K/Akt Signaling Pathway. *Lab. Invest.* 100 (8), 1042–1056. doi:10.1038/s41374-020-0425-4

Gevrenova, R., Kondeva-Burdina, M., Denkov, N., and Zheleva-Dimitrova, D. (2015). Flavonoid Profiles of Three Bupleurum Species and in Vitrohepatoprotective Activity of Bupleurum Flavum Forsk. *Phcog Mag.* 11 (41), 14–23. doi:10.4103/0973-1296.149680

Gfeller, D., Grosdidier, A., Wirth, M., Daina, A., Michielin, O., and Zoete, V. (2014). SwissTargetPrediction: a Web Server for Target Prediction of Bioactive Small Molecules. *Nucleic Acids Res.* 42 (Web Server issue), W32–W38. doi:10.1093/nar/gku293

Guo, X., Zhu, C., Liu, X., Ge, Y., Jiang, X., and Zhao, W. (2019). Hyperoside Protects against Heart Failure-Induced Liver Fibrosis in Rats. *Acta Histochem.* 121 (7), 804–811. doi:10.1016/j.acthis.2019.07.005

Hafez, M. M., Al-Harbi, N. O., Al-Hoshani, A. R., Al-Hosaini, K. A., Al Shrari, S. D., Al Rejaie, S. S., et al. (2015). Hepato-protective Effect of Rutin via IL-6/STAT3 Pathway in CCl4-Induced Hepatotoxicity in Rats. *Biol. Res.* 48 (1), 30. doi:10.1186/s40659-015-0022-y

Higashi, T., Friedman, S. L., and Hoshida, Y. (2017). Hepatic Stellate Cells as Key Target in Liver Fibrosis. *Adv. Drug Deliv. Rev.* 121, 27–42. doi:10.1016/j.addr.2017.05.007

Hopkins, A. L. (2008). Network Pharmacology: the Next Paradigm in Drug Discovery. *Nat. Chem. Biol.* 4 (11), 682–690. doi:10.1038/nchembio.118

Hu, Y. B., Peng, J. B., Gu, S., Pei, J. F., and Zou, Z. M. (2012). Molecular Docking in Xin-Ke-Shu Preparation's Multi-Target Effect on Coronary Heart Disease. *Acta Phys. -Chim. Sin.* 28 (05), 1257–1264. doi:10.3866/PKU.WHXB201202212

Hu, W.-B., Ouyang, K.-H., Wu, G.-Q., Chen, H., Xiong, L., Liu, X., et al. (2018). Hepatoprotective Effect of Flavonoid-Enriched Fraction from Cyclocarya Paliurus Leaves on LPS/D-GalN-induced Acute Liver Failure. *J. Funct. Foods* 48, 337–350. doi:10.1016/j.jff.2018.07.031

Jaeschke, H. (2006). Mechanisms of Liver Injury. II. Mechanisms of Neutrophil-Induced Liver Cell Injury during Hepatic Ischemia-Reperfusion and Other Acute Inflammatory Conditions. *Am. J. Physiol.-Gastrointest. Liver Physiol.* 290 (6), G1083–G1088. doi:10.1152/ajpgi.00568.2005

Jiang, X.-P., Ai, W.-B., Wan, L.-Y., Zhang, Y.-Q., and Wu, J.-F. (2017). The Roles of microRNA Families in Hepatic Fibrosis. *Cell Biosci.* 7, 34. doi:10.1186/s13578-017-0161-7

Kang, J.-W., Yoon, S.-J., Sung, Y.-K., and Lee, S.-M. (2012). Magnesium Chenoursodeoxycholic Acid Ameliorates Carbon Tetrachloride-Induced Liver Fibrosis in Rats. *Exp. Biol. Med. (Maywood)* 237 (1), 83–92. doi:10.1258/ebm.2011.011219

Kubes, P., and Jenne, C. (2018). Immune Responses in the Liver. *Annu. Rev. Immunol.* 36, 247–277. doi:10.1146/annurev-immunol-051116-052415

Kwan, S. Y., Jiao, J., Qi, J., Wang, Y., Wei, P., McCormick, J. B., et al. (2020). Bile Acid Changes Associated with Liver Fibrosis and Steatosis in the Mexican-American Population of South Texas. *Hepatol. Commun.* 4 (4), 555–568. doi:10.1002/hep4.1490

Kwo, P. Y., Cohen, S. M., and Lim, J. K. (2017). ACG Clinical Guideline: Evaluation of Abnormal Liver Chemistries. *Am. J. Gastroenterol.* 112 (1), 18–35. doi:10.1038/ajg.2016.517

Lai, W.-Y., Wang, J.-W., Huang, B.-T., Lin, E. P.-Y., and Yang, P.-C. (2019). A Novel TNF-α-Targeting Aptamer for TNF-α-Mediated Acute Lung Injury and Acute Liver Failure. *Theranostics* 9 (6), 1741–1751. doi:10.7150/thno.30972

Lee, T.-Y., Chen, F.-Y., Chang, H.-H., and Lin, H.-C. (2009). The Effect of Capillarisin on Glycochenodeoxycholic Acid-Induced Apoptosis and Heme Oxygenase-1 in Rat Primary Hepatocytes. *Mol. Cel. Biochem.* 325 (1-2), 53–59. doi:10.1007/s11010-008-0019-8

Lee, S., Lee, J., Lee, H., and Sung, J. (2019). Relative Protective Activities of Quercetin, Quercetin-3-glucoside, and Rutin in Alcohol-induced Liver Injury. *J. Food Biochem.* 43 (11), e13002. doi:10.1111/jfbc.13002

Lei, F., Liu, Y. M., Zhou, F., Qin, J. J., Zhang, P., Zhu, L., et al. (2020). Longitudinal Association between Markers of Liver Injury and Mortality in COVID-19 in China. *Hepatology* 72 (2), 389–398. doi:10.1002/hep.31301

Li, C. X., Lo, C. M., Lian, Q., Ng, K. T.-P., Liu, X. B., Ma, Y. Y., et al. (2016). Repressor and Activator Protein Accelerates Hepatic Ischemia Reperfusion Injury by Promoting Neutrophil Inflammatory Response. *Oncotarget* 7 (19), 27711–27723. doi:10.18632/oncotarget.8509

Li, C., Chen, Y., Yuan, X., He, L., Li, X., Huang, S., et al. (2020). Vitexin Ameliorates Chronic Stress Plub High Fat Diet-Induced Nonalcoholic Fatty Liver Disease by Inhibiting Inflammation. *Eur. J. Pharmacol.* 882, 173264. doi:10.1016/j.ejphar.2020.173264

Liu, X., and Zhao, X. (2017). Scoparone Attenuates Hepatic Stellate Cell Activation through Inhibiting TGF-β/Smad Signaling Pathway. *Biomed. Pharmacother.* 93, 57–61. doi:10.1016/j.biopha.2017.06.006

Liu, H., Wang, R. B., Xie, Y. M., Li, Y. Y., Liao, X., Liu, S. N., et al. (2019). Expert Consensus Statement on Hugan Tablets in Clinical Practice *China J. Chin. Mater. Med.* 44 (14), 2943–2946. doi:10.19540/j.cnki.cjcmm.20190528.502

Niu, C., Ma, M., Han, X., Wang, Z., and Li, H. (2017). Hyperin Protects against Cisplatin-Induced Liver Injury in Mice. *Acta Cir. Bras.* 32 (8), 633–640. doi:10.1590/s0102-865020170080000005

Puche, J. E., Saiman, Y., and Friedman, S. L. (2013). Hepatic Stellate Cells and Liver Fibrosis. *Compr. Physiol.* 3 (4), 1473–1492. doi:10.1002/cphy.c120035

Rao, S. N., Head, M. S., Kulkarni, A., and LaLonde, J. M. (2007). Validation Studies of the Site-Directed Docking Program LibDock. *J. Chem. Inf. Model.* 47 (6), 2159–2171. doi:10.1021/ci6004299

Rosmorduc, O., and Housset, C. (2010). Hypoxia: a Link between Fibrogenesis, Angiogenesis, and Carcinogenesis in Liver Disease. *Semin. Liver Dis.* 30 (3), 258–270. doi:10.1055/s-0030-1255355

Ru, J., Li, P., Wang, J., Zhou, W., Li, B., Huang, C., et al. (2014). TCMSP: a Database of Systems Pharmacology for Drug Discovery from Herbal Medicines. *J. Cheminform.* 6 (1), 13. doi:10.1186/1758-2946-6-13

Shi, H., Shi, A., Dong, L., Lu, X., Wang, Y., Zhao, J., et al. (2016). Chlorogenic Acid Protects against Liver Fibrosis *In Vivo* and *In Vitro* through Inhibition of Oxidative Stress. *Clin. Nutr.* 35 (6), 1366–1373. doi:10.1016/j.clnu.2016.03.002

Szklarczyk, D., Morris, J. H., Cook, H., Kuhn, M., Wyder, S., Simonovic, M., et al. (2017). The STRING Database in 2017: Quality-Controlled Protein-Protein Association Networks, Made Broadly Accessible. *Nucleic Acids Res.* 45 (D1), D362–D368. doi:10.1093/nar/gkw937

Tan, X.-j., Li, Q., Chen, X.-h., Wang, Z.-w., Shi, Z.-y., Bi, K.-s., et al. (2008). Simultaneous Determination of 13 Bioactive Compounds in Herba Artemisiae Scopariae (Yin Chen) from Different Harvest Seasons by HPLC-DAD. *J. Pharm. Biomed. Anal.* 47 (4-5), 847–853. doi:10.1016/j.jpba.2008.04.010

Tao, G.-Z., Lehwald, N., Jang, K. Y., Baek, J., Xu, B., Omary, M. B., et al. (2013). Wnt/β-Catenin Signaling Protects Mouse Liver against Oxidative Stress-Induced Apoptosis through the Inhibition of Forkhead Transcription Factor FoxO3. *J. Biol. Chem.* 288 (24), 17214–17224. doi:10.1074/jbc.M112.445965

Tasneem, S., Yang, Y., Liu, B., Choudhary, M. I., and Wang, W. (2021). Cytotoxicity of Schisandronic Acid from Kadsura Coccinea by Activation of Caspase-3, Cleavage of Poly-Adp Ribose Polymerase, and Reduction of Oxidative Stress. *Rev. Bras. Farmacogn.* 31 (5), 51–58. doi:10.1007/s43450-021-00136-7

Townsend, N., Wilson, L., Bhatnagar, P., Wickramasinghe, K., Rayner, M., and Nichols, M. (2019). Corrigendum to: Cardiovascular Disease in Europe: Epidemiological Update 2016. *Eur. Heart J.* 40 (2), 189. doi:10.1093/eurheartj/ehy342

Wang, X., Wang, Q., Burczynski, F. J., Kong, W., and Gong, Y. (2013). Saikosaponin A of Bupleurum Chinense (Chaihu) Elevates Bone Morphogenetic Protein 4 (BMP-4) during Hepatic Stellate Cell Activation. *Phytomedicine* 20 (14), 1330–1335. doi:10.1016/j.phymed.2013.07.010

Wang, Y., Tang, C., and Zhang, H. (2015). Hepatoprotective Effects of Kaempferol 3-O-Rutinoside and Kaempferol 3-O-Glucoside from Carthamus tinctorius L. On CCl4-Induced Oxidative Liver Injury in Mice. *J. Food Drug Anal.* 23 (2), 310–317. doi:10.1016/j.jfda.2014.10.002

Wang, F., Zhang, Q., Lu, Z., Wang, Q., Wang, M., Liu, Y., et al. (2016). Identification of Chemical Constituents in Traditional Chinese Medicine Formula Using HPLC Coupled with Linear Ion Trap-Orbitrap MS from High Doses of Medicinal Materials to Equivalent Doses of Formula: Study on Xiang-Sha-Liu-Jun-Zi-Jia-Jian Granules. *J. Sep. Sci.* 39 (9), 1619–1627. doi:10.1002/jssc.201501223

Wang, M. L., Zhang, Q. Q., Fu, S., Liu, Y. H., Liang, C. L., Chen, N., et al. (2017). Characterization of morinda Officinalis How. By UPLC-Q-TOF MS^E Coupled with UNIFI Database Filter. *J. Chin. Mass. Spectrom. Soc.* 38, 75–82. doi:10.7538/zpxb.2017.38.01.0075

Wu, S.-J., Lin, Y.-H., Chu, C.-C., Tsai, Y.-H., and Chao, J. C.-J. (2008). Curcumin or Saikosaponin a Improves Hepatic Antioxidant Capacity and Protects against CCl4-Induced Liver Injury in Rats. *J. Med. Food* 11 (2), 224–229. doi:10.1089/jmf.2007.555

Xiao, P., Huang, H., Chen, J., and Li, X. (2014). *In Vitro* antioxidant and Anti-inflammatory Activities of Radix Isatidis Extract and Bioaccessibility of Six Bioactive Compounds after Simulated Gastro-Intestinal Digestion. *J. Ethnopharmacol.* 157, 55–61. doi:10.1016/j.jep.2014.09.005

Xie, W., Wang, M., Chen, C., Zhang, X., and Melzig, M. F. (2016). Hepatoprotective Effect of Isoquercitrin against Acetaminophen-Induced Liver Injury. *Life Sci.* 152, 180–189. doi:10.1016/j.lfs.2016.04.002

Xing, T. T., Zhao, X. J., Zhang, Y. D., and Li, Y. F. (2017). Fast Separation and Sensitive Quantitation of Polymethoxylated Flavonoids in the Peels of Citrus Using UPLC-Q-TOF-MS. *J. Agric. Food Chem.* 65 (12), 2615–2627. doi:10.1021/acs.jafc.6b05821

Yao, X., Xia, F., Tang, W., Xiao, C., Yang, M., and Zhou, B. (2018). Isobaric Tags for Relative and Absolute Quantitation (iTRAQ)-Based Proteomics for the Investigation of the Effect of Hugan Qingzhi on Non-alcoholic Fatty Liver Disease in Rats. *J. Ethnopharmacol.* 212, 208–215. doi:10.1016/j.jep.2017.09.016

Zhang, C., An, R., Bao, Y.-W., Meng, X.-M., Wang, T.-Q., Sun, H.-N., et al. (2019). Inhibitory Effects of Octreotide on the Progression of Hepatic Fibrosis via the Regulation of Bcl-2/Bax and PI3K/AKT Signaling Pathways. *Int. Immunopharmacol.* 73, 515–526. doi:10.1016/j.intimp.2019.05.055

Zhao, Y., Geng, C.-A., Ma, Y.-B., Huang, X.-Y., Chen, H., Cao, T.-W., et al. (2014). UFLC/MS-IT-TOF Guided Isolation of Anti-HBV Active Chlorogenic Acid Analogues from Artemisia Capillaris as a Traditional Chinese Herb for the Treatment of Hepatitis. *J. Ethnopharmacol.* 156, 147–154. doi:10.1016/j.jep.2014.08.043

Zhu, H., Chen, L., Yu, J., Cui, L., Ali, I., Song, X., et al. (2020). Flavonoid Epimers from Custard Apple Leaves, a Rapid Screening and Separation by HSCCC and Their Antioxidant and Hypoglycaemic Activities Evaluation. *Sci. Rep.* 10 (1), 8819. doi:10.1038/s41598-020-65769-5

13

Prediction of Drug Positioning for Quan-Du-Zhong Capsules Against Hypertensive Nephropathy Based on the Robustness of Disease Network

Feifei Guo[1], *Wen Zhang*[1,2], *Jin Su*[1], *Haiyu Xu*[1*] *and Hongjun Yang*[1*]

[1] *Institute of Chinese Materia Medica, China Academy of Chinese Medical Sciences, Beijing, China,* [2] *College of Ethnic Medicine, Chengdu University of Traditional Chinese Medicine, Chengdu, China*

Correspondence:
Haiyu Xu
hy_xu627@163.com
Hongjun Yang
hjyang@icmm.ac.cn

Hypertensive nephropathy (HN) is a medical condition in which chronic high blood pressure causes different kidney damage, including vascular, glomerular and tubulointerstitial lesions. For HN patients, glomerular and tubulointerstitial lesions occur in different renal structure with distinct mechanisms in the progression of renal damage. As an extraction of *Eucommia ulmoides*, Quan-du-zhong capsule (QDZJN) has the potential to treat HN due to antihypertensive and renal protective activities. Complicated mechanism of HN underlying various renal lesions and the "multi-component and multi-target" characteristics of QDZJN make identifying drug positioning for various renal lesions of HN complex. Here, we proposed an approach based on drug perturbation of disease network robustness, that is used to assess QDZJN positioning for various HN lesions. Topological characteristics of drug-attacked nodes in disease network were used to evaluated nodes importance to network. To evaluate drug attack on the whole disease network of various HN lesions, the robustness of disease networks before/after drug attack were assessed and compared with null models generated from random networks. We found that potential targets of QDZJN were specifically expressed in the kidneys and tended to participate in the "inflammatory response," "regulation of blood pressure," and "response to LPS and hypoxia," and they were also key factors of HN. Based on network robustness assessment, QDZJN may specifically target glomeruli account to the stronger influence on glomerular network after removal of its potential targets. This prediction strategy of drug positioning is suitable for multi-component drugs based on drug perturbation of disease network robustness for two renal compartments, glomeruli and tubules. A stronger influence on the disease network of glomeruli than of tubules indicated that QDZJN may specifically target glomerular lesion of HN patients and will provide more evidence for precise clinical application of QDZJN against HN. Drug positioning approach we proposed also provides a new strategy for predicting precise clinical use of multi-target drugs.

Keywords: hypertensive nephropathy, *Eucommia ulmoides*, drug positioning, network robustness, network pharmacology

---

Abbreviations: APL, average length of shortest path; CC_{net}, clustering coefficient; CC_{node}, closeness centrality; CFDA, China's Food and Drug Administration; DEGs, differentially expressed genes; EU, *Eucommia ulmoides*; HN, hypertensive nephropathy; PUFAs, polyunsaturated fatty acids; QDZJN, Quan-du-zhong capsule; RAAS, renin-angiotensin-aldosterone system; ROS, reactive oxygen species.

INTRODUCTION

Hypertension is a disease that leads to organ damage. Renal damage is a common lesion induced by hypertension due to the interaction of multiple factors, including blood pressure, endothelial dysfunction, the RAAS, ROS, and inflammation (Imig et al., 2018). Hypertensive nephropathy (HN) is a medical condition in which chronic high blood pressure causes kidney damage, including damage to two renal compartments, the glomerular and tubulointerstitial compartments. Exploration of interactions between glomerular and tubulointerstitial compartments contributing to HN creates opportunities to find better therapeutic strategies for renal protection against organ damage in hypertension. For HN patients, glomerulosclerosis and tubulointerstitial fibrosis occur in different renal structure with distinct mechanisms in the progression of renal damage. At the level of the tubulointerstitial compartment, it constitutes 95% of the total kidney mass (Berthier et al., 2012). Early tubular injury is caused by renovascular hypertension, leading to tubular cell proliferation and deposition of matrix proteins primarily within the interstitium which extends far beyond the glomeruli (Mai et al., 1993). In some hypertension patients, circulating antibodies and immunoglobin G deposit along the tubular basement membranes (Mai et al., 1993). Thus, tubulointerstitial change is regarded as a determinative factor in the development of renal damage (Nath, 1992) and may be the important initial site of injury (Mai et al., 1993). At the level of the glomeruli, increased blood pressure leads to increased capillary pressure which results in capillary stretching, endothelial damage, and breakdown of the capillary barrier (Folkow et al., 1977' Bidani and Griffin, 2004). This leads to increased glomerular protein filtration that causes segmental necrosis and glomerulosclerosis (Shankland, 2006). Glomerular sclerosis and preglomerular vascular structural alterations can cause a further reduction in renal blood flow and enhance the progression of hypertensive renal injury (Folkow et al., 1977; Campese et al., 1991; Shankland, 2006; Hemmelgarn et al., 2010).

Numerous drugs are used to control blood pressure, including β-blockers, vasodilators, renin-angiotensin system inhibitors and diuretics. The clinical strategy for treatment of HN is to achieve and maintain blood pressure using minimal drug combinations with minimal side effects (Halbach, 2018). However, in later periods, hypertension patients become less responsive to drugs, and drug combinations are associated with significant side effects (Yusuf et al., 2008; Parving et al., 2012; Fried et al., 2013). It is a challenge to find the best treatment for HN patients that can balance the positive and negative effects of drugs. In China, EU has been widely used to treat hypertension and has also been used in Chinese traditional medicine as a folk drink and functional food for several thousand years (Hussain et al., 2016). EU is a plant containing various chemical constituents such as lignans, iridoids, phenolics, steroids, flavonoids, and other compounds; these components of EU possess various medicinal properties, such as antioxidant, anti-inflammatory, and anti-allergic properties, as well as blood pressure control (Kulomaa et al., 1997; Yen and Hsieh, 1998; Hsieh and Yen, 2000; Park et al., 2006; Bonghyun et al., 2009). *Eucommia* bark extract is a vasorelaxant used for antihypertensive formulations (Kwan et al., 2003; Luo et al., 2010; Greenway et al., 2011). Extract of EU has also been reported to reduce the concentration of hydrogen peroxide in the kidneys and to protect against renal injury (Park et al., 2006; Liu et al., 2012). Thus, EU has the potential to treat HN because of its antihypertensive and renal protective activities with fewer side effects.

However, multicomponents and various medicinal properties make it complex to illustrate the effect of EU on renal protection and blood pressure control. More importantly, the architecture of the kidney increases the complexity. It is difficult to elucidate the mechanisms of EU in treating HN because this involves connecting a multi-component drug with various properties to a complex disease with various risk factors. Based on the "multi-component and multi-target" principle, network robustness methods can be learned from network sciences to identify drug positioning for various HN lesions. Complex systems of disease can be described by networks, in which gene interactions in specific disease conditions are represented by vertices and edges between vertices. Drug disturbance can be presented as an attack on the disease network. Drug effects on system robustness can be addressed by analyzing how the network architecture changes as drug-attacked vertices are removed. In the field of network science, network robustness against perturbations provides a standard of measurement for assessing multi-drug attacks on disease network. Health systems are generally robust against various perturbations but can be fragile when faced with perturbations for which the system has not been optimized (e.g., disease conditions) (Kitano, 2007). Drug attacks with stronger effects on the reduction of the robustness of the disease network suggest that this drug maybe more effective for this disease or pathological process.

Based on the various lesions of HN and the genes expressed in different compartments of kidneys of HN patients, we proposed an approach based on the drug perturbation of disease network robustness of two renal compartments, which is suitable for the assessment of multicomponent drug positioning. The drug perturbation of two different disease networks, renal glomeruli and tubules, will be helpful in describing clinical features and applications of drugs. As an example of a multicomponent drug, an extraction of EU called the QDZJN, which is approved by CFDA, was used in our study. We found that potential targets of QDZJN were specifically expressed in the kidneys and tended to participate in the inflammatory response, regulation of blood pressure, and response to LPS and hypoxia, which were also key factors of HN. Based on network robustness assessment, QDZJN may specifically target glomeruli, suggested by its stronger influence on the glomerular network after removal of its potential targets. QDZJN may be used for HN patients with glomerular injury for better pharmaceutical effects. These finding will provide more evidence for the precise clinical application of QDZJN against HN. This approach we proposed maybe helpful for the precision clinical use of multi-target drugs against HN and other complex diseases.

MATERIALS AND METHODS

Literature Mining of Component Compounds of QDZJN

QDZJN is a CFDA-approved drug that is the extraction of EU. The 84 identified component compounds of QDZJN were retrieved by literature mining of research papers about the bioactive constituents of EU. "*Eucommia ulmoides,*" "du zhong," "compounds," "chemical" and related synonyms were used to retrieve relevant literatures. Information on the component compounds collected from the literature was tidied and reorganized. The molecular structure files of all the component compounds of QDZJN were downloaded from the ChemSpider database[1] and saved in InChI format. Detailed information on the constituent components of QDZJN is provided in **Supplementary Table S1**.

Target Prediction of QDZJN's Component Compounds

Target prediction of the component compounds was executed by BATMAN-TCM (Liu et al., 2016), which is a web service for discovering the therapeutic mechanisms of multicomponent drug (Liu et al., 2016). In BATMAN-TCM, potential drug-target interactions were sorted based on possibility scores from largest to smallest. Possibilities of drug-target interactions were predicted according to their similarities to known drug-target interactions that were previously published and validated (Liu et al., 2016). Three types of validation methods, including "leave-one-interaction-out" cross-validation, "leave-one-drug-out" cross-validation and validation of the independent test set, were applied to measure the performances. Th results showed that BATMAN-TCM had satisfactory performance for target prediction. In this study, potential targets of 84 compounds for QDZJN were predicted with possibility scores larger than 20.

Annotation Enrichment Analysis of Gene Tissue Specificity and Biological Function

Tissue specificity of potential targets of QDZJN was analyzed by the DAVID functional annotation of tissue expression ("Uniprot Tissue") and GO functional enrichment analysis of DAVID was used to detect enriched biological processes of genes (Dennis et al., 2003), both based on the hypergeometric cumulative distribution test. Annotation terms with p-values < 0.05 and fold enrichment larger than 1 were considered statistically significant.

Disease Genes of Hypertension and HN

1409 disease genes related to hypertension were downloaded from DisGeNET Database via MeSH term D006973 (Piñero et al., 2017). And 57 disease genes related to HN were downloaded from DisGeNET via MeSH terms D006977 and D006978 (downloaded on December 3rd, 2018).

[1]http://www.chemspider.com/

Differentially Expressed Genes From Renal Compartments of HN Patients

Transcriptome data were collected from tubulointerstitial and glomerular compartments from kidney biopsies of HN patients ($n = 15$) and healthy living donors ($n = 27$) in Berthier's study (Berthier et al., 2012). In this study, 12,025 human genes were expressed above the 27 Poly-A Affymetrix control expression baseline (negative controls) in the glomerular and tubulointerstitial compartments and were used for further analyses. Microarray data from HN patients will be available on the GEO web site under accession numbers GSE37455 (tubulointerstitial) and GSE37460 (glomeruli). For the microarray data, unpaired statistical analyses for each comparison between the relevant study groups were performed using the significance analysis of microarrays method. DEGs of glomeruli and tubules compared to those of healthy samples were defined by a p-value < 0.05 and with a fold change ≥ 1.1 for the upregulated genes and ≤ 0.91 for the downregulated genes, which were considered significant and used for further transcriptional and pathway analyses.

Construction of Disease Networks for Two Renal Compartments

Disease networks consisted of DEGs and interactions between DEGs. Protein interactions from STRING (Szklarczyk et al., 2017) (version 10) whose confidence scores were larger than 0.4 were used to separately construct protein–protein interaction networks of DEGs of glomerular and tubulointerstitial compartments of HN patients (downloaded on March 19, 2018). Cytoscape (version 3.4.0) was utilized to visualize the networks and calculate the topological characteristics of nodes, including degree, APL, and CC_{node} (Su et al., 2014). Node size is correlated with node degree in networks. Nodes with degrees twofold larger than the median degree of all nodes were defined as hub nodes. Some nodes were also potential targets of QDZJN, these were marked by red edges and ere regarded as nodes attacked by the drug.

Network Robustness Represented by Topological Characteristics of Nodes

First, two characteristics of nodes were used to evaluate the importance of drug-attacked nodes in networks, including APL and CC_{node} of node. Average length of shortest path (APL_{node}) is a characteristic of network nodes that provides a more sophisticated view than the node degree of local connections by also considering the degree of a node's neighbors. This approach accounts for the fact that all edges are not equal: connections to a highly connected node may render a node more significant or influential (Baldassano and Bassett, 2016). The shorter the path length is, the more important the node is.

The average shortest path length of source node is

$$APL_{\text{node}(s)} = \sum_{t \in V} \frac{d(s,t)}{n},$$

where V is the set of nodes in G, $d(s, t)$ is the shortest path from s to t, and s is the source node. n is the number of nodes in G.

Closeness centrality of a node s is the reciprocal of the sum of the shortest path distances from v to all $n-1$ other connected nodes. Since the sum of distances depends on the number of nodes connected with source node s, closeness is normalized by the sum of minimum possible distances $n-1$,

$$CC_{\text{node}(s)} = \frac{n-1}{\sum_{v=1}^{n-1} d(s, v)},$$

where $d(s, v)$ is the shortest-path distance between s and v, and n is the number of nodes connected with s in the graph. The larger the CC_{node} is, the more important the node is.

Here, a comparison of drug-attacked nodes and other nodes in disease network provides a more comparative view of drug-attacked node topological networks, and a unpaired t-test was used to assess differences between two kinds of nodes; a p-value < 0.05 was considered significant.

Network Robustness Represented by Topological Characteristics of Networks

Drug attack on networks were evaluated by changes of network's topological characteristics after removal of the drug target. The Average path length (APL_{net}) is one of the most robust measures of network topology, along with its CC_{net}.

The average shortest path length of a whole network is

$$APL_{\text{net}} = \sum_{s,t \in V} \frac{d(s, t)}{n(n-1)},$$

where V is the set of nodes in G, $d(s, t)$ is the shortest path from s to t, and n is the number of nodes in G.

The clustering of a node v is the fraction of possible triangles through that node that exist,

$$C_v = \frac{2T(v)}{\deg(v)\left(\deg(v) - 1\right)},$$

where $T(v)$ is the number of triangles through node v and $deg(v)$ is the degree of v. The CC_{net} for the graph G is the average,

$$CC_{\text{net}} = \frac{1}{n} \sum_{v \in G} C_v,$$

where n is the number of nodes in G.

In our study, these two indicators were used to evaluated network robustness, including the APL and the CC_{net} of the whole network. First, the average path length distinguishes a stable network from one, with a shorter average path length being more robust. Therefore, the quotient of the APL before/after attack was used to evaluate the influence of drug attack on the disease network. The larger the APL was, the less stable the network and, the larger the influence made by the drug. Similarly, the quotient of the CC_{net} before/after attack was also used to evaluate network robustness after a drug attack. A smaller network CC_{net} indicated a less stable network and a larger drug influence.

Null Model of Random Network and Permutation Test of Real and Random Networks

To assess drug attack effects on network robustness, the network robustness indicators (RI) of random networks were generated as a null model. Drug attack to a real disease network was compared with null models with these two indicators (APL_{net} and CC_{net}) to investigate whether there were significant differences of network robustness between real network and random network after same drug attack. Null models were generated for the disease networks through randomization of network with preserved node and edge numbers of real network. 1,000 random networks were generated as a benchmark, and 1,000 indicators were generated after the same drug attack on random networks as a null distribution for the permutation test (Baldassano and Bassett, 2016). The indicator of a real network out of a 95% confidence interval of null distribution was regarded as having a significant difference (p-value < 0.05 of permutation test). Comparing to the null distribution generated from 1,000 random networks, drug attack that make a significant disturbance in the real disease network was significative. The p-value of drug attack on a real network can be used as a network robustness index for comparison. Smaller p-values indicate larger network disturbance drug attacks.

Construction of Hierarchical Network for QDZJN Compounds, DEGs of Glomeruli and HN Related Process

A hierarchical network of chemical compounds, potential targets and pathological processes was constructed, including component compounds and potential targets of QDZJN, HN related biological processes, drug-target interactions predicted by BATMAN-TCM, relationships between targets and pathological processes of HN retrieved from literatures. Potential targets of QDZJN were also DEGs of glomeruli, namely, drug-attacked nodes in the glomerular network.

RESULTS

QDZJN's Potential Targets Were Upregulated in the Kidney and May Have Anti-hypertension Activity Based on Functional Enrichment Analysis

QDZJN is a CFDA approved drug for hypertension. As multicomponent drug extracted from EU, 84 component compounds of QDZJN were collected via literature mining, including 26 lignans, 17 iridoids, 22 phenylpropanoids, 13 flavonoid, and 8 other kinds of compounds. The structures and other detailed information of the component compounds of QDZJN are shown in the **Supplementary Table S1**. The 427 potential targets of 84 compounds were predicted by BATMAN-TCM (Liu et al., 2016).

Tissue specific expression of potential targets was investigated to explore target tissue attacked by QDZJN. Enriched tissue terms within the UP_Tissue ("Uniprot Tissue") were detected

A

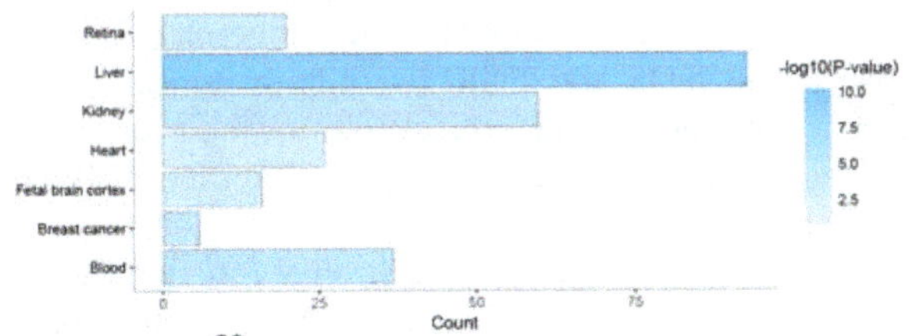

B

	Drug target		Percentage	P-value
	Yes	No		
HN	11	46	19.3%/80.7%	6.80×10^{-6} ****
Hypertension	124	1285	8.8%/91.2%	
Total	135	1331		

C

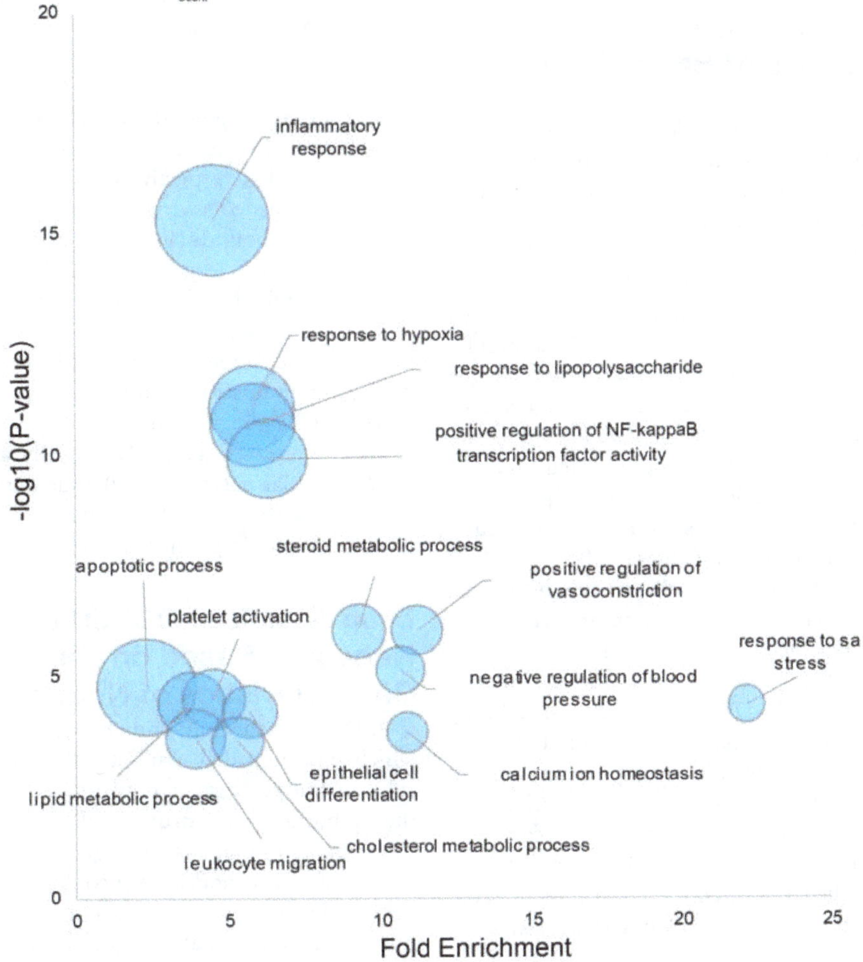

FIGURE 1 | Tissue enrichment and functional enrichment of potential targets of QDZJN. **(A)** Histogram of possible target tissue of QDZJN's potential targets by tissue expression enrichment in DAVID. *X*-axis is the count of targets, and color gradient of bar is related with *p*-value of enrichment analysis. **(B)** Chi-square test table for comparison of the distribution of QDZJN's targets in disease gene of hypertension and HN. **(C)** Bubble diagram of enriched GO terms of QDZJN's targets. *X*-axis is fold enrichment, *Y*-axis is related with *p*-value of enrichment analysis. Bubble size changes with the count of targets in this term.

using DAVID functional annotation of tissue expression (Dennis et al., 2003). Interestingly, potential targets of QDZJN were enriched in UP_TISSUE terms including liver and kidney, among which 60 potential targets were expressed in a high level in normal kidney tissue (**Figure 1A**). Besides, 1409 disease genes related to hypertension and 57 disease genes related to HN were downloaded from DisGeNet Database. A chi-square test was used to compare the distribution of drug target in disease gene of hypertension and HN. A small *P*-value indicates that potential drug targets of QDZJN are enriched in disease genes in HN than hypertension (*p*-value = 6.80×10^{-6}, **Figure 1B**). Even though more drug targets are also hypertensive genes, there are 19.3% disease genes of HN targeted by QDZJN which significantly larger than this proportion in hypertension. This result suggests that kidney may be one of the target organs of QDZJN and HN may be a proper indication of QDZJN than hypertension which was in agreement with the renal protection activity of EU. Functional enrichment analysis of GO terms showed that QDZJN potential targets were enriched in biological processes including "inflammatory response," "response to hypoxia," "response to LPS," "regulation of vasoconstriction and blood pressure" (**Figure 1C**). Consistent with this finding, EU has been reported to exhibit anti-oxidant, anti-hypertensive, and anti-inflammatory activity.[18,30, 31] According to the above result, QDZJN has the potential to prevent kidney damage induced by hypertension, as well as hypertension. Of note, a randomized controlled study of QDZJN showed that this drug was effective for the treatment of renal hypertension (Zhen and Liang, 2012; Jing et al., 2015).

Differentially Expressed Genes in Glomeruli and Tubules of HN Patients

Glomerular and tubulointerstitial lesion are two common types of kidney damage induced by hypertension. To investigate the relationship between QDZJN and two kidney compartments, gene expression data were collected from kidney tubules and glomerular samples of HN patients and healthy living donors in Berthier's study (Berthier et al., 2012). DEGs were identified from comparing the kidneys of human with HN with healthy kidneys, as the kidney maybe QDZJN's target organ. Kidneys from HN patients demonstrated 325 glomerular and 147 tubulointerstitial genes with significantly changed mRNA expression compared with healthy kidneys (**Figure 2A**). A total of 131 upregulated and 194 downregulated genes were identified in glomeruli, and 90 upregulated and 57 downregulated genes were identified in tubule (**Figure 2A**). There were 53 genes differentially expressed in both glomerular and tubulointerstitial compartments (**Figure 2B**). Result of enrichment analysis showed that glomeruli and tubules shared some pathways, e.g., "inflammatory and immune response," "apoptotic process," "angiogenesis," and "response to oxidative stress" (**Figure 2C**) which are key factors in renal damage induced by hypertension (Imig et al., 2018). DEGs in glomeruli specifically participate in the regulation of blood pressure and cholesterol homeostasis which is related to hypothalamic-pituitary-adrenal (HPA) axis. Similar to DEGs, biological processes related to "inflammatory response,""response to hypoxia," and "regulation of blood pressure" were also enriched in QDZJN's potential targets. This finding implied that QDZJN intervenes in renal damage by controlling responses to inflammation, oxidative stress and blood pressure.

Construction of Disease Networks of Kidney Glomeruli and Tubules

Disease networks based on DEGs in glomeruli and tubules were constructed to exhibit the interaction between DEGs in two kidney compartments and to assess the drug perturbation of disease networks. The glomerular disease network consisted of DEGs in the glomerulus and interactions between DEGs from STRING database, containing 234 nodes with 836 edges (**Figure 3A**). The tubule disease network contained 109 nodes with 280 edges (**Figure 3B**). Node size is relevant to the degree of node in the disease network, which is defined as the number of edges connected to that node (see "Materials and Methods" section). Hubs are important in the disease network. After the hub is attacked by drug, it broadcasts the effect to the nodes to which it is linked. Nodes with degree two-fold larger than median of degrees of all nodes were defined as hub nodes which play important roles. There were 15 and 44 hub nodes in tubular and glomerular networks, respectively. ALB, FOS and EGR1 were both hub nodes in two networks, these genes play critical roles in the progression of HN. Based on previous studies, urinary albumin (ALB) had the potential to be a marker for hypertension (Takase et al., 2015). EGR1 deficiency protects against renal function by attenuating NF-κB and TGFβ-mediated renal inflammation/fibrosis (Ho et al., 2016, 1). However, most hub nodes were specifically expressed in single renal compartment.

To investigate the importance of drug-attacked nodes in the disease network, potential targets were marked with red edges in **Figure 3**. In the glomerular and tubulointerstitial network, 6 and 22 nodes, respectively, were potential targets of QDZJN and were regarded as drug-attacked nodes that were attacked by QDZJN's compounds (**Figure 3**). In the glomerular network, hub node PPARG was targeted by QDZJN, it has been reported to be a new target for the treatment of hypertension as well as pivotal in vascular muscle as a regulator of vascular structure, vascular function, and blood pressure (Leibovitz and Schiffrin, 2007). In both tubulointerstitial and glomerular networks, LTF was a key node that has been verified to be an antihypertensive peptide (Ruiz-Giménez et al., 2012). QDZJN attacked 8 hub nodes in the glomerular network, but 0 node in the tubular network. This result suggested that potential targets of QDZJN may play more important roles in glomerular network.

Drug Attack of QDZJN on Disease Networks Based on Topological Characteristics of Nodes

QDZJN affected eight hub nodes of the glomerular network which indicated that drug-attacked nodes may play important roles in the glomerular network. To comprehensively evaluate the importance of drug-attacked nodes in glomerular and tubulointerstitial disease network, two more topological features of drug-attacked nodes were compared with other nodes in the disease network, including average path length and CC_{node} of node. The average path length of node (APL_{node}) is defined as the average number of steps along the shortest paths for all nodes connected to that node. It is a measure of the efficiency of information or mass transport on a network. CC_{node} of a node is a measure of centrality in a network, calculated as the sum of the length of the shortest paths between the node and all other nodes in the graph. The more central a node is, the closer it is to all other nodes. In glomerular network, drug-attacked nodes have relative shorter APL_{node} and larger CC_{node} than other nodes in the glomerular network with statistically significant difference ($p_{apl} = 1.42 \times 10^{-2}$; $p_{cc} = 2.75 \times 10^{-2}$) indicating that drug-attacked nodes tend to connect closely to nodes in the network (**Figures 4A,B**). However, APL_{node} and CC_{node} of drug-attacked nodes in tubulointerstitial network had no significant differences with other nodes (**Figures 4A,B**). Comparing drug-attacked node in these two different disease networks, drug-attacked nodes in the glomerular network had more important position and attacks to these nodes will more greatly influence linked nodes and whole

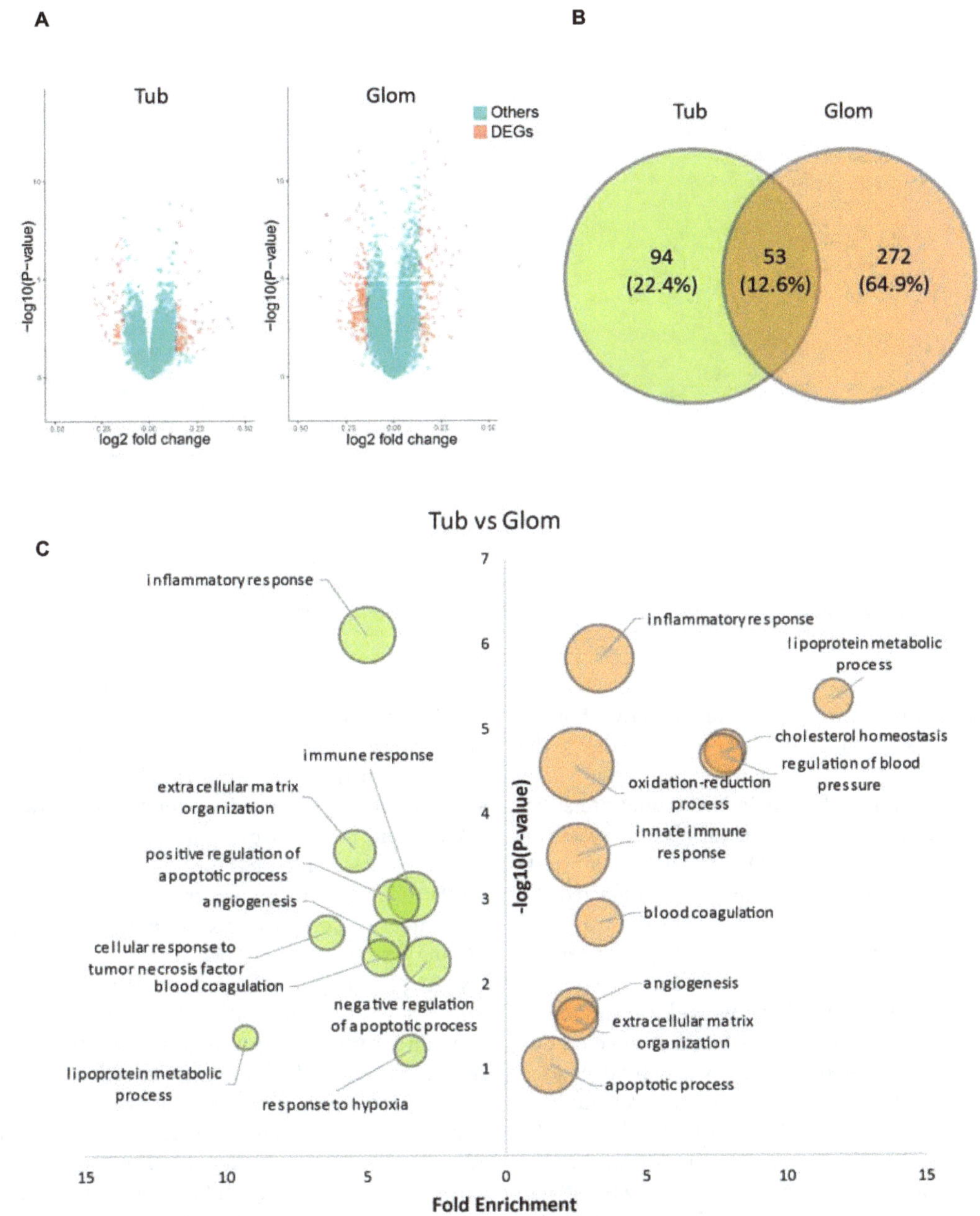

FIGURE 2 | Differentially expressed genes (DEGs) in tubules and glomeruli of HN patients. **(A)** Volcano plot of differentially expressed genes in tubules and glomeruli. **(B)** Venn diagram of DEGs in tubules (green) and glomeruli (orange). **(C)** Bubble plot of enriched GO terms of DEGs of tubules (green) and glomeruli (orange). *X*-axis is fold enrichment, *Y*-axis is related with *p*-value of enrichment analysis. Bubble size changes with the count of targets in this term.

network robustness, but there was no sizeable difference in the tubulointerstitial network.

QDZJN Tent to Disturb Glomerular Network of HN Patients Based on Network Robustness

Next, the robustness of whole networks against drug attack was assessed to evaluate QDZJN attack on the disease network of glomeruli and tubules (**Figure 4C**). Here, two of the most robust measures of network topology, average length of shortest path (APL_{net}) and CC_{net}, were used. The results showed that overall network structure in the tubulointerstitial network was more robust than that of the random network after drug attack with minimal change in APL_{net} and CC_{net} (**Figures 4D,E**). However, the network structure of glomerular network was less robust than that of the random network under drug attack with bigger change in APL_{net} and CC_{net} (**Figures 4D,E**). This finding indicated that drug attack on the disease networks of two renal regions result in a different reaction of genes connection in glomeruli

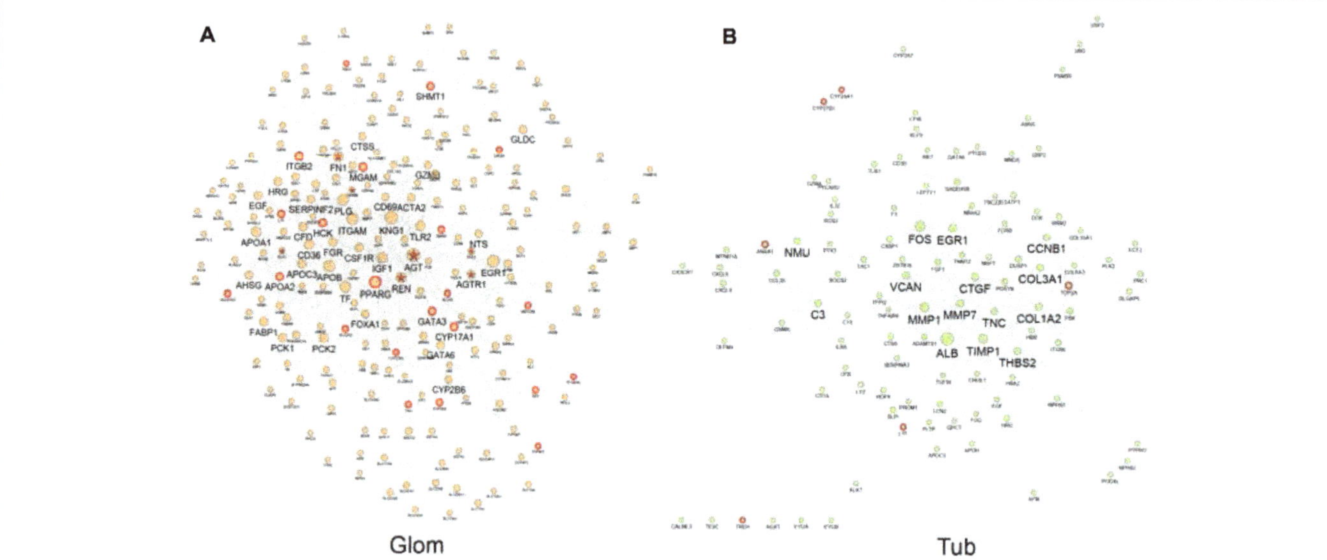

FIGURE 3 | Interaction network of DEGs in glomeruli **(A)** and tubules **(B)**. Node size changes with the node degree in network. The hub nodes were marked with big name labels and potential drug targets of QDZJN were marked with red edges. Nodes with red star label were disease genes related to HN from DisGeNET database.

and tubules: the glomerular network was more sensitive, but the tubulointerstitial network remained stable in structure due to the removal of drug targets.

Interestingly, APL_{net} was decreased in the tubulointerstitial network (p-value < 0.001 by permutation test) but increased in the glomerular network (p-value < 0.001 by permutation test) after drug attack. The different change in APL_{net} reflected the underlying difference in network organization for the two renal regions; drug attack on the glomerulus system was characterized by greater rich-club organization, and increasing dependence on hub nodes, resulting in greater fragility under drug attack. In contrast, the tubulointerstitial network was less affected due to its redundant structure. Moreover, CC_{net} was only decreased in the glomerular network (p-value < 0.001 by permutation test), but not in the tubulointerstitial network (p-value > 0.05 by permutation test). The different change in CC_{net} implies that the glomerular system is more sensitive to QDZJN attack. Overall structure changes of glomerular and tubulointerstitial networks after drug attack show that QDZJN specifically targeted glomeruli, as shown by the increased APL_{net} and decreased CC_{net} after removal of drug targets.

Mechanism of Drug Protection Against Glomerular Damage Induced by Hypertension

To illustrate the mechanism of QDZJN against glomerular damage induced by hypertension, a hierarchical network of chemical compounds common targets of QDZJN and DEGs from glomeruli, and pathological processes related to HN was constructed, including drug-target interactions and relationships between targets and HN pathological processes (**Figure 5**). This network shows that 13 drug-attacked nodes in the glomerular network were related to hypertensive pathological processes and 21 chemical compounds of QDZJN interacted with these drug-attacked nodes. These 13 drug-attacked nodes belonged to four key pathways of HN, e.g., RAAS, lipid metabolism, immune response, and inflammatory response. PAH interacts with DCC to regulate dopamine synthesis from tyrosine. Recent studies show that the intrarenal dopaminergic system indirectly inhibits renal renin expression (Zhang et al., 2005). Specifically, CYP3A4, CYP27B1, and SNAI2 play important roles in vitamin D metabolism, and evidence has been collected to indicate that vitamin D may interact with renin to represses the RAAS system and reduce the loss of glomerular filtration rate (Santoro et al., 2015). Some drug-attacked nodes maintain lipid metabolic homeostasis (specifically, metabolism of cholesterol and PUFAs, adipogenesis). As a synthesis enzyme of cholesterol, CYP3A4 closely connects to high blood pressure. The SNP genotypes of APOA2, ALOX5, and CYP4F2 were associated with the content of PUFAs (Tagetti et al., 2015; Ballester et al., 2016) which is associated with significant improvement in vascular function and lower blood pressure (Colussi et al., 2016). Epidemiological studies show that circulating PUFAs contribute to preserving renal function (Syren et al., 2017). PPARG influences adipogenesis in glomeruli and knock down of PPARG can lead to glomerular hypertrophy (Toffoli et al., 2017). GATA3, and ITGB2 participated in different immune responses, glomerular immunoglobin A deposition (Yamanaka et al., 2016) and leukocyte recruitment to the inflamed glomerulus (Kuligowski et al., 2006), respectively. In glomerular injury, upregulation of ALOX5 promotes inflammation (Hao and Breyer, 2007), but LTF (Drago-Serrano et al., 2017) and PTGER2 suppress it. As the prostaglandin E2 receptor, activation of PTGER2 accentuates chronic inflammation and protects

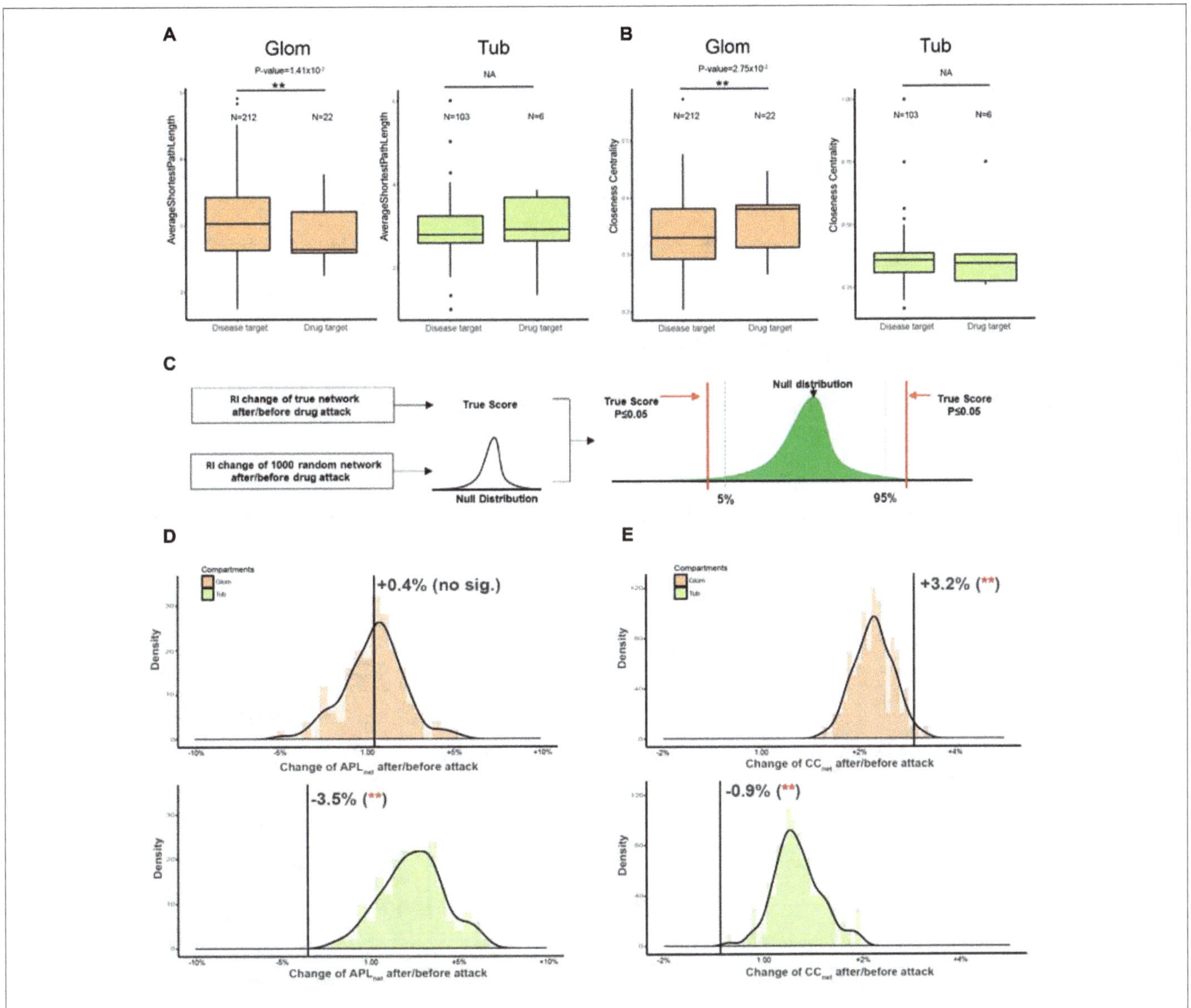

FIGURE 4 | Comparison of topological features of drug-attacked node in tubulointerstitial and glomerular network. **(A,B)** Boxplot of APL_{node} **(A)** and CC_{node} **(B)** of drug-attacked nodes and other nodes in tubulointerstitial and glomerular network. **p-value < 0.05. **(C)** Schematic diagram of Permutation test. Network topological features were used as robustness indicators (RI) of networks. Null distribution of RI of 1000 random network was generated to maintain the same edge number of the true network and randomize interactions between nodes. Comparing with the null distribution, statistical significance of RI of true network can be calculated. **(D,E)** Robustness (APL_{net} for **D**, CC_{net} for **E**) of glomerular and tubulointerstitial network versus random network (green distribution for tubules and orange distribution for glomeruli). *X*-axis is the percentage change of robustness indicators before/after attack. **p-value < 0.05.

against angiotensin II-induced hypertension via inhibition of oxidative stress (Jia et al., 2008; Jiang and Dingledine, 2013). Vitamin D also preserves kidney function via attenuating the inflammatory response during lipopolysaccharide-induced acute kidney injury (Xu et al., 2015). Among these drug-attacked nodes, LTF, PPARG, and APOA2 have been proven to be targets for hypertension treatment (Ruiz-Giménez et al., 2012; Ballester et al., 2016; Toffoli et al., 2017). Eight out of 21 possible active compounds have been already found to have anti-hypertension or glomerular protection activity, including ursolic acid (Somova et al., 2003; Zhou et al., 2010), β-sitosterol (Olaiya et al., 2014), ascorbic acid (Duffy et al., 1999), gallic acid (Jin et al., 2017), protocatechuic acid (Safaeian et al., 2016), pyrogallol (Lai and Spector, 1978), epicatechin (Galleano et al., 2013), and catechin (Rhee et al., 2002; Bhardwaj and Khanna, 2013).

DISCUSSION

As the leading cause of cardiovascular mortality, hypertension also leads to damage of various organs, especially renal damage. As a multicomponent drug, QDZJN was widely used to control blood pressure and protect renal function. In our study,

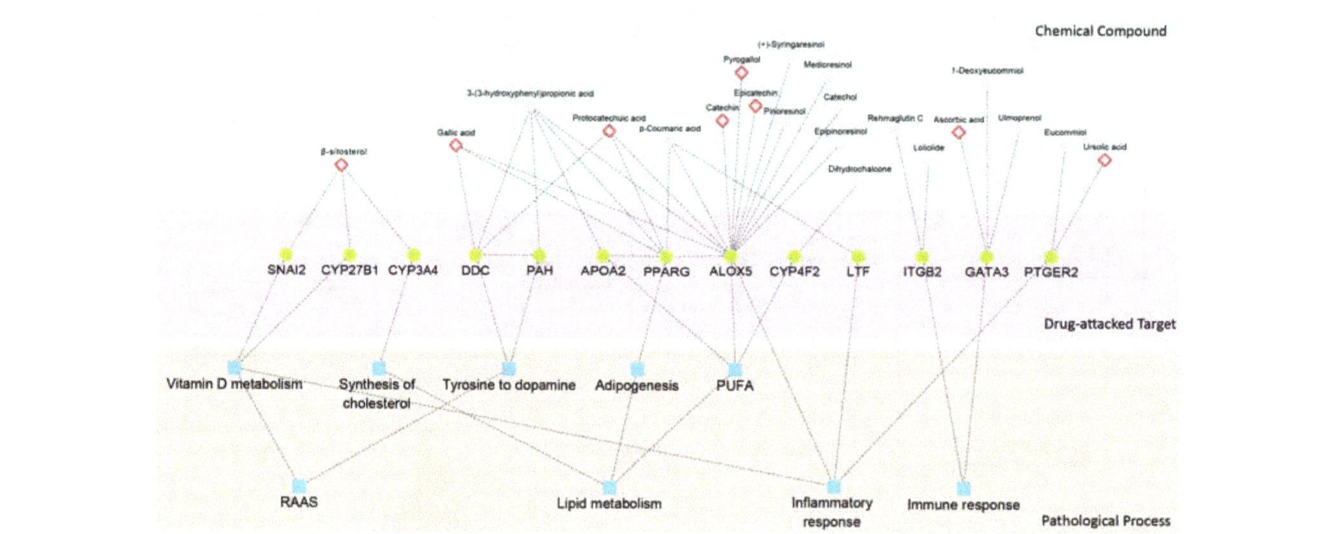

FIGURE 5 | Hierarchy network of chemical compound, drug-attacked nodes in the glomerular network and HN related pathological processes. Compounds with red edge represent drug with anti-hypertensive activity.

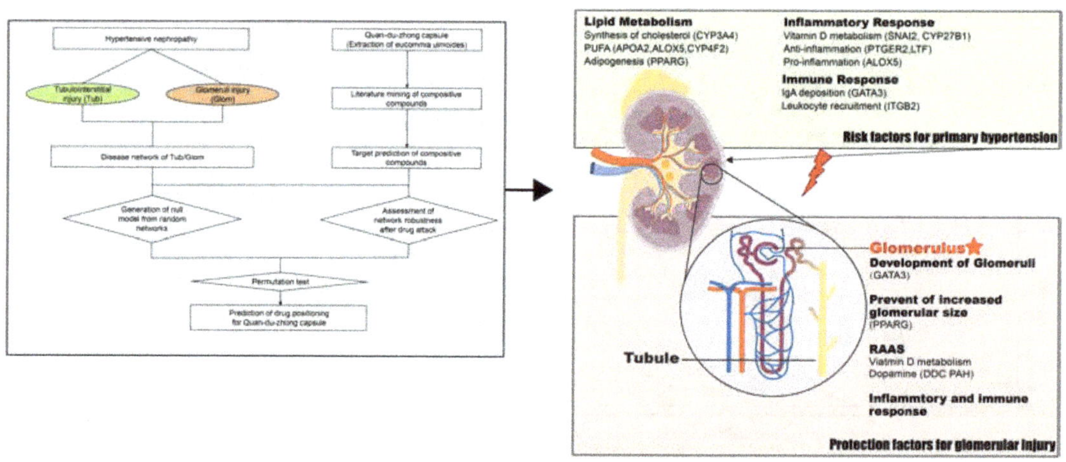

FIGURE 6 | QDZJN against HN via renal protection and reduction of hypertension risk. Left part is the schematic diagram of tissue location of drug based on network robustness. Possible mechanism of QDZJN protect against glomerular injury of HN was summarized in right part.

QDZJN was found to specifically target glomerular damage of HN patients.

Hypertensive nephropathy is a medical condition in which chronic high blood pressure causes kidney damage, including vascular, glomerular, and tubulointerstitial lesions. Glomeruli and tubules play different roles in HN. Thus, tubulointerstitial changes are regarded as a major determinant in the progression of renal damage and may be the important initial sites of injury. Then, an increase in capillary pressure causes segmental necrosis and glomerulosclerosis. Finally, glomerulosclerosis and preglomerular vascular structural alterations can cause a further reduction in renal blood flow. Based on transcriptome data from Berthier's study, DEGs in glomeruli specifically participate in pathways related to blood pressure control and cholesterol homeostasis. Glomeruli and tubules also share some pathways, including oxidative stress, angiogenesis, inflammatory response and immune response.

Because of the anti-oxidant, anti-hypertensive, and anti-inflammatory activities of QDZJN, it has the potential to treat HN. Moreover, potential targets of QDZJN were specifically expressed in renal tissue, which provides more evidence to support QDZJN positioning to HN. If QDZJN has the potential to prevent renal damage, question include how and on which part QDZJN will intervene. To discovery the precise target sub-organ position of QDZJN, the robustness of disease networks from glomeruli and tubules was evaluated under QDZJN attack (**Figure 6**). Drug-attacked nodes in the glomerular network had more important positions in disease network with larger CC_{node} and smaller shortest path length, which implies that attack to these nodes will more strongly influence network robustness.

Overall structural change in the glomerular and tubulointerstitial networks after QDZJN attack show that QDZJN specifically target glomeruli, as indicated by the increased shortest path length and decreased CC_{net} of the whole network after removal of drug targets.

A hierarchical network of 21 chemical compounds of QDZJN, 13 drug-attacked nodes in the glomerular network, and pathological processes related to HN was constructed to clarify the relationship between drug and disease. And all these 21 possible active compounds may target on 13 genes specifically expressed in glomeruli which were related to RAAS, lipid metabolism, immune response, and inflammatory response. These biological processes can be divided into two categories, primary hypertension factors and kidney protection factors (**Figure 6**). Specifically, lipid metabolism is a critical pathway in primary hypertension and plays important roles in renal damage. CYP3A4, APOA2, PPARG, ALOX, and CYP4F2, proteins related to lipid homeostasis affect the occurrence of hypertension, and PTGER2, ALOX5, LTF, ITGB, and GATA3 relate to the inflammatory and immune response in glomeruli. For kidney protection, GATA3 and PPARG both have protective effects on glomeruli. GATA3 was specifically expressed in glomeruli and is related to renal aplasia (Moriguchi et al., 2016, 3). PPARG influences adipogenesis in glomeruli, and knock down of PPARG can lead to glomerular hypertrophy (Toffoli et al., 2017). SNAI2, CYP27B1, DDC, and PAH inhibits the RAAS system to reserve glomerular function by regulating concertation of vitamin D and dopamine. In summary, QDZJN can preserve renal function and reduce hypertensive risk factor by anti-inflammation, antioxidation and regulation of metabolic homeostasis.

Similar to QDZJN, most multicomponent drugs have various medicinal properties, making it a challenge to maximize the efficacy of drugs and to find optimum indications. Based on the "multi-component and multi-target" principle, multiple attacks on network can simulate multicomponent drug effects to disease network. Evaluation of network robustness can assess the strength of drug attacks on network. In previous studies, network robustness has been used in drug discovery, and cancer biology. In this study, we innovatively proposed a strategy to precisely position the clinical application of drug based on network robustness which can be applied to the precise clinical positioning of other multi-target drugs. This strategy suggests a new approach for multicomponent drug discovery. For multi-target drugs, including monomers with many targets, and multicomponent drugs, approaches based on network robustness can be applied to many research topics, such as, the best indication for a drug and, upon which part of a complex disease does the drug work. In our study, QDZJN was repositioned to HN, especially glomeruli, which is also a new finding about QDZJN and needs further experimental verification. Prediction of precise position for drug is very helpful for drug clinical applications, QDZJN may be used for patients with glomerular injury for better pharmaceutical effects.

AUTHOR CONTRIBUTIONS

FG, HX, and HY conceived the study and wrote the manuscript. FG and WZ performed the data analysis. JS collected the component of QDZJN. All authors reviewed and approved the final manuscript.

FUNDING

The authors acknowledge support from the National Major Scientific and Technological Special Project for "Significant New Drugs Development" (2018ZX09201009), the National Natural Science Foundation of China (81703951), the Fundamental Research Funds for the Central Public Welfare Research Institutes (ZXKT17058), and Jiangxi Prozin Pharmaceutical Co., Ltd.

REFERENCES

Baldassano, S. N., and Bassett, D. S. (2016). Topological distortion and reorganized modular structure of gut microbial co-occurrence networks in inflammatory bowel disease. *Sci. Rep.* 6:26087. doi: 10.1038/srep26087

Ballester, M., Revilla, M., Puig-Oliveras, A., Marchesi, J. A., Castelló, A., Corominas, J., et al. (2016). Analysis of the porcine APOA2 gene expression in liver, polymorphism identification and association with fatty acid composition traits. *Anim. Genet.* 47, 552–559. doi: 10.1111/age.12462

Berthier, C. C., Bethunaickan, R., Gonzalez-Rivera, T., Nair, V., Ramanujam, M., Zhang, W., et al. (2012). Cross-species transcriptional network analysis defines shared inflammatory responses in murine and human lupus nephritis. *J. Immunol.* 189, 988–1001. doi: 10.4049/jimmunol.1103031

Bhardwaj, P., and Khanna, D. (2013). Green tea catechins: defensive role in cardiovascular disorders. *Chin. J. Nat. Med.* 11, 345–353. doi: 10.1016/S1875-5364(13)60051-5

Bidani, A. K., and Griffin, K. A. (2004). Pathophysiology of hypertensive renal damage: implications for therapy. *Hypertension* 44, 595–601. doi: 10.1161/01.HYP.0000145180.38707.84

Bonghyun, K., Kyoungsik, P., and Chang, I. M. (2009). Elucidation of anti-inflammatory potencies of *Eucommia ulmoides* bark and *Plantago asiatica* seeds. *J. Med. Food* 12, 764–769. doi: 10.1089/jmf.2008.1239

Campese, V. M., Parise, M., Karubian, F., and Bigazzi, R. (1991). Abnormal renal hemodynamics in black salt-sensitive patients with hypertension. *Hypertension* 18, 805–812.

Colussi, G., Catena, C., Novello, M., Bertin, N., and Sechi, L. A. (2016). Impact of omega-3 polyunsaturated fatty acids on vascular function and blood pressure: relevance for cardiovascular outcomes. *Nutr. Metab. Cardiovasc. Dis.* 27, 191–200. doi: 10.1016/j.numecd.2016.07.011

Dennis, G., Sherman, B. T., Hosack, D. A., Yang, J., Gao, W., Lane, H. C., et al. (2003). DAVID: database for annotation, visualization, and integrated discovery. *Genome Biol.* 4:R60. doi: 10.1186/gb-2003-4-9-r60

Drago-Serrano, M. E., Campos-Rodríguez, R., Carrero, J. C., and de la Garza, M. (2017). Lactoferrin: balancing ups and downs of inflammation due to microbial infections. *Int. J. Mol. Sci.* 18:E501. doi: 10.3390/ijms18030501

Duffy, S. J., Gokce, N., Holbrook, M., Huang, A., Frei, B., Duffy, J. F. Jr., et al. (1999). Treatment of hypertension with ascorbic acid. *Lancet* 354, 2048–2049. doi: 10.3390/ijms18030501

Folkow, B., Göthberg, G., Lundin, S., and Ricksten, S. E. (1977). Structural "resetting" of the renal vascular bed in spontaneously hypertensive rats (SHR). *Acta Physiol. Scand.* 100, 270–272. doi: 10.1111/j.1748-1716.1977.tb05949.x

Fried, L. F., Emanuele, N., Zhang, J. H., Brophy, M., Conner, T. A., Duckworth, W., et al. (2013). Combined angiotensin inhibition for the treatment of diabetic nephropathy. *N. Engl. J. Med.* 369, 1892–1903. doi: 10.1111/j.1748-1716.1977.tb05949.x

Galleano, M., Bernatova, I., Puzserova, A., Balis, P., Sestakova, N., Pechanova, O., et al. (2013). Epicatechin reduces blood pressure and improves vasorelaxation in spontaneously hypertensive rats by NO-mediated mechanism. *Iubmb Life* 65, 710–715. doi: 10.1002/iub.1185

Greenway, F., Liu, Z., Yu, Y., and Gupta, A. (2011). A clinical trial testing the safety and efficacy of a standardized *Eucommia ulmoides* oliver bark extract to treat hypertension. *Altern. Med. Rev.* 16, 338–347. doi: 10.1002/iub.1185

Halbach, S. M. (2018). *Hypertension in Chronic Kidney Disease.* Available at: http://www.researchgate.net/publication/322967523_Hypertension_in_Chronic_Kidney_Disease [accessed July 10, 2018].

Hao, C.-M., and Breyer, M. D. (2007). Physiologic and pathophysiologic roles of lipid mediators in the kidney. *Kidney Int.* 71, 1105–1115. doi: 10.1038/sj.ki.5002192

Hemmelgarn, B. R., Manns, B. J., Lloyd, A., James, M. T., Klarenbach, S., Quinn, R. R., et al. (2010). Relation between kidney function, proteinuria, and adverse outcomes. *JAMA* 303, 423–429. doi: 10.1001/jama.2010.39

Ho, L.-C., Sung, J.-M., Shen, Y.-T., Jheng, H.-F., Chen, S.-H., Tsai, P.-J., et al. (2016). Egr-1 deficiency protects from renal inflammation and fibrosis. *J. Mol. Med.* 94, 933–942. doi: 10.1007/s00109-016-1403-6

Hsieh, C. L., and Yen, G. C. (2000). Antioxidant actions of du-zhong (*Eucommia ulmoides Oliv.*) toward oxidative damage in biomolecules. *Life Sci.* 66, 1387–1400. doi: 10.1016/S0024-3205(00)00450-1

Hussain, T., Tan, B., Liu, G., Oladele, O. A., Rahu, N., Tossou, M. C., et al. (2016). Health-promoting properties of *Eucommia ulmoides*: a review. *Evid. Based Complement. Alternat. Med.* 2016:5202908. doi: 10.1155/2016/5202908

Imig, J. D., Khan, M. A. H., and El-Meanawy, A. (2018). "Molecular Pathways in Hypertensive Renal Damage," in *Disorders of Blood Pressure Regulation Updates in Hypertension and Cardiovascular Protection*, eds A. E. Berbari and G. Mancia (Cham: Springer), 445–463. doi: 10.1007/978-3-319-59918-2_26

Jia, Z., Guo, X., Zhang, H., Wang, M. H., Dong, Z., and Yang, T. (2008). Microsomal prostaglandin synthase-1–derived prostaglandin E2 protects against angiotensin II–induced hypertension via inhibition of oxidative stress. *Hypertension* 52, 952–959. doi: 10.1161/HYPERTENSIONAHA.108.111229

Jiang, J. J., and Dingledine, R. (2013). Prostaglandin receptor EP2 in the crosshairs of anti-inflammation, anti-cancer, and neuroprotection. *Trends Pharmacol. Sci.* 34, 413–423. doi: 10.1016/j.tips.2013.05.003

Jin, L., Piao, Z. H., Sun, S., Liu, B., Kim, G. R., Seok, Y. M., et al. (2017). Gallic acid reduces blood pressure and attenuates oxidative stress and cardiac hypertrophy in spontaneously hypertensive rats. *Sci. Rep.* 7:15607. doi: 10.1038/s41598-017-15925-1

Jing, X., Huang, W.-H., Tang, Y.-J., Wang, Y.-Q., Li, H., Tian, Y.-Y., et al. (2015). *Eucommia ulmoides* Oliv. *(Du-Zhong)* lignans inhibit angiotensin ii-stimulated proliferation by affecting P21, P27, and bax expression in rat mesangial cells. *Evid. Based Complement. Alternat. Med.* 2015:987973. doi: 10.1155/2015/987973

Kitano, H. (2007). A robustness-based approach to systems-oriented drug design. *Nat. Rev. Drug Discov.* 6, 202–210. doi: 10.1038/nrd2195

Kuligowski, M. P., Kitching, A. R., and Hickey, M. J. (2006). Leukocyte recruitment to the inflamed glomerulus: a critical role for platelet-derived P-selectin in the absence of rolling. *J. Immunol.* 176, 6991–6999. doi: 10.4049/jimmunol.176.11.6991

Kulomaa, A., Sirén, H., and Riekkola, M. L. (1997). Identification of antioxidative compounds in plant beverages by capillary electrophoresis with the marker index technique. *J. Chromatogr. A* 781, 523–532. doi: 10.1016/S0021-9673(97)00357-9

Kwan, C. Y., Chen, C. X., Deyama, T., and Nishibe, S. (2003). Endothelium-dependent vasorelaxant effects of the aqueous extracts of the *Eucommia ulmoides* Oliv. leaf and bark: implications on their antihypertensive action. *Vasc. Pharmacol.* 40:229–235. doi: 10.1016/j.vph.2003.09.001

Lai, F. M., and Spector, S. (1978). The potentiating effect of clorgyline and pyrogallol on the blood pressure responses to norepinephrine. *Arch. Int. Pharmacodyn. Thér.* 234:279–286.

Leibovitz, E., and Schiffrin, E. L. (2007). PPAR activation: a new target for the treatment of hypertension. *J. Cardiovasc. Pharmacol.* 50, 120–125. doi: 10.1097/FJC.0b013e318062153b

Liu, E., Han, L., Wang, J., He, W., Shang, H., Gao, X., et al. (2012). *Eucommia ulmoides* bark protects against renal injury in cadmium-challenged rats. *J. Med. Food* 15, 307–314. doi: 10.1089/jmf.2011.1756

Liu, Z., Guo, F., Wang, Y., Li, C., Zhang, X., Li, H., et al. (2016). BATMAN-TCM: a bioinformatics analysis tool for molecular mechanism of traditional chinese medicine. *Sci. Rep.* 6:21146. doi: 10.1038/srep21146

Luo, L. F., Wu, W. H., Zhou, Y. J., Yan, J., Yang, G. P., and Ouyang, D. S. (2010). Antihypertensive effect of *Eucommia ulmoides* Oliv. extracts in spontaneously hypertensive rats. *J. Ethnopharmacol.* 129, 238–243. doi: 10.1016/j.jep.2010.03.019

Mai, M., Geiger, H., Hilgers, K. F., Veelken, R., Mann, J. F., Dämmrich, J., et al. (1993). Early interstitial changes in hypertension-induced renal injury. *Hypertension* 22, 754–765. doi: 10.1161/01.HYP.22.5.754

Moriguchi, T., Yu, L., Otsuki, A., Ainoya, K., Lim, K.-C., Yamamoto, M., et al. (2016). Gata3 hypomorphic mutant mice rescued with a yeast artificial chromosome transgene suffer a glomerular mesangial cell defect. *Mol. Cell. Biol.* 36, 2272–2281. doi: 10.1128/MCB.0017316

Nath, K. A. (1992). Tubulointerstitial changes as a major determinant in the progression of renal damage. *Am. J. Kidney Dis.* 20, 1–17. doi: 10.1016/S0272-6386(12)80312-X

Olaiya, C. O., Esan, A. M., and Alabi, T. D. (2014). Ameliorative effects of β-sitosterol on some biochemical indices of hypertension in wistar albino rats. *Afr. J. Med. Med. Sci.* 43:157–166.

Park, S. A., Choi, M.-S., Jung, U. J., Kim, M.-J., Kim, D. J., Park, H.-M., et al. (2006). *Eucommia ulmoides* Oliver leaf extract increases endogenous antioxidant activity in type 2 diabetic mice. *J. Med. Food* 9, 474–479. doi: 10.1089/jmf.2006.9.474

Parving, H. H., Brenner, B. M., Mcmurray, J. J., De, Z. D., Haffner, S. M., Solomon, S. D., et al. (2012). Cardiorenal end points in a trial of aliskiren for type 2 diabetes. *N. Engl. J. Med.* 367, 2204–2213. doi: 10.1056/NEJMoa1208799

Piñero, J., Bravo, À, Queralt-Rosinach, N., Gutiérrez-Sacristán, A., Deu-Pons, J., Centeno, E., et al. (2017). DisGeNET: a comprehensive platform integrating information on human disease-associated genes and variants. *Nucleic Acids Res.* 45, D833–D839. doi: 10.1093/nar/gkw943

Rhee, S.-J., Kim, M.-J., and Kwag, O.-G. (2002). Effects of green tea catechin on prostaglandin synthesis of renal glomerular and renal dysfunction in streptozotocin-induced diabetic rats. *Asia Pac. J. Clin. Nutr.* 11, 232–236. doi: 10.1046/j.1440-6047.2002.00312.x

Ruiz-Giménez, P., Salom, J. B., Marcos, J. F., Vallés, S., Martínez-Maqueda, D., Recio, I., et al. (2012). Antihypertensive effect of a bovine lactoferrin pepsin hydrolysate: identification of novel active peptides. *Food Chem.* 131, 266–273. doi: 10.1016/j.foodchem.2011.08.076

Safaeian, L., Hajhashemi, V., Haghjoo, J. S., and Sanaye, N. H. (2016). The effect of protocatechuic acid on blood pressure and oxidative stress in glucocorticoid-induced hypertension in rat. *Iran. J. Pharm. Res.* 15, 83–91.

Santoro, D., Caccamo, D., Lucisano, S., Buemi, M., Sebekova, K., Teta, D., et al. (2015). Interplay of Vitamin D, erythropoiesis, and the renin-angiotensin system. *Biomed. Res. Int.* 2015:145828. doi: 10.1155/2015/145828

Shankland, S. J. (2006). The podocyte's response to injury: role in proteinuria and glomerulosclerosis. *Kidney Int.* 69, 2131–2147. doi: 10.1038/sj.ki.5000410

Somova, L. O., Nadar, A., Rammanan, P., and Shode, F. O. (2003). Cardiovascular, antihyperlipidemic and antioxidant effects of oleanolic and ursolic acids in experimental hypertension. *Phytomedicine* 10, 115–121. doi: 10.1078/094471103321659807

Su, G., Morris, J. H., Demchak, B., and Bader, G. D. (2014). Biological network exploration with cytoscape 3. *Curr. Protoc. Bioinformatics* 47, 8.13.1–8.13.24. doi: 10.1002/0471250953.bi0813s47

Syren, M. L., Turolo, S., Marangoni, F., Milani, G. P., Edefonti, A., Montini, G., et al. (2017). The polyunsaturated fatty acid balance in kidney health and disease: a review. *Clin. Nutr.* 37(6 Pt A), 1829–1839. doi: 10.1016/j.clnu.2017.11.019

Szklarczyk, D., Morris, J. H., Cook, H., Kuhn, M., Wyder, S., Simonovic, M., et al. (2017). The STRING database in 2017: quality-controlled protein-protein association networks, made broadly accessible. *Nucleic Acids Res.* 45, D362–D368. doi: 10.1093/nar/gkw937

Tagetti, A., Ericson, U., Montagnana, M., Danese, E., Almgren, P., Nilsson, P., et al. (2015). Intakes of omega-3 polyunsaturated fatty acids and blood pressure change over time: possible interaction with genes involved in 20-HETE and EETs metabolism. *Prostaglandins Other Lipid Mediat.* 120, 126–133. doi: 10.1016/j.prostaglandins.2015.05.003

Takase, H., Sugiura, T., Ohte, N., and Dohi, Y. (2015). Urinary albumin as a marker of future blood pressure and hypertension in the general population. *Medicine* 94:e511. doi: 10.1097/MD.0000000000000511

Toffoli, B., Gilardi, F., Winkler, C., Soderberg, M., Kowalczuk, L., Arsenijevic, Y., et al. (2017). Nephropathy in pparg-null mice highlights PPARγ systemic activities in metabolism and in the immune system. *PLoS One* 12:e0171474. doi: 10.1371/journal.pone.0171474

Xu, S., Chen, Y. H., Tan, Z. X., Xie, D. D., Zhang, C., Zhang, Z. H., et al. (2015). Vitamin D3 pretreatment regulates renal inflammatory responses during lipopolysaccharide-induced acute kidney injury. *Sci. Rep.* 5:18687. doi: 10.1038/srep18687

Yamanaka, T., Tamauchi, H., Suzuki, Y., Suzuki, H., Horikoshi, S., Terashima, M., et al. (2016). Release from Th1-type immune tolerance in spleen and enhanced production of IL-5 in Peyer's patch by cholera toxin B induce the glomerular deposition of IgA. *Immunobiology* 221, 577–585. doi: 10.1016/j.imbio.2015.12.001

Yen, G. C., and Hsieh, C. L. (1998). Antioxidant activity of extracts from du-zhong (*Eucommia ulmoides*) toward various lipid peroxidation models in vitro. *J. Agric. Food Chem.* 46, 3952–3957. doi: 10.1021/jf9800458

Yusuf, S., Teo, K. K., Pogue, J., Dyal, L., Copland, I., Schumacher, H., et al. (2008). Yusuf, S. et al. for the ONTARGET investigators. telmisartan, ramipril, or both in patients at high risk for vascular events. *N. Engl. J. Med.* 358, 1547–1559. doi: 10.1056/NEJMoa0801317

Zhang, M.-Z., Yao, B., McKanna, J. A., and Harris, R. C. (2005). Cross talk between the intrarenal dopaminergic and cyclooxygenase-2 systems. *Am. J. Physiol. Renal Physiol.* 288, F840–F845. doi: 10.1152/ajprenal.00240.2004

Zhen, W. Z., and Liang, L. F. (2012). *The Randomized Controlled Study of Quanduzhong Capsule Jiont Levamlodipine to Cure Renal Hypertension for Ganshenyinxu.* Available at: http://en.cnki.com.cn/Article_en/CJFDTOTAL-SYZY201210023.htm [accessed May 29, 2018].

Zhou, Y., Li, J. S., Zhang, X., Wu, Y. J., Huang, K., and Zheng, L. (2010). Ursolic acid inhibits early lesions of diabetic nephropathy. *Int. J. Mol. Med.* 26, 565–570. doi: 10.3892/ijmm_00000500

14

In Silico and In Vivo Studies on the Mechanisms of Chinese Medicine Formula (Gegen Qinlian Decoction) in the Treatment of Ulcerative Colitis

Xiaolu Liu[1,2], Yuling Fan[2], Lipeng Du[2], Zhigang Mei[1,2] and Yang Fu[3]**

[1]Institute of Basic Theory for Integrated Traditional Chinese and Western Medicine, College of Integrated Traditional Chinese and Western Medicine, Hunan University of Chinese Medicine, Changsha, China, [2]Third-Grade Pharmacological Laboratory on Chinese Medicine Approved by State Administration of Traditional Chinese Medicine, Medical College of China Three Gorges University, Yichang, China, [3]Xiangyang Hospital of Traditional Chinese Medicine, Xiangyang, China

***Correspondence:**
Zhigang Mei
meizhigang@hnucm.edu.cn
Yang Fu
fuyangtcm@aliyun.com

Ulcerative colitis (UC) is a chronic inflammatory bowel disease, and Gegen Qinlian Decoction (GQD), a Chinese botanical formula, has exhibited beneficial efficacy against UC. However, the mechanisms underlying the effect of GQD still remain to be elucidated. In this study, network pharmacology approach and molecular docking in silico were applied to uncover the potential multicomponent synergetic effect and molecular mechanisms. The targets of ingredients in GQD were obtained from Traditional Chinese Medicine Systems Pharmacology Database and Analysis Platform (TCMSP) and Bioinformatics Analysis Tool for Molecular mechANism of TCM (BATMAN-TCM) database, while the UC targets were retrieved from Genecards, therapeutic target database (TTD) and Online Mendelian Inheritance in Man (OMIM) database. The topological parameters of Protein-Protein Interaction (PPI) data were used to screen the hub targets in the network. The possible mechanisms were investigated with gene ontology (GO) enrichment analysis and Kyoto Encyclopedia of Genes and Genomes (KEGG) pathway enrichment analysis. Molecular docking was used to verify the binding affinity between the active compounds and hub targets. Network pharmacology analysis successfully identified 77 candidate compounds and 56 potential targets. The targets were further mapped to 20 related pathways to construct a compound-target-pathway network and an integrated network of GQD treating UC. Among these pathways, PI3K-AKT, HIF-1, VEGF, Ras, and TNF signaling pathways may exert important effects in the treatment of UC via inflammation suppression and anti-carcinogenesis. In the animal experiment, treatment with GQD and sulfasalazine (SASP) both ameliorated inflammation in UC. The

---

Abbreviations: UC, ulcerative colitis; GQD, gegen qinlian decoction; TCMSP, traditional chinese medicine systems pharmacology database and analysis platform; BATMAN-TCM, bioinformatics analysis tool for molecular mechANism of TCM; TTD, therapeutic target database; OMIM, online mendelian inheritance in man; PPI, protein-protein interaction; GO, dene ontology; KEGG, kyoto encyclopedia of genes and genomes; SASP, sulfasalazine; IBD, inflammatory bowel disease; TCM, traditional chinese medicine; GG, *pueraria lobata (Willd.) ohwi* (Ge-Gen in Chinese); HQ, *scutellaria baicalensis georgi* (Huang-Qin in Chinese); HL, *coptis chinensis franch* (Huang-Lian in Chinese); GC, *glycyrrhiza uralensis fisch* (Gan-Cao in Chinese); OB, oral bioavailability; Caco-2, Caco-2 cell permeability; DL, drug-likeness; DAVID, database for annotation, visualization, and integrated discovery; DSS, dextran sulfate sodium; HPLC, high-performance liquid chromatography; TNF-α, tumor necrosis factor-α; IL-1β, interleukin-1 beta; IL-6, interleukin-6; EGFR, epidermal growth factor receptor erbB1; PI3K, phosphoinositide 3-kinase; AKT, serine/threonine-protein kinase akt-1; Q-marker, quality marker.

proinflammatory cytokines (TNF-α, IL-1β, and IL-6) induced by UC were significantly decreased by GQD and SASP. Moreover, the protein expression of EGFR, PI3K, and phosphorylation of AKT were reduced after GQD and SASP treatment, and there was no significance between the GQD group and SASP group. Our study systematically dissected the molecular mechanisms of GQD on the treatment of UC using network pharmacology, as well as uncovered the therapeutic effects of GQD against UC through ameliorating inflammation via downregulating EGFR/PI3K/AKT signaling pathway and the pro-inflammatory cytokines such as TNF-α, IL-1β and IL-6.

Keywords: gegen qinlian decoction (GQD), network pharmacology, molecular docking, inflammatory bowel disease, ulcerative colitis

INTRODUCTION

Ulcerative colitis (UC), a subcategory of inflammatory bowel disease (IBD), is an idiopathic chronic inflammatory disorder of intestinal mucosa or lamina propria (Torres, et al., 2012). The cardinal symptom of this disease can range from mild to severe with many characteristics, including abdominal pain, diarrhea, rectal urgency, and bloody stool (Head and Jurenka, 2003). In recent years, the overall incidence and prevalence of UC is reported to be increased per year (Shivashankar et al., 2017). However, the occurrence and development of UC are connected to the etiology and pathology of multiple factors in human body, such as age, sex, genetics, environmental factors and autoimmunity, which makes UC a complex disease (Ordás et al., 2012). Notably, with continuous infiltration of immune cells and repeated stimulation of epithelial cells in intestinal mucosa, a risk of tumor initiation on UC also has dramatically increased (Rubin et al., 2012). Effective treatment is still lacking in clinic, the traditional drug, such as sulfasalazine (SASP) and glucocorticoids, have severe side effects, which restrict their widespread use in clinic. Currently, the options of medication depend on the severity of disease, while 5-Aminosalicylate and corticosteroids are recommended for mild to moderate UC (Bressler et al., 2015). For the patients with moderate to severe UC, calcineurin inhibitors or biologic agent should be selected (Lv et al., 2014). Although there are optimized medical management to choose, some patients still require colectomy, which is an option for decreasing risk of neoplasia and improvement in health-related quality of life (Gallo et al., 2018). Therefore, up to now no regular method is fit for every patient, and patients may require multiple and integral treatment modalities to achieve best therapeutic effect. Fortunately, this happened to coincide with the theory of traditional Chinese medicine (TCM) based on the comprehensive and individual medicinal system.

TCM has been used clinically in Asia for more than 2000 years, and numerous Chinese botanical medicines can be adopted as an auxiliary treatment for UC (Sałaga et al., 2014). Gegen Qinlian decoction (GQD), a well-known Chinese medicinal formula, was originally invented by Zhongjing Zhang, an eminent herbalist in Eastern Han dynasty in China, and it has been clinically applied to treat diarrhea and dysentery for approximately 2000 years. According to the *Chinese pharmacopoeia*, GQD consists of four botanical drugs, namely *Pueraria lobata (Willd.) Ohwi* (Ge-Gen in Chinese, GG), *Scutellaria baicalensis Georgi* (Huang-Qin in Chinese, HQ), *Coptis chinensis Franch* (Huang-Lian in Chinese, HL), and *Glycyrrhiza uralensis Fisch* (Gan-Cao in Chinese, GC) at the ration of 8:3:3:2. Our previous study and clinical studies have revealed that GQD possessed amazing curative effects in the treatment of UC (Shijun, 2010; Yan et al., 2012; Fan et al., 2019). However, researches on GQD were limited to single pharmacological activity, such as alleviating the gastrointestinal function, anti-inflammatory and antibacterial properties, the overall relationships between compounds and pharmacological mechanisms of GQD have not been clarified in depth (Yu et al., 2005; Xu et al., 2015). Systems network pharmacology is a newly prominent field that combines multiple disciplines and techniques and attempts to probe potential molecular mechanisms and relationships by constructing biological network models (Huang et al., 2014; Kim et al., 2018a). At present, the network pharmacology analysis has been largely applied for several TCM formulae pharmacological research such as the Sini powder for the treatment of chronic hepatitis, the Banxia Xiexin decoction against irritable bowel syndrome, and the antidiabetic activity of GQD in the treatment of type 2 diabetes, as well as the potential mechanisms underlying the formulae effect have also been systematically illuminated (Li et al., 2014; Shu et al., 2018; Li et al., 2019). Thus, in current study, the newly network pharmacology-based approach was employed to integrate active compounds, targets and pathways prediction, and network analysis, which may provide novel insights into the therapeutic effects and molecular mechanisms of GQD. In addition, *in vivo* experiment was also conducted to reveal the underlying mechanisms of GQD in the treatment for UC.

MATERIALS AND METHODS

Chemical Ingredients Database Construction

All components of the four Chinese botanical drugs in GQD were retrieved from the Traditional Chinese Medicine Systems Pharmacology Database and Analysis Platform (TCMSP, http://lsp.nwu.edu.cn/) (Ru et al., 2014) and Bioinformatics

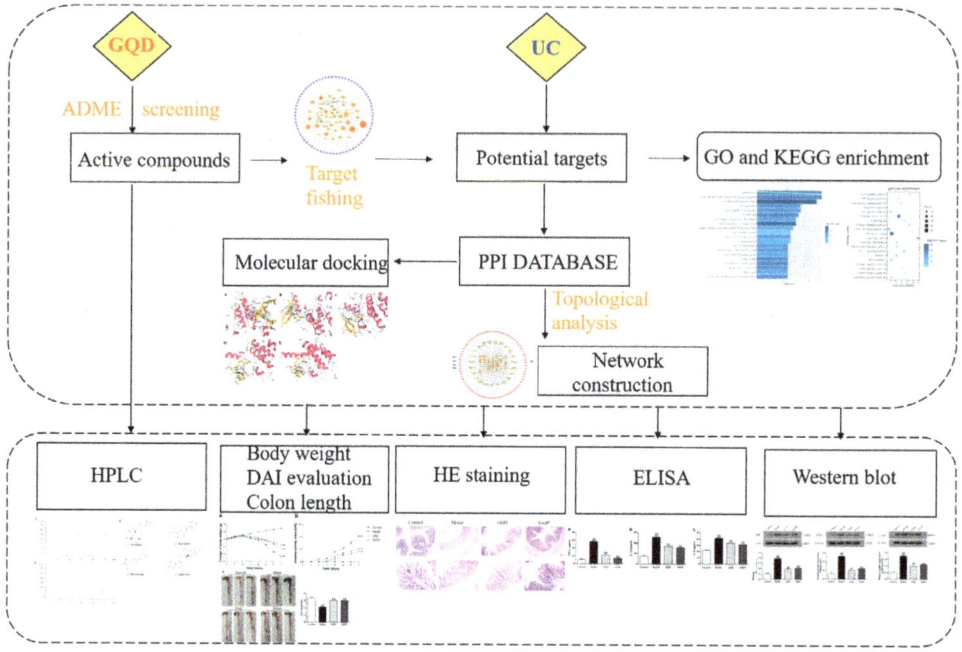

FIGURE 1 | The flowchart of network pharmacology and molecular docking-based strategy for deciphering the underlying mechanisms of GQD on the treatment of UC.

Analysis Tool for Molecular mechANism of TCM (BATMAN-TCM, http://bionet.ncpsb.org/batman-tcm) (Liu et al., 2016). Then we screen out the compounds which might not be matched with the criterion but were important components by a wide-scale text mining. The framework of this study was shown in **Figure 1**.

Pharmacokinetic Selection

To verify the pharmacokinetic characteristics of drugs, a compound screening model provided by the TCMSP data platform, including the evaluation of oral bioavailability (OB), Caco-2 cell permeability (Caco-2) and drug-likeness (DL) were employed. And the three parameters above were clarified as following. OB refers to the rate of an orally administered drugs of unmodified drug that delivers to circulatory system, which is considered predictive of bioactive molecule indicators as therapeutic agents (Xu et al., 2012; Chow, 2014). According to the recommended drug screening criteria, the compounds of which the threshold of OB $\geq$ 30% in this research could be qualified as a candidate ingredient. Caco-2 is another important parameter generally used as a model to predict the intestinal drug absorption in pre-clinical investigations (Artursson and Karlsson, 1991). And the application of this model employed in screening potential botanical-drug interactions is gaining popularity (Awortwe et al., 2014). In this study, to make sure the putative ingredients of GQD have high permeability via the intestinal membrane enterocytes, we increased the threshold values to Caco-2 $\geq$ 0.4. DL is a qualitative concept used in drug design for an estimate on how "drug-like" a prospective compound is, which helps to optimize pharmacokinetic and pharmaceutical properties, such as solubility and chemical stability (Tao et al., 2013). The "drug-like" level of the compounds is 0.18, which is used as a selection criterion to filter out molecules with undesirable properties in traditional Chinese botanical drugs (Tian et al., 2015). Consequently, ingredients in database of which the parameters' information meets the above screening criteria were opted to the next step.

Potential Targets Fishing

The protein targets of the candidate substances in GQD were retrieved from The Swiss Target Prediction database (http://www.swisstargetprediction.ch/), which can be mined automatically to retrieve specific information for a large number of molecules (Gfeller et al., 2014). In Swiss Target Prediction database, query molecules can be import either as SMILES structure format or drawn in 2D. And the molecular structure information of candidate compounds was derived from PubChem (https://pubchem.ncbi.nlm.nih.gov/), which is a pivotal chemistry resource served as an archive of chemical substance description and structure standardization (Kim et al., 2018b). Then, the target name was mapped to the disease target predictive database to find the disease associated with the protein and retrieved the diseases about UC. UC-related human genes were collected from three resources, which consist of Genecards (http://www.genecards.org), therapeutic target database (TTD) (http://db.idrblab.net/ttd/) and Online Mendelian Inheritance in Man (OMIM) database (http://omim.org/).

Protein-Protein Interaction

The protein-protein interaction (PPI) of each target were generated from STRING database (http://string-db.org/, ver.

11) with the species limited to "Homo sapiens" and a confidence score > 0.7 (Szklarczyk et al., 2019). Because of the complexity of the original network generated in STRING database, we imported the PPI data into the network visualization software Cytoscape (version 3.7.2) to reconstruct the network for better visualization, and screen out the hub targets.

Gene Ontology and Kyoto Encyclopedia of Genes and Genomes Pathway Enrichment Analysis

To systematically explore the concerned biological processes of GQD as a therapy against UC, we performed GO and KEGG enrichment analysis by the functional annotation tool DAVID (database for annotation, visualization, and integrated discovery; http://david.abcc.ncifcrf.gov). GO terms and KEGG pathways with p value less than 0.05 according to Fisher's exact test were considered statistically significant and subjected to further analyses.

Network Construction

To comprehensive understand the molecular mechanisms of GQD to UC, the networks including compound-target-pathway network were constructed using Cytoscape version 3.7.2. The construction of the network was based on the binding of active ingredients to the correlative targets and the signaling pathways, which uncover the underlying interactions between botanical drugs and the disease. In this graphical network, nodes represent the compounds, targets, or signaling pathways by different shapes, and the interactions between them were signified by edges. The degree of a node was marked by different color or size, which was defined as the number of edges relate to it. Moreover, the topological properties were analyzed by the plugin Network Analyzer of Cytoscape (Shannon et al., 2003).

Molecular Docking

Molecular docking of the critical active compounds with hub targets was performed by CB-Dock (http://cao.labshare.cn/cb-dock/), a web used for predicting the binding sites and affinity with a popular docking program, Autodock Viana (Liu et al., 2020). CB-Dock is a new blind docking tool, which focus on enhancing the docking accuracy. PDB formats of the proteins and a ligand file in the MOL2 or SDF were input to CB-dock to generate a set of points to represent the solvent-accessible surface, and the cavities were ranked according to their sizes. Then a docking box for the following computation was customized, and irrelevant poses was excluded as many as possible. Then we predicted the binding sites, calculated the centers and sizes with a novel curvature-based cavity detection approach, and performed ligand docking with Autodock Vina, and obtained the binding activities and the Vina score, which represents the binding affinity. The more negative the Vina score is, the more stable the ligand-receptor binding (Liu et al., 2020). Ball and stick and cartoon chain represented the ligand and protein, respectively.

Animals

A total of 60 male C57BL/6 mice weighing about 18–22 g were purchased from the Laboratory Animal Center of China Tree Gorges University (Yichang, China). All mice were randomly assigned to four groups (n = 15/group): control group, model group, GQD group and SASP group. All animals were maintained under a 12 h light/dark cycle environment. The room temperature was controlled at (22 ± 1)°C, with (60 ± 5) % humidity, and adequate food and water were provided. The animal experiments were approved by the Laboratory Animal Ethical Committee of Three Gorges University, China (No. 20180904C, approved at 2018-9-11).

Drugs and Reagents

The botanical formula GQD is comprised of four medicinal botanical drugs: *Pueraria lobata (Willd.) Ohwi* (Batch No: 202011027, Hubei Tianji Pharmaceutical Co. Ltd.), *Scutellaria baicalensis Georgi* (Batch No: 20201103, Hubei Tianji Pharmaceutical Co. Ltd.), *Coptis chinensis Franch* (Batch No: 202011019, Hubei Tianji Pharmaceutical Co. Ltd.), and *Glycyrrhiza uralensis Fisch* (Batch No: 202012018, Hubei Tianji Pharmaceutical Co. Ltd.). All the botanical drugs were purchased from Yichang Hospital of Traditional Chinese Medicine, Hubei province, China. Dextran sulfate sodium (DSS; molecular weight: 36–50 kDa) was obtained from MP Biomedicals (Santa Ana, CA, United States). EGFR antibody, and PI3K antibody were obtained from Proteintech Group (Chicago, United States); p-AKT antibody was purchased from Affinity Biologicals (Yarker, Canada), and β-actin antibody was obtained from Boster Biological Technology (Wuhan, China).

Preparation of Gegen Qinlian Decoction Extract

For the extraction of GQD, *Pueraria lobata (Willd.) Ohwi* (24 g), *Scutellaria baicalensis Georgi* (9 g), *Coptis chinensis Franch* (9 g), and *Glycyrrhiza uralensis Fisch* (6 g) were soaked in 75% ethanol at eightfold volume overnight and then boiled for 1.5 h, the first decoction was thus obtained. Then the residue was boiled a second time with an addition of sixfold volume of 75% ethanol for 1 h to obtain the second decoction. Finally, the first and second decoction were mixed, filtered through gauze, and evaporated to dryness under reduced pressure, and then the extractum was freeze drying to powder.

Component Analysis of Gegen Qinlian Decoction With High-Performance Liquid Chromatography

The analytical standards were purchased from Push Bio-technology Co., Ltd. (Chengdu, China), and the analysis of GQD was performed on Agilent 1,260 Infinity II HPLC system (Agilent Technologies, Santa Clara, CA, United States) equipped with a Diode Array Detector (DAD). A reversed phase Welch Ultimate XB C18 (25 × 4.6 mm, 5 μm) was used and kept at 30°C. The mobile phase consisted of aqueous solution of phosphoric acid and methanol with a gradient elution at a flow rate of 1.0 ml/min. And the detection wavelength was set at 250, 350, 280, and 250 nm.

Treatment Protocol for Dextran Sulfate Sodium-Induced Colitic Mice

Mice were randomly allocated to four groups (n = 15/group): control group, model group, GQD group, and SASP group. All mice except the control group were induced by administration of 3% DSS dissolved in drinking water continuously for 7 days. And the mice in normal group received distilled water without DSS throughout the entire experimental period. According to clinical administration dose, the mice in GQD group and SASP group were administered with GQD enema (0.68 g/kg per day) or SASP enema (0.5 g/kg per day), respectively. Meanwhile, the mice in control group and model group were administrated with saline by enemata. The animals were monitored once a day for body weight, stool consistency, and presence of blood in the feces and the anus. At day 7, mice were anesthetized and sacrificed by cervical dislocation, and the colon samples were collected immediately. Then the colon length was measured and stored for subsequently experiments.

Evaluation of Disease Activity and Colon Length

To assess the severity of colitis, the disease activity index (DAI) was calculated as the average of body weight loss score, diarrhea score, and fecal blood score. DAI evaluation was calculated under the guidance of previously established scoring system (Yan et al., 2018b; Hassan and Hassan, 2018), and the scoring criteria was based on the following parameters: 1) body weight loss (0, no loss; 1, 1–5% loss; 2, 5–10% loss; 3, 10–20% loss; 4, over 20% loss); 2) diarrhea (0, normal; 2, loose stools; 4, watery diarrhea); and 3) hematochezia (0, no bleeding; 2, slight bleeding; 4, gross bleeding). Body weight gain was expressed as the difference from the initial body weight. Colon length was regarded as an indirect marker of inflammation, thereby, the length of colons from the ileocecal junction to the anal verge was measured.

Histopathological Analysis

Colon tissues were collected and fixed in 4% paraformaldehyde overnight, then dehydrated at gradient concentrations of ethanol, and embedded in paraffin. Tissues were sectioned at 4 μm thickness with a paraffin and stained with hematoxylin and eosin (HE). The images of the tissues were obtained using Image-Pro Plus 5.0 system.

Enzyme-Linked Immunosorbent Assay

To test the anti-inflammatory effects of GQD on ulcerative colitis, colon homogenate supernatants of all the experimental groups were collected, and the expression of TNF-α, IL-1β, and IL-6 was measured by ELISA kits (USCN Cloud-Clone Corp, Wuhan, China) according to the manufacturer's instructions.

Western Blotting Analysis

The total protein of colon tissue was extracted using RIPA lysis buffer with the protease inhibitor cocktail (Beyotime Biotechnology, China), and protein concentration was measured using the BCA protein assay kit (Beyotime Biotechnology) according to the manufacturer's instructions. Equivalent amounts of protein (20 μg) were separated by SDS-PAGE and then transferred onto 0.45 μm PVDF membranes (Millipore, Billeria, MA, United States). The membranes were then blocked in 5% nonfat milk in TBST buffer for 1 h at room temperature, followed by incubation with primary antibodies at 4°C overnight. Then membranes were washed with TBST and incubated with secondary antibody for 1 h at room temperature, proteins were detected using ECL reagent (Applygen, China). The antibodies used were as follows: EGFR (1:2,000), PI3K (1:1,000), *p*-AKT (1:1,000), and β-actin (1:500).

Statistical Analysis

All the experimental data were analyzed using SPSS 20.0 statistical software (IBM Corp., Armonk, NY, United States). GraphPad Prism 6.0 software (GraphPad Software Inc., San Diego, CA, United States) was used for the calculations. All results are expressed as means ± standard error of the mean (SEM). Multigroup comparisons were performed using one-way analysis of variance (ANOVA) and post hoc Statistical least significant difference (LSD) test. p value < 0.05 was considered statistically significant.

RESULTS

Identification of Candidate Compounds in Gegen Qinlian Decoction

After the absorption, distribution, metabolism, elimination (ADME) parameters screening (OB ≥ 30%, DL ≥ 0.18, Caco-2 ≥ 0.4), 75 potential components of the four botanical medicines were collected from database and relate literatures. Among them, 3 ingredients belong to GG, 9 belong to HL, 20 belong to HQ, and 47 belong to GC. It is worth mentioning that formononetin (OB = 69.67%, Caco-2 = 0.78, DL = 0.21) as an important component existed in both GG and GC. Additionally, beta-sitosterol (OB = 39.91%, Caco-2 = 1.32, DL = 0.75), exhibited good ADME properties, can be collected from GG and HQ. Both coptisine (OB = 30.67%, Caco-2 = 1.21, DL = 0.86) and epiberberine (OB = 43.09%, Caco-2 = 1.17, DL = 0.78) are common ingredients found in HQ and HL. Additionally, two compounds, puerarin and daidzein, did not meet the three criteria were taken into consideration as their obvious bioactivities (Qi et al., 2004). Consequently, after removing redundancy, a total of 77 compounds were identified as candidate compounds for further analysis. All the compounds identified from GQD and their concreted predicted OB, DL, and Caco-2 values are showed in **Table 1**.

Targets Identification of Gegen Qinlian Decoction on Ulcerative Colitis

Based on The Swiss Target Prediction database, a total of 740 targets related to the 77 compounds were obtained in GQD. In order to explore the relevance and underlying mechanism of these targets specific to GQD in the development of UC, A total of 3785 UC-related genes were retrieved from the GeneCards,

TABLE 1 | Information for the candidate bioactive compounds of GQD.

ID	Chemical	OB (%)	Caco-2	DL	Herb
C01	Puerarin	24.03	−1.15	0.69	GG
C02	Formononetin	69.67	0.78	0.21	GG GC
C03	Daidzein	19.44	0.59	0.19	GG
C04	Beta-sitosterol	36.91	1.32	0.75	GG HQ
C05	3′-methoxydaidzein	48.57	0.56	0.24	GG
C06	Coptisine	30.67	1.21	0.86	HQ HL
C07	Epiberberine	43.09	1.17	0.78	HQ HL
C08	Berberine	36.86	1.24	0.78	HL
C09	Berberrubine	35.74	1.07	0.73	HL
C10	(R)-canadine	55.37	1.04	0.77	HL
C11	Berlambine	36.68	0.97	0.82	HL
C12	Palmatine	64.60	1.33	0.65	HL
C13	Worenine	45.83	1.22	0.87	HL
C14	Moupinamide	86.71	0.55	0.26	Hl
C15	5,2′,6′-trihydroxy-7,8-dimethosyflavone	45.05	0.48	0.33	HQ
C16	5,2′-dihydroxy-6,7,8-trimethoxyflavone	31.71	0.93	0.35	HQ
C17	5,7,4′-trihydroxy-6-methoxyflavanone	36.63	0.43	0.27	HQ
C18	Acacetin	34.97	0.67	0.24	HQ
C19	Baicalein	33.52	0.63	0.21	HQ
C20	Dihydrobaicalin	40.04	0.56	0.21	HQ
C21	Dihydrooroxylin	66.06	0.67	0.23	HQ
C22	Moslosooflavone	44.09	1.01	0.25	HQ
C23	Norwogonin	39.40	0.60	0.21	HQ
C24	Oroxylin a	41.37	0.76	0.23	HQ
C25	Panicolin	76.26	0.84	0.29	HQ
C26	Rivularin	37.94	0.65	0.37	HQ
C27	Salvigenin	49.07	0.86	0.33	HQ
C28	Skullcapflavone II	69.51	0.68	0.44	HQ
C29	Stigmasterol	43.83	1.44	0.76	HQ
C30	Supraene	33.55	2.08	0.42	HQ
C31	Wogonin	30.68	0.79	0.23	HQ
C32	1-Methoxyphaseollidin	69.98	1.01	0.64	GC
C33	3′-hydroxy-4′-O-Methylglabrindin	43.71	1.00	0.57	GC
C34	3′-methoxyglabridin	46.16	0.94	0.57	GC
C35	7-Acetoxy-2-methylisoflavone	38.92	0.74	0.26	GC
C36	7-Methoxy-2-methylisoflavone	42.56	1.16	0.20	GC
C37	Calycosin	47.75	0.52	0.24	GC
C38	DFV	32.76	0.51	0.18	GC
C39	Eurycaprin A	43.28	0.43	0.37	GC
C40	Gancaonin A	51.08	0.80	0.40	GC
C41	Gancaonin B	48.79	0.58	0.45	GC
C42	Gancaonin G	60.44	0.78	0.39	GC
C43	Glabranin	52.90	0.97	0.31	GC
C44	Glabrene	46.27	0.99	0.44	GC
C45	Glabridin	53.25	0.97	0.47	GC
C46	Glabrone	52.51	0.59	0.50	GC
C47	Glepidotin A	44.72	0.79	0.35	GC
C48	Glyasperin B	65.22	0.47	0.44	GC
C49	Glyasperin C	45.56	0.71	0.40	GC
C50	Glyasperin F	75.84	0.43	0.54	GC
C51	Glycyrin	52.61	0.59	0.47	GC
C52	Glycyrol	90.78	0.71	0.67	GC
C53	Glypallichalcone	61.60	0.76	0.19	GC
C54	HMO	38.37	0.79	0.21	GC
C55	Inermine	75.18	0.89	0.54	GC
C56	Inflacoumarin A	39.71	0.73	0.33	GC
C57	Isoglycyrol	44.70	0.91	0.84	GC
C58	Isolicoflavonol	45.17	0.54	0.42	GC
C59	Isotrifoliol	31.94	0.53	0.42	GC
C60	Jaranol	50.83	0.61	0.29	GC
C61	Kanzonols W	50.48	0.63	0.52	GC
C62	Licoagrocarpin	58.81	1.23	0.58	GC
C63	Licoagroisoflavone	57.28	0.71	0.49	GC
C64	Licochalcone A	40.79	0.82	0.29	GC

(Continued on following page)

TABLE 1 | (*Continued*) Information for the candidate bioactive compounds of GQD.

ID	Chemical	OB (%)	Caco-2	DL	Herb
C65	Licochalcone B	76.76	0.47	0.19	GC
C66	Licochalcone G	49.25	0.64	0.32	GC
C67	Licoisoflavone B	38.93	0.46	0.55	GC
C68	Licoricone	63.58	0.53	0.47	GC
C69	Lupiwighteone	51.64	0.68	0.37	GC
C70	Mairin	55.38	0.73	0.78	GC
C71	Medicarpin	49.22	1.00	0.34	GC
C72	Odoratin	49.95	0.42	0.30	GC
C73	Phaseol	78.77	0.76	0.58	GC
C74	Phaseolinisoflavan	32.01	1.01	0.45	GC
C75	Semilicoisoflavone B	48.78	0.45	0.55	GC
C76	Shinpterocarpin	80.30	1.10	0.73	GC
C77	Vestitol	74.66	0.86	0.21	GC

OB, oral bioavailability; Caco-2, Caco-2 cell permeability; DL, drug-likeness.

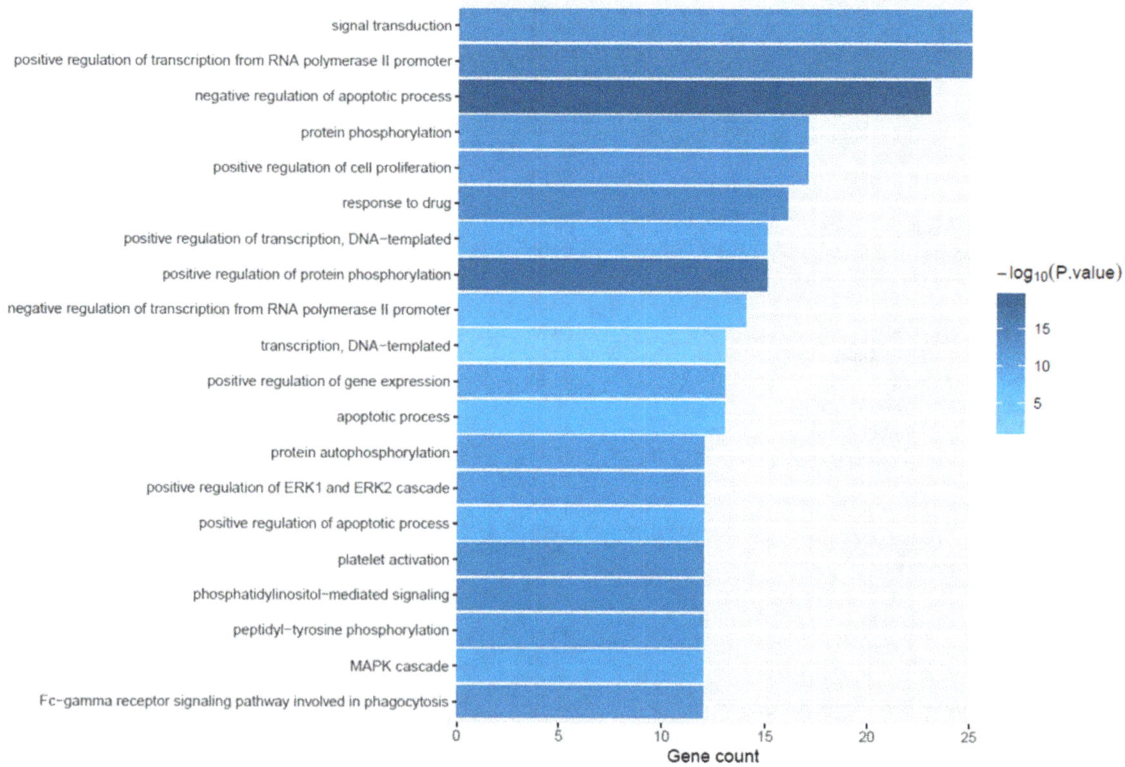

FIGURE 2 | The results of gene ontology (GO) biological process analysis. The X-axis represents gene count, while the Y-axis represents the categories of biological process (p-value ≤ 0.05).

OMIM, and TTD databases by employing a keyword-based search. After eliminating the overlaps, 287 targets were shared between 740 compound-related targets and 3785 UC-related targets. PPI network of these 287 targets were established in STRING database and visualized by Cytoscape software. There were 287 nodes and 4,490 edges in this interaction network. According to previous study, a node would be defined as a hub target when the degree was more than twofold the median degree of all nodes in the network (Li et al., 2007). Eventually, 59 major hub targets were considered to be the effective therapeutic targets of UC. Topological analysis indicated that serine/threonine-protein kinase AKT (AKT1, degree = 165), vascular endothelial growth factor A (VEGFA, degree = 151), epidermal growth factor receptor erbB1 (EGFR, degree = 141), MAP kinase ERK1 (MAPK3, degree = 141), TNF-alpha (TNF, degree = 136), signal transducer and activator of transcription3

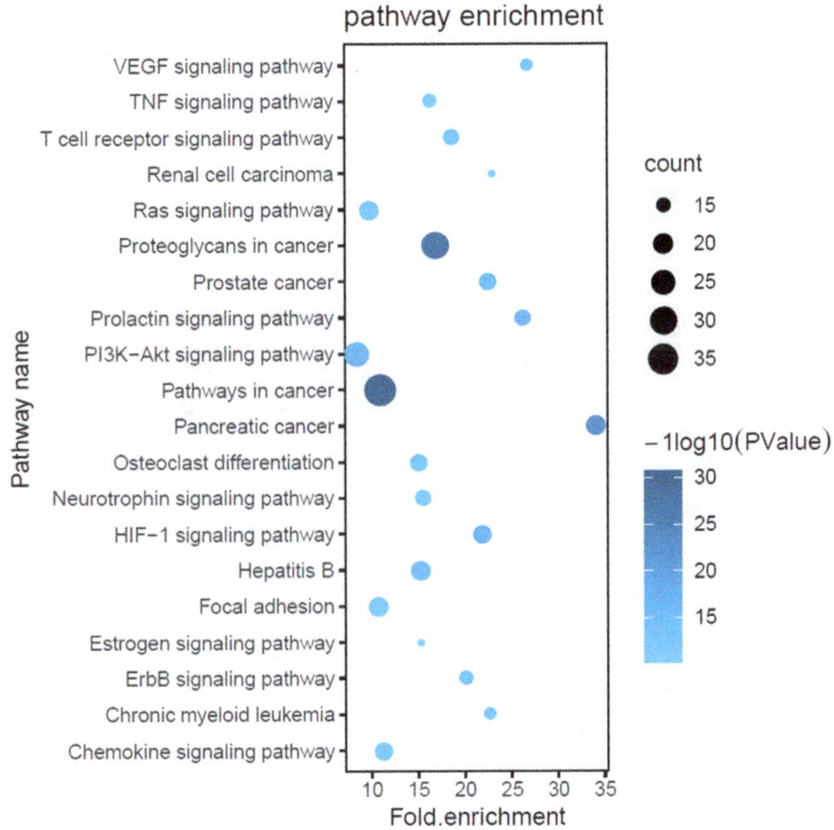

FIGURE 3 | Kyoto Encyclopedia of Genes and Genomes (KEGG) enrichment analysis. The X-axis represents the enrichment rate of these genes in total genes, while the Y-axis represents the enrichment pathways of the target genes (p-value ≤ 0.05). The depth of the color represents the size of the value, and the size of circle represents the enrichment counts of these pathways.

(STAT3, degree = 128), tyrosine-protein kinase SRC (SRC, degree = 126), cyclooxygenase-2 (PTGS2, degree = 113) were the top hub targets based on degree centrality.

Gene Ontology and Pathway Enrichment Analysis

To explore the biological processes of the 59 putative targets of GQD on UC, GO and pathway enrichment analysis was further performed. As shown in **Figure 2**, the top 20 most significantly enriched GO terms were exhibited with their p-value and gene count. These targets were obviously enriched in negative regulation of apoptotic process, protein phosphorylation, cell proliferation, MAPK cascade and inflammatory response, which have a strongly correlation with the pathogenesis of UC. These results indicated the multiple synergies of GQD on biological processes. To further reveal the potential mechanisms of the therapeutic effects of GQD, we conducted KEGG pathway enrichment analysis on 59 targets, and screened out 20 pathways based on the threshold of p-value < 0.05. The top 20 significantly enriched pathways contained pathways in cancer, HIF-1 signaling pathway, PI3K-AKT signaling pathway, TNF signaling pathway, VEGF signaling pathway and Ras signaling pathway (**Figure 3**).

Compound-Target-Pathway Network Analysis

To further elucidate the underlying pharmacological mechanisms of the candidate compounds for the treatment of GQD, the compound-target network and compound-target-pathway network were constructed based on the protein targets and the corresponding pathway enrichment analysis. As shown in **Figure 4**, the compound-target network was composed of 132 nodes and 684 edges, and the average degree value of hub targets was 9.03. The epiberberine (C07, degree = 26) from HQ and HL, acacetin (C18, degree = 18) and the baicalein (C19, degree = 16) from HQ, berberine (C08, degree = 13) from HL, wogonin (C31, degree = 13) from HQ, glabridin (C45, degree = 12) from GC were identified as relatively high-degree active compounds, which indicated that the six compounds play more important roles in the pathological processes of ulcerative colitis. According to previous studies, puerarin, one of the most important constituents in GG, has been widely used in the treatment of UC by inhibiting inflammatory response (Jeon et al., 2020). Therefore, we hypothesize that epiberberine, acacetin, baicalein, berberine, wogonin, glabridin and puerarin may account for the essential therapeutic effects of GQD on UC. Then we selected four representative compounds of each of the four botanical drugs for molecular docking and HPLC analysis.

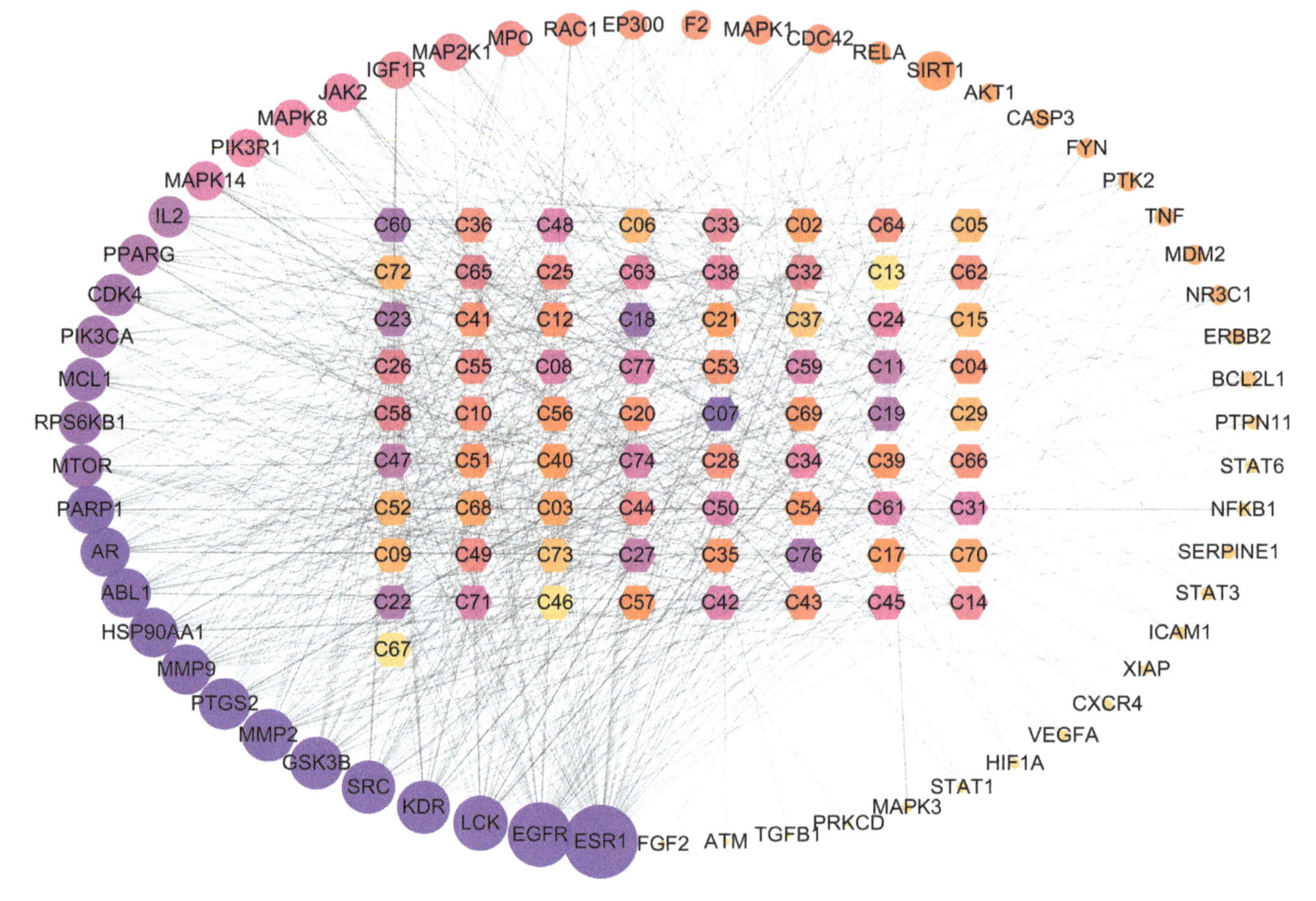

FIGURE 4 | The interaction network between compounds and hub targets. The hexagon represents the herbal compounds, the circles stand for the potential targets, and the edges represent the interactions between them. The depth of color and the size of circle are proportional to their degree value. The ID of the compounds was elaborated in **Table 1**.

Among these compounds, puerarin from GG, baicalein from HQ, berberine from HL, and glabridin from GC were taken into consideration. In the meantime, the 59 hubs with higher degree scores, such as estrogen receptor alpha (ESR1, degree = 47), epidermal growth factor receptor erbB1 (EGFR, degree = 38), tyrosine-protein kinase SRC (SRC, degree = 27), matrix metalloproteinase 2 (MMP2, degree = 26), glycogen synthase kinase-3 beta (GSK3B, degree = 26), cyclooxygenase-2 (PTGS2, degree = 25) possessed highly connection with compounds and pathways (**Figure 5**). Detailed information about the hub targets is provided in **Table 2**. Furthermore, an investigation at the relationship between 59 targets and 20 remarkably enriched pathways was conducted based on the compound-target-pathway network, and the average degree value of hub targets per pathway was 18.39. These pathways probably attributed to the therapeutic effect of GQD on UC.

Molecular Docking

To further verify the results of network pharmacology screening, the four crucial active compounds in GQD were docked with the hub target EGFR via CB-dock. It is generally believed that the vina score indicates the binding affinity between the ligand and the receptor, and the more negative the vina score is, the more stable the compounds bind to the hub target. As shown in **Figure 6**, the crucial active components in GQD, which consist of puerarin, baicalein, berberine and glabridin, all possessed good binding activities to EGFR. And puerarin exhibited the best binding affinity with EGFR, which was higher than the positive control drug SASP.

High-Performance Liquid Chromatography Analysis of Gegen Qinlian Decoction

As shown in **Figure 7**, HPLC analysis indicated the retention time of standards puerarin (15.429 min), baicalein (25.764 min), berberine (41.765 min) and glabridin (49.096 min), respectively, in **Figure 6A**. Moreover, comparison with mixed check samples were performed, and external method was used to calculate the concentrations. The contents of puerarin, baicalein, berberine and glabridin were 1,290.93 μg/g (2.52%), 6,616.57 μg/g (11.35%), 1,129.38 μg/g (2.8%) and 5.49 μg/g (0.57%), respectively. The results showed that GQD contained the four active components. In addition, there were many peaks from

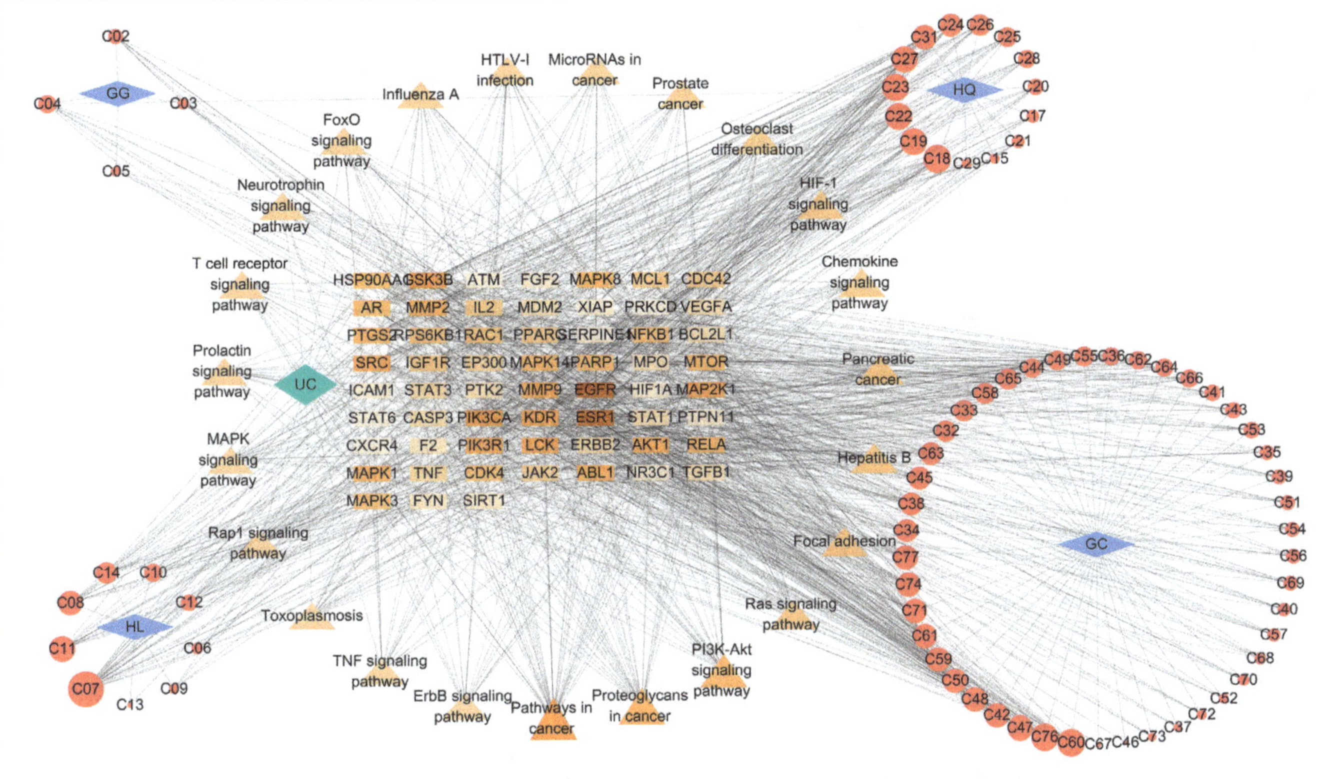

FIGURE 5 | Compound–target–pathway network. The rectangle, triangle and circle represent the potential targets, major pathways and botanical compounds, respectively. The rhombus represents the four botanical drugs in GQD. Edges represent the interaction between them. For the potential targets and pathways, the change in color depth reflect the degree value. For the botanical compounds, the circle size is proportional to their degree value. GG, *Pueraria lobata (Willd.) Ohwi*; HQ, *Scutellaria baicalensis Georgi*; HL, *Coptis chinensis Franch*; GC, *Glycyrrhiza uralensis Fisch*.

more concentrated compounds that were not analyzed quantitatively or qualitatively in the chromatograms of GQD. It has been demonstrated that the glycyrrhizic acid and baicalin, which belong to triterpene saponins and *O*-glycosides, respectively, possess protective effects against non-alcoholic fatty liver disease and diabetes (Wang et al., 2016; Yan et al., 2018a; Qiao et al., 2018). Therefore, the high concentrated compounds in HPLC chromatogram may be the compounds mentioned above.

Gegen Qinlian Decoction Ameliorated Dextran Sulfate Sodium-Induced Ulcerative Colitis in Mice

To explore the protective effects of GQD on UC, the mouse model of acute ulcerative colitis was established by administrating mice with 5% DSS for 7 days. SASP was served as a positive control in this study. The therapeutic effect of GQD on UC was assessed preliminary by body weight loss, colon length and DAI score. On the 3rd day of DSS induction, body weight of model group was markedly decreased compared to sham group, with a continuous daily decrease thereafter. And administration of GQD and SASP significantly blunted the body weight loss induced by DSS compared with model group ($p < 0.01$, **Figure 8A**). Meanwhile, DSS administration for 7 days led to severe diarrhea, blood in stool and body weight loss integrated as remarkably high disease activity index compared with normal group ($p < 0.01$), while this elevation was relieved by GQD and SASP treatment ($p < 0.01$, **Figure 8B**). In addition, after the establishment of UC model, DSS resulted in a significant shortening of the colon length, while GQD and SASP treatment markedly reduced DSS-induced colon shortening compared with model group ($p < 0.01$, **Figure 8C**). Collectively, we assessed preliminary effect of GQD on UC, and the results suggested that GQD exerted protective effects in UC treatment.

Effects of Gegen Qinlian Decoction on Histopathological Changes in Colon Tissues

The diarrhea and stool blood caused by daily DSS administration were accompanied by inflammation in colonic tissues and damage to the intestinal wall. HE staining was applied to observe the pathological changes of intestinal tissue in each group. As shown in **Figure 9**, the colonic mucosa was intact, and the intestinal epithelial cells and glands were arranged neatly in control group. And severe epithelial cell necrosis, crypt

TABLE 2 | Potential targets of GQD on UC.

Gene name	Target	Uniprot ID	Degree
ESR1	Estrogen receptor alpha	P03372	47
EGFR	Epidermal growth factor receptor erbB1	P00533	38
LCK	Tyrosine-protein kinase LCK	P06239	29
SRC	Tyrosine-protein kinase SRC	P12931	27
KDR	Vascular endothelial growth factor receptor 2	P35968	27
MMP2	Matrix metalloproteinase 2	P08253	26
GSK3β	Glycogen synthase kinase-3 beta	P49841	26
PTGS2	Cyclooxygenase-2	P35354	25
MMP9	Matrix metalloproteinase 9	P14780	24
HSP90AA1	Heat shock protein HSP 90-alpha	P07900	23
AR	Androgen receptor	P10275	23
ABL1	Tyrosine-protein kinase ABL	P00519	23
PARP1	Poly [ADP-ribose] polymerase-1	P09874	22
MTOR	Serine/threonine-protein kinase mTOR	P42345	17
MCL1	Induced myeloid leukemia cell differentiation protein Mcl-1	Q07820	17
RPSKB1	Ribosomal protein S6 kinase 1	P23443	17
PIK3CA	PI-kinase p110-alpha subunit	P42336	16
CDK4	Cyclin-dependent kinase 4	P11802	16
PPARG	Peroxisome proliferator-activated receptor gamma	P37231	15
IL2	Interleukin-2	P60568	14
MAPK14	MAP kinase p38 alpha	Q16539	13
MAPK8	c-Jun N-terminal kinase 1	P45983	12
PIK3R1	PI3-kinase p85-alpha subunit	P27986	12
JAK2	Tyrosine-protein kinase IAK2	O60674	12
MAPK2K1	Dual specificity mitogen-activated protein kinase 1	Q02750	11
IGF1R	Insulin-like growth factor 1 receptor	P08069	11
MPO	Myeloperoxidase	P05164	10
RAC1	Ras-related C3 botulinum toxin substrate 1	P63000	9
MAPK1	MAP kinase ERK2	P28482	8
EP300	Histone acetyltransferase p300	Q09472	8
CDC42	Cell division control protein 42 homolog	P60953	8
F2	Thrombin	P00734	8
SIRT1	NAD-dependent control protein 42 homolog	Q96EB6	6
RELA	Nuclear factor NF-kappa-B p65 subunit	Q04206	6
AKT1	Serine/threonine-protein kinase AKT	P31749	5
TNF	Tumor necrosis factor	P01375	5
CASP3	Caspase-3	P42574	5
MDM2	P53-binding protein Mdm-2	Q00987	5
FYN	Tyrosine-protein kinase fyn	P06241	5
NR3C1	Glucocorticoid receptor	P04150	5
PTK2	Focal adhesion kinase 1	Q05397	5
ERBB2	Receptor protein-tyrosine kinase erbB-2	P04626	4
BCL2L1	Apoptosis regulator Bcl-X	Q07817	4
STAT3	Signal transducer and activator pf transcription 3	P40763	3
ICAM1	Intercellular adhesion molecule-1	P05362	3
NFκB	Nuclear factor NF-kappa-B p105 subunit	P19838	3
PTPN11	Protein-tyrosine phosphatase 2C	Q06124	3
SERPPINE1	Plasminogen activator inhibitor-1	P05121	3
STAT6	Signal transducer and activator of transcription 6	P42226	3
VEGFA	Vascular endothelial growth factor A	P15692	2
MAPK3	MAP kinase ERK1	P27361	2
CXCR4	C-X-C chemokine receptor type 4	P61073	2
STAT1	Signal transducer and activator of transcription 1 alpha/beta	P42224	2
HIF1A	Hypoxia-inducible factor 1 alpha	Q16665	2
XIAP	Inhibitor of apoptosis protein 3	P98170	2
FGF2	Basic fibroblast growth factor	P09038	1
ATM	Serine-protein kinase ATM	Q13315	1
TGFB1	Transforming growth factor	P01137	1
PRKCD	Protein kinase C delta	Q05655	1

destruction and inflammatory cell infiltration were observed in DSS-treated mice. However, both GQD and SASP treatment could attenuate the histopathological manifestation of colitis. Mild epithelial cells degeneration or necrosis, and a small number of inflammatory cells could be observed in GQD and SASP group.

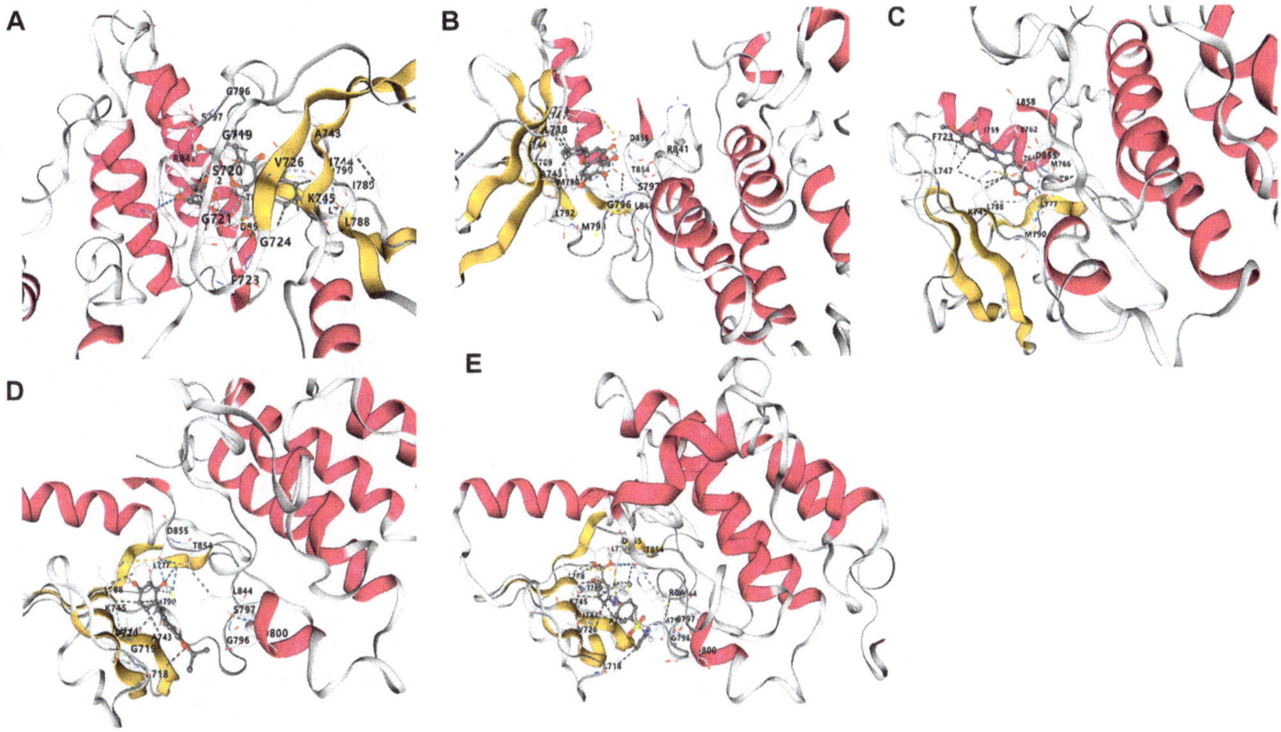

FIGURE 6 | Molecular docking analysis of the binding affinity of the four active compounds toward to the hub target EGFR. **(A)** Puerarin, vina score = −8.4; **(B)** Baicalein, vina score = −7.8; **(C)** Berberine, vina score = −7.8; **(D)** Glabridin, vina score = −7.9. **(E)** SASP, vina score = −8.2.

Gegen Qinlian Decoction-Treatment Inhibited the Pro-Inflammatory Cytokines in Colon Tissues

As pro-inflammatory factors play important roles in the pathogenesis and progress of UC, we investigated whether GQD possess the anti-inflammatory effect in UC. ELISA essay was performed in colonic samples of all the experimental groups. As shown in **Figure 10**, DSS significantly evoked the expression of pro-inflammatory cytokines including TNF-α, IL-1β, and IL-6 compared with those in sham group ($p < 0.01$). However, the administration of GQD and SASP inhibited the content of TNF-α, IL-1β, and IL-6 significantly than that of the model group ($p < 0.01$). These data demonstrated that GQD and SASP could inhibit the inflammatory reaction induced by DSS in UC.

Gegen Qinlian Decoction Ameliorated Dextran Sulfate Sodium-Induced Inflammation Through EGFR/PI3K/AKT Signaling Pathway

Based on numerous studies and the network pharmacology analysis, inflammation plays an essential role in the pathogenesis and process of UC, and the inflammatory response may partially mediate by EGFR/PI3K/AKT signaling pathway (Neurath, 2014). Thereby, we investigated whether GQD could exert therapeutic effects on UC by inhibiting inflammation via regulating the expression of EGFR, PI3K, and *p*-AKT. As shown in **Figure 11**, western blotting results showed that DSS induced a remarkably increase in the protein expression of EGFR, PI3K, and *p*-AKT in colon tissue, which indicates the activation of EGFR/PI3K/AKT signaling pathway in UC. Notably, the elevation of these protein targets was blocked by GQD treatment. Similarly, administration of SASP downregulated the protein expression of EGFR, PI3K, and *p*-AKT as well. These results demonstrated that GQD protects against UC partially through inhibiting the activation of EGFR/PI3K/AKT signaling pathway.

DISCUSSION

UC is a common intestinal inflammatory disease. Presently, numerous studies have demonstrated that GQD, as a classical complementary and alternative TCM prescription, exerted acclaimed therapeutic effects against UC (Xu et al., 2015; Li et al., 2016). Whereas, these clinical or experimental trials were designed on the basis of traditional research model of "one drug, one target", ignoring the complexity of biological systems. It is well known that botanical medicines usually contain a large group of chemical components, which may act synergistically to achieve the therapeutic effects (Qiao et al., 2016). Thus, to uncover the underlying mechanisms of the therapeutic effects of GQD on UC in a systemic perspective, the present study employed network pharmacological strategy. By means of active compounds screening, drug targeting, and pathway enrichment analysis,

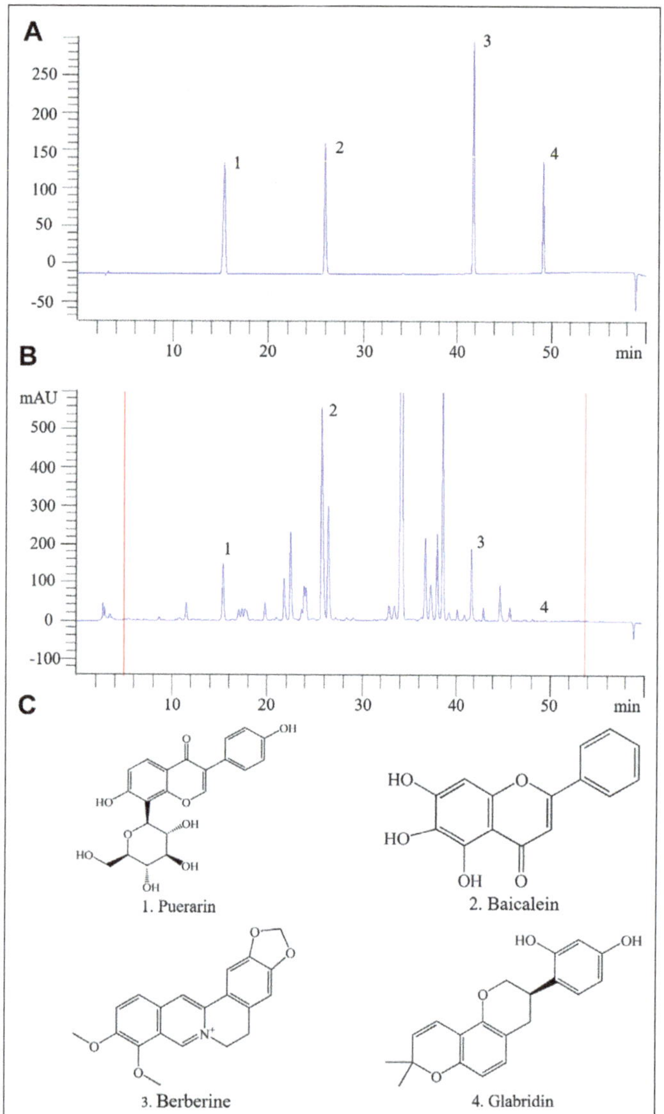

FIGURE 7 | HPLC profiles of the main active components of GQD. **(A)** The mixed standard sample. **(B)** The four active components. **(C)** The chemical formula of the four active compounds. 1. puerarin; 2. baicalein; 3. berberine; 4. glabridin.

network pharmacological analysis of GQD identified four botanical drugs, 77 compounds, and 59 hub targets, which were significantly enriched in several pathways related to UC such as HIF-1 signaling pathway, PI3K-AKT signaling pathway and TNF signaling pathway. In addition, molecular docking results demonstrated that the crucial active compounds in GQD exhibited good binding affinity to the hub target. The putative active components and multi-targets mechanisms of GQD in the treatment of UC were comprehensively elucidated in the present study, which provided theoretic evidence for the clinical application of GQD on UC treatment.

Among the identified compounds linked to the network, most chemical ingredients in GQD related to UC could be classified into flavonoids, alkaloids, and triterpenoid saponins. Baicalein and wogonin (a flavonoid), the major bioactive compounds isolated from HQ, had a better absorption effect. It has been reported that baicalein possesses potent anti-inflammatory and anti-colitis effect via suppressing the activity of TNF-α and interleukin IL-1β (He et al., 2015; Luo et al., 2017), as well as inhibiting the expression of NF-κB and STAT3 signaling pathways (Dong et al., 2015), while the wogonin exerts a dramatically preventive effect on colitis-associated cancer with its anti-angiogenesis activity through inhibiting secretion of VEGF and accelerated the degradation of HIF-1α (Song et al., 2013; Sun et al., 2015). Additionally, formononetin (an isoflavone) was also recognized as one of potential ingredients in the treatment of UC, which might possess the prominent anti-inflammation and antiproliferative effect on human colorectal cancer by downregulating the expression of HIF-1α and inflammatory cytokines (Huang et al., 2015; Ong et al., 2019), such as TNF-α, NF-κB (Wang et al., 2012). Glabridin, another isoflavonoid retrieved from GC, associated with a wide range of biological properties such as antioxidant, anti-inflammatory and antibacterial activities (Simmler et al., 2013). In addition, berberine possessed relatively high bioactivity and showed the high degree number of interactions linked to hub targets. It was a quaternary ammonium alkaloid from HL that exerted beneficial effects against UC via suppressing the IL-6/STAT3/NF-κB signaling pathway *in vivo* (Zhang et al., 2017; Zhu et al., 2019). According to previous research, the anti-inflammatory effect of berberine was mediated through COX-2 regulation (Kuo et al., 2004). Epiberberine is also a protoberberine alkaloid with antibacterial activities and synergistic effects for berberine (Luo et al., 2013; Tan et al., 2017). Moreover, puerarin, one of the main isoflavonoid components in *Pueraria lobata (Willd.) Ohwi*, has been known to possess anti-inflammatory and antioxidant effects in UC via down-regulating the expression of nuclear factor-κB and the secretion of pro-inflammatory mediators (Jeon et al., 2020). Overall, the above findings indicate that multi-compounds of GQD may conjointly execute the beneficial effects for UC. And the HPLC results in the present study also showed the existence and contents of puerarin, baicalein, berberine, and glabridin in GQD, which provided the pharmacological evidence for GQD to be used as an agent in the UC treatment. Besides the therapeutic effects of important compounds mentioned above, multiple actions and pharmacological efficacy of comprehensive ingredients in GQD have not been well evaluated yet, which is a challenge in pharmacology study due to the complex composition of compounds, synergetic effects and multi-targets of compounds in botanical drugs (Heinrich et al., 2020). And in the present study, numerous targets and pathways were identified to be relate to multiple compounds from different botanical drugs in GQD, which revealed the synergistic property of the compounds in GQD for the treatment of UC.

Among the main putative target mapped to compounds in the C-T network, many targets (ESR1, EGFR, SRC, MMP2, GSK3B, and PTGS2) with higher degree to compound might play a crucial role in the process of UC treatment. ESR1, an estrogen receptor, has been identified as a potential marker for identifying individuals at increased risk of neoplasia among those with

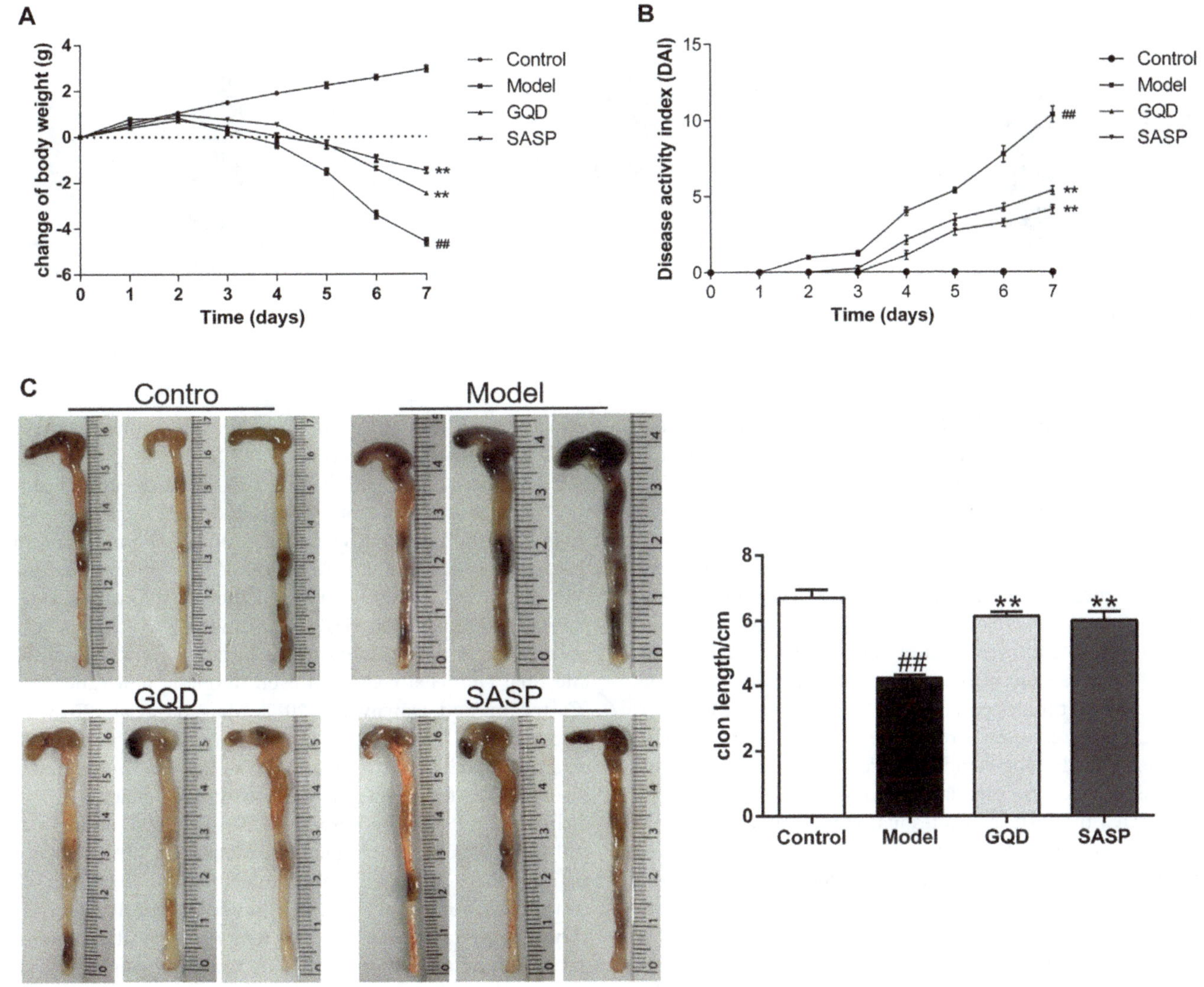

FIGURE 8 | GQD ameliorated DSS-induced body weight loss, DAI score and colonic shortening. **(A)** Change of body weight in four groups. **(B)** DAI score during experimental colitis. **(C)** Colon length in four groups. Values presented as mean ± SEM. $^{##}p < 0.01$ vs. control; $^{**}p < 0.01$ vs. model.

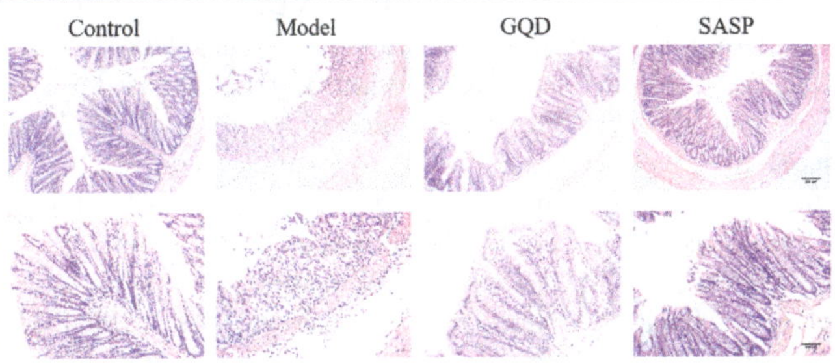

FIGURE 9 | Representative images of colonic tissues with HE staining (× 100 and × 200 magnification).

long-standing and extensive UC (Principi et al., 2014). EGFR, the epidermal growth factor receptor, is one of the major proteins regulating cell proliferation and survival on gut mucosal (Yarden and Pines, 2012). The binding of EGF at the enterocyte surface induces the dimerization of EGFR and tyrosine autophosphorylation, of which the formation initiates several intracellular signaling pathways including PI3K/AKT signaling pathway, and Ras/ERK signaling pathway (Wang, 2017). The GSK3B, as the components of the PI3K pathway, also can be initiated by chronic inflammation and the increased turnover of epithelial cells in the development of UC (Rogler, 2014; Setia et al., 2014). And the expression level of main target MMP2 also has been found to be closely related with TNF-α in colonic mucosa subjected to UC inflammation (Mao et al., 2012). In this study, we speculated that above targets closely related to GQD may be important functional targets for the treatment of UC. Besides, according to GO enrichment and KEGG pathway enrichment, the network analysis revealed that the GQD may exert a therapeutic effect to UC via many cellular processes, such as the regulation of inflammatory response, cell proliferation,

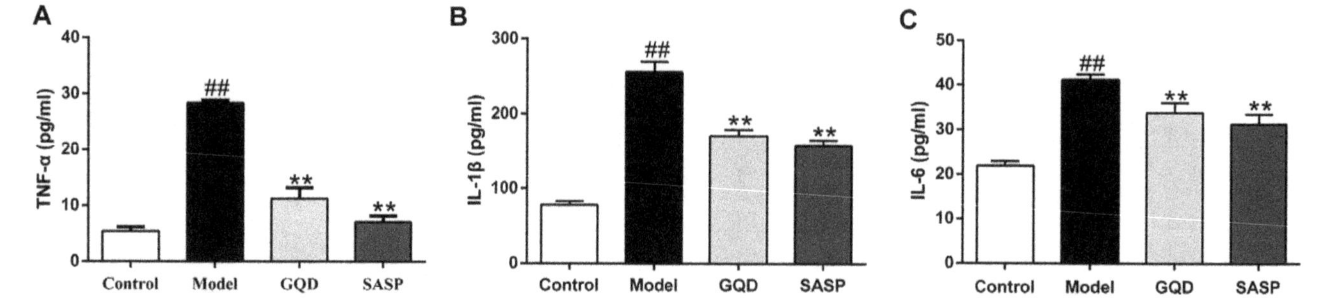

FIGURE 10 | The influence of GQD and SASP on proinflammatory cytokines TNFα **(A)**, IL-1β **(B)**, and IL-6 **(C)** in the colonic tissues. Values presented as mean ± SEM. $^{\#\#}p < 0.01$ vs. control; $^{**}p < 0.01$ vs. model.

angiogenesis and apoptosis. Moreover, among the enriched pathways linked to the hub targets, multiple pathways, such as PI3K-AKT signaling pathway, HIF-1 signaling pathway, VEGF signaling pathway, TNF signaling pathway, and Ras signaling pathway may be closely related to the pathogenesis of UC.

Dysregulated inflammatory response has been demonstrated to play a crucial role in the initiation, development, and progression of UC (Neurath, 2014). Inflammation and inflammatory cytokine in intestinal epithelial cells, and inflammatory cells were recognized as a risk factor for chronic inflammation to tumorigenesis (Yao et al., 2019). Moreover, colorectal cancer is a well-recognized complication of UC. And patients with long-standing chronic inflammation have an increased risk of potential carcinogenesis (Rubin et al., 2012). In UC, the disturbed intestinal epithelial cell generated the mucosal barrier dysfunction and the development of ulcers, leading to cancer occurrence (Yang et al., 2009). In the network pharmacology study, we found that many active components, prediction targets and pathways related to GQD were involved in the inflammation, angiogenesis, cell proliferation and apoptosis, which are closely related to cell carcinogenesis in UC. Specifically, the role of EGFR in inflammatory pathologies of colon is well known, and the expression of EGFR has been found upregulate in experimental colitis and patients with UC, then regulates cytokines production and intestinal inflammation (Lu et al., 2014). Moreover, PI3K is one of the EGFR targets, and the abnormality of PI3K/AKT signaling pathway is considered to be related to the onset of UC, as well as UC-induced colon cancer (Jiang et al., 2019). PI3K-AKT pathway is tightly related to the regulation of inflammatory response in the progression of UC. The abnormal activation of PI3K/AKT signaling pathway in UC has been demonstrated to enhance the expression and secretion of proinflammatory cytokines, such as TNF-α, IL-1β, and IL-6 (Wu et al., 2013; Jiang et al., 2019). However, TNF-a is a pro-inflammatory cytokine central to the pathogenesis of UC, which has a direct effect on the expression and organization of tight junction proteins, resulting in loss of tight junction functions, increased epithelial permeability and the induction of an inflammatory response (Leppkes et al., 2014). Hence, anti-TNF therapies is widely used in clinic as an appropriate way in the management of UC (Lawrance, 2015). Especially, TNF signaling pathway exerts a broad spectrum of activities, including regulation of inflammation and the migration of intestinal epithelial cells (Armaka et al., 2008; Schliemann et al., 2011), and it has been confirmed that ErbB signaling can be activated by the phosphorylation of TNF-α-induced receptor, which modulates the intestinal wound healing of inflammatory bowel disease (Frey et al., 2009). And PI3K/AKT signaling pathway is active in cells infiltrating inflamed human colon tissue via the participation of PTEN, GSK3B and mTOR, which may lead to over-transcription of downstream target genes, proliferation of intestinal epithelial cells, and even dysplasia and cancerization (Castellano and Downward, 2011; Matsuda et al., 2013; Chen et al., 2015). In addition, HIF-1, a transcription factor that regarded as the master regulator of oxygen homeostasis, is involved in the expression of a broad genetic program, including toll-like receptors (TLR)-mediated inflammatory pathway, which can trigger the activation of transcription factors (such as NF-κB) and induce TNF-a secretion (Jung et al., 2003; Kim et al., 2012). It has been reported that HIF-1 play an important role in vascular remodeling at sites of intestinal injury and inflammation of IBD, by regulating angiogenic genes such as VEGF (Feinman et al., 2010; Bakirtzi et al., 2014), a major paracrine growth factor involved in blood vessel development, which has been unregulated in active UC and UC-associated cancer (Tolstanova et al., 2009). Meanwhile, the fundamental regulator of angiogenesis and vascular permeability of VEGF has been found, which indicates that VEGF may also has proinflammatory properties (Chidlow et al., 2006). VEGF signaling pathway can be promoted by increased many inflammatory cells infiltrating ulcerative mucosa. And the increased leukocyte infiltration would contribute to inflammation initiation and subsequent tissue damage which is a characteristic feature of UC (Goebel et al., 2006). Therefore, we hypothesize that GQD may exert its therapeutic effects on UC by decreasing the inflammation response via regulating EGFR/PI3K/AKT signaling pathway.

To examine the effect of GQD on the inflammatory response in UC, as well as the role of EGFR-regulated PI3K/AKT signaling pathway in DSS-induced UC, we evaluated colon inflammation and injury in mice administrated with DSS. DSS-treated mice in model group exhibited more severe injury and acute colitis, while these abnormalities were ameliorated by GQD or SASP administration. We found that

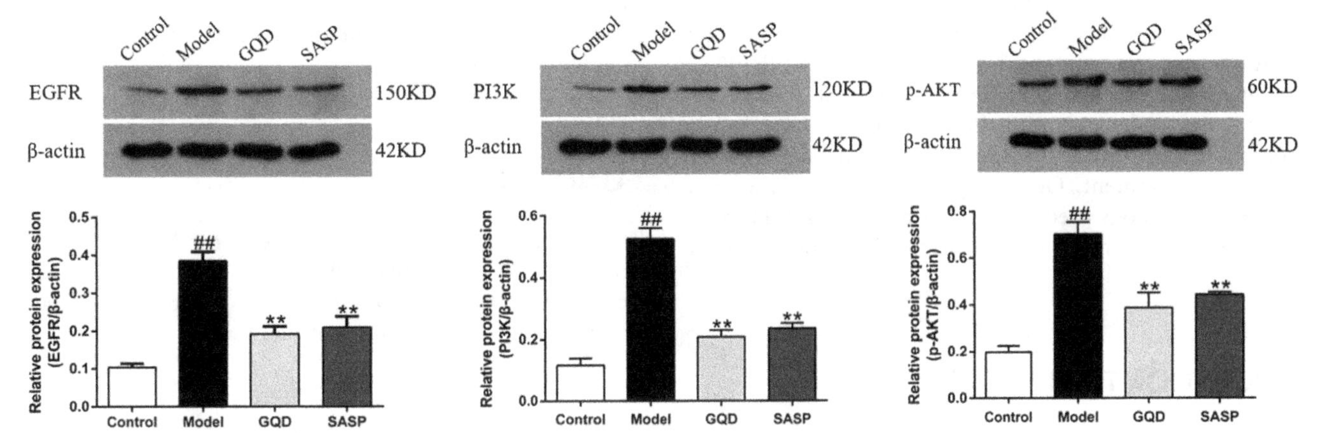

FIGURE 11 | Western blot and quantitative analysis of EGFR, PI3K and *p*-AKT in the colon tissues. Values presented as mean ± SEM. $^{\#\#}p < 0.01$ vs. control; $^{**}p < 0.01$ vs. model.

GQD and SASP could alleviate the shortening of the colon length, the DAI parameters, the pathological changes and the secretion of inflammatory cytokines. Moreover, the results indicated that EGFR/PI3K/AKT signaling pathway was activated abnormally in model group and played an important role in inflammation, consequently, a series of inflammatory responses and mucosal damage occurs, resulting in the development of UC. However, the expression of EGFR, PI3K and *p*-AKT in the colon tissues was significantly decreased in the GQD and SASP groups compared to model group, suggesting the protective effects of GQD and SASP in the treatment of UC. From the integrated drug target prediction, pathway enrichment analysis and *in vivo* experiment, the results demonstrated that the effective downregulation of the expression of EGFR, PI3K, and *p*-AKT by the administration of GQD and SASP may contribute to ameliorating UC.

The limitation of this study is lacking standardization of active compounds in GQD. However, it has been demonstrated that the governing authorities' rules on market entry of TCM products is primarily focused on the quality, safety and efficacy of TCM (Li et al., 2018). Compared with chemical drugs and biological products, the quality control of TCM is much more complicated and difficult because of the extremely large amounts of bioactive components and diverse synergistic effects. Standardization of TCM is an essential part of the modernization of TCM, which has been a topic of discussion over the past few decades in China with the goal to promote advances in TCM (Song et al., 2011). With regards to quality, international consensus is that all the TCM products must meet certain qualitative and quantitative quality standards that demonstrated authentication, identification and chemical composition (Qu et al., 2019), and several national standards of TCM has been proposed in China over the past few decades, *Chinese Pharmacopoeia* is the cornerstone of national standards for TCM (Song et al., 2011). The considerations for quality control should mainly include the following aspects: the source control of natural raw material, standardization of decoction pieces processing, in-process control of manufacturing, and specification that fit the characteristics of TCM. In addition, for the selection of quantitative control indicators, the active ingredients that relate to clinical function indications is considered, and when the active ingredients are unclear, representative components should be chosen (Qu et al., 2019). Development of the qualitative and quantitative analytic method to capture the fingerprint and content information of multiple chemical markers is the basis for standardization of TCM. Recently, a concept of "quality marker" (Q-marker) was proposed. Q-marker-base fingerprint and multi-component determination could contribute to the construction of more scientific quality control system of TCM (Yang et al., 2017). TCM standardization is an inevitable trend for the purpose of comprehensive development of TCM, and many measures should be taken to further promote the standardization of TCM.

Most recently, the draft of *Network Pharmacology Evaluation Method Guidance* was proposed, which addressed the data collection, network analysis, experiment verification principles, procedures, and evaluation indicators in network pharmacology research (Li, 2021). According to the guidance, there are multiple problems in the current network pharmacology studies, such as uneven research quality, lack of data standardization, and insufficient scientific verification. Here, we use the evaluation methods from three aspects–reliability, standardization, and rationality to assess the quality of our present study and find that it basically meets the evaluation requirement. Biological functional prediction is an important part in network pharmacology. The inflammatory response, regulation of apoptotic process, protein phosphorylation, and cell proliferation have been identified as important biological functions according to our prediction, while we mainly focused on inflammatory response in this paper, and in the future we will carry out further experiments to probe other possible predicted functions and mechanisms.

CONCLUSION

In summary, the combination of network pharmacological analysis in silico and *in vivo* experiment indicated that

GQD could effectively ameliorate DSS-induced colitis, and the therapeutic effect of GQD was associated with its synergic modulation on inflammation suppression via EGFR/PI3K/AKT signaling pathway. Therefore, we suggest that GQD could be developed as a promising therapy for UC, and it provided novel indications for further mechanistic studies of GQD on UC treatment. Our study also suggested that the network pharmacology prediction may exert as a useful tool to characterize the pharmacological mechanisms of TCM in detail.

AUTHOR CONTRIBUTIONS

ZM and YF conceived and designed the study; XL and YF performed the study, analyzed the data; XL and ZM drafted the manuscript; LD provided some positive suggestions and amended the final manuscript; XL and LD contributed to molecular docking analysis; ZM and YF contributed to revising the manuscript and improving the language in the final version of manuscript.

FUNDING

This work was supported by the fund for Youth Top Talent Project of Hubei Provincial Health and Family Planning Commission (EWT-2019-48), and Key Projects of Hunan Province Education Department (20A366).

ACKNOWLEDGMENTS

Special thanks to Xiang Guo and Tong Yang for the assistance in the network pharmacology approach and molecular docking analysis.

REFERENCES

Armaka, M., Apostolaki, M., Jacques, P., Kontoyiannis, D. L., Elewaut, D., and Kollias, G. (2008). Mesenchymal Cell Targeting by TNF as a Common Pathogenic Principle in Chronic Inflammatory Joint and Intestinal Diseases. *J. Exp. Med.* 205, 331–337. doi:10.1084/jem.20070906

Artursson, P., and Karlsson, J. (1991). Correlation between Oral Drug Absorption in Humans and Apparent Drug Permeability Coefficients in Human Intestinal Epithelial (Caco-2) Cells. *Biochem. Biophysical Res. Commun.* 175, 880–885. doi:10.1016/0006-291x(91)91647-u

Awortwe, C., Fasinu, P. S., and Rosenkranz, B. (2014). Application of Caco-2 Cell Line in Herb-Drug Interaction Studies: Current Approaches and Challenges. *J. Pharm. Pharm. Sci.* 17, 1–19. doi:10.18433/j30k63

Bakirtzi, K., West, G., Fiocchi, C., Law, I. K. M., Iliopoulos, D., and Pothoulakis, C. (2014). The Neurotensin-HIF-1α-Vegfα Axis Orchestrates Hypoxia, Colonic Inflammation, and Intestinal Angiogenesis. *Am. J. Pathol.* 184, 3405–3414. doi:10.1016/j.ajpath.2014.08.015

Bressler, B., Marshall, J. K., Bernstein, C. N., Bitton, A., Jones, J., Leontiadis, G. I., et al. (2015). Clinical Practice Guidelines for the Medical Management of Nonhospitalized Ulcerative Colitis: The Toronto Consensus. *Gastroenterology* 148, 1035–1058. doi:10.1053/j.gastro.2015.03.001

Castellano, E., and Downward, J. (2011). RAS Interaction with PI3K: More Than Just Another Effector Pathway. *Genes. Cancer* 2, 261–274. doi:10.1177/1947601911408079

Chen, J., Shao, R., Li, F., Monteiro, M., Liu, J.-P., Xu, Z. P., et al. (2015). PI3K/Akt/mTOR Pathway Dual Inhibitor BEZ235 Suppresses the Stemness of colon Cancer Stem Cells. *Clin. Exp. Pharmacol. Physiol.* 42, 1317–1326. doi:10.1111/1440-1681.12493

Chidlow, J. H., Langston, W., Greer, J. J. M., Ostanin, D., Abdelbaqi, M., Houghton, J., et al. (2006). Differential Angiogenic Regulation of Experimental Colitis. *Am. J. Pathol.* 169, 2014–2030. doi:10.2353/ajpath.2006.051021

Chow, S.-C. (2014). Bioavailability and Bioequivalence in Drug Development. *Wiley Interdiscip. Rev. Comput. Stat.* 6, 304–31. doi:10.1002/wics.1310

Dong, S.-j., Zhong, Y.-q., Lu, W.-t., Li, G.-h., Jiang, H.-l., and Mao, B. (2015). Baicalin Inhibits Lipopolysaccharide-Induced Inflammation through Signaling NF-Kb Pathway in HBE16 Airway Epithelial Cells. *Inflammation* 38, 1493–1501. doi:10.1007/s10753-015-0124-2

Fan, Y., Yi, W., Huang, H., Mei, Z., and Feng, Z. (2019). Efficacy of Herbal Medicine (Gegen Qinlian Decoction) on Ulcerative Colitis. *Medicine (Baltimore)* 98 (52), e18512. doi:10.1097/MD.0000000000018512

Feinman, R., Deitch, E. A., Watkins, A. C., Abungu, B., Colorado, I., Kannan, K. B., et al. (2010). HIF-1 Mediates Pathogenic Inflammatory Responses to Intestinal Ischemia-Reperfusion Injury. *Am. J. Physiology-Gastrointestinal Liver Physiol.* 299, G833–G843. doi:10.1152/ajpgi.00065.2010

Frey, M. R., Edelblum, K. L., Mullane, M. T., Liang, D., and Polk, D. B. (2009). The ErbB4 Growth Factor Receptor Is Required for colon Epithelial Cell Survival in the Presence of TNF. *Gastroenterology* 136, 217–226. doi:10.1053/j.gastro.2008.09.023

Gallo, G., Kotze, P. G., and Spinelli, A. (2018). Surgery in Ulcerative Colitis: when? How?. *Best Pract. Res. Clin. Gastroenterol.* 32-33, 71–78. doi:10.1016/j.bpg.2018.05.017

Gfeller, D., Grosdidier, A., Wirth, M., Daina, A., Michielin, O., and Zoete, V. (2014). SwissTargetPrediction: a Web Server for Target Prediction of Bioactive Small Molecules. *Nucleic Acids Res.* 42, W32–W38. doi:10.1093/nar/gku293

Goebel, S., Huang, M., Davis, W. C., Jennings, M., Siahaan, T. J., Alexander, J. S., et al. (2006). VEGF-A Stimulation of Leukocyte Adhesion to Colonic Microvascular Endothelium: Implications for Inflammatory Bowel Disease. *Am. J. Physiology-Gastrointestinal Liver Physiol.* 290, G648–G654. doi:10.1152/ajpgi.00466.2005

Hassan, S. M., and Hassan, A. H. (2018). The Possibility of Using Shogaol for Treatment of Ulcerative Colitis. *Iran J. Basic Med. Sci.* 21, 943–949. doi:10.22038/IJBMS.2018.28616.6932

He, X., Wei, Z., Zhou, E., Chen, L., Kou, J., Wang, J., et al. (2015). Baicalein Attenuates Inflammatory Responses by Suppressing TLR4 Mediated NF-Kb and MAPK Signaling Pathways in LPS-Induced Mastitis in Mice. *Int. Immunopharmacology* 28, 470–476. doi:10.1016/j.intimp.2015.07.012

Head, K. A., and Jurenka, J. S. (2003). Inflammatory Bowel Disease Part 1: Ulcerative Colitis-Ppathophysiology and Conventional and Alternative Treatment Options. *Altern. Med. Rev.* 8, 247–283. doi:10.1046/j.1360-0443.2003.00426.x

Heinrich, M., Appendino, G., Efferth, T., Fürst, R., Izzo, A. A., Kayser, O., et al. (2020). Best Practice in Research - Overcoming Common Challenges in Phytopharmacological Research. *J. Ethnopharmacology* 246, 112230. doi:10.1016/j.jep.2019.112230

Huang, C., Zheng, C., Li, Y., Wang, Y., Lu, A., and Yang, L. (2014). Systems Pharmacology in Drug Discovery and Therapeutic Insight for Herbal Medicines. *Brief Bioinform* 15, 710–733. doi:10.1093/bib/bbt035

Huang, J., Xie, M., Gao, P., Ye, Y., Liu, Y., Zhao, Y., et al. (2015). Antiproliferative Effects of Formononetin on Human Colorectal Cancer via Suppressing Cell Growth *In Vitro* and *In Vivo*. *Process Biochem.* 50, 912–917. doi:10.1016/j.procbio.2015.03.001

Jeon, Y.-D., Lee, J.-H., Lee, Y.-M., and Kim, D.-K. (2020). Puerarin Inhibits Inflammation and Oxidative Stress in Dextran Sulfate Sodium-Induced Colitis Mice Model. *Biomed. Pharmacother.* 124, 109847. doi:10.1016/j.biopha.2020.109847

Jiang, W., Han, Y. P., Hu, M., Bao, X. Q., Yan, Y., and Chen, G. (2019). A Study on Regulatory Mechanism of miR-223 in Ulcerative Colitis through PI3K/Akt-mTOR Signaling Pathway. *Eur. Rev. Med. Pharmacol. Sci.* 23, 4865–4872. doi:10.26355/eurrev_201906_18074

Jung, Y.-J., Isaacs, J. S., Lee, S., Trepel, J., and Neckers, L. (2003). IL-1β Mediated Up-regulation of HIF-lα via an NFkB/COX-2 Pathway Identifies HIF-1 as a Critical Link between Inflammation and Oncogenesis. *FASEB. J.* 17, 1–22. doi:10.1096/fj.03-0329fje

Kim, D.-S., Kim, S.-J., Kim, M.-C., Jeon, Y.-D., Um, J.-y., and Hong, S.-H. (2012). The Therapeutic Effect of Chelidonic Acid on Ulcerative Colitis. *Biol. Pharm. Bull.* 35, 666–671. doi:10.1248/bpb.35.666

Kim, J., Yoo, M., Shin, J., Kim, H., Kang, J., and Tan, A. C. (2018b). Systems Pharmacology-Based Approach of Connecting Disease Genes in Genome-wide Association Studies with Traditional Chinese Medicine. *Int. J. Genomics* 2018, 1–11. doi:10.1155/2018/7697356

Kim, S., Shoemaker, B. A., Bolton, E. E., and Bryant, S. H. (2018a). Finding Potential Multitarget Ligands Using PubChem. *Methods Mol. Biol.* 1825, 63–91. doi:10.1007/978-1-4939-8639-2_2

Kuo, C.-L., Chi, C.-W., and Liu, T.-Y. (2004). The Anti-inflammatory Potential of Berberine *In Vitro* and *In Vivo*. *Cancer Lett.* 203, 127–137. doi:10.1016/j.canlet.2003.09.002

Lawrance, I. C. (2015). Early Investigational TNF Receptor Antagonists for the Treatment of Ulcerative Colitis. *Expert Opin. Investig. Drugs* 24, 761–768. doi:10.1517/13543784.2015.1020371

Leppkes, M., Roulis, M., Neurath, M. F., Kollias, G., and Becker, C. (2014). Pleiotropic Functions of TNF- in the Regulation of the Intestinal Epithelial Response to Inflammation. *Int. Immunol.* 26, 509–515. doi:10.1093/intimm/dxu051

Li, B., Rui, J., Ding, X., and Yang, X. (2019). Exploring the Multicomponent Synergy Mechanism of Banxia Xiexin Decoction on Irritable Bowel Syndrome by a Systems Pharmacology Strategy. *J. Ethnopharmacology* 233, 158–168. doi:10.1016/j.jep.2018.12.033

Li, H., Zhao, L., Zhang, B., Jiang, Y., Wang, X., Guo, Y., et al. (2014). A Network Pharmacology Approach to Determine Active Compounds and Action Mechanisms of Ge-Gen-Qin-Lian Decoction for Treatment of Type 2 Diabetes. *Evidence-Based Complement. Altern. Med.* 2014, 1–12. doi:10.1155/2014/495840

Li, J., Zhu, J., Hu, H., Harnett, J. E., Lei, C. I., Chau, K. Y., et al. (2018). Internationalization of Traditional/Complementary Medicine Products: Market Entry as Medicine. *Chin. Med.* 13, 50. doi:10.1186/s13020-018-0209-6

Li, R., Chen, Y., Shi, M., Xu, X., Zhao, Y., Wu, X., et al. (2016). Gegen Qinlian Decoction Alleviates Experimental Colitis via Suppressing TLR4/NF-Kb Signaling and Enhancing Antioxidant Effect. *Phytomedicine* 23, 1012–1020. doi:10.1016/j.phymed.2016.06.010

Li, S. (2021). Network Pharmacology Evaluation Method Guidance - Draft. *World J. Tradit Chi Med.* 7, 146–154. doi:10.4103/wjtcm.wjtcm_11_21

Li, S., Zhang, Z. Q., Wu, L. J., Zhang, X. G., Wang, Y. Y., and Li, Y. D. (2007). Understanding ZHENG in Traditional Chinese Medicine in the Context of Neuro-Endocrine-Immune Network. *IET Syst. Biol.* 1, 51–60. doi:10.1049/iet-syb:20060032

Liu, Y., Grimm, M., Dai, W.-t., Hou, M.-c., Xiao, Z.-X., and Cao, Y. (2020). CB-dock: a Web Server for Cavity Detection-Guided Protein-Ligand Blind Docking. *Acta Pharmacol. Sin* 41, 138–144. doi:10.1038/s41401-019-0228-6

Liu, Z., Guo, F., Wang, Y., Li, C., Zhang, X., Li, H., et al. (2016). BATMAN-TCM: a Bioinformatics Analysis Tool for Molecular mechANism of Traditional Chinese Medicine. *Sci. Rep.* 6, 21146. doi:10.1038/srep21146

Lu, N., Wang, L., Cao, H., Liu, L., Van Kaer, L., Washington, M. K., et al. (2014). Activation of the Epidermal Growth Factor Receptor in Macrophages Regulates Cytokine Production and Experimental Colitis. *J. Immunol.* 192, 1013–1023. doi:10.4049/jimmunol.1300133

Luo, J., Yan, D., Yang, M., Dong, X., and Xiao, X. (2013). Multicomponent Therapeutics of Berberine Alkaloids. *Evidence-Based Complement. Altern. Med.* 2013, 1–10. doi:10.1155/2013/545898

Luo, X., Yu, Z., Deng, C., Zhang, J., Ren, G., Sun, A., et al. (2017). Baicalein Ameliorates TNBS-Induced Colitis by Suppressing TLR4/MyD88 Signaling cascade and NLRP3 Inflammasome Activation in Mice. *Sci. Rep.* 7, 16374. doi:10.1038/s41598-017-12562-6

Lv, R., Qiao, W., Wu, Z., Wang, Y., Dai, S., Liu, Q., et al. (2014). Tumor Necrosis Factor Alpha Blocking Agents as Treatment for Ulcerative Colitis Intolerant or Refractory to Conventional Medical Therapy: a Meta-Analysis. *PLoS One* 9, e86692. doi:10.1371/journal.pone.0086692

Mao, J.-W., Tang, H.-Y., Tan, X.-Y., and Wang, Y.-D. (2012). Effect of Etiasa on the Expression of Matrix Metalloproteinase-2 and Tumor Necrosis Factor-α in a Rat Model of Ulcerative Colitis. *Mol. Med. Rep.* 6, 996–1000. doi:10.3892/mmr.2012.1021

Matsuda, S., Nakanishi, A., Wada, Y., and Kitagishi, Y. (2013). Roles of PI3K/AKT/PTEN Pathway as a Target for Pharmaceutical Therapy. *Tomcj* 7, 23–29. doi:10.2174/1874104501307010023

Neurath, M. F. (2014). Cytokines in Inflammatory Bowel Disease. *Nat. Rev. Immunol.* 14, 329–342. doi:10.1038/nri3661

Ong, S., Shanmugam, M., Fan, L., Fraser, S., Arfuso, F., Ahn, K., et al. (2019). Focus on Formononetin: Anticancer Potential and Molecular Targets. *Cancers* 11, 611. doi:10.3390/cancers11050611

Ordás, I., Eckmann, L., Talamini, M., Baumgart, D. C., and Sandborn, W. J. (2012). Ulcerative Colitis. *The Lancet* 380, 1606–1619. doi:10.1016/S0140-6736(12)60150-0

Principi, M., Barone, M., Pricci, M., De Tullio, N., Losurdo, G., Ierardi, E., et al. (2014). Ulcerative Colitis: from Inflammation to Cancer. Do Estrogen Receptors Have a Role?. *World. J. Gastroentrol.* 20, 11496–11504. doi:10.3748/wjg.v20.i33.11496

Qi, L., Kai, D., An, M. A., and Jia, L. (2004). Analysis of Puerarin and Daidzein in Gegen Qinlian Preparations by High Performance Capillary Electrophoresis. *Chin. J. Pharm. Anal.* 24, 11–13. doi:10.1016/S0898-6568(03)00096-2

Qiao, X., Wang, Q., Wang, S., Kuang, Y., Li, K., Song, W., et al. (2018). A 42-Markers Pharmacokinetic Study Reveals Interactions of Berberine and Glycyrrhizic Acid in the Anti-diabetic Chinese Medicine Formula Gegen-Qinlian Decoction. *Front. Pharmacol.* 9, 622. doi:10.3389/fphar.2018.00622

Qiao, X., Wang, Q., Wang, S., Miao, W.-j., Li, Y.-j., Xiang, C., et al. (2016). Compound to Extract to Formulation: a Knowledge-Transmitting Approach for Metabolites Identification of Gegen-Qinlian Decoction, a Traditional Chinese Medicine Formula. *Sci. Rep.* 6, 39534. doi:10.1038/srep39534

Qu, J., Zhang, T., Liu, J., Su, Y., and Wang, H. (2019). Considerations for the Quality Control of Newly Registered Traditional Chinese Medicine in China: A Review. *J. AOAC Int.* 102, 689–694. doi:10.5740/jaoacint.18-0301

Rogler, G. (2014). Chronic Ulcerative Colitis and Colorectal Cancer. *Cancer Lett.* 345, 235–241. doi:10.1016/j.canlet.2013.07.032

Ru, J., Li, P., Wang, J., Zhou, W., Li, B., Huang, C., et al. (2014). TCMSP: a Database of Systems Pharmacology for Drug Discovery from Herbal Medicines. *J. Cheminform* 6, 13. doi:10.1186/1758-2946-6-13

Rubin, D. C., Shaker, A., and Levin, M. S. (2012). Chronic Intestinal Inflammation: Inflammatory Bowel Disease and Colitis-Associated colon Cancer. *Front. Immun.* 3, 107. doi:10.3389/fimmu.2012.00107

Sałaga, M., Zatorski, H., Sobczak, M., Chen, C., and Fichna, J. (2014). Chinese Herbal Medicines in the Treatment of IBD and Colorectal Cancer: a Review. *Curr. Treat. Options. Oncol.* 15, 405–420. doi:10.1007/s11864-014-0288-2

Schliemann, M., Bullinger, E., Borchers, S., Allgöwer, F., Findeisen, R., and Scheurich, P. (2011). Heterogeneity Reduces Sensitivity of Cell Death for TNF-Stimuli. *BMC Syst. Biol.* 5, 204. doi:10.1186/1752-0509-5-204

Setia, S., Nehru, B., and Sanyal, S. N. (2014). Upregulation of MAPK/Erk and PI3K/Akt Pathways in Ulcerative Colitis-Associated colon Cancer. *Biomed. Pharmacother.* 68, 1023–1029. doi:10.1016/j.biopha.2014.09.006

Shannon, P., Markiel, A., Ozier, O., Baliga, N. S., Wang, J. T., Ramage, D., et al. (2003). Cytoscape: a Software Environment for Integrated Models of Biomolecular Interaction Networks. *Genome Res.* 13, 2498–2504. doi:10.1101/gr.1239303

Shijun, Z. (2010). Clinical Research of Gegenqinlian Decoction in Treating Dampess and Heat Ulcerative Colitis. *China J. Chin. Med.* 25, 970–971. doi:10.16368/j.issn.1674-8999.2010.05.052

Shivashankar, R., Tremaine, W. J., Harmsen, W. S., and Loftus, E. V. (2017). Incidence and Prevalence of Crohn's Disease and Ulcerative Colitis in Olmsted County, Minnesota from 1970 through 2010. *Clin. Gastroenterol. Hepatol.* 15, 857–863. doi:10.1016/j.cgh.2016.10.039

Shu, Z., He, W., Shahen, M., Guo, Z., Shu, J., Wu, T., et al. (2018). Clarifying of the Potential Mechanism of Sinisan Formula for Treatment of Chronic Hepatitis by Systems Pharmacology Method. *Biomed. Pharmacother.* 100, 532–550. doi:10.1016/j.biopha.2018.02.047

Simmler, C., Pauli, G. F., and Chen, S.-N. (2013). Phytochemistry and Biological Properties of Glabridin. *Fitoterapia* 90, 160–184. doi:10.1016/j.fitote.2013.07.003

Song, P., Gao, J., Kokudo, N., and Tang, W. (2011). Standardization of Traditional Chinese Medicine and Evaluation of Evidence from its Clinical Practice. *Drug. Discov. Ther.* 5 (6), 261–265. doi:10.5582/ddt.2011.v5.6.261

Song, X., Yao, J., Wang, F., Zhou, M., Zhou, Y., Wang, H., et al. (2013). Wogonin Inhibits Tumor Angiogenesis via Degradation of HIF-1α Protein. *Toxicol. Appl. Pharmacol.* 271, 144–155. doi:10.1016/j.taap.2013.04.031

Sun, Y., Zhao, Y., Yao, J., Zhao, L., Wu, Z., Wang, Y., et al. (2015). Wogonoside Protects against Dextran Sulfate Sodium-Induced Experimental Colitis in Mice by Inhibiting NF-Kb and NLRP3 Inflammasome Activation. *Biochem. Pharmacol.* 94, 142–154. doi:10.1016/j.bcp.2015.02.002

Szklarczyk, D., Gable, A. L., Lyon, D., Junge, A., Wyder, S., Huerta-Cepas, J., et al. (2019). STRING V11: Protein-Protein Association Networks with Increased Coverage, Supporting Functional Discovery in Genome-wide Experimental Datasets. *Nucleic Acids Res.* 47 (D1), D607–D613. doi:10.1093/nar/gky1131

Tan, L., Li, C., Chen, H., Mo, Z., Zhou, J., Liu, Y., et al. (2017). Epiberberine, a Natural Protoberberine Alkaloid, Inhibits Urease of *Helicobacter pylori* and jack Bean: Susceptibility and Mechanism. *Eur. J. Pharm. Sci.* 110, 77–86. doi:10.1016/j.ejps.2017.02.004

Tao, W., Xu, X., Wang, X., Li, B., Wang, Y., Li, Y., et al. (2013). Network Pharmacology-Based Prediction of the Active Ingredients and Potential Targets of Chinese Herbal Radix Curcumae Formula for Application to Cardiovascular Disease. *J. Ethnopharmacology* 145, 1–10. doi:10.1016/j.jep.2012.09.051

Tian, S., Wang, J., Li, Y., Li, D., Xu, L., and Hou, T. (2015). The Application of In Silico Drug-Likeness Predictions in Pharmaceutical Research. *Adv. Drug Deliv. Rev.* 86, 2–10. doi:10.1016/j.addr.2015.01.009

Tolstanova, G., Khomenko, T., Deng, X., Chen, L., Tarnawski, A., Ahluwalia, A., et al. (2009). Neutralizing Anti-vascular Endothelial Growth Factor (VEGF) Antibody Reduces Severity of Experimental Ulcerative Colitis in Rats: Direct Evidence for the Pathogenic Role of VEGF. *J. Pharmacol. Exp. Ther.* 328, 749–757. doi:10.1124/jpet.108.145128

Torres, J., Billioud, V., Sachar, D. B., Peyrin-Biroulet, L., and Colombel, J.-F. (2012). Ulcerative Colitis as a Progressive Disease: the Forgotten Evidence. *Inflamm. Bowel Dis.* 18, 1356–1363. doi:10.1002/ibd.22839

Wang, C., Duan, X., Sun, X., Liu, Z., Sun, P., Yang, X., et al. (2016). Protective Effects of Glycyrrhizic Acid from Edible Botanical glycyrrhiza Glabra against Non-alcoholic Steatohepatitis in Mice. *Food Funct.* 7, 3716–3723. doi:10.1039/c6fo00773b

Wang, Y., Zhu, Y., Gao, L., Yin, H., Xie, Z., Wang, D., et al. (2012). Formononetin Attenuates IL-1β-Induced Apoptosis and NF-Kb Activation in INS-1 Cells. *Molecules* 17, 10052–10064. doi:10.3390/molecules170910052

Wang, Z. (2017). ErbB Receptors and Cancer. *Methods Mol. Biol.* 1652, 3–35. doi:10.1007/978-1-4939-7219-7_1

Wu, X.-F., Xu, R., Ouyang, Z.-J., Qian, C., Shen, Y., Wu, X.-D., et al. (2013). Beauvericin Ameliorates Experimental Colitis by Inhibiting Activated T Cells via Downregulation of the PI3K/Akt Signaling Pathway. *PLoS One* 8, e83013, doi:10.1371/journal.pone.0083013

Xu, B.-L., Zhang, G.-J., and Ji, Y.-B. (2015). Active Components Alignment of Gegenqinlian Decoction Protects Ulcerative Colitis by Attenuating Inflammatory and Oxidative Stress. *J. Ethnopharmacology* 162, 253–260. doi:10.1016/j.jep.2014.12.042

Xu, X., Zhang, W., Huang, C., Li, Y., Yu, H., Wang, Y., et al. (2012). A Novel Chemometric Method for the Prediction of Human Oral Bioavailability. *Int. J. Mol. Sci.* 13, 6964–6982. doi:10.3390/ijms13066964

Yan, M. W., Mei, Q. K., Yan, B. C., Zhi, X. X., and Rui, F. W. (2012). Clinical Study of Internal and External Treatment of Gegen Qinlian Wutan Decoction in Active Ulcerative Colitis. *Chin. J. Exp. Traditional Med. Formulae* 18, 267–270. doi:10.13422/j.cnki.syfjx.2012.17.005

Yan, Y.-x., Shao, M.-j., Qi, Q., Xu, Y.-s., Yang, X.-q., Zhu, F.-h., et al. (2018b). Artemisinin Analogue SM934 Ameliorates DSS-Induced Mouse Ulcerative Colitis via Suppressing Neutrophils and Macrophages. *Acta Pharmacol. Sin* 39, 1633–1644. doi:10.1038/aps.2017.185

Yan, Y., Du, C., Li, Z., Zhang, M., Li, J., Jia, J., et al. (2018a). Comparing the Antidiabetic Effects and Chemical Profiles of Raw and Fermented Chinese Ge-Gen-Qin-Lian Decoction by Integrating Untargeted Metabolomics and Targeted Analysis. *Chin. Med.* 13, 54. doi:10.1186/s13020-018-0208-7

Yang, G.-Y., Taboada, S., and Liao, J. (2009). Inflammatory Bowel Disease: a Model of Chronic Inflammation-Induced Cancer. *Methods Mol. Biol.* 511, 193–233. doi:10.1007/978-1-59745-447-6_9

Yang, W., Zhang, Y., Wu, W., Huang, L., Guo, D., and Liu, C. (2017). Approaches to Establish Q-Markers for the Quality Standards of Traditional Chinese Medicines. *Acta Pharmaceutica Sinica B* 7, 439–446. doi:10.1016/j.apsb.2017.04.012

Yao, D., Dong, M., Dai, C., and Wu, S. (2019). Inflammation and Inflammatory Cytokine Contribute to the Initiation and Development of Ulcerative Colitis and its Associated Cancer. *Inflamm. Bowel Dis.* 25, 1595–1602. doi:10.1093/ibd/izz149

Yarden, Y., and Pines, G. (2012). The ERBB Network: at Last, Cancer Therapy Meets Systems Biology. *Nat. Rev. Cancer* 12, 553–563. doi:10.1038/nrc3309

Yu, L. Z., Wu, J. Y., Luo, J. B., Huang, X. G., Lin, H., and Xing, Y. L. (2005). Experimental Study on Anti-diarrhae Effect of Gegenqinlian Decoction and its Compounds. *Chin. Traditional Patent Med.* 27, 300–304.

Zhang, L.-C., Wang, Y., Tong, L.-C., Sun, S., Liu, W.-Y., Zhang, S., et al. (2017). Berberine Alleviates Dextran Sodium Sulfate-Induced Colitis by Improving Intestinal Barrier Function and Reducing Inflammation and Oxidative Stress. *Exp. Ther. Med.* 13, 3374–3382. doi:10.3892/etm.2017.4402

Zhu, L., Gu, P., and Shen, H. (2019). Protective Effects of Berberine Hydrochloride on DSS-Induced Ulcerative Colitis in Rats. *Int. Immunopharmacology* 68, 242–251. doi:10.1016/j.intimp.2018.12.036

15

Comparative Network Pharmacology Analysis of Classical TCM Prescriptions for Chronic Liver Disease

Zikun Chen[1], Xiaoning Wang[2], Yuanyuan Li[3], Yahang Wang[3], Kailin Tang[1], Dingfeng Wu[1], Wenyan Zhao[1], Yueming Ma[3], Ping Liu[2,4]* and Zhiwei Cao[1]**

[1] Department of Gastroenterology, Shanghai Tenth People's Hospital, School of Life Sciences and Technology, Tongji University, Shanghai, China, [2] Institute of Interdisciplinary Integrative Medicine Research, Shanghai University of Traditional Chinese Medicine, Shanghai, China, [3] Department of Pharmacology, Shanghai University of Traditional Chinese Medicine, Shanghai, China, [4] Key Laboratory of Liver and Kidney Diseases of Ministry of Education of China, Institute of Liver Diseases, Shuguang Hospital, Shanghai University of Traditional Chinese Medicine, Shanghai, China

***Correspondence:**
Yueming Ma
mayueming@shutcm.edu.cn
Ping Liu
liuliver@vip.sina.com
Zhiwei Cao
zwcao@tongji.edu.cn

Chronic liver disease (CLD) has become a major global health problem while herb prescriptions are clinically observed with significant efficacy. Three classical Traditional Chinese Medicine (TCM) formulae, Yinchenhao Decoction (YCHT), Huangqi Decoction (HQT), and Yiguanjian (YGJ) have been widely applied in China to treat CLD, but no systematic study has yet been published to investigate their common and different mechanism of action (MOA). Partial limitation may own to deficiency of effective bioinformatics methods. Here, a computational framework of comparative network pharmacology is firstly proposed and then applied to herbal recipes for CLD disease. The analysis showed that, the three formulae modulate CLD mainly through functional modules of immune response, inflammation, energy metabolism, oxidative stress, and others. On top of that, each formula can target additional unique modules. Typically, YGJ ingredients can uniquely target the ATP synthesis and neurotransmitter release cycle. Interestingly, different formulae may regulate the same functional module in different modes. For instance, YCHT and YGJ can activate oxidative stress-related genes of SOD family while HQT are found to inhibit SOD1 gene. Overall, our framework of comparative network pharmacology proposed in our work may not only explain the MOA of different formulae treating CLD, but also provide hints to further investigate the biological basis of CLD subtypes.

Keywords: network comparative analysis, TCM, chronic liver disease, Yinchenhao Decoction, Huangqi Decoction, Yiguanjian

INTRODUCTION

With increasing alcohol consumption and viral infection, chronic liver disease (CLD) has become a worldwide health concern. Chronic liver disease in the clinical context is a disease process of the liver that involves a process of progressive destruction and regeneration of the liver parenchyma leading to fibrosis and cirrhosis. "Chronic liver disease" refers to disease of the liver that lasts over a period of six months. It consists of a wide range of liver pathologies covering inflammation (chronic hepatitis), liver cirrhosis, and hepatocellular carcinoma.

According to causes, chronic liver diseases can be classified as viral disease, toxic and drug-related disease, metabolic disease, autoimmune-response disease, and so on. While the nucleotide analogues (NUCs) and pegylated-interferon (Peg-IFN) therapies are effective, patients may not tolerate their adverse effects in lifelong treatment. In the meantime, most of CLD patients seek medical help from herbal medicine for its significant efficacy and low side effects. Recently, several meta-studies of randomized, controlled, clinical trials (RCTs) suggested that herbal remedies have a similar and even better effects compared to western drug therapy in dealing with CLD (Peng et al., 2016; Chen et al., 2019).

According to Guidelines for the diagnosis and treatment of liver fibrosis in integrative medicine practice of China, three classical formulae, Yinchenhao Decoction (YCHT), Huangqi Decoction (HQT), and Yiguanjian (YGJ) have been recommended to treat different subtypes of CLD according to "Zheng" differentiation, which classifies the pathological state of a patient at system level leading to individualized treatments. Syndrome Differentiation and Treatment (SDAT) is the basis of clinical application of traditional Chinese Medicine prescription. A chronic liver disease can be treated with the different efficacy TCM prescription based on its different TCM syndrome. Formula YCHT is suggested to treat "damp-heat" type of patients featured by jaundice, inflammation, and abnormal fatty acids metabolism (Yan et al., 2017), and the therapeutic characteristic of Yinchenhao decoction is to clear heat and drain dampness. Clinically, it is applied mainly to treat patients who have acute jaundice hepatitis, hepatitis B, cholelithiasis, cholecystitis, leptospirosis, typhoid fever, pneumonia, hemolytic jaundice caused by favism, and so on (Yan et al., 2017), while formula HQT, with the proportion of Huangqi [*Astragalus mongholicus* Bge.] and Zhigancao [*Glycyrrhiza uralensis* Fisch.] at 6:1, is recommended for those "Qi-deficiency" patients with weak body, black and yellowish complexion, palpitations and vexations in the chest, dry lips and mouths, pale complexion and lack of appetite. The therapeutic characteristic of HQT is tonifying qi. HQT is applied clinically to treat CLD patients who have liver fibrosis or cirrhosis, heart failure, constipation, type 2 diabetes, and diabetic peripheral neuropathy with "Qi-blood deficiency" (Wang et al., 2015). Additionally, HQT alleviated DMN-induced liver fibrosis (Song et al., 2016). As the therapeutic characteristic of YGJ is nourishing liver and kidney, it is applied clinically to treat those who have chronic liver diseases, chronic gastritis, gastric and duodenal ulcer, intercostal neuralgia, and neurosis with "Yin-deficiency" (Wang et al., 2015).

Studies have investigated the liver-protective activity of above formula. For instance, being composed of Yinchen [*Artemisia capillaris* Thunb.], Zhizi [*Gardenia jasminoides* J. Ellis], and Dahuang [*Rheum palmatum* L.], YCHT demonstrated variable ability of liver protection in treating cholestasis, liver fibrosis, hepatitis, biliary cirrhosis, and cholesteric liver diseases (Yan et al., 2017). The liver protection of YCHT was also confirmed by histopathology and biochemical experiments (Sun et al., 2019), and YCHD treatment could reverse the damage by DMN-induced in liver function (Cai et al., 2018). According to literature validation, pharmacological research revealed that YCHT showed function of anti-oxidative stress, inhibiting apoptosis. Also, it was validated to regulate cellular inflammation and lipid metabolism (Wang et al., 2015). Kupffer cells (KC) activation of inflammatory response and abnormal fatty acid metabolism were found to be the main pathological basis in the early inflammation for YCHT Syndrome (Xu-Dong et al., 2014).

Through literature searching, HQT decoction was reported to downregulate the expressions of PDGF genes, collagen genes (COL1A1, COL1A2, COL5A2), and THBS1, inhibiting TGF-beta and PDGF signaling pathways, followed by verification *via* qRT-PCR (Zhang et al., 2015). Also, it was noticed to promote Kupffer cell activation (Du et al., 2012; Liu et al., 2012; Zhang et al., 2015; Song et al., 2016), inhibit Notch signaling pathway (Wang et al., 2015), and alleviate oxidative stress and lipid peroxidation injury. In an animal experiment, HQT was found to significantly reduce alpha-naphthylisothiocyanate-induced cholestasis in mice (Wu et al., 2017). At herb level, herb Huangqi in HQT were reported with anti-oxidative and immune regulating effects (Shahzad et al., 2016; Li et al., 2019).

YGJ decoction has 6 herbs: Beishashen [*Glehnia littoralis* F. Schmidt ex Miq.], Maidong [*Ophiopogon japonicus* (Thunb.) Ker Gawl.], Danggui [*Angelica sinensis* (Oliv.) Diels], Shengdihuang [*Rehmannia glutinosa* (Gaertn.) DC.], Gouqizi [*Lycium barbarum* L.], and Chuanlianzi [*Melia azedarach* L.]. Research indicates the hepatoprotective, anti-fibrogenic, anti-angiogenesis effects of YGJ in hepatic injury mice models (Tian et al., 2016). In rat model of liver fibrosis, YGJ was found to alleviate the hepatic collagen hyperplasia and deteriorated hepatic function (Tao et al., 2009). Also, YGJ can reduce the liver oxidative stress and lipid peroxidation injury while inhibiting angiogenesis and induce cell differentiation (Zhou et al., 2015). In a rat model of liver cirrhosis, YGJ was reported with repairing function of liver cirrhosis, and the key mechanism was suggested as relating to the regulation of macrophage activation state (Xu et al., 2018).

Above studies showed the biological activity of formulae, but it would be interesting to know the detailed MOA difference or similarities between the three formulae under the same background of CLD disease. As TCM formulae are believed to produce efficacy in a holistic way, the difficulty in detecting the MOA similarities and differences lie in the inherent complexity of multi-ingredients and multi-targets for TCM formulae.

With the development of systems biology and accumulated herbal targets information, the emerging method of network pharmacology makes it possible for MOA analysis of herbal ingredients. Coupled with transcriptomics validation, a latest article provided an excellent model adopting network pharmacology to predict the active components and regulation mechanisms of YCHT against liver fibrosis (Cai et al., 2019). Until now, network pharmacology has been applied to study individual ingredients, herbs, or formulae. One reason causing the difficulty is the lack of effective bioinformatics methods. Here, we developed a computational framework aiming to compare the MOA between formulae for same disease, taking the YCHT, HQT, and YGJ as an example.

The results indicated that although different formulae have different molecular targeting profile, they are commonly involved in a group of functional modules, indicating the CLD disease background. In addition to that, each formula was detected with unique function modules in MOA analysis. More interestingly, even on the same functional module, different regulating modes were found for different formulae agreeing with observed "Zheng" classification of CLD subtyping.

MATERIALS AND METHODS

Dataset

Formulae, Herbs, Ingredients, and Targets

For each of the three formulae, herb components, ingredients and targets of each ingredients were collected from HIT (Ye et al., 2011), NPASS (Zeng et al., 2018b), TCMDB (Chen, 2011) and TCM-ID (Huang et al., 2018) databases respectively.

Method

Disease Network, Disease Modules and Function Annotation

Targets of herbal active ingredients were obtained from HIT (Ye et al., 2011) and NPASS (Zeng et al., 2018b) database for target network construction. Potential protein-protein interaction (PPI) network of disease is generated *via* Reactome database (Croft et al., 2014) based on combined unique targets from 3 formulae *via* step size 1 (one bridging node). Then, the disease network was modularized through ReactomeFIViz (Wu and Haw, 2017). Genecards database (Safran et al., 2010) was used for function annotation of each module because of its high level of function annotation. Disease network and modularization were displayed *via* Cytoscape (Shannon et al., 2003). KEGG (Kanehisa, 2002) and GO Biological Process (Ashburner et al., 2000; Mi et al., 2017; The Gene Ontology, 2017) databases were used for biological function annotation for targets of each formula.

Statistic Enrichment of Functional Modules

For the given number of formula targets, we tested whether it is significantly enriched in a specific module A, comparing to a randomly picked module with equal size of A, from nodes of disease network background. To make the variation comparable in statistics, we repeated the picking for 5000 times. And each time, half the number of given targets were randomly picked. T-test statistics was made between the hitting of tested targets on specific module and the random module equally sized. According to above, different number of targets for each formula were enriched respectively into the functional modules of disease.

Effect of Kaempferol on the Absorption of Astragalosides

To investigate the effect of kaempferol on the absorption of astragalosides, experiments of verted rat sac was performed as previously described (Yan et al., 2015). Briefly, the everted intestinal sacs were prepared by rapidly removing the small intestine from starved rats euthanized under carbon dioxide (CO_2) anesthesia. Then, four intestinal segments (the duodenum, upper jejunum, bottom jejunum, and ileum) were excised, flushed several times with saline solution at room temperature, and then placed immediately into oxygenated buffer solution at 37°C. Intestine segments from four rats were divided into four groups treated with astragalosides without or with kaempferol at three different concentrations (1, 3, 10M) using a 4 × 4 Latin square design (Gressley et al., 2016).

4 × 4-latin square design.

Rat	Duodenum	Upper jejunum	Bottom jejunum	Ileum
1	A	B	C	D
2	B	C	D	A
3	C	D	A	B
4	D	A	B	C

A: Astragalosides + 1μM kaempferol;
B: Astragalosides + 3μM kaempferol;
C: Astragalosides + 10μM kaempferol;
D: Astragalosides.

The concentration of Astragaloside solutions was set at 8 mg/mL based on the gastrointestinal concentration after oral administration of Huangqi [*Astragalus mongholicus* Bge.] decoction to rats, and the concentration of the additional kaempferol was 1, 3, and 10 μM. Then, aliquots of the sac fluid sample (200 μL) were removed, and the same volume of buffer solution was added at 0, 0.5, 1, and 2 h. The area of each sac was calculated closely. Furthermore, each sac was weighed before and after fluid collection to calculate accurately the volume inside the sac. The samples were analyzed using UPLC-LTQ-Orbitrap in both positive and negative ionization mode as previously described. The proposed method could be used to determine the 10 compounds in astragalosides simultaneously with high precision, sensitivity, and accuracy (Zeng et al., 2018a). A multivariate analysis of variance (ANOVA) was performed using the SPSS ver. 13.0 software while p-values < 0.05 were considered statistically significant.

RESULTS

Computational Framework of Comparative Network Pharmacology

The idea of comparative network pharmacology is to construct a background disease network covering all the targets of different formulae, and then analyze the common and different modules or regulations. The framework of comparative network pharmacology is proposed as below (**Figure 1**): 1. Disease network construction and modularization of combined targets; 2. Comparative analysis of formulae on disease module network; 3. Detailed regulation comparison between formulae.

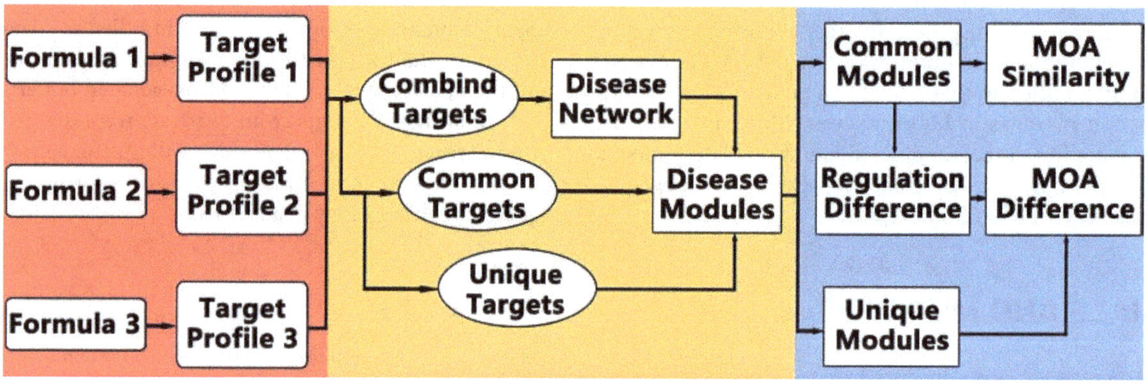

FIGURE 1 | Computational Framework of comparative network pharmacology.

Accordingly, the computational framework works like this: 1. Retrieve targets of each formula for same disease; 2. Construct the disease network based on combined targets of all formulae; 3. Partition and annotate the disease network into function modules; 4. Calculate the enriched modules for common targets among all formulae and unique targets for each formula; 5. Analyze the MOA similarities and differences.

Disease Network and Function Modules

The known ingredients with experimental target evidence from literatures were retrieved from databases and summarized into **Supplementary Table 1** for each herb and formula. Though different formulae are composed of different number of herbs, the overall known targets for each formula is roughly similar ranging from 120 to 140 genes. A total of 293 non-redundant targets were combined for all 3 formulae.

Targets of each formula was firstly enriched into KEGG and GO database for function annotation. The results show that all the three formulae are primarily targeting pathway of Hepatitis B, suggesting their common therapeutic effects in liver disease, but the enriched pathway lists are heavily overlapping (**Supplementary Table 2**). Similarly, mapping to GO databases also shows similar pathways profiles and GO terms. This suggests that the commonly used bioinformatics analysis of KEGG and GO annotation is good at inferring the MOA similarities, rather than the MOA differences for different formulae.

After running the pipeline of comparative network pharmacology, we proposed the biggest connected subnetwork containing 244 targets (83.28% of total) as the CLD disease background network.

This CLD network was initially clustered into 16 modules by ReactomeFIViz (Wu and Haw, 2017). After removing the two modules fully composed of background bridging nodes, we kept the remaining 14 modules for further analysis.

Common and Unique Functional Modules for TCM Formulae

Since active ingredient list is often an arguable issue for herbs, consensus has not been reached particularly for those commonly found among herbs, such as kaempferol, vitamins, or quercetins. Despite the molecular activity *in vitro*, the low bioavailability was often reported (Barve et al., 2009). Under the complexity of multi-ingredients context of herbs, their potential ADME effect to known active ingredients deserves further investigation. Taking kaempferol as an example, we tested the effects of kaempferol on the absorption of astragalosides in Huangqi herb *via* verted rat sac method under 4 different dosages. In the preliminary test, it was found that there were significant differences in the absorption of astragalosides in different rats and different gut segments. Then, Latin square was adopted to exclude the influence of different rats and intestinal segments. As the detailed results shown in **Supplementary Table 3**, under the concentration range of 1-10μM, kaempferol was observed with no significant effect on the absorption of 10 components in astragalosides in verted rat sac model.

As such, the active ingredient list was perturbed from full to shortlist by removing kaempferol, vitamin C, and vitamin E one by one. The module enrichment results were summarized in **Supplementary Table 1** (Sheet name: results of enrichment). Despite the perturbation, all formulae share 3 consensus modules and one conditional module, and each formula own two unique modules. Ten modules covered 236 targets, and their functional annotation are shown in **Table 1** by GeneCards (Safran et al., 2010).

Through the computational framework, the MOA similarity and differences are illustrated in **Figure 2** as shown below in the background of disease modules. The four common modules cover 167 targets, mainly involving oxidative stress, drug metabolism, DNA damage, NFAT and Cardiac Hypertrophy, Jak-STAT signaling and inflammation, etc. Further details of modules are shown in **Figure 3**. These common processes of oxidative stress, inflammation, and corresponding signaling pathways are highly involved in the pathological basis of CLD. For instance, oxidative stress, caused by imbalance between production and consumption by antioxidants, is a prominent feature in the pathophysiology of CLD (Vuppalanchi et al., 2011). Once oxidative stress is initiated, continuous cycle of cellular damage and release of proinflammatory cytokines will move on leading to hepatic inflammation, fibrosis, and cirrhosis (Comporti et al., 2009).

TABLE 1 | List of functional modules for CLD disease network derived from three TCM formulae.

Module ID	Module Function
1	Immune Response (lectin induced complement pathway)
2	ECM-receptor interaction; Leukocyte trans-endothelial migration Fluid shear stress and atherosclerosis; Cell adhesion
3	ATP Binding (LKB1 signaling events)
4	CDK-mediated phosphorylation and removal of Cdc6
5	ATP synthesis; Doxorubicin Pathway (Cardiomyocyte Cell), Respiratory electron transport
6	Neurotransmitter Release Cycle
7	Drug metabolism - cytochrome P450 Oxidative Stress
8	DNA Damage Oxidative Stress
9	NFAT and Cardiac Hypertrophy
10	Jak-STAT signaling; Cytokine-cytokine receptor interaction IL-17 signaling; Inflammatory mediator regulation of TRP channels

In view of literature report, consistent mechanistic evidences have been found between our computing analysis and independent validation. Modules 8 and 7 are involved with anti-oxidative stress. All three formulae can target these two common modules, indicating their common anti-oxidative function. Furthermore, module 10 is mainly involved with inflammation, and all three formulae were predicted to interact with a wide variety of inflammation factors. For instance, YCHT can target IL1B, IL4, and IL6; HQT can target IL6 and IL10; and YGJ can target more factors of IL1B, IL2, IL4, IL5, IL6, IL10, and IL13. At molecular level, our predictive results gained support from previous validation in that TGF-beta was targeted by HQT, and collagen genes (COL1A1, COL4A2, and COL7A1) were targeted by YGJ.

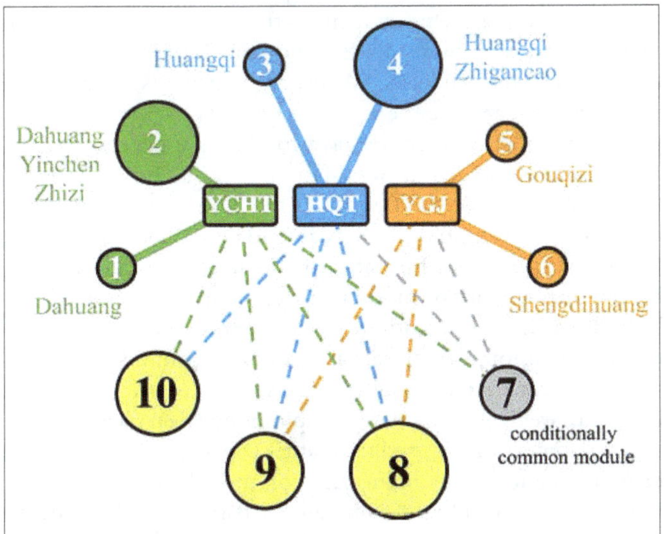

FIGURE 2 | Common and unique functional modules between the three formulae. Each cycle represents a functional module, and the size of each cycle is correlated to the number of genes in each module. Modules 8, 9, and 10 are illustrated as common module, while module 7 is meant as conditional common module. Herbs are labelled as well indicating that their ingredients can target unique module.

Meanwhile, each formula can significantly target two unique modules as illustrated in **Figure 2**. YCHT can significantly target modules 1 and 2. Module 1 is specifically involved with immune response of lectin induced complement pathway, where Dahuang herb can uniquely interact with it. Module 2 is related to leukocyte trans-endothelial migration and cell membrane interaction or adhesion, where all herbs in YCHT can target this module. HQT compounds can interact with CDK-mediated phosphorylation and removal of Cdc6, together with ATP binding in LKB1 signaling events (modules 3 and 4). Most interestingly, YGJ ingredients can directly and uniquely target the ATP synthesis (Kamanna et al., 2013) and neurotransmitter release cycle (modules 5 and 6), implying the potential modulation of ATP energy and neuron alertness.

Different Regulation Modes in the Same Functional Module

It is noted that, despite the unique modules for different formulae, the majority of targets are still involving the same functional modules. We investigated the regulation modes of herbal ingredients in each formula on the same module and found that a substantial number of targets are differently regulated by different formulae. It's realized that the information of regulation modes on targets is highly precious, where only a few databases such as HIT collected the sparse evidences. Details of regulation modes on three consensus modules can be found in **Table 2**.

For the module of DNA Damage and Oxidative Stress (Module 8), we can see that YCHT and YGJ ingredients can activate the antioxidant-related genes SOD families, while HQT compounds inhibit SOD1 genes. This actually agrees well with previous literature results for HQT (Wang et al., 2008). On Module 9 of NFAT and Cardiac Hypertrophy, YCHT ingredient can inhibit ESR1 target and HQT ingredient has inverse action, while YGJ shows mixed function. The 10th Module contains a list of inflammation factors. Generally, all formulae inhibit a wide range of pro-inflammation factors, such as IL1, IL2, IL4, IL5, etc.

Previous studies have shown that YCHT can regulate Kupffer cells; inhibit the release of proinflammatory cytokines, such as TNF-α, IL-1β, and IL-6; and promote the release of anti-inflammatory and anti-fibrogenic factors, IFN-γ and IL-10 (Zhang et al., 2013). Palmitic acid contained in herb Zhizi can inhibit the cytokines involved in various inflammatory processes as an antagonist of CASP1 (Xu et al., 2016). Further, the active ingredients in YCHT, such as salicylic acid, rottlerin, and garlic acid can also reduce the expression of NOS2, TNF, and RELA, and then inhibit the inflammation (Hee Sun et al., 2008). Among the cytokines, IL10 is well known for its balanced function of inflammation-inhibition. On this particular gene of IL10, HQT shows negative effects, while YGT ingredients show positive effects. It is noted that only individual ingredients were

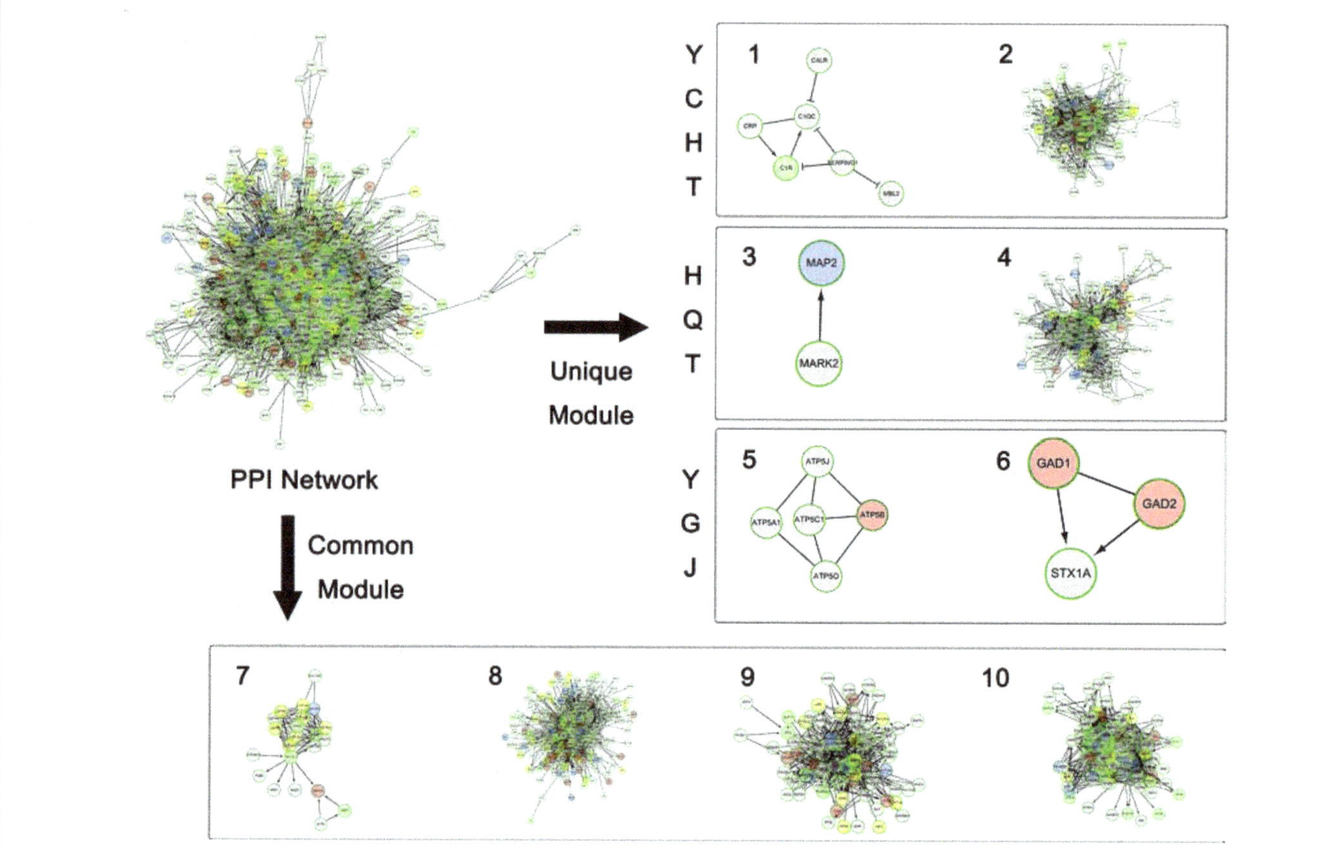

FIGURE 3 | The overall network modularization. Green nodes indicate unique targets of YCHT; blue nodes indicate unique targets of HQT; pink nodes indicate unique targets of YGJ; and yellow nodes indicate overlapping targets from 2 or 3 formulae.

reported with activating/inhibiting effect on molecular targets; the final *in vivo* effects may depend on the relative content and bioavailability of multiple ingredients in formula.

DISCUSSION

Highly personalized prescriptions of different formulae are frequently applied to treat one same disease in different states. Comparing the MOA similarities and differences between formulae for same disease will provide us a good opportunity to study the pathogenesis of disease subtypes. However, as shown in this study, the commonly simple adoption of KEGG or GO annotation often gives more similarities than differences because the pathway maps or GO terms have been strictly predefined while they are actually densely cross-talked. We thus set up a computational framework of comparative network pharmacology for this purpose and illustrated an example to reveal MOA details of 3 herbal recipes for CLD disease.

In applying this framework to other formulae, there are some suggestions to get better understanding of the method. First, instead of the predicted targets, we strongly support to collect those clearly validated ingredients and targets with regulation modes. One reason is that the prediction error may expand and mess up the modularization part during the subsequent analysis. Another reason is, regulation modes are normally deficient in the results of computational prediction. That is why we have to abandon several elegant TCM databases, such as SymMap (Wu et al., 2018), TCMSP (Ru et al., 2014), or YaTCM (Li et al., 2018). Secondly, other databases or household PPI list can also be adopted to generate PPI network if the information in Reactome is not enough. Lastly, the statistics of module enrichment is elaborated here by comparing with a randomly picked module with equal size of targeting groups in disease network background.

The comparative analysis finds the MOA difference correlates well with the Zheng symptoms between the formulae. As we know, YCHT is used to treat CLD patients with jaundice or inflammation. The unique function module of YCHT is just related to lectin-induced complement pathway and leukocyte trans-endothelial migration, which might mobilize extra anti-inflammation factors to deal with "damp-heat" symptoms. Another interesting finding here is that YGJ can directly target ATP synthesis and neurotransmitter release, which may promote ATP supply and increase the alertness of neuro systems.

TABLE 2 | Different regulation modes of different formulae on the same functional module. Information of regulation modes is collected from HIT database (Ye et al., 2011).

8	YCHT	da huang	rottlerin	Activate	SOD3	P08294
		yin chen	salicylic acid	Activate	SOD1	P00441
	HQT	huang qi	acetic acid	Inhibit	SOD1	P00441
		huang qi	lupeol	Inhibit	SOD1	P00441
	YGJ	chuan lian zi	oleic acid	Activate	SOD1	P00441
		dang gui	z-ligustilide	Activate	SOD1	P00441
9	YCHT	da huang	emodin	Inhibit	ESR1	P03372
	HQT	huang qi	lupeol	Activate	ESR1	P03372
	YGJ	bei sha shen	apigenin	Inhibit	ESR1	P03372
		bei sha shen	psoralen	Activate	ESR1	P03372
10	YCHT	da huang	emodin	Activate	IL1B	P01584
		da huang	emodin	Inhibit	IL1B	P01584
		da huang	rottlerin	Inhibit	IL6	P05231
		yin chen	salicylic acid	Inhibit	IL4	P05112
	HQT	huang qi	acetic acid	Inhibit	IL10	P22301
		huang qi	saikosaponin-d	Inhibit	IL6	P05231
	YGJ	bei sha shen	apigenin	Inhibit	IL4	P05112
		bei sha shen	apigenin	Inhibit	IL13	P35225
		bei sha shen	apigenin	Inhibit	IL2	P60568
		bei sha shen	lauric acid	Activate	IL6	P05231
		bei sha shen	methyl palmitate	Activate	IL10	P22301
		bei sha shen	methyl palmitate	Activate	IL6	P05231
		bei sha shen	methyl palmitate	Inhibit	IL10	P22301
		bei sha shen	sesamol	Activate	IL10	P22301
		bei sha shen	styrene	Inhibit	IL4	P05112
		bei sha shen	styrene	Activate	IL4	P05112
		bei sha shen	styrene	Activate	IL5	P05113
		bei sha shen	styrene	Activate	IL13	P35225
		chuan lian zi	ginkgolide b	Inhibit	IL1B	P01584
		dang gui	palmitic acid	Activate	IL10	P22301
		sheng di huang	gamma-aminobutyric acid	Inhibit	IL6	P05231

In our previous study, YGJ was found with ability to modulate the abnormal energy metabolism (Yan et al., 2017). This unique MOA of YGJ agrees well with its clinical application to treat "Yin deficiency" patients with extreme fatigue and weakness.

Yet, most of the time, disease subtypes of TCM Zheng are classified by highly summarized concepts of tongue color, pulse feeling, and personal overall phenotypes. While the Zheng research is still at beginning stage, our comparison framework from formula's perspective may provide alternative views to study their material basis. In addition to above, more consistent evidence may be proposed in future with both the progress in herbal target information and the TCM Zheng study.

Lastly, interaction between compounds and protein targets plays an important role in modulating the biological process and activity. We collected only those compounds with target information and activity evidence for network analysis. Yet, what ingredients are actually pharmacologically active deserves further investigation for these formulae. Correspondingly, perturbation tests are necessary to reach consensus conclusion. In fact, the list of active compounds may be affected by multiple factors such as the quantities in herbs, herb dosage, conjugated forms, compound interactions, biotransformation, dietary usage, bioavailability, other ADME issues (Dabeek and Marra, 2019).

To summarize, the comparative network pharmacology can detect a list of functional modules inferring the potential mechanisms of different formulae and provide functional insights for the subsequent exploration for not only formulae, but also disease subtyping. It's aware that all the information in the framework is collected from public database. Thus, the analysis results may be influenced by the abundancy and accuracy of related information. In the future, with more herbal experimental evidences accumulated, MOA comparison between different formulae is expected to be refreshed quantitatively and highlighted.

ETHICS STATEMENT

The experimental procedures involving the use of animals were approved by the Committee on the Use of Live Animals for Teaching and Research of the Shanghai University of Traditional Chinese Medicine and all experiments were performed in accordance with the guidelines of this committee.

AUTHOR CONTRIBUTIONS

ZKC conducted the project and wrote the manuscript. YL and YW finished the experimental verification. XW, KT, and DW collected the data and interpreted the results. WZ modified the manuscript. YM, PL, and ZWC designed and supervised the project. All authors read, critically reviewed, and approved the final manuscript.

FUNDING

This work was supported in part by National Key R&D Program of China (grant number 2017YFC1700200 and 2017YFC0908400), the National Natural Science Foundation of China (31671379, 81573873, 81774196).

SUPPLEMENTARY MATERIAL

SUPPLEMENTARY TABLE 1 | The detailed results of targets and ingredients.

SUPPLEMENTARY TABLE 2 | The detailed results of Enrichment in KEGG and GO.

SUPPLEMENTARY TABLE 3 | The detailed results of the everted intestinal sacs experiment.

REFERENCES

Ashburner, M., Ball, C. A., Blake, J. A., Botstein, D., Butler, H., Cherry, J. M., et al. (2000). Gene ontology: tool for the unification of biology. The gene ontology Consortium. *Nat. Genet.* 25 (1), 25–29. doi: 10.1038/75556

Barve, A., Chen, C., Hebbar, V., Desiderio, J., Saw, C. L., and Kong, A. N. (2009). Metabolism, oral bioavailability and pharmacokinetics of chemopreventive kaempferol in rats. *Biopharm. Drug Dispos.* 30 (7), 356–365. doi: 10.1002/bdd.677

Cai, F. F., Wu, R., Song, Y. N., Xiong, A. Z., Chen, X. L., Yang, M. D., et al. (2018). Yinchenhao decoction alleviates liver fibrosis by regulating bile acid metabolism and TGF-beta/Smad/ERK signalling pathway. *Sci. Rep.* 8 (1), 15367. doi: 10.1038/s41598-018-33669-4

Cai, F. F., Bian, Y. Q., Wu, R., Sun, Y., Chen, X. L., Yang, M. D., et al. (2019). Yinchenhao decoction suppresses rat liver fibrosis involved in an apoptosis regulation mechanism based on network pharmacology and transcriptomic analysis. *BioMed. Pharmacother.* 114, 108863. doi: 10.1016/j.biopha.2019.108863

Chen, G., Huang, C., Lu, J., Huang, R., Zhang, J., Chen, Z., et al. (2019). Efficacy and safety of Yinchen Sini decoction in treating biliary atresia patients after Kasai portoenterostomy: a systematic review and meta-analysis protocol. *Med. (Baltimore)* 98 (2), e13935. doi: 10.1097/MD.0000000000013935

Chen, C. Y. (2011). TCM Database@Taiwan: the world's largest traditional Chinese medicine database for drug screening in silico. *PloS One* 6 (1), e15939. doi: 10.1371/journal.pone.0015939

Comporti, M., Arezzini, B., Signorini, C., Vecchio, D., and Gardi, C. (2009). Oxidative stress, isoprostanes and hepatic fibrosis. *Histol. Histopathol.* 24 (7), 893–900. doi: 10.14670/HH-24.893

Croft, D., Mundo, A. F., Haw, R., Milacic, M., Weiser, J., Wu, G., et al. (2014). The Reactome pathway knowledgebase. *Nucleic Acids Res.* 42 (Database issue), D472–D477. doi: 10.1093/nar/gkt1102

Dabeek, W. M., and Marra, M. V. (2019). Dietary Quercetin and Kaempferol: bioavailability and potential cardiovascular-related bioactivity in humans. *Nutrients* 11 (10), 2288. doi: 10.3390/nu11102288

Du, J. X., Sun, M. Y., Du, G. L., Li, F. H., Liu, C., Mu, Y. P., et al. (2012). Ingredients of Huangqi decoction slow biliary fibrosis progression by inhibiting the activation of the transforming growth factor-beta signaling pathway. *BMC Complement. Altern. Med.* 12, 33. doi: 10.1186/1472-6882-12-33

Gressley, T. F., Davison, K. A., Macies, J., Leonardi, C., McCarthy, M. M., Nemec, L. M., et al. (2016). Effect of abomasal carbohydrates and live yeast on measures of postruminal fermentation. *J. Anim. Sci.* 94 (1), 284–296. doi: 10.2527/jas.2015-9324

Hee Sun, B., Minho, W., Kyeong Ah, P., Young-Rae, K., Byung Lyul, C., Hyunji, L., et al. (2008). Prevention of TNF-induced necrotic cell death by rottlerin through a Nox1 NADPH oxidase. *Exp. Mol. Med.* 40 (2), 186. doi: 10.3858/emm.2008.40.2.186

Huang, L., Xie, D., Yu, Y., Liu, H., Shi, Y., Shi, T., et al. (2018). TCMID 2.0: a comprehensive resource for TCM. *Nucleic Acids Res.* 46 (D1), D1117–D1120. doi: 10.1093/nar/gkx1028

Kamanna, V. S., Ganji, S. H., and Kashyap, M. L. (2013). Recent advances in niacin and lipid metabolism. *Curr. Opin. In Lipidol.* 24 (3), 239–245. doi: 10.1097/MOL.0b013e3283613a68

Kanehisa, M. (2002). The KEGG database. *Novartis Found Symp.* 247, 91–101. doi: 10.1002/0470857897.ch8

Li, B., Ma, C., Zhao, X., Hu, Z., Du, T., Xu, X., et al. (2018). YaTCM: yet another traditional Chinese medicine database for drug discovery. *Comput. Struct. Biotechnol. J.* 16, 600–610. doi: 10.1016/j.csbj.2018.11.002

Li, W. K., Wang, G. F., Wang, T. M., Li, Y. Y., Li, Y. F., Lu, X. Y., et al. (2019). Protective effect of herbal medicine Huangqi decoction against chronic cholestatic liver injury by inhibiting bile acid-stimulated inflammation in DDC-induced mice. *Phytomedicine* 62, 152948. doi: 10.1016/j.phymed.2019.152948

Liu, C., Wang, G., Chen, G., Mu, Y., Zhang, L., Hu, X., et al. (2012). Huangqi decoction inhibits apoptosis and fibrosis, but promotes Kupffer cell activation in dimethylnitrosamine-induced rat liver fibrosis. *BMC Complement. Altern. Med.* 12, 51. doi: 10.1186/1472-6882-12-51

Mi, H., Huang, X., Muruganujan, A., Tang, H., Mills, C., Kang, D., et al. (2017). PANTHER version 11: expanded annotation data from Gene ontology and reactome pathways, and data analysis tool enhancements. *Nucleic Acids Res.* 45 (D1), D183–D189. doi: 10.1093/nar/gkw1138

Peng, H., He, Y., Zheng, G., Zhang, W., Yao, Z., and Xie, W. (2016). Meta-analysis of traditional herbal medicine in the treatment of nonalcoholic fatty liver disease. *Cell Mol. Biol. (Noisy-le-grand)* 62 (4), 88–95. doi: 10.14715/cmb/2016.62.4.16

Ru, J., Li, P., Wang, J., Zhou, W., Li, B., Huang, C., et al. (2014). TCMSP: a database of systems pharmacology for drug discovery from herbal medicines. *J. Cheminform.* 6, 13. doi: 10.1186/1758-2946-6-13

Safran, M., Dalah, I., Alexander, J., Rosen, N., Iny Stein, T., Shmoish, M., et al. (2010). GeneCards Version 3: the human gene integrator. *Database (Oxford)* 2010, baq020. doi: 10.1093/database/baq020

Shahzad, M., Shabbir, A., Wojcikowski, K., Wohlmuth, H., and Gobe, G. C. (2016). The antioxidant effects of Radix Astragali (Astragalus membranaceus and related species) in protecting tissues from injury and disease. *Curr. Drug Targets* 17 (12), 1331–1340. doi: 10.2174/1389450116666150907104742

Shannon, P., Markiel, A., Ozier, O., Baliga, N. S., Wang, J. T., Ramage, D., et al. (2003). Cytoscape: a software environment for integrated models of biomolecular interaction networks. *Genome Res.* 13 (11), 2498–2504. doi: 10.1101/gr.1239303

Song, Y. N., Zhang, G. B., Lu, Y. Y., Chen, Q. L., Yang, L., Wang, Z. T., et al. (2016). Huangqi decoction alleviates dimethylnitrosamine-induced liver fibrosis: an analysis of bile acids metabolic mechanism. *J. Ethnopharmacol.* 189, 148–156. doi: 10.1016/j.jep.2016.05.040

Sun, H., Zhang, A. H., Yang, L., Li, M. X., Fang, H., Xie, J., et al. (2019). High-throughput chinmedomics strategy for discovering the quality-markers and potential targets for Yinchenhao decoction. *Phytomedicine* 54, 328–338. doi: 10.1016/j.phymed.2018.04.015

Tao, Q., Sun, M. Y., and Feng, Q. (2009). Syndrome identification of CCl4 induced liver fibrosis model rats based on syndrome detecting from recipe used. *Chin. J. Integr. Tradit. Western Med.* 29 (3), 246–250. doi: CNKI:SUN:ZZXJ.0.2009-03-020

The Gene Ontology, C. (2017). Expansion of the Gene Ontology knowledgebase and resources. *Nucleic Acids Res.* 45 (D1), D331–D338. doi: 10.1093/nar/gkw1108

Tian, M., Liu, W., You, H., Zhao, Q., Ouyang, L., Gao, B., et al. (2016). Protective effect of Yiguanjian decoction against DNA damage on concanavalin A-induced liver injury mice model. *J. Tradit. Chin. Med.* 36 (4), 471–478. doi: 10.1016/s0254-6272(16)30064-4

Vuppalanchi, R., Juluri, R., Bell, L. N., Ghabril, M., Kamendulis, L., Klaunig, J. E., et al. (2011). Oxidative stress in chronic liver disease: relationship between peripheral and hepatic measurements. *Am. J. Med. Sci.* 342 (4), 314–317. doi: 10.1097/MAJ.0b013e31821d9905

Wang, L., Liu, P., and Wang, C. S. (2008). Effects of 5 classical recipes on anti-oxidative stress in rat liver with cirrhosis. *Zhongguo Zhong Xi Yi Jie He Za Zhi* 28 (5), 435. doi: CNKI:SUN:ZZXJ.0.2008-05-023

Wang, X., Xie, G., Wang, X., Zhou, M., Yu, H., Lin, Y., et al. (2015). Urinary metabolite profiling offers potential for differentiation of liver-kidney yin deficiency and dampness-heat internal smoldering syndromes in posthepatitis B cirrhosis patients. *Evid Based Complement. Alternat. Med.* 2015, 464969. doi: 10.1155/2015/464969

Wu, G., and Haw, R. (2017). Functional interaction network construction and analysis for disease discovery. *Methods Mol. Biol.* 1558, 235–253. doi: 10.1007/978-1-4939-6783-4_11

Wu, J. S., Li, Y. F., Li, Y. Y., Dai, Y., Li, W. K., Zheng, M., et al. (2017). Huangqi decoction alleviates Alpha-Naphthylisothiocyanate induced intrahepatic cholestasis by reversing disordered bile acid and glutathione homeostasis in mice. *Front. Pharmacol.* 8, 938. doi: 10.3389/fphar.2017.00938

Wu, Y., Zhang, F., Yang, K., Fang, S., Bu, D., Li, H., et al. (2018). SymMap: an integrative database of traditional Chinese medicine enhanced by symptom mapping. *Nucleic Acids Res.* 47 (D1), D1110–D1117. doi: 10.1093/nar/gky1021

Xu, W., Guo, Y. B., Li, X., He, M. R., and Liu, S. D. (2016). [Palmitic acid induces hepatocellular oxidative stress and activation of inflammasomes]. *Nan Fang Yi Ke Da Xue Xue Bao* 36 (5), 655–659. doi: 10.3969/j.issn.1673-4254.2016.05.11

Xu, Y., Fan, W. W., Xu, W., Jiang, S. L., Chen, G. F., Liu, C., et al. (2018). Yiguanjian decoction enhances fetal liver stem/progenitor cell-mediated repair of liver cirrhosis through regulation of macrophage activation state. *World J. Gastroenterol.* 24 (42), 4759–4772. doi: 10.3748/wjg.v24.i42.4759

Xu-Dong, H. U., Ting-Jie, Y. E., Wang, X. L., Bo-Qin, L. I., Liu, P., and Biology, D. O. (2014). The prevention and treatment effect of Yin-chen-hao decoction on Concanavalin A-induced acute mice hepatitis by inhibiting the activation of Kupffer cells. *Lishizhen Med. Materia Med. Res.* 25 (06), 1340-1343. doi: 10.3969/j.issn.1008-0805.2014.06.022

Yan, D., Ma, B., Shi, R., Wang, T., and Ma, Y. (2015). Involvement of herb-herb interactions in the influences of Radix Scutellaria and Coptis Chinensis on the bioavailability of the anthraquinones form Rhei Rhizoma in rats. *Eur. J. Drug Metab. Pharmacokinet.* 40 (1), 103–110. doi: 10.1007/s13318-014-0188-7

Yan, J., Xie, G., Liang, C., Hu, Y., Zhao, A., Huang, F., et al. (2017). Herbal medicine Yinchenhaotang protects against α-naphthylisothiocyanate-induced cholestasis in rats. *Sci. Rep.* 7 (1), 4211. doi: 10.1038/s41598-017-04536-5

Ye, H., Ye, L., Kang, H., Zhang, D., Tao, L., Tang, K., et al. (2011). HIT: linking herbal active ingredients to targets. *Nucleic Acids Res.* 39 (Database issue), D1055–D1059. doi: 10.1093/nar/gkq1165

Zeng, J. K., Li, Y. Y., Wang, T. M., Zhong, J., Wu, J. S., Liu, P., et al. (2018a). Simultaneous quantification of multiple components in rat plasma by UPLC-MS/MS and pharmacokinetic study after oral administration of Huangqi decoction. *BioMed. Chromatogr.* 32 (5), e4178. doi: 10.1002/bmc.4178

Zeng, X., Zhang, P., He, W., Qin, C., Chen, S., Tao, L., et al. (2018b). NPASS: natural product activity and species source database for natural product research, discovery and tool development. *Nucleic Acids Res.* 46 (D1), D1217–D1222. doi: 10.1093/nar/gkx1026

Zhang, Y. Q., Tang, X. D., Wang, F. Y., Yang, B., Liu, Y. L., Guo, P., et al. (2013). [Effect of ronggan mixture on immunoregulation and hepatocyte apoptosis-related factors in concanavalin A induced acute immunological liver injury mice]. *Zhongguo Zhong Xi Yi Jie He Za Zhi* 33 (11), 1500–1506. doi: 10.7661/CJIM.2013.11.1500

Zhang, G. B., Song, Y. N., Chen, Q. L., Dong, S., Lu, Y. Y., Su, M. Y., et al. (2015). Actions of Huangqi decoction against rat liver fibrosis: a gene expression profiling analysis. *Chin. Med.* 10, 39. doi: 10.1186/s13020-015-0066-5

Zhou, Y. N., Mu, Y. P., Fu, W. W., Ning, B. B., Du, G. L., Chen, J. M., et al. (2015). Yiguanjian decoction and its ingredients inhibit angiogenesis in carbon tetrachloride-induced cirrhosis mice. *BMC Complement. Altern. Med.* 15, 342. doi: 10.1186/s12906-015-0862-6

16

Investigation of the Multi-Target Mechanism of Guanxin-Shutong Capsule in Cerebrovascular Diseases: A Systems Pharmacology and Experimental Assessment

Juanli Zhang[1,2†], Jiaxin Zhao[1†], Yang Ma[1†], Wenjun Wang[1†], Shaojie Huang[1], Chao Guo[1], Kai Wang[1], Xiaomei Zhang[3], Wei Zhang[1], Aidong Wen[1], Ming Shi[2*] and Yi Ding[1*]*

[1]Department of Pharmacy, Xijing Hospital, Fourth Military Medical University, Xi'an, China, [2]Department of Neurology, Xijing Hospital, Fourth Military Medical University, Xi'an, China, [3]Basic Medical School, Yunnan University of Traditional Chinese Medicine, Kunming, China

***Correspondence:**
Aidong Wen
adwen-2004@hotmail.com
Ming Shi
biomidas@163.com
Yi Ding
dingyi.007@163.com

†These authors have contributed equally to this work

Guanxin-Shutong capsule (GXSTC), a combination of Mongolian medicines and traditional herbs, has been clinically proven to be effective in treating cerebrovascular diseases (CBVDs). However, the underlying pharmacological mechanisms of GXSTC in CBVDs remain largely unknown. In this study, a combination of systems pharmacology and experimental assessment approach was used to investigate the bioactive components, core targets, and possible mechanisms of GXSTC in the treatment of CBVDs. A total of 15 main components within GXSTC were identified using high-performance liquid chromatography coupled with diode array detector (HPLC-DAD) and a literature research. Fifty-five common genes were obtained by matching 252 potential genes of GXSTC with 462 CBVD-related genes. Seven core components in GXSTC and 12 core genes of GXSTC on CBVDs were further determined using the protein-protein interaction (PPI) and component-target-pathway (C-T-P) network analysis. Gene Ontology (GO) and Kyoto Encyclopedia of Genes and Genomes (KEGG) pathway enrichment analysis results predicted that the molecular mechanisms of GXSTC on CBVDs were mainly associated with the regulation of the vascular endothelial function, inflammatory response, and neuronal apoptosis. Molecular docking results suggested that almost all of core component-targets have an excellent binding activity (affinity < -5 kcal/mol). More importantly, in middle cerebral artery occlusion (MCAO) -injured rats, GXSTC significantly improved the neurological function, reduced the infarct volume, and decreased the percentage of impaired neurons in a dose-dependent manner. Western blotting results indicated that GXSTC markedly upregulated the expression of vascular endothelial growth factor A (VEGFA) and endothelial nitric oxide synthase (eNOS), while downregulating the expression of cyclooxygenase-2 (COX-2) and transcription factor AP-1 (c-Jun) in MCAO-injured rats. These findings confirmed our prediction that GXSTC exerts a multi-target synergetic mechanism in CBVDs by maintaining vascular endothelial function, inhibiting neuronal apoptosis and inflammatory processes. The results of this study may provide a theoretical basis for GXSTC research and the clinical application of GXSTC in CBVDs.

Keywords: guanxin-shutong capsule, multi-target mechanism, cerebrovascular diseases, systems pharmacology, experimental assessment

INTRODUCTION

Cerebrovascular diseases, characterized by stroke and other forms of neurological dysfunction and degeneration, are among the most common causes of morbidity and mortality worldwide, seriously affecting human health and life (Collaborators., G.B.D.N., 2019). Until now, intravenous thrombolysis with recombinant tissue plasminogen activator (rt-PA) has been the main treatment option for acute CBVDs. However, owing to the limited therapeutic window (<4.5 h after symptom onset) and the hemorrhagic complications induced by rt-PA, only a small number of stroke patients can benefit from this treatment (Hankey, 2017). In addition, most neuroprotective drugs have been demonstrated to be effective in animal experimental studies but their effectiveness could not be demonstrated in clinical trials (Zhou et al., 2018). Therefore, there is a pressing need to develop safer and more effective drugs for CBVDs.

Traditional Chinese medicine (TCM) has been used for thousands of years to prevent and treat CBVDs. Guanxin-Shutong capsule, a combination of Mongolian medicines and traditional herbs, has been commonly used to treat angina pectoris and coronary heart diseases in China (Li et al., 2019); it consists of *Choerospondias axillaris* (Roxb.) B.L.Burtt and A.W.Hill [*Anacardiaceae; Choerospondiatis fructus*], *Salvia miltiorrhiza Bunge* [*Lamiaceae; Radix Salviae miltiorrhizae*], *Syzigium aromaticum* (L.) Merr. and L.M.Perry [Myrtaceae; *Caryophylli flos*], *Dryobalanops aromatica* C.F.Gaertn [Dipterocarpaceae; *Bomeolum*], and *Bambusa textilis* McClure [Poaceae; *Concretio silicea bambusae*] (Rivera et al., 2014) at a weight ratio of 16:8:2:1:1 by weight. The major active components of GXSTC include phenolic acids, tanshinones, saponins, and others (Gao et al., 2017). In recent years, several clinical trials have further demonstrated that GXSTC has a significant clinical effect in treating ischemic stroke, and could markedly improve the nerve function of stroke patients (Wu, 2015; Shao, 2018). However, the effective components and potential mechanisms of action of GXSTC against CBVDs remain unclear.

Systems pharmacology is an effective tool for drug-target analysis with the advantages of a low cost, short cycle, and providing more comprehensive information. Moreover, it has gradually promoted the paradigm shift from the "one-target, one-drug" mode to a "network-targets, multiple-components" approach in drug discovery (Kibble et al., 2015; Zhang et al., 2019). Coincidentally, the holistic strategy of systems pharmacology is in accordance with the combinatorial therapeutic strategies of TCM. Therefore, it has been widely used to investigate the complex pharmacological mechanisms of TCM (Yuan et al., 2017). Several studies have successfully revealed the mystery of TCM formulae for treating CBVDs based on systems pharmacology, such as Danhong injections (Wei et al., 2016), Shuxuening injections (Cui et al., 2020), and Naoxintong capsules (Xu et al., 2016).

In this study, the mechanisms of action of GXSTC on CBVDs were investigated by combining systems pharmacology and experimental assessment. The detailed workflow is shown in **Figure 1**. First, the main components of GXSTC were identified by using HPLC-DAD to determine standard samples. The potential targets of these components and therapeutic targets related to CBVDs were collected from multiple databases. Subsequently, 55 common targets were identified by matching the potential targets of GXSTC with the CBVD-related targets. On this basis, network construction and enrichment analysis were performed to systematically investigate the underlying interactions between bioactive components, key targets, and pathways. The interactions between the core components and the corresponding core targets were evaluated using molecular docking. Finally, an animal model of ischemic stroke was used to investigate the molecular mechanism of GXSTC in CBVDs.

MATERIALS AND METHODS

Chemicals and Materials

GXSTC was supplied by Buchang Pharmaceuticals (Xianyang, China). The reference standards of gallic acid, ellagic acid, tanshinone IIA, cryptotanshinone, protocatechuic acid, and eugenol were obtained from the National Institute for the Control of Pharmaceutical and Biological Products (Beijing, China). The reference standards of danshensu, 5-hydroxymethylfurfural, protocatechualdehyde, rosmarinic acid, salvianolic acid A, salvianolic acid B, tanshinone I, and dihydrotanshinone I were purchased from Baoji Chenguang Biotechnology Co. Ltd. Deionized water was purified by a Milli-Q water purification system (Millipore, MA, United States). Acetonitrile and methanol (HPLC-grade) were purchased from Fisher Scientific (Fair Lawn, NJ, United States). 2,3,5-triphenyltetrazolium chloride (TTC, purity > 98.0%) was obtained from Sigma-Aldrich (St. Louis, MO). A bicinchoninic acid (BCA) protein assay kit and a sodium dodecyl sulfate polyacrylamide gel electrophoresis (SDS-PAGE) kit were bought from Dingguo Changsheng Biotechnology (Beijing, China). The running buffer (pH: 8.4–8.6), transfer buffer (pH: 8.4), and Tris-buffered saline (TBS) were purchased from Servicebio (Wuhan, China). Anti-VEGFA (ab46154) were bought from Abcam (Cambridge, MA, United States). Anti-β-actin (13E5) and anti-c-Jun (60A8) rabbit mAbs were bought from Cell Signaling Technology (CST, Beverly, MA, United States of America). Anti-eNOS (GB11086) and anti-COX2 (GB11077-2) rabbit polyclonal antibodies were obtained from Servicebio. HRP-conjugated AffiniPure goat anti-rabbit IgG (H + L, SA00001-2) was purchased from ProteinTech Group (Chicago, IL, United States). Anti-β-tubulin and other reagents were supplied by other Chinese suppliers.

Determination of the Main Components of GXSTC

The GXSTC powder (0.5 g), and a mixture of 14 reference standards were dissolved in 50 ml methanol, respectively. After sonication for 30 min, the samples were filtered through 0.22 μm

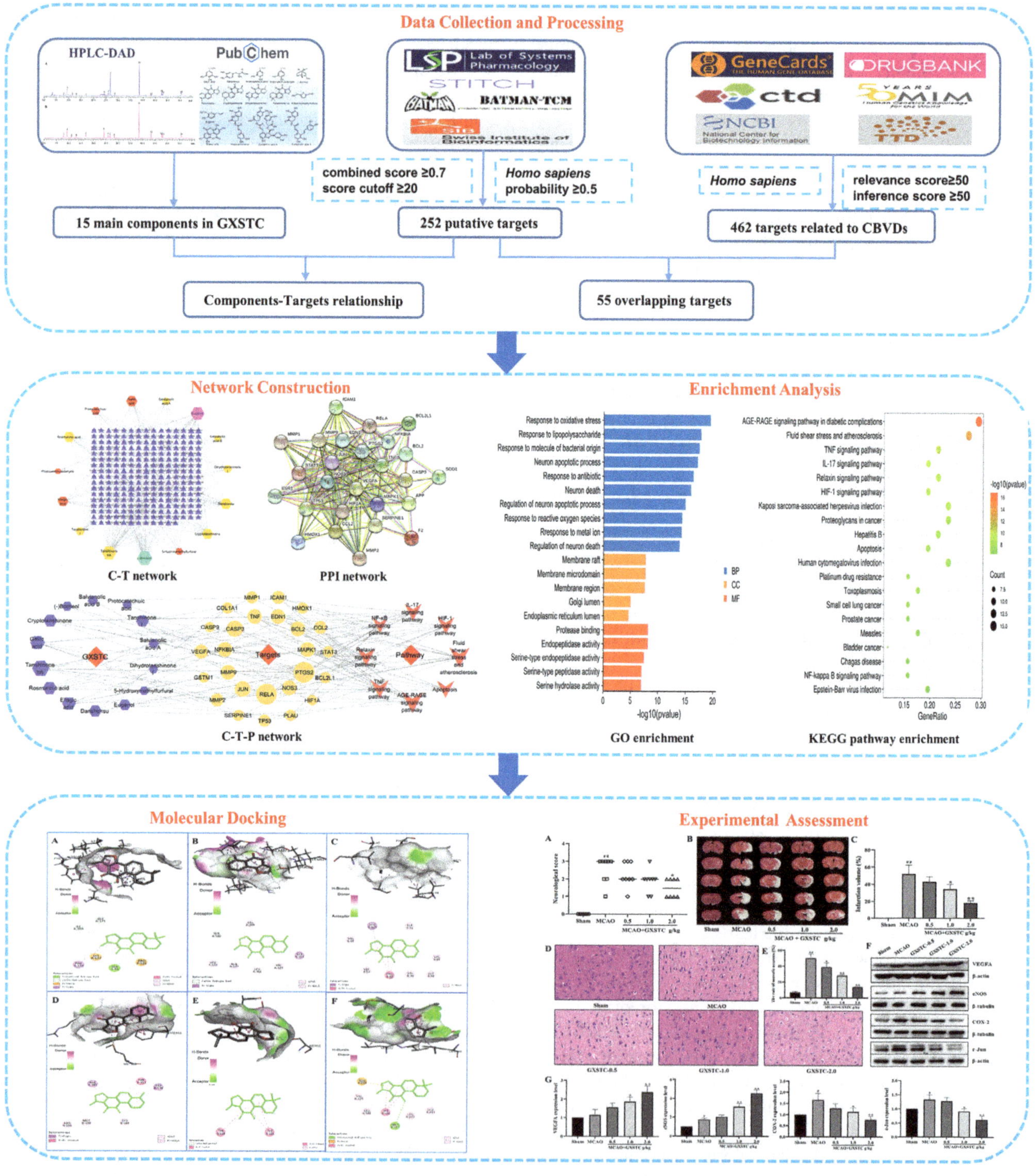

FIGURE 1 | Workflow of systems pharmacology analysis and experimental assessment.

syringe filter, and 20 μL filtrate was injected into the HPLC-DAD system for analysis. HPLC analysis of GXSTC was performed by LC-20AT HPLC system (Shimadzu, Kyoto, Japan) with an Agilent TC-C_{18} column (4.6 × 250 mm, 5 μm). The mobile phase was composed of solvent A (acetonitrile) and solvent B (water containing 0.05% phosphoric acid) and the gradient procedure was set as follows: 0–15 min, 5–20% A; 15–18 min, 20–34% A; 18–30 min, 34–40% A; 30–35 min, 40–50% A; 35–40 min, 50–65% A; 40–60 min, 65–75% A; the UV detection wavelength was set at 274 nm.

Target Prediction of GXSTC Components

First, we obtained the molecular structures and canonical SMILES codes of all the components from PubChem (https://pubchem.ncbi.nlm.nih.gov/) (Kim et al., 2019). Next, the targets related to these components were collected by using TCMSP (http://tcmspw.com/tcmsp.php, ver. 2.3) (Ru et al., 2014), BATMAN-TCM (http://bionet.ncpsb.org/batman-tcm/, ver. 2016) (Liu et al., 2016), STITCH (http://stitch.embl.de/, ver. 5.18) (Kuhn et al., 2008), and Swiss Target Prediction (http://www.swisstargetprediction.ch/, ver. 2019) (Daina et al., 2019) databases with the species limited to "*Homo sapiens*". In these databases, the predicted interactions between components and targets were attributed to "score cutoff," "combined score," or "probability" with a higher score indicating a stronger interaction. In the present study, only the targets with a score cutoff ≥20 in BATMAN-TCM, a combined score ≥0.7 in STITCH, and a probability ≥0.5 in Swiss Target Prediction databases were selected.

Candidate Target Collection of CBVDs

The targets related to CBVDs were acquired from six databases, which aimed to shed light on the relationship between targets and diseases from different perspectives. "cerebrovascular diseases" or "cerebrovascular" was used as a keyword to search the OMIM (http://omim.org/) (Amberger and Hamosh, 2017), GeneCards (https://www.genecards.org/) (Stelzer et al., 2016), NCBI Gene (https://www.ncbi.nlm.nih.gov/gene/) (Brown et al., 2015), TTD (http://bidd.nus.edu.sg/group/cjttd/) (Wang et al., 2020), and Drugbank (https://www.drugbank.ca) (Wishart et al., 2006) databases. "Cerebrovascular disorders" was used as a keyword to search the CTD (http://ctdbase.org/) (Davis et al., 2019). To ensure the reliability of target prediction, we only chose the targets with a relevance score ≥50 in GeneCards and an inference score ≥50 in the CTD database, respectively. Finally, all the protein names were standardized into official gene symbols and IDs using UniProtKB (https://www.uniprot.org/) (Bateman et al., 2019) database by confining the species to "*Homo sapiens*." After removing the duplicate targets, the common targets related to CBVDs and the candidate components were identified as the candidate targets.

C-T and PPI Network Construction

To understand the complicated interactions between components and their corresponding targets, the component-target (C-T) network was established by using Cytoscape (https://cytoscape.org/, ver. 3.7.2) (Franz et al., 2016). In addition, the candidate targets were uploaded to the STRING database (https://string-db.org/, ver. 11.0) (Szklarczyk et al., 2019) to obtain the PPI data by confining the species to "*Homo sapiens*" and a high confidence score ≥0.7. The PPI data were obtained, and the PPI network was constructed through Cytoscape. Moreover, the degree values of nodes were calculated in the network, and the targets with a degree above their median were selected as key targets of the PPI network.

GO Functional and KEGG Pathway Enrichment Analysis

To investigate the potential molecular mechanisms of GXSTC on CBVDs, candidate targets were analyzed for GO functional and KEGG pathway enrichment analysis based on the "cluster profiler" and "org.Hs.eg.db packages" of the R project (https://www.r-project.org/, ver. 3.6.2) (Mair et al., 2015). The enrichment *p*-value was calculated, and a $p < 0.05$ was considered to be statistically significant. Finally, a component-target-pathway (C-T-P) network was constructed to investigate the reciprocity of the components, targets and pathways by using Cytoscape.

Molecular Docking Studies

To evaluate the reliability of the predicted interactions between the core components and their corresponding targets, molecular docking was performed by using AutoDock Vina 1.1.2 (Trott and Olson, 2010). First, the 3D structures of core components (ligands) were downloaded from PubChem and stored in a PDB file format, and then converted to MOL2 files by using ChemBioDraw Ultra 14.0. The crystal structures of the core targets were obtained from the RCSB Protein Data Bank (https://www.rcsb.org/) (Rose et al., 2017). Then, the components and target proteins for docking were prepared by using PyMOL 1.7.2.1, and they were saved as PDBQT files using AutoDockTools 1.5.6. Finally, a docking simulation was performed under AutoDock program, and the lower affinity score for the component-target was selected for further analysis. The action modes of the core components with their corresponding targets were analyzed and visualized by using Discovery Studio Visualizer.

Experimental Assessment

Experimental Design

Adult male Sprague-Dawley rats with a body weight of 250–280 g were supplied by the Experimental Animal Center of the Fourth Military Medical University. Rats were housed under controlled conditions with a 12 h light/dark cycle at 25 ± 2°C and 50 ± 10% humidity. The experimental protocols were approved by the Ethics Committee for Animal Experimentation of the Fourth Military Medical University and were performed according to the National Institutes of Health Guide for the Care and Use of Laboratory Animals. Rats were randomly divided into five groups ($n = 8$ in each group): sham, middle cerebral artery occlusion, and MCAO + GXSTC pretreatment (0.5, 1.0, and 2.0 g/kg per day). These doses were chosen based on the dosage of GXSTC in clinical practice (0.3 g/capsule, 3 capsules once, 3 times a day) (Li et al., 2019) and previous studies (0.5–2.0 g/kg in rats) (Zhuo et al., 2012; Zhu et al., 2020). Rats in the sham and MCAO groups were pretreated with 0.9% saline solution, and rats in the GXSTC groups were pretreated with GXSTC (0.5, 1.0, and 2.0 g/kg per day, respectively) via intragastric administration for 7 days. The rats were then anesthetized, and a MCAO was established as previously described (Guo et al., 2017). After 2.0 h of MCAO, the filament was withdrawn to allow reperfusion for 24 h. The sham group underwent the same surgical procedure except that the filament was not inserted into the internal carotid artery.

Neurological Deficit Score

After reperfusion, the neurological deficits were scored using a 5-point scale scoring system, as described previously (Longa et al., 1989). The detailed scoring criteria were as follows: 0, no deficit; 1, failure to fully extend the left forepaw; 2, circling to the left; 3, falling to the left; and 4, no spontaneous walking with a depressed level of consciousness.

Infarct Volume Assessment

After reperfusion, the rats were deeply anesthetized and decapitated. The brains were rapidly removed and stored on ice for 15 min. The brains were cut into 2 mm coronal slices, stained with 2% TTC solution for 30 min, and then fixed with 4% paraformaldehyde solution at 4°C overnight. After staining, the slices were arranged in groups and photographed, and the infarct volume of each slice was measured by using Image Pro Plus 6.0. To exclude the confounding effect of brain edema, the corrected infarct volumes were calculated through the following formula:

$$\text{Measured infarct volume} \times \left(1 - \frac{\text{ipsilateral hemisphere volume} - \text{contralateral hemisphere volume}}{\text{contralateral hemisphere}}\right)$$

Finally, the infarct volume (%) in each group was expressed as the percentage of contralateral hemispheric volume.

Histological Observation

To evaluate the histological damage, rats were deeply euthanized and sacrificed at 24 h after reperfusion. Subsequently, the brains were quickly removed and immediately immersed in 4% paraformaldehyde. After fixation for 24 h, the brain tissues were dehydrated, embedded in paraffin and cut into 5 μm coronal slides. Finally, the brain slides were stained with H&E, and the histopathological changes were observed by using light microscopy at a ×400 magnification.

Western Blot Analysis

After 24 h of reperfusion, the right brain tissues were pooled and homogenized via sonication in RIPA lysis buffer (Beyotime, China) containing protease and phosphatase inhibitors (Vazyme Biotech, Nanjing, China). The total protein concentration in each sample was measured by a BCA protein assay kit according to the manufacturer's instructions. Equal amounts of protein samples (30–60 μg per sample) were separated by using 8–10% SDS-PAGE gels and transferred to PVDF membranes. The membranes were blocked with 5% nonfat milk in TBS containing 0.1% TWEEN (TBST) at room temperature for 1 h, and then incubated with the following primary antibodies: anti-VEGFA (1:1,000), e-NOS (1: 500), c-Jun (1:1,000), COX-2 (1:1,000), β-actin (1:1,000), and β-tubulin (1:1,000) at 4°C overnight. Next, the membranes were rinsed in TBST for 10 min three times, and then incubated with HRP-labeled secondary antibody (goat anti-rabbit IgG, 1:10,000) for 1 h at room temperature. Finally, the blots were visualized by using an enhanced chemiluminescence method (Diyibio, Shanghai, China) and were analyzed using the ImageJ software (version 1.46r, National Institutes of Health, United States).

Statistical Analysis

Statistical analysis was performed using GraphPad Prism 8.0.1 for Windows. All data, except for the neurologic score values, were expressed as mean ± standard deviation. Statistical differences between the various groups were analyzed using one-way analysis of variance (ANOVA). Statistical significance was set at $p < 0.05$, and a significant statistical significance was set at $p < 0.01$.

RESULTS

HPLC Profile of GXSTC

A total of 14 main components in GXSTC were unambiguously identified by comparing the retention time with those of standard samples (**Figure 2**). Based on the TCMSP databases and on literature research, five components were primarily derived from *Choerospondiatis fructus*, eight components were primarily produced by *Radix Salviae miltiorrhizae*, and two components were derived from *Salviae miltiorrhizae*. However, only tanshinone IIA, salvianolic acid B, and borneol were used as marker components for the quality control of GXSTC in the Chinese Pharmacopeia. Among them, borneol was the most important constituent in *Bomeolum* and had a neuroprotective effect on cerebral ischemia, but it can hardly be detected by using HPLC. Therefore, borneol was also included as a candidate component for further analyses in this study. Detailed information and structures of these components are provided in **Supplementary Table S1**.

C-T Network Analysis

According to the predefined screening conditions, 252 targets related to the GXSTC components were collected (**Supplementary Table S2**). A visual C-T network with 267 nodes and 422 edges was established by using Cytoscape (**Figure 3**). The "degree" value of a node, is defined as the number of edges that connect to it in the network, representing the significance of the node in the network. Therefore, we calculated the degree value of all nodes in the C-T network, and eight components with degree values above the median value were identified, including borneol, eugenol, tanshinone IIA, danshensu, gallic acid, cryptotanshinone, rosmarinic acid, and ellagic acid.

PPI Network Analysis

A total of 462 CBVD-related targets were collected from six public databases (**Supplementary Table S3**). After marching the targets related to CBVDs with putative targets of GXSTC, 55 common targets were identified as candidate targets (**Supplementary Table S4**). Subsequently, the PPI network was constructed and visualized by using Cytoscape 3.7.2 (**Figure 4**). A network analyzer was performed, and the 26 genes with a degree above the median were identified as key genes in the PPI network (**Supplementary Table S5**). Among them, the top 10 targets with higher degree values were mitogen-activated protein kinase 1 (MAPK1), cellular tumor antigen p53 (TP53), tumor necrosis factor (TNF), beta-amyloid/A4 protein precursor (APP), transcription factor AP-1 (JUN), vascular endothelial growth factor A (VEGFA), signal transducer activator of transcription 3 (STAT3), matrix metalloproteinase-9 (MMP9), prostaglandin-endoperoxide synthase 2 (PTGS2), and endothelin-1 (EDN1).

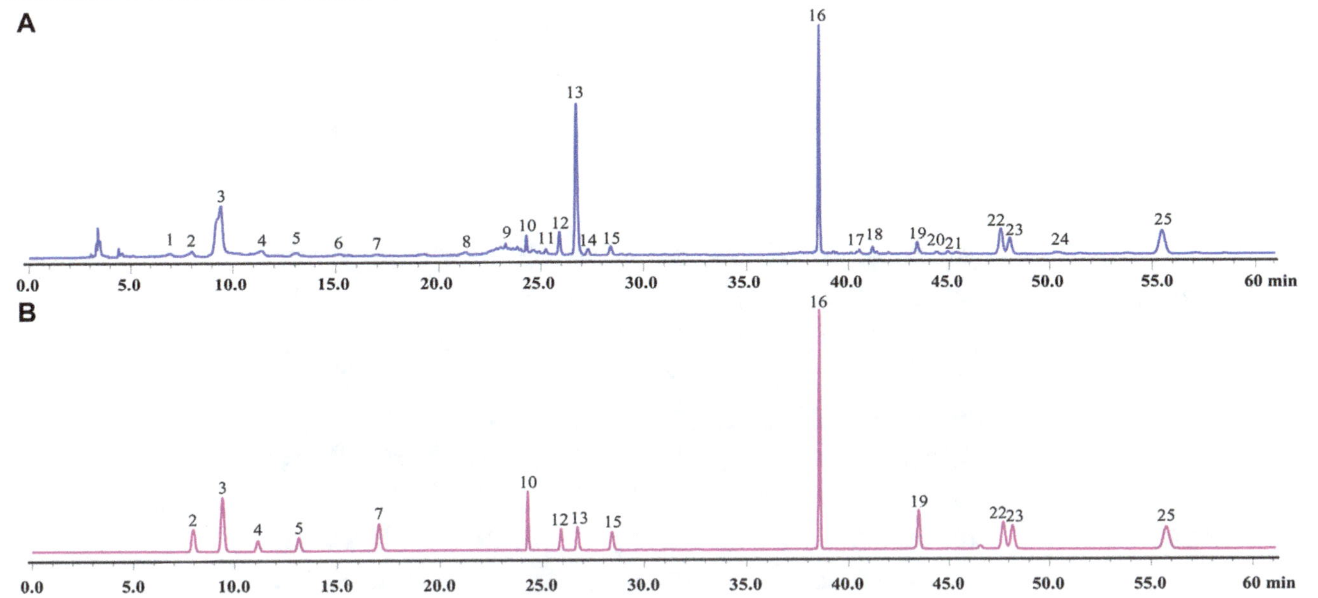

FIGURE 2 | HPLC chromatograms of GXSTC **(A)** and mixed standard sample **(B)** at 274 nm. Mixed standard sample was consisted of gallic acid (2), 5-Hydroxymethylfurfural (3), danshensu (4), protocatechuic acid (5), protocatechualdehyde (7), ellagic acid (10), rosmarinic acid (12), salvianolic acid B (13), salvianolic acid A (15), eugenol (16), dihydrotanshinone I (19), cryptotanshinone (22), tanshinone I (23), tanshinone IIA (25).

GO Functional and KEGG Pathway Enrichment Analysis

GO enrichment results were divided into biological process (BP), molecular function (MF) and cellular component (CC). According to the screening criteria of $p < 0.05$, a total of 1,515 BPs, 47 CCs, 64 MFs, and 112 pathways were obtained (**Supplementary Table S6**), and the top 10 BPs, top 5 MFs, top 5 CCs and top 20 KEGG items are shown in **Figure 5**. GO enrichment analysis indicated that the BPs of GXSTC on CBVDs were related to the regulation of oxidative stress, lipopolysaccharide, and neuronal apoptotic processes. CCs were related to membrane raft, membrane microdomain, Golgi lumen, among others. MFs were involved in protease binding, serine-type endopeptidase and peptidase activity. KEGG enrichment analysis revealed that the pathways of GXSTC on CBVDs were predominantly involved in AGE-RAGE, HIF-1, TNF, IL-17 signaling pathways, fluid shear stress, atherosclerosis, and apoptosis etc.

C-T-P Network Analysis

Based on the KEGG enrichment analysis results, we established a C-T-P network to systematically explain the mechanism of GXSTC on CBVDs. The network includes 48 nodes and 147 edges. The blue octagon represent 14 bioactive components of GXSTC, the orange ellipses represent 26 corresponding targets of components, and the rose-red V shapes represent the pathways related to CBVDs in the top 20 pathways (**Figure 6**). Seven core components with degree values above the median were identified as tanshinone IIA, cryptotanshinone, gallic acid, rosmarinic acid, ellagic acid, tanshinone I, and danshensu. Similarly, 12 core targets were identified as transcription factor p65 (RELA), PTGS2, Caspase-3 (CASP3), JUN, endothelial nitric oxide synthase (NOS3), MMP9, NF-κB inhibitor alpha (NFKBIA), TNF, EDN1, B-cell lymphoma 2 (BCL2), MAPK1, and VEGFA. These targets were selected as core targets because they play an essential role in the C-T-P network, and they are also key targets of the PPI network; therefore, these targets may be the center of the regulatory network of GXSTC against CBVDs.

Docking Results Analysis

The docking analysis between the seven core components and their corresponding core targets was carried out by using AutoDock Vina. Among them, EDN1 could not be docked because there is currently no suitable protein crystal structure available. Therefore, a total of 28 pairs of docking results were obtained, with an affinity ranging from −4.8 to −10.3 kcal/mol (**Table 1**). Affinity values were used to evaluate the binding interactions. The binding interaction was stronger when the docking score was lower. Usually, it is believed that an affinity < −5 kcal/mol represents a good binding activity between the component and target, and an affinity < −7 kcal/mol represents a stronger binding activity (Xia et al., 2020). In this study, there were 27 pairs of docking results satisfied the criteria of an affinity < −5 kcal/mol, and 15 pairs (15/28) met the criteria of an affinity < −7 kcal/mol. The results indicated that these core component-targets had a strong binding activity, and further confirmed the reliability of the interactions predicted by using systemic pharmacology. Among the docking results, the six pairs with the higher docking scores were selected for 3D and 2D visualization (**Figures 7A–F**).

Experimental Assessment

GXSTC Improves the Neurological Deficits and Reduces the Infarct Volume in MCAO-Induced Rats

No neurological deficits were detected in the sham group, while severe neurological deficits were observed in the MCAO group ($p < 0.01$, vs. sham group). The pretreatment with GXSTC (2.0 g/kg) significantly

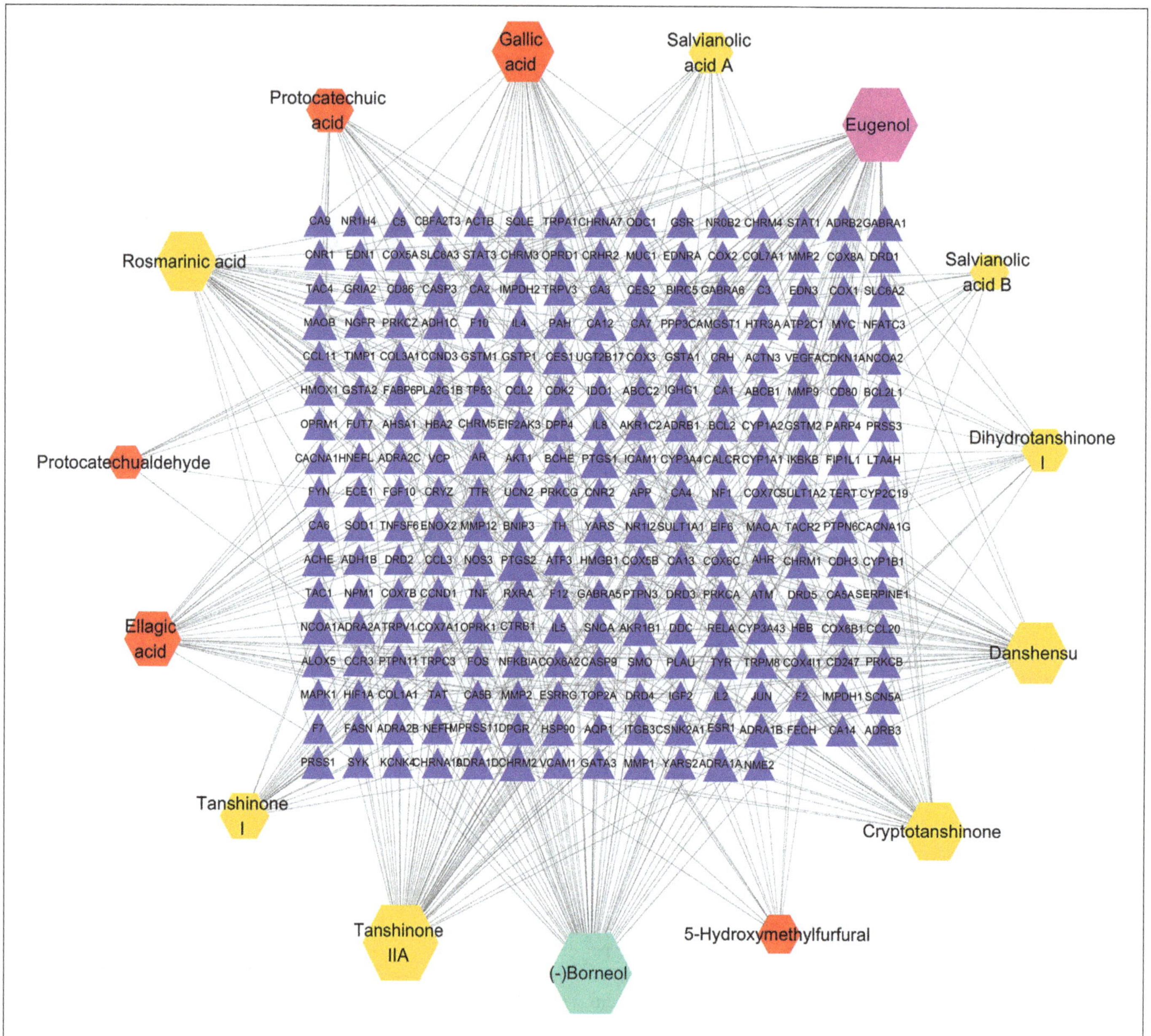

FIGURE 3 | The C-T network of GXSTC, the hexagons represent the components of *Choerospondiatis fructus* (red), *Radix Salviae miltiorrhizae* (orange), *Salviae miltiorrhizae* (purple) and *Borneolum* (blue); the blue triangles represent the targets of GXSTC components.

reduced the neurological deficits score ($p < 0.05$, vs. MCAO group; **Figure 8A**). Similarly, there was no detectable infarct volume in the sham group, but a large infarct volume was observed in the MCAO group ($p < 0.01$), which suggested that the MCAO model was successfully established. Furthermore, the pretreatment with GXSTC (2.0 g/kg) significantly reduced the cerebral infarct volume from 38.19 to 18.56% ($p < 0.05$, **Figures 8B,C**).

GXSTC Decreases the Rates of Necrotic Neurons After MCAO

The neuroprotective effect of GXSTC on brain injury was further confirmed by using H and E staining. As shown in **Figures 8D,E**, in the sham group, the neurons displayed a regular cell arrangement with a clear cell outline, and their nuclei were in the center of the cells. However, the percentage of necrotic neurons with shrunken nucleus pulposus was significantly increased in the MCAO group ($p < 0.01$, vs. sham group). After pretreatment with GXSTC at doses of 1.0 and 2.0 g/kg, the rates of necrotic neurons were markedly decreased ($p < 0.01$, vs. MCAO group).

GXSTC Promotes the Expression of VEGFA, e-NOS, While Inhibiting the Expression of COX-2 and c-Jun After MCAO

Because the core targets were mainly associated with inflammatory responses, regulation of vascular endothelial function, and neuronal apoptosis, we chose VEGFA, e-NOS (NOS3), COX-2 (PTGS2), and

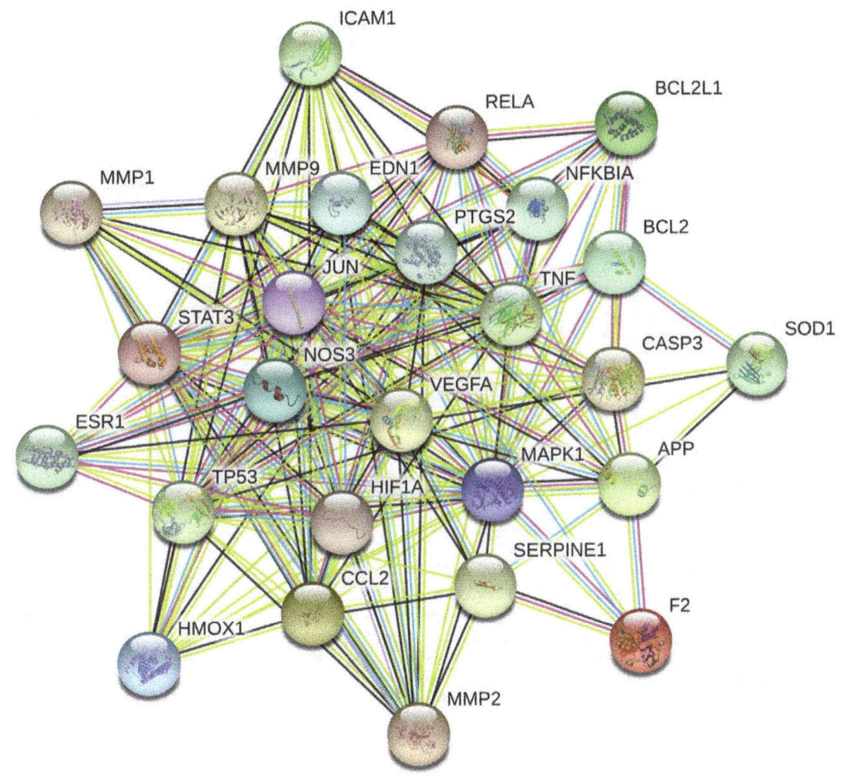

FIGURE 4 | The PPI network of key targets, the different colored nodes represent different proteins; filled nodes represent some 3D structure is known or predicted; wathet and purple lines represent known protein-protein interactions; red lines represent predicted protein-protein interactions; green, black and lilac lines represent textmining, co-expression and protein homology, respectively.

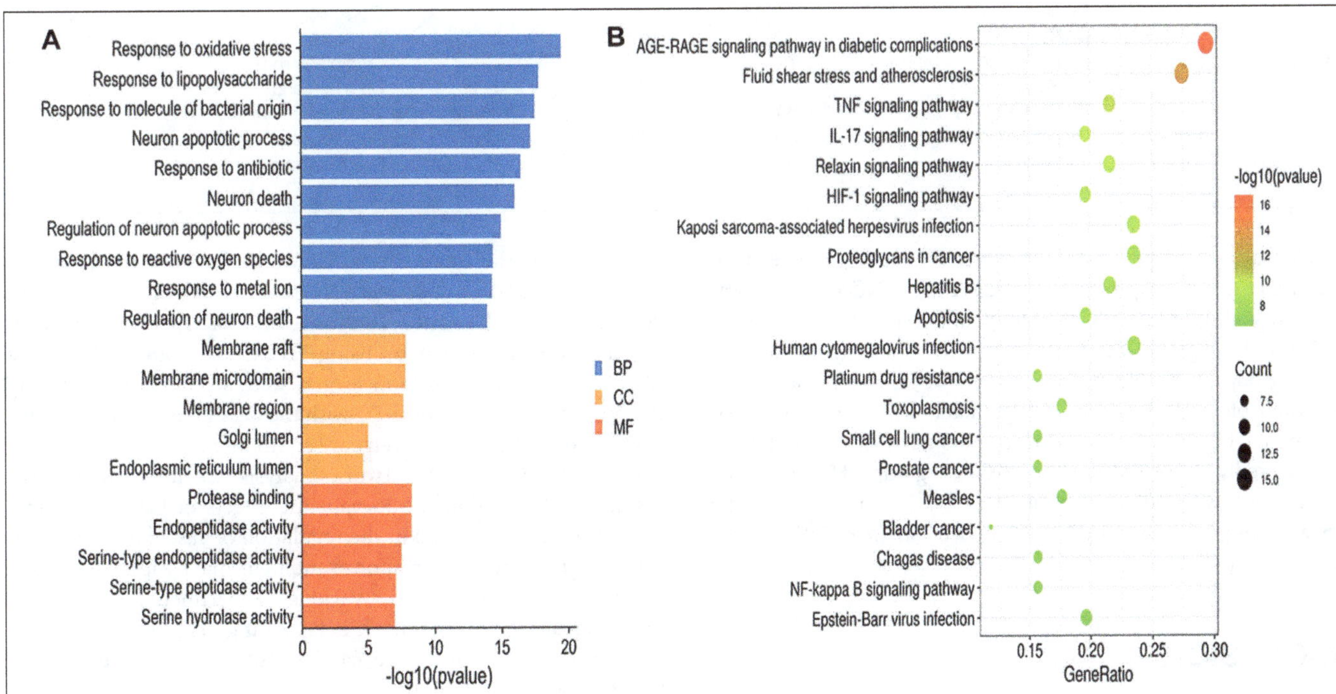

FIGURE 5 | GO functional **(A)** and KEGG pathway **(B)** enrichment analysis.

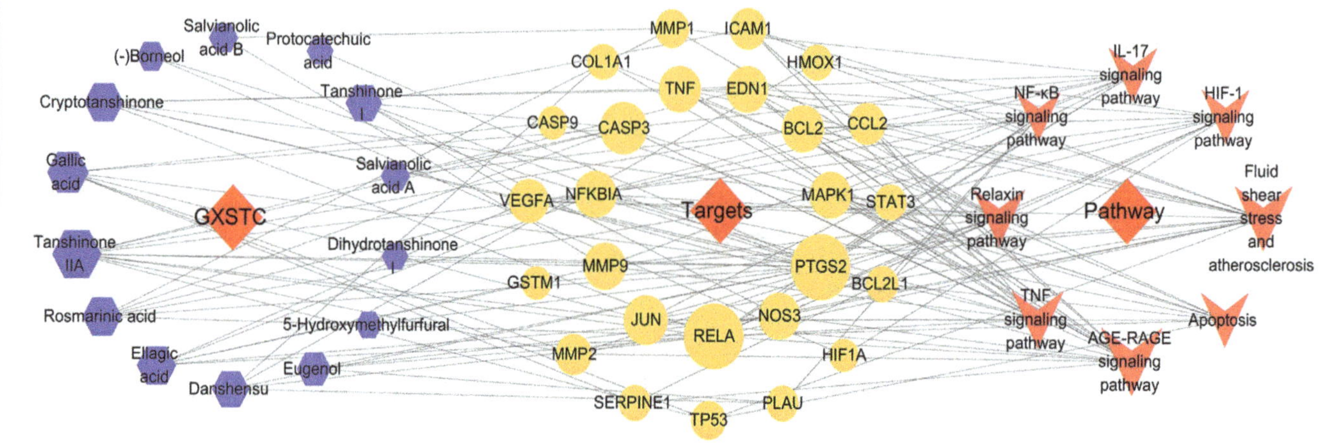

FIGURE 6 | The C-T-P network of GXSTC against CBVDs. The nodes represent components (blue hexagons), targets (orange ellipses), and pathways (rose-red V shapes).

TABLE 1 | Docking scores between seven core components and their corresponding core targets.

Core target	PDB ID	GXSTC component	Affinity (kcal/mol)	Core target	PDB ID	GXSTC component	Affinity (kcal/mol)
RELA	6NV2	Original ligand	-6.4	JUN	1JNM	Tanshinone IIA	-6.1
		Tanshinone IIA	-7.3			Gallic acid	-5.4
		Cryptotanshinone	-7.1	CASP3	3H0E	Original ligand	-7.3
		Ellagic acid	-6.7			Ellagic acid	-7.3
		Rosmarinic acid	-6.6			Gallic acid	-4.8
		Danshensu	-5.3			Rosmarinic acid	-6.4
PTGS2	5KIR	Original ligand	-10.2			Tanshinone I	-7.2
		Tanshinone I	-9.3	MMP9	5CUH	Original ligand	-9.5
		Tanshinone IIA	-8.7			Tanshinone IIA	-10.3
		Cryptotanshinone	-8.3			Ellagic acid	-6.9
		Rosmarinic acid	-8.3	NFKBIA	1NFI	Tanshinone IIA	-6.4
		Danshensu	-6.8			Ellagic acid	-6.2
		Gallic acid	-6.1	TNF	2AZ5	Original ligand	-8.2
VEGFA	4QAF	Original ligand	-7.5			Cryptotanshinone	-9.2
		Tanshinone I	-10.1	BCL2	4IEH	Original ligand	-8.2
		Ellagic acid	-6.7			Tanshinone IIA	-8.0
NOS3	6PP4	Original ligand	-9.1	MAPK1	1TVO	Original ligand	-9.4
		Tanshinone I	-9.9			Rosmarinic acid	-7.9
		Ellagic acid	-7.7				

c-Jun for further investigation. As shown in **Figure 9**, compared with the sham group, the expression of VEGFA and e-NOS proteins was increased slightly in the MCAO group, and markedly increased in the 1.0 and 2.0 g/kg GXSTC pretreatment groups ($p < 0.05$, vs. MCAO group). With the increase in the GXSTC concentration, the expression of VEGFA and e-NOS gradually increased. Moreover, compared with the sham group, the expression of COX-2 and c-Jun was markedly increased in the MCAO group. However, the pretreatment with 1.0 and 2.0 g/kg GXSTC could significantly decreased the expression of COX-2 and c-Jun ($p < 0.01$, vs. the MCAO group).

DISCUSSION

GXSTC, which is derived from a Mongolian medicine formulation, has been clinically proven to be an effective and safe TCM for the treatment of CBVDs. However, the bioactive components and multi-target mechanisms of GXSTC have not yet been clearly elucidated. In this study, 15 active components in GXSTC were identified by using HPLC-DAD and a literature research. Fifty-five common targets were screened by matching the potential targets of GXSTC with the CBVD-associated targets. Twelve core targets and seven core components were identified by using PPI and C-T-P network analysis. Enrichment analysis results predicted that the therapeutic effects of GXSTC against CBVDs may be involved in the regulation of vascular endothelial function, inflammatory response and neuronal apoptosis. Finally, molecular docking and various experiments (including neurological scale scoring, TTC staining, H and E staining, and western blotting) were carried out to assess the systems pharmacology prediction.

The chemical components of TCM are characterized by complex, various types, and a constant or trace composition

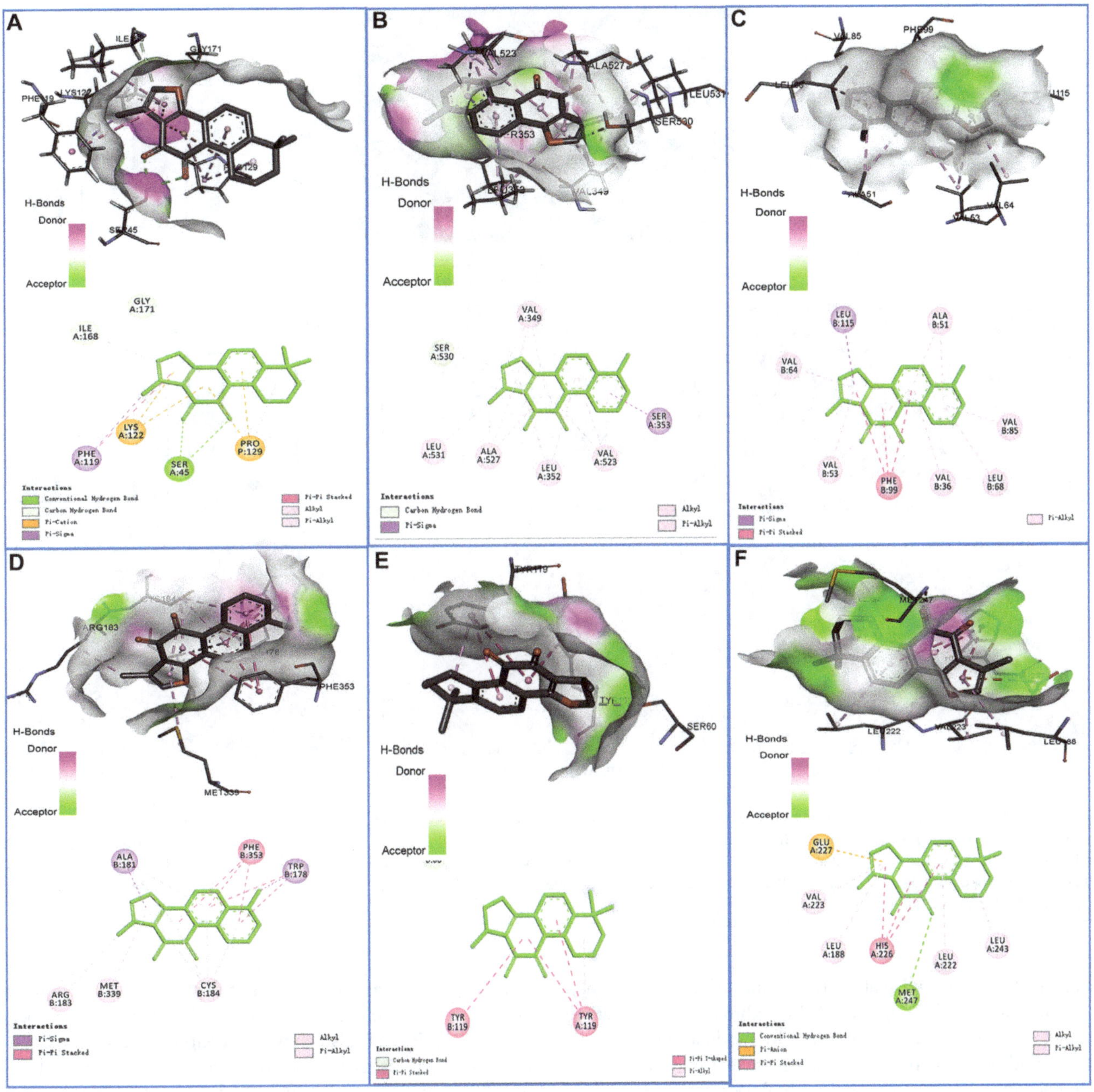

FIGURE 7 | Schematic diagrams (3D and 2D) of the binding modes of representative component-targets. **(A)** Tanshinone IIA with RELA; **(B)** Tanshinone I with PTGS2; **(C)** Tanshinone I with VEGFA; **(D)** Tanshinone I with NOS3; **(E)** Tanshinone IIA with MMP9; **(F)** Cryptotanshinone with TNF.

coexistence, but the main components of TCM are often the material basis of their efficacy. In this study, we identified 15 main components of GXSTC by using HPLC-DAD combined with a literature research, which was consistent with the results of previous studies (Zhou et al., 2016). Moreover, 13 of them had a high oral bioavailability (OB) in the TCMSP database, and their OB values are listed in **Supplementary Table S1**. Several studies have elucidated and identified the GXSTC components using liquid chromatography/mass spectrometry (LC/MS) *in vitro* and *in vivo* (Gao et al., 2017; Liu et al., 2018). According to their findings, the 15 main components we identified were also determined using LC/MS *in vitro*, and 12 of 15 main components were identified in rat plasma. These findings further suggested that these main components may be the key substances via which GXSTC exerts its efficacy *in vivo*.

The results of the topological analysis of the C-T-P network indicated seven core components with the higher degree values: tanshinone IIA, cryptotanshinone, gallic acid, rosmarinic acid, ellagic acid, tanshinone I, and danshensu. Several previous studies, including our own, have shown that phenolic acids,

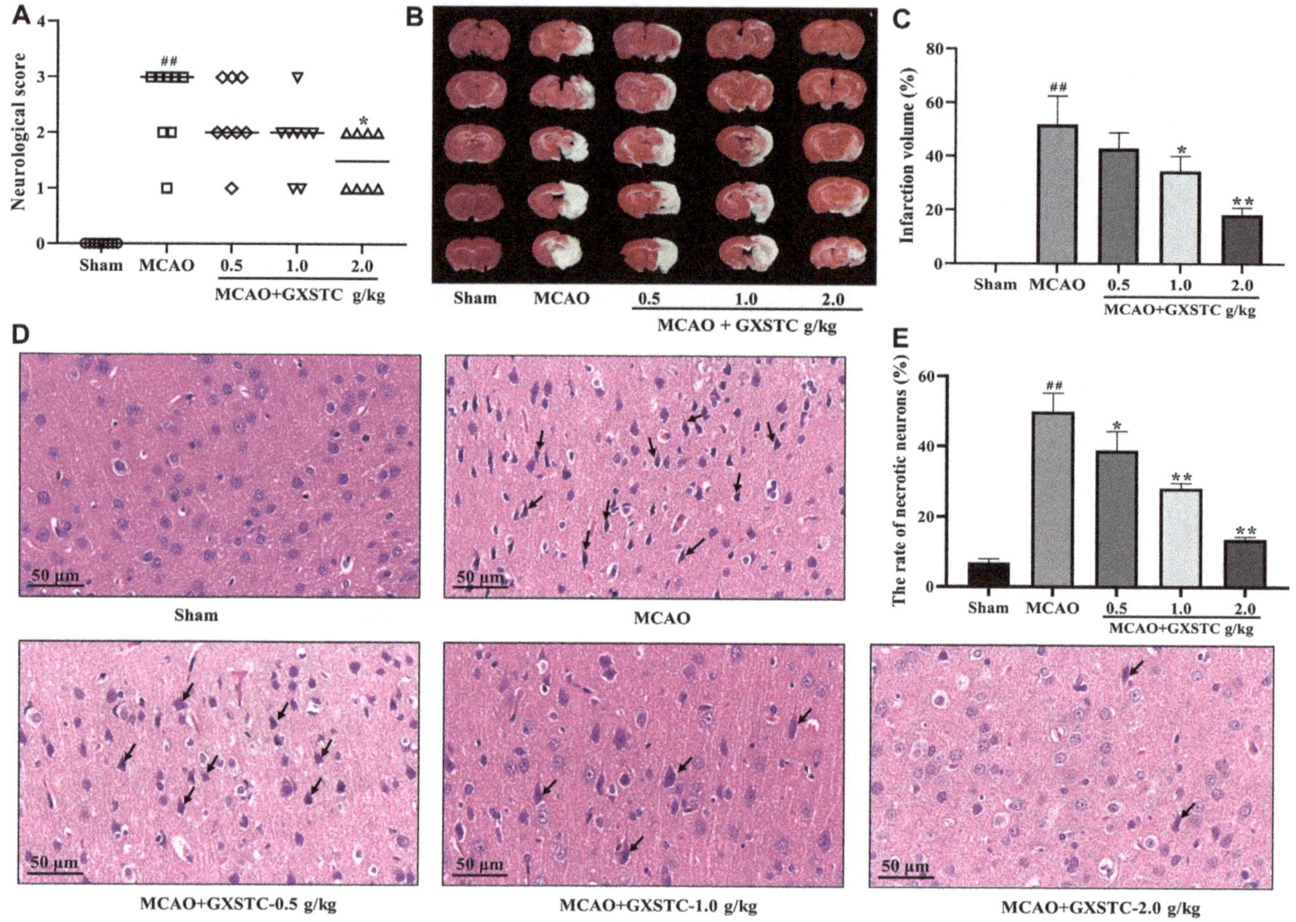

FIGURE 8 | GXSTC alleviates MCAO-induced brain injury **(A)** Scatterplot of the neurological deficits in the sham, MCAO, 0.5, 1.0, 2.0 g/kg GXSTC pretreatment groups (data were expressed as median, $n = 8$) **(B)** The cerebral infarct volume of rats in each group **(C)** Statistical analysis of the rate of infarct volume in each group **(D)** H and E staining of coronal slices of the ischemic cerebral cortex, and the black arrow points to necrotic neurons **(E)** Statistical analysis results of the rate of necrotic neurons in each group. All data, except for neurologic score, were expressed as mean ± SD; $^{\#\#}p < 0.01$, compared with the sham group; $^{*}p < 0.05$ or $^{**}p < 0.01$, compared with the MCAO group.

such as gallic acid (Nabavi et al., 2016), rosmarinic acid (Cui et al., 2018), and ellagic acid (Ding et al., 2014), exhibit neuroprotective effects against cerebral ischemic injury by modulating oxidative stress. In addition, our previous study indicated that danshensu has a neuroprotective effect on cerebral ischemia/reperfusion injury, and the mechanism may inhibit the apoptosis process by regulating the PI3K/Akt pathway (Guo et al., 2015). Tanshinone IIA, cryptotanshinone, and tanshinone I are major lipid-soluble components of *Radix Salviae miltiorrhizae* that can attenuate permanent cerebral ischemia by inhibiting thrombosis formation, platelet aggregation, and by activating the PLC/PKC pathway in rats (Fei et al., 2017). Taken together, these findings indicate that the core components of GXSTC are effective in treating CBVDs.

In addition, we identified 12 core targets of GXSTC on CBVDs using network analysis, and these targets were primarily related to inflammatory responses (RELA, PTGS2, NFKBIA, JUN, TNF, and MMP9), neuronal apoptosis (CASP3, JUN, BCL2, and MAPK1), and vascular endothelial function (VEGFA, NOS3, and EDN1). Inflammation is a hallmark of stroke pathology and contributes to the aggravation of brain injury (Lambertsen et al., 2012). PTGS2, also known as cyclooxygenase-2 (COX-2), is the principal isozyme responsible for the production of inflammatory prostaglandins, and its inhibition may help improve the enlargement of the infarction after CBVDs. In addition, PTGS2 can be linked to six core components of GXSTC and multiple signaling pathways; thus, it may play an essential role in GXSTC against CBVDs (Jiang et al., 2011). JUN (c-Jun), which is a subunit of the AP-1 transcription factor, plays an essential role in neuronal apoptosis and inflammation. Generally, c-Jun can be highly activated after cerebral ischemia, and the expression level of c-Jun is significantly increased in the cerebral cortex (Raivich and Behrens., 2006). MMP-9 belongs to the subfamily of MMPs that play a key role in blood-brain barrier injury and inflammatory processes after cerebral ischemia. Previous research has suggested that GXSTC can downregulate the expression of MMP-9 receptor protein in ischemic tissues (Fernández-Cadenas et al., 2012).

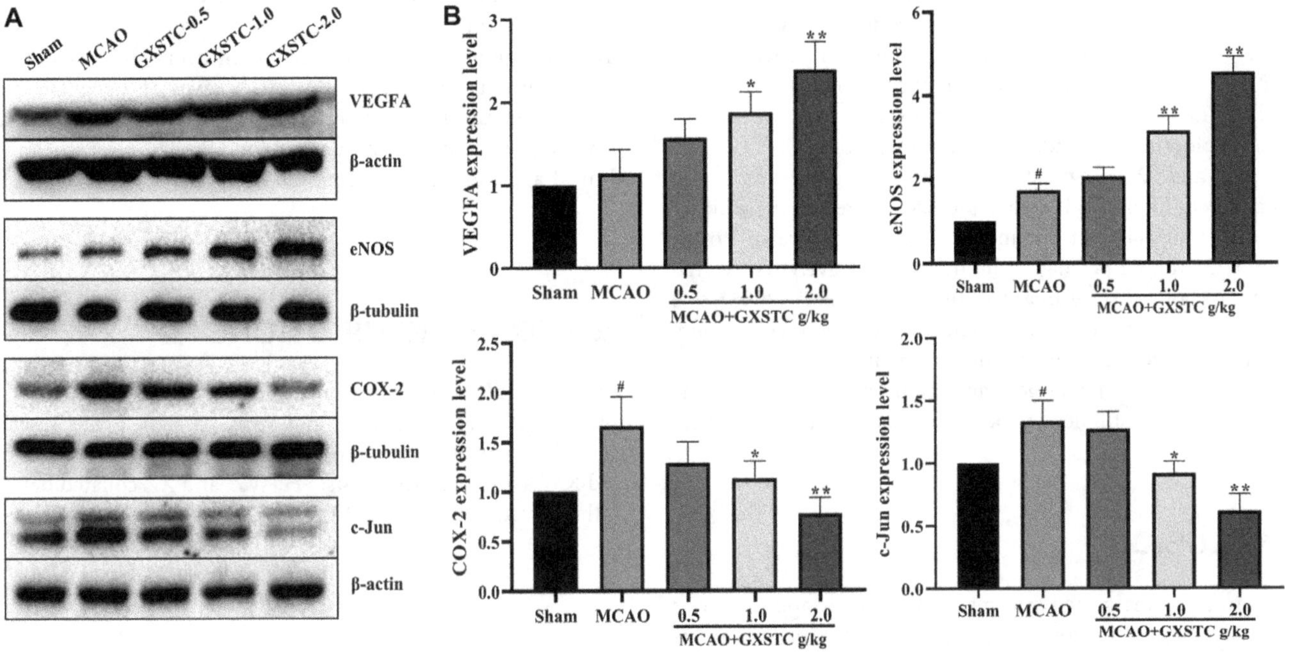

FIGURE 9 | Relative expression of VEGFA, e-NOS, COX-2, and c-Jun in the cerebral cortex of the sham, MCAO, 0.5, 1.0, 2.0 g/kg GXSTC pretreatment groups were detected by using Western blot analysis. Representative bands exhibited the relative expression of VEGFA, e-NOS, COX-2 and c-JUN **(A)**; Statistical analysis results of detected proteins in each group **(B)**. Data were presented as mean ± SD. $\#p < 0.05$, compared with the sham group; $^{*}p < 0.05$ or $^{**}p < 0.01$, compared with the MCAO group.

VEGFA, a main proangiogenic factor, plays a central role in vasculogenesis and neurogenesis and is associated with neurological function in stroke recovery. When cerebral ischemia occurs, VEGFA is markedly upregulated in the ischemic penumbra area. Therefore, therapeutic angiogenesis by VEGFA is advocated as a promising treatment strategy for CBVDs (Geiseler and Morland, 2018). NOS3, also known as eNOS, plays a vital role in maintaining vascular homeostasis. When the expression of eNOS is increased, it can relax the blood vessels and prevent thrombosis (Endres et al., 2004).

GO functional and KEGG pathway enrichment analyses were performed to better understand the reciprocity of these common targets. The enriched results suggested that the molecular mechanisms of GXSTC on CBVDs were predominately involved in AGE-RAGE, HIF-1, TNF, IL-17, and the apoptosis signaling pathway. These results are consistent with those of previous studies showing that the above pathways play important roles in the progression and development of CBVDs (Wang et al., 2019). Among them, the HIF-1 signaling pathway is a major regulator of angiogenesis after CBVDs; it is observed to participate in vascular formation maintenance of vascular tension through synergistic correlations with other proangiogenic factors, such as VEGFA, eNOS, and EDN1. Therefore, the HIF-1 signaling pathway may play a crucial role in GXSTC against CBVDs (Hong et al., 2019). In addition, TNF signaling is the best-researched inflammatory pathway related to CBVDs, in which TNF-α mediates the microglial activation and triggers the activation of multiple pathways, including the NF-κB and MAPK pathways (Bradley, 2008). IL-17, which is a signature cytokine secreted by Th17 cells, is another typical pro-inflammatory cytokine involved in CBVDs, and the IL-17 pathway also plays a vital role in the inflammatory injury processes of CBVDs (Swardfager et al., 2013).

To further investigate the interactions between the core components and their corresponding core targets, molecular docking studies were performed to elucidate the binding modes. The results indicated that almost all of core components-targets had a good binding activity (affinity < −5 kcal/mol), and more than half of them had a stronger binding activity (affinity < −7 kcal/mol), which further confirmed the reliability of the systemic pharmacology prediction. More importantly, in MCAO-injured rats, GXSTC significantly improved the neurological function, reduced the infarct volume, and decreased the rate of impaired neurons in a dose-dependent manner. In addition, we selected vascular function-related proteins (VEGFA and eNOS), inflammation-related proteins (COX-2, c-Jun), neuronal apoptosis-related protein (c-Jun) from 12 core targets to further assess the molecular mechanisms. These proteins were also enriched in the HIF-1, TNF, and IL-17 signaling pathways, and may be the center of the regulatory network of GXSTC against CBVDs. Western blot analyses indicated that GXSTC markedly upregulated the expression of VEGFA and e-NOS, and downregulated the expression of COX-2 and c-Jun in MCAO-induced rats. These findings provide the evidence that GXSTC exerts a multi-target synergetic effect on CBVDs by maintaining vascular endothelial function, inhibiting neuronal apoptosis and inflammatory processes. However, identifying the core components by using network pharmacological analysis alone has some limitations, such as that it neither reflect the effect intensity against CBVDs of these core components, nor illuminate the correlation between their concentration and efficacy. Therefore, these core components are worthy of further exploration. In addition, the three doses of GXSTC (0.5, 1.0, and 2.0 g/kg per day) used in this study are comparatively high and it remains unclear whether these doses will result in artefacts in our model. They are equivalent to 80, 160, and 320 mg/kg per day in humans, respectively (converted by using the body surface area) (Administration, F. D., 2005), so a lower dose range needs to be studied in further investigation. Also, the specific neuroprotection mechanisms of GXSTC in CBVDs, as well as the targets and pathways acting with the active components still need to be further confirmed in follow-up studies.

CONCLUSION

In this study, an integrated systems pharmacology approach was used to investigate the bioactive components, therapeutic targets and explore the pharmacological mechanisms of GXSTC in treating CBVDs. The results suggested that the multi-target synergetic mechanism of GXSTC in CBVDs mainly involved three therapeutic modules, including maintaining vascular endothelial function, inhibiting neuronal apoptosis and inflammatory processes. Then, we selected the rat MCAO/reperfusion model to evaluate the protective effects of GXSTC on CBVDs and chosen several core proteins to assess the predicted molecular mechanisms, confirming the reliability of our method. In conclusion, our study gives an insight into the multi-target mechanisms by systems pharmacology approach, providing a scientific foundation for GXSTC research and its clinical application in treating CBVDs.

AUTHOR CONTRIBUTIONS

AW, MS, YD, and JuZ conceived the idea and revised the manuscript. JuZ, JiZ, YM, and WW designed the research, carried out most of the experiments and wrote the paper. CG and KW assisted experiments; SH, WZ, and XZ collated data. All authors read and approved the final manuscript.

FUNDING

The study was supported by the National Natural Science Foundation of China (No. 82074321, 82071464, 21662048), the key research and development plan of Shaanxi Province (2019SF-118).

REFERENCES

Administration, F. D. (2005). Guidance for Industry: Estimating the maximum safe starting dose in initial clinical trials for therapeutics in adult healthy volunteers. in *Pharmacology and Toxicology*, 1–27. Available at: https://www.fda.gov/regulatory-information/search-fda-guidance-documents/estimating-maximum-safe-starting-dose-initial-clinical-trials-therapeutics-adult-healthy-volunteers.

Amberger, J. S., and Hamosh, A. (2017). Searching Online Mendelian Inheritance in Man (OMIM): A Knowledgebase of Human Genes and Genetic Phenotypes. *Curr. Protoc. Bioinformatics* 58, 1.2.1–1.2.12. doi:10.1002/cpbi.27

Bateman, A., Martin, M. J., Orchard, S., Magrane, M., Alpi, E., Bely, B., et al. (2019). UniProt: a Worldwide Hub of Protein Knowledge. *Nucleic Acids Res.* 47 (D1), D506–D515. doi:10.1093/nar/gky1049

Bradley, J. (2008). TNF-mediated Inflammatory Disease. *J. Pathol.* 214 (2), 149–160. doi:10.1002/path.2287

Brown, G. R., Hem, V., Katz, K. S., Ovetsky, M., Wallin, C., Ermolaeva, O., et al. (2015). Gene: a Gene-Centered Information Resource at NCBI. *Nucleic Acids Res.* 43 (Database issue), D36–D42. doi:10.1093/nar/gku1055

Collaborators., G.B.D.N. (2019). Global, Regional, and National Burden of Neurological Disorders, 1990-2016: a Systematic Analysis for the Global Burden of Disease Study 2016. *Lancet Neurol.* 18 (5), 459–480. doi:10.1016/S1474-4422(18)30499-X

Cui, H. Y., Zhang, X. J., Yang, Y., Zhang, C., Zhu, C. H., Miao, J. Y., et al. (2018). Rosmarinic Acid Elicits Neuroprotection in Ischemic Stroke via Nrf2 and Heme Oxygenase 1 Signaling. *Neural Regen. Res.* 13 (12), 2119–2128. doi:10.4103/1673-5374.241463

Cui, Q., Zhang, Y.-L., Ma, Y.-H., Yu, H.-Y., Zhao, X.-Z., Zhang, L.-H., et al. (2020). A Network Pharmacology Approach to Investigate the Mechanism of Shuxuening Injection in the Treatment of Ischemic Stroke. *J. Ethnopharmacol.* 257, 112891. doi:10.1016/j.jep.2020.112891

Daina, A., Michielin, O., and Zoete, V. (2019). SwissTargetPrediction: Updated Data and New Features for Efficient Prediction of Protein Targets of Small Molecules. *Nucleic Acids Res.* 47 (W1), W357–W364. doi:10.1093/nar/gkz382

Davis, A. P., Grondin, C. J., Johnson, R. J., Sciaky, D., Mcmorran, R., Wiegers, J., et al. (2019). The Comparative Toxicogenomics Database: Update 2019. *Nucleic Acids Res.* 47 (D1), D948–D954. doi:10.1093/nar/gky868

Ding, Y., Zhang, B., Zhou, K., Chen, M., Wang, M., Jia, Y., et al. (2014). Dietary Ellagic Acid Improves Oxidant-Induced Endothelial Dysfunction and Atherosclerosis: Role of Nrf2 Activation. *Int. J. Cardiol.* 175 (3), 508–514. doi:10.1016/j.ijcard.2014.06.045

Endres, M., Laufs, U., Liao, J. K., and Moskowitz, M. A. (2004). Targeting eNOS for Stroke Protection. *Trends Neurosciences* 27 (5), 283–289. doi:10.1016/j.tins.2004.03.009

Fei, Y.-x., Wang, S.-q., Yang, L.-j., Qiu, Y.-y., Li, Y.-z., Liu, W.-y., et al. (2017). *Salvia miltiorrhiza* Bunge (Danshen) Extract Attenuates Permanent Cerebral Ischemia through Inhibiting Platelet Activation in Rats. *J. Ethnopharmacol.* 207, 57–66. doi:10.1016/j.jep.2017.06.023

Fernández-Cadenas, I., del Río-Espínola, A., Carrera, C., Domingues-Montanari, S., Mendióroz, M., Delgado, P., et al. (2012). Role of the MMP9 Gene in Hemorrhagic Transformations after Tissue-type Plasminogen Activator Treatment in Stroke Patients. *Stroke* 43 (5), 1398–1400. doi:10.1161/STROKEAHA.111.639823

Franz, M., Lopes, C. T., Huck, G., Dong, Y., Sumer, O., and Bader, G. D. (2016). Cytoscape.js: a Graph Theory Library for Visualisation and Analysis. *Bioinformatics* 32 (2), 309–311. doi:10.1093/bioinformatics/btv557

Gao, X., Mu, J., Li, Q., Guan, S., Liu, R., Du, Y., et al. (2017). Comprehensive Identification of Guan-Xin-Shu-Tong Capsule via a Mass Defect and Fragment Filtering Approach by High Resolution Mass Spectrometry: *In Vitro* and *In Vivo* Study. *Molecules* 22 (6), 1007. doi:10.3390/molecules22061007

Geiseler, S., and Morland, C. (2018). The Janus Face of VEGF in Stroke. *Int J Mol Sci.* 19 (5), 1362. doi:10.3390/ijms19051362

Guo, C., Ma, Y., Ma, S., Mu, F., Deng, J., Duan, J., et al. (2017). The Role of TRPC6 in the Neuroprotection of Calycosin against Cerebral Ischemic Injury. *Sci. Rep.* 7 (1), 3039. doi:10.1038/s41598-017-03404-6

Guo, C., Yin, Y., Duan, J., Zhu, Y., Yan, J., Wei, G., et al. (2015). Neuroprotective Effect and Underlying Mechanism of Sodium Danshensu [3-(3,4-dihydroxyphenyl) Lactic Acid from Radix and Rhizoma *Salviae miltiorrhizae* = Danshen] against Cerebral Ischemia and Reperfusion Injury in Rats. *Phytomedicine* 22 (2), 283–289. doi:10.1016/j.phymed.2014.12.001

Hankey, G. J. (2017). Stroke. *Lancet* 389, 641–654. doi:10.1016/S0140-6736(16)30962-X

Hong, M., Shi, H., Wang, N., Tan, H.-Y., Wang, Q., and Feng, Y. (2019). Dual Effects of Chinese Herbal Medicines on Angiogenesis in Cancer and Ischemic Stroke Treatments: Role of HIF-1 Network. *Front. Pharmacol.* 10, 696. doi:10.3389/fphar.2019.00696

Jiang, C., Cui, K., Wang, J., and He, Y. (2011). Microglia and Cyclooxygenase-2: Possible Therapeutic Targets of Progesterone for Stroke. *Int. Immunopharmacol.* 11 (11), 1925–1931. doi:10.1016/j.intimp.2011.08.001

Kibble, M., Saarinen, N., Tang, J., Wennerberg, K., Mäkelä, S., and Aittokallio, T. (2015). Network Pharmacology Applications to Map the Unexplored Target Space and Therapeutic Potential of Natural Products. *Nat. Prod. Rep.* 32 (8), 1249–1266. doi:10.1039/c5np00005j

Kim, S., Chen, J., Cheng, T., Gindulyte, A., He, J., He, S., et al. (2019). PubChem 2019 Update: Improved Access to Chemical Data. *Nucleic Acids Res.* 47 (D1), D1102–D1109. doi:10.1093/nar/gky1033

Kuhn, M., Von Mering, C., Campillos, M., Jensen, L. J., and Bork, P. (2008). STITCH: Interaction Networks of Chemicals and Proteins. *Nucleic Acids Res.* 36 (Database issue), D684–D688. doi:10.1093/nar/gkm795

Lambertsen, K. L., Biber, K., and Finsen, B. (2012). Inflammatory Cytokines in Experimental and Human Stroke. *J. Cereb. Blood Flow Metab.* 32 (9), 1677–1698. doi:10.1038/jcbfm.2012.88

Li, Y., Zhang, L., Lv, S., Wang, X., Zhang, J., Tian, X., et al. (2019). Efficacy and Safety of Oral Guanxinshutong Capsules in Patients with Stable Angina Pectoris in China: a Prospective, Multicenter, Double-Blind, Placebo-Controlled, Randomized Clinical Trial. *BMC Complement. Altern. Med.* 19 (1), 363. doi:10.1186/s12906-019-2778-z

Liu, F., Du, X., Su, R., Sun, Y. H., and Zhang, Y. M. (2018). Screening and Analysis of Key Active Constituents in GuanxinShutong Capsule by Using Mass Spectrum and Integrative Network Pharmacology. *Chin. J. Nat. Med.* 16 (3), 302–312. doi:10.3724/SP.J.1009.2018.000010.1016/s1875-5364(18)30060-8

Liu, Z., Guo, F., Wang, Y., Li, C., Zhang, X., Li, H., et al. (2016). BATMAN-TCM: a Bioinformatics Analysis Tool for Molecular mechanism of Traditional Chinese Medicine. *Sci. Rep.* 6, 21146. doi:10.1038/srep21146

Longa, E. Z., Weinstein, P. R., Carlson, S., and Cummins, R. (1989). Reversible Middle Cerebral Artery Occlusion without Craniectomy in Rats. *Stroke* 20 (1), 84–91. doi:10.1161/01.str.20.1.84

Mair, P., Hofmann, E., Gruber, K., Hatzinger, R., Zeileis, A., and Hornik, K. (2015). Motivation, Values, and Work Design as Drivers of Participation in the R Open Source Project for Statistical Computing. *Proc. Natl. Acad. Sci. USA.* 112 (48), 14788–14792. doi:10.1073/pnas.1506047112

Nabavi, S., Habtemariam, S., Di Lorenzo, A., Sureda, A., Khanjani, S., Nabavi, S., et al. (2016). Post-stroke Depression Modulation and In Vivo Antioxidant Activity of Gallic Acid and its Synthetic Derivatives in a Murine Model System. *Nutrients* 8 (5), 248. doi:10.3390/nu8050248

Raivich, G., and Behrens, A. (2006). Role of the AP-1 Transcription Factor C-Jun in Developing, Adult and Injured Brain. *Prog. Neurobiol.* 78 (6), 347–363. doi:10.1016/j.pneurobio.2006.03.006

Rivera, D., Allkin, R., Obón, C., Alcaraz, F., Verpoorte, R., and Heinrich, M. (2014). What Is in a Name? the Need for Accurate Scientific Nomenclature for Plants. *J. Ethnopharmacol.* 152, 393–402. doi:10.1016/j.jep.2013.12.022

Rose, P. W., Prlić, A., Altunkaya, A., Bi, C., Bradley, A. R., Christie, C. H., et al. (2017). The RCSB Protein Data Bank: Integrative View of Protein, Gene and 3D Structural Information. *Nucleic Acids Res.* 45 (D1), D271–D281. doi:10.1093/nar/gkw1000

Ru, J., Li, P., Wang, J., Zhou, W., Li, B., Huang, C., et al. (2014). TCMSP: a Database of Systems Pharmacology for Drug Discovery from Herbal Medicines. *J. Cheminform* 6, 13. doi:10.1186/1758-2946-6-13

Shao, G. (2018). Effect of Dan Hong Injection Combined with Guan Xin Shu Tong Capsule in the Treatment of Ischemic Stroke. *Chin. Community Doctors* 034 (025), 106. doi:10.3969/j.issn.1007-614x.2018.25.066

Stelzer, G., Rosen, N., Plaschkes, I., Zimmerman, S., Twik, M., Fishilevich, S., et al. (2016). The GeneCards Suite: From Gene Data Mining to Disease Genome Sequence Analyses. *Curr. Protoc. Bioinformatics* 54, 1.30.1–1.30.33. doi:10.1002/cpbi.5

Swardfager, W., Winer, D. A. D., Herrmann, N., Winer, S. K., and Lanctôt, K. L. (2013). Interleukin-17 in Post-stroke Neurodegeneration. *Neurosci. Biobehav. Rev.* 37 (3), 436–447. doi:10.1016/j.neubiorev.2013.01.021

Szklarczyk, D., Gable, A. L., Lyon, D., Junge, A., Wyder, S., Huerta-Cepas, J., et al. (2019). STRING V11: Protein-Protein Association Networks with Increased Coverage, Supporting Functional Discovery in Genome-wide Experimental Datasets. *Nucleic Acids Res.* 47 (D1), D607–D613. doi:10.1093/nar/gky1131

Trott, O., and Olson, A. J. (2009). AutoDock Vina: Improving the Speed and Accuracy of Docking with a New Scoring Function, Efficient Optimization, and Multithreading. *J. Comput. Chem.* 31 (2), 455–461. doi:10.1002/jcc.21334

Wang, P., Dai, L., Zhou, W., Meng, J., Zhang, M., Wu, Y., et al. (2019). Intermodule Coupling Analysis of Huang-Lian-Jie-Du Decoction on Stroke. *Front. Pharmacol.* 10, 1288. doi:10.3389/fphar.2019.01288

Wang, Y., Zhang, S., Li, F., Zhou, Y., Zhang, Y., Wang, Z., et al. (2020). Therapeutic Target Database 2020: Enriched Resource for Facilitating Research and Early Development of Targeted Therapeutics. *Nucleic Acids Res.* 48 (D1), D1031–D1041. doi:10.1093/nar/gkz981

Wei, J., Zhang, Y., Jia, Q., Liu, M., Li, D., Zhang, Y., et al. (2016). Systematic Investigation of Transcription Factors Critical in the Protection against Cerebral Ischemia by Danhong Injection. *Sci. Rep.* 6, 29823. doi:10.1038/srep29823

Wishart, D. S., Knox, C., Guo, A. C., Shrivastava, S., Hassanali, M., Stothard, P., et al. (2006). DrugBank: a Comprehensive Resource for In Silico Drug Discovery and Exploration. *Nucleic Acids Res.* 34 (Database issue), D668–D672. doi:10.1093/nar/gkj067

Wu, X. (2015). Guanxin Shutong Capsule Combined with Danhong Injection in the Treatment of Ischemic Stroke for 40 Cases. *Chin. Med. Mod. Distance Education China* 20, 47–48. doi:10.3969/j.issn.1672-2779.2015.20.024

Xia, Q. D., Xun, Y., Lu, J. L., Lu, Y. C., Yang, Y. Y., Zhou, P., et al. (2020). Network Pharmacology and Molecular Docking Analyses on Lianhua Qingwen Capsule Indicate Akt1 Is a Potential Target to Treat and Prevent COVID-19. *Cell Prolif* 53 (12), e12949. doi:10.1111/cpr.12949

Xu, H. Y., Shi, Y., Zhang, Y. Q., Jia, Q., Li, D. F., Zhang, Y., et al. (2016). Identification of Key Active Constituents of Buchang Naoxintong Capsules with Therapeutic Effects against Ischemic Stroke by Using an Integrative Pharmacology-Based Approach. *Mol. Biosyst.* 12 (1), 233–245. doi:10.1039/c5mb00460h

Yuan, H., Ma, Q., Cui, H., Liu, G., Zhao, X., Li, W., et al. (2017). How Can Synergism of Traditional Medicines Benefit from Network Pharmacology? *Molecules* 22 (7), 1135. doi:10.3390/molecules22071135

Zhang, R., Zhu, X., Bai, H., and Ning, K. (2019). Network Pharmacology Databases for Traditional Chinese Medicine: Review and Assessment. *Front. Pharmacol.* 10, 123. doi:10.3389/fphar.2019.00123

Zhou, F., Zhang, L., Gu, L., Zhang, Y., Hou, C., Bi, K., et al. (2016). Simultaneous Quantification of 13 Compounds in Guanxin Shutong Capsule by HPLC Method. *J. Chromatogr. Sci.* 54 (6), 971–976. doi:10.1093/chromsci/bmw029

Zhou, Z., Lu, J., Liu, W.-W., Manaenko, A., Hou, X., Mei, Q., et al. (2018). Advances in Stroke Pharmacology. *Pharmacol. Ther.* 191, 23–42. doi:10.1016/j.pharmthera.2018.05.012

Zhu, J., Zhou, H., Li, C., He, Y., Pan, Y., Shou, Q., et al. (2020). Guanxinshutong Capsule Ameliorates Cardiac Function and Architecture Following Myocardial Injury by Modulating Ventricular Remodeling in Rats. *Biomed. Pharmacother.* 130, 110527. doi:10.1016/j.biopha.2020.110527

Zhuo, L., Li-Feng, L., Tian-Ming, Y., Yu, H., and Ya-Ling, H. (2012). Cardioprotective Effects of Guanxinshutong (GXST) against Myocardial Ischemia/reperfusion Injury in Rats. *J. Geriatr. Cardiol.* 9 (2), 130–136. doi:10.3724/SP.J.1263.2011.11261

Permissions

All chapters in this book were first published by Frontiers; hereby published with permission under the Creative Commons Attribution License or equivalent. Every chapter published in this book has been scrutinized by our experts. Their significance has been extensively debated. The topics covered herein carry significant findings which will fuel the growth of the discipline. They may even be implemented as practical applications or may be referred to as a beginning point for another development.

The contributors of this book come from diverse backgrounds, making this book a truly international effort. This book will bring forth new frontiers with its revolutionizing research information and detailed analysis of the nascent developments around the world.

We would like to thank all the contributing authors for lending their expertise to make the book truly unique. They have played a crucial role in the development of this book. Without their invaluable contributions this book wouldn't have been possible. They have made vital efforts to compile up to date information on the varied aspects of this subject to make this book a valuable addition to the collection of many professionals and students.

This book was conceptualized with the vision of imparting up-to-date information and advanced data in this field. To ensure the same, a matchless editorial board was set up. Every individual on the board went through rigorous rounds of assessment to prove their worth. After which they invested a large part of their time researching and compiling the most relevant data for our readers.

The editorial board has been involved in producing this book since its inception. They have spent rigorous hours researching and exploring the diverse topics which have resulted in the successful publishing of this book. They have passed on their knowledge of decades through this book. To expedite this challenging task, the publisher supported the team at every step. A small team of assistant editors was also appointed to further simplify the editing procedure and attain best results for the readers.

Apart from the editorial board, the designing team has also invested a significant amount of their time in understanding the subject and creating the most relevant covers. They scrutinized every image to scout for the most suitable representation of the subject and create an appropriate cover for the book.

The publishing team has been an ardent support to the editorial, designing and production team. Their endless efforts to recruit the best for this project, has resulted in the accomplishment of this book. They are a veteran in the field of academics and their pool of knowledge is as vast as their experience in printing. Their expertise and guidance has proved useful at every step. Their uncompromising quality standards have made this book an exceptional effort. Their encouragement from time to time has been an inspiration for everyone.

The publisher and the editorial board hope that this book will prove to be a valuable piece of knowledge for researchers, students, practitioners and scholars across the globe.

List of Contributors

Linglong Liu
College of Integrative Medicine, Fujian University of Traditional Chinese Medicine, Fuzhou, China

Limei Xu
College of Integrative Medicine, Fujian University of Traditional Chinese Medicine, Fuzhou, China
Academy of Integrative Medicine, Fujian University of Traditional Chinese Medicine, Fuzhou, China

Xiaoning Wang
College of Integrative Medicine, Fujian University of Traditional Chinese Medicine, Fuzhou, China
Academy of Integrative Medicine, Fujian University of Traditional Chinese Medicine, Fuzhou, China
Institute of Interdisciplinary Integrative Medicine Research, Shanghai University of Traditional Chinese Medicine, Shanghai, China

Shengjie Wang
College of Pharmacy Science, Fujian University of Traditional Chinese Medicine, Fuzhou, China

Lili Wang, Huifeng Xu and Hongzhi Ye
Academy of Integrative Medicine, Fujian University of Traditional Chinese Medicine, Fuzhou, China
Fujian Key Laboratory of Integrative Medicine on Geriatrics, Fuzhou, China

Xihai Li
College of Integrative Medicine, Fujian University of Traditional Chinese Medicine, Fuzhou, China
Fujian Key Laboratory of Integrative Medicine on Geriatrics, Fuzhou, China

Yin Xiong and Xiuming Cui
Faculty of Life Science and Technology, Kunming University of Science and Technology, Kunming, China
Yunnan Key Laboratory of Panax Notoginseng, Kunming, China
Laboratory of Sustainable Utilization of Panax Notoginseng Resources, State Administration of Traditional Chinese Medicine, Kunming, China

Yupiao Hu, Lijuan Chen, Zejun Zhang and Yiming Zhang
Faculty of Life Science and Technology, Kunming University of Science and Technology, Kunming, China

Ming Niu
China Military Institute of Chinese Materia Medica, 302 Military Hospital of China, Beijing, China

Jian Gao, Qiming Wang, Yuwei Huang and Zhiwei Cao
Shanghai 10th People's Hospital, School of Life Sciences and Technology, Tongji University, Shanghai, China

Kailin Tang
Shanghai 10th People's Hospital, School of Life Sciences and Technology, Tongji University, Shanghai, China
Department of Gastroenterology, Shanghai Tenth People's Hospital, School of Life Sciences and Technology, Tongji University, Shanghai, China

Xue Yang
Department of Traditional Chinese Medicine, Yangpu Hospital, School of Medicine, TongJi University, Shanghai, China

Zhi-Yi Yan
School of Traditional Chinese Medicine, Beijing University of Chinese Medicine, Beijing, China
Dongfang Hospital Affiliated to Beijing University of Chinese Medicine, Beijing, China

Hai-Yan Jiao, Jian-Bei Chen, Kai-Wen Zhang, Xi-Hong Wang, You-Ming Jiang, Yue-Yun Liu and Zhe Xue
School of Traditional Chinese Medicine, Beijing University of Chinese Medicine, Beijing, China

Qing-Yu Ma and Xiao-Juan Li
Formula-pattern Research Center, School of Traditional Chinese Medicine, Jinan University, Guangzhou, China

Jia-Xu Chen
School of Traditional Chinese Medicine, Beijing University of Chinese Medicine, Beijing, China
Formula-pattern Research Center, School of Traditional Chinese Medicine, Jinan University, Guangzhou, China

Joaquim Olivés
Research Group on Systems Pharmacology, Research Programme on Biomedical Informatics (GRIB), IMIM Hospital del Mar Medical Research Institute, Barcelona, Spain

Jordi Mestres
Research Group on Systems Pharmacology, Research Programme on Biomedical Informatics (GRIB), IMIM Hospital del Mar Medical Research Institute, Barcelona, Spain
Department of Experimental and Health Sciences, University Pompeu Fabra, Barcelona, Spain

Ao Du, Yumin Xie, Hao Ouyang, Bin Lu, Wangya Jia, Hong Xu and Lili Ji
The MOE Key Laboratory for Standardization of Chinese Medicines, Shanghai Key Laboratory of Compound Chinese Medicines and The SATCM Key Laboratory for New Resources and Quality Evaluation of Chinese Medicines, Institute of Chinese Materia Medica, Shanghai University of Traditional Chinese Medicine, Shanghai, China

Saisai Tian and Jian Yang
School of Pharmacy, The Second Military Medical University, Shanghai, China

Pengli Huang and Yu Gu
Institute of Interdisciplinary Complex Research, Shanghai University of Traditional Chinese Medicine, Shanghai, China

Jing Zhao
Institute of Interdisciplinary Complex Research, Shanghai University of Traditional Chinese Medicine, Shanghai, China
Division of Nephrology, Affiliated Hospital of Nanjing University of Chinese Medicine, Jiangsu Province Hospital of Chinese Medicine, Nanjing, China

Ran Wu
Shanghai Tenth People's Hospital, Tongji University, Shanghai, China

Ai-Jun Liu
School of Pharmacy, The Second Military Medical University, Shanghai, China
Department of Pharmacy, Shanghai Pulmonary Hospital, Shanghai, China

Weidong Zhang
School of Pharmacy, The Second Military Medical University, Shanghai, China
Institute of Interdisciplinary Complex Research, Shanghai University of Traditional Chinese Medicine, Shanghai, China

Jianxiong Wu, Xietao Ye, Songhong Yang, Huan Yu, Lingyun Zhong and Qianfeng Gong
School of Pharmacy, Jiangxi University of Traditional Chinese Medicine, Nanchang, China

Nani Wang and Pingcui Xu
Department of Medicine, Tongde Hospital of Zhejiang Province, Hangzhou, China
School of Pharmacy, Zhejiang Chinese Medical University, China

Hailiang Xin
School of Pharmacy, Second Military Medical University, China

Zhongming Yu and Dan Shou
Department of Medicine, Tongde Hospital of Zhejiang Province, Hangzhou, China

Chen Yong, Guoshun Huang, Yang Yang, Yiye Zhu, Qijing Wu, Zhongchi Xu, Chong Chen, Kun Gao and Enchao Zhou
Division of Nephrology, Affiliated Hospital of Nanjing University of Chinese Medicine, Jiangsu Province Hospital of Chinese Medicine, Nanjing, China

Zhengchun Zhang
Division of Nephrology, JiangYan Hospital affiliated to Nanjing University of Chinese Medicine, Taizhou, China

Leilei Qian
Division of Nephrology, The People's Hospital of Rugao, Rugao, China

Fang Tian and Li Liu
Research Center of Chinese Medicine, Jiangsu Province Hospital of Chinese Medicine, Nanjing, China

Yan-Fang Yang, Bo Liu, Zhong-Zhu Ai, Peng-Tao You and He-Zhen Wu
Faculty of Pharmacy, Hubei University of Chinese Medicine, Wuhan, China
Key Laboratory of Traditional Chinese Medicine Resources and Chemistry of Hubei Province, Wuhan, China
Collaborative Innovation Center of Traditional Chinese Medicine of New Products for Geriatrics Hubei Province, Wuhan, China

Song-Tao Wu, Zhou-Tao Xie, Wei-Chen Xiong, Peng-Fei Hao, Wen-Ping Xiao and Yuan Sun
Faculty of Pharmacy, Hubei University of Chinese Medicine, Wuhan, China

Shujing Lv, Honghong Yu, Xinyue Liu and Xiaoyan Gao
School of Chinese Materia Medica, Beijing University of Chinese Medicine, Beijing, China

Feifei Guo, Jin Su, Haiyu Xu and Hongjun Yang
Institute of Chinese Materia Medica, China Academy of Chinese Medical Sciences, Beijing, China

Wen Zhang
Institute of Chinese Materia Medica, China Academy of Chinese Medical Sciences, Beijing, China
College of Ethnic Medicine, Chengdu University of Traditional Chinese Medicine, Chengdu, China

Yang Fu
Xiangyang Hospital of Traditional Chinese Medicine, Xiangyang, China

Xiaolu Liu and Zhigang Mei
Institute of Basic Theory for Integrated Traditional Chinese and Western Medicine, College of Integrated Traditional Chinese and Western Medicine, Hunan University of Chinese Medicine, Changsha, China
Third-Grade Pharmacological Laboratory on Chinese Medicine Approved by State Administration of Traditional Chinese Medicine, Medical College of China Three Gorges University, Yichang, China

Yuling Fan and Lipeng Du
Third-Grade Pharmacological Laboratory on Chinese Medicine Approved by State Administration of Traditional Chinese Medicine, Medical College of China Three Gorges University, Yichang, China

Zikun Chen, Dingfeng Wu, Wenyan Zhao and Zhiwei Cao
Department of Gastroenterology, Shanghai Tenth People's Hospital, School of Life Sciences and Technology, Tongji University, Shanghai, China

Yuanyuan Li, Yahang Wang and Yueming Ma
Department of Pharmacology, Shanghai University of Traditional Chinese Medicine, Shanghai, China

Ping Liu
Institute of Interdisciplinary Integrative Medicine Research, Shanghai University of Traditional Chinese Medicine, Shanghai, China
Key Laboratory of Liver and Kidney Diseases of Ministry of Education of China, Institute of Liver Diseases, Shuguang Hospital, Shanghai University of Traditional Chinese Medicine, Shanghai, China

Juanli Zhang
Department of Pharmacy, Xijing Hospital, Fourth Military Medical University, Xi'an, China
Department of Neurology, Xijing Hospital, Fourth Military Medical University, Xi'an, China

Jiaxin Zhao, Yang Ma, Wenjun Wang, Shaojie Huang, Chao Guo, Kai Wang, Wei Zhang, Aidong Wen and Yi Ding
Department of Pharmacy, Xijing Hospital, Fourth Military Medical University, Xi'an, China

Xiaomei Zhang
Basic Medical School, Yunnan University of Traditional Chinese Medicine, Kunming, China

Ming Shi
Department of Neurology, Xijing Hospital, Fourth Military Medical University, Xi'an, China

Index

www.ingramcontent.com/pod-product-compliance
Lightning Source LLC
LaVergne TN
LVHW082206200926
848484LV00008B/2219